Wally Zollman MD
1976

SURGICAL DISORDERS OF THE PERIPHERAL NERVES

SURGICAL DISORDERS OF THE PERIPHERAL NERVES

SIR HERBERT SEDDON, C.M.G.

Honorary Consulting Surgeon, Royal National Orthopaedic Hospital, London. Honorary Fellow, Worcester College, Oxford. Sometime Nuffield Professor of Orthopaedic Surgery, Oxford and Professor of Orthopaedic Surgery, London

SECOND EDITION

CHURCHILL LIVINGSTONE
EDINBURGH LONDON AND NEW YORK 1975

CHURCHILL LIVINGSTONE
Medical Division of Longman Group Limited

Distributed in the United States of America by Longman Inc., New York and by associated companies, branches and representatives throughout the world.

First edition 1972
Second edition 1975

ISBN 0 443 01264 4

Library of Congress Cataloging in Publication Data

Seddon, Sir Herbert.
Surgical disorders of the peripheral nerves.

Bibliography: p.
Includes indexes.
1. Nerves, Peripheral—Surgery. 2. Nerves, Peripheral—Wounds and injuries. I. Title.
[DNLM: 1. Peripheral nerves—Injuries. 2. Peripheral nerves—Surgery. WL500 S447s]
RD595.S33 1975 617′.483 75-9991

PRINTED IN GREAT BRITAIN

IN MEMORIAM

HUGH CAIRNS
1896-1952

Nuffield Professor of Surgery, Oxford

GEORGE RIDDOCH
1888-1947

Physician: the London Hospital and the
National Hospital for Nervous Diseases

Preface to the Second Edition

ALTHOUGH only three years have elapsed since the publication of the first edition of this book it has needed revision. Never before in peacetime has there been such widespread interest in peripheral nervous disorders. What the French so aptly call electrology has come of age, as is evident in the three volumes edited by Desmedt that appeared in 1973. Manipulative ingenuity has been very great. It is becoming almost indecent not to use an operating microscope, and epineural suture is becoming old-fashioned.

An impressive report is the Proceedings of the 13th Congress of the Spanish Orthopaedic Association, held in 1972, which is devoted entirely to the surgery of peripheral nerves. But the most important recent work is that published under the direction of those giants of peripheral nerve surgery Michon and Moberg: *Les Lésions Traumatiques des Nerfs Périphériques*, 1973. (An English edition entitled *Traumatic Nerve Lesions of the Upper Limb* has, most happily, been published this year by Churchill Livingstone.) What distinguishes this collection of essays is an underlying and healthy discontent, nowhere expressed better than by Eric Moberg in his *espoirs d'avenir*. If, for example, the recording of sensory recovery can be better defined—and generally adopted—it will be a great step forward.

Kindly critics have pointed out a number of errors and omissions which I have endeavoured to correct. Professor P. K. Thomas has once again been a wise counsellor, and, striving as he always does for perfection, has replaced some of the electron-micrographs in Chapters 1 and 2.

The burden of secretarial work on the manuscript has been cheerfully borne by Miss Carole Easton, the most willing and capable secretary I have ever met. The librarian of the Institute of Orthopaedics, Mr C. Davenport, has never once failed to produce a paper or book I wished to consult. Proof-reading has again been shared with my long-suffering wife. Churchill Livingstone has changed its name, but not its image as a publishing house of the highest standard, combined with extraordinary felicity in its personal relationships with an author. To all I express my deep gratitude.

Stanmore, 1975 H. J. SEDDON

Preface to the First Edition

Of the various disorders of the peripheral nerves that excite the interest of surgeons, injuries eclipse all the rest put together. The commonest cause of injury is an open wound, particularly that produced by a missile; thus surgery of the peripheral nerves is a child of war, and it was born a century ago.

The first organized investigation of nerve injuries was undertaken during the American Civil War, at the instigation of W. A. Hammond, Surgeon General to the Federal Armies. Work began in May 1863 at an army hospital in Turner's Lane, Philadelphia, with Silas Weir Mitchell in charge. After fifteen months he and his co-workers published a little book that is the foundation stone of our knowledge of nerve injuries. Another and a more complete work appeared in 1872.[1] Weir Mitchell was a man of such remarkable ability and versatility that he would undoubtedly have made valuable observations on such patients as came to him in the ordinary course of military hospital practice; but the foresight of his chief provided him with opportunities that would otherwise have been lost.

In Britain, a policy of concentration was adopted, though not immediately, during the First World War and throughout the Second World War.

The wound that injures a nerve often damages neighbouring structures—bones, joints, blood vessels and tendons—and it is, therefore, desirable that the surgeon choosing (or in times of war ordered) to devote himself particularly to the surgery of peripheral nerves should have a wide range of skills. Moreover, reconstructive operations are sometimes necessary if a nerve cannot be mended or fails to recover satisfactorily after repair.[2]

As in the management of traumatic paraplegia—in which diverse skills are also required—the organization should be such that the patient is never in doubt about who is looking after him. And as in some other disorders of the locomotor system a precise programme of treatment is all-important: the man who draws it up is the one to whom the patient knows he belongs. Moreover, the commitment has no time limit. Ideally, the arrangements should be immune from disruption by administrative machinery. In Britain, during the Second World War, great pains were taken to ensure that this was so; and despite the hazards of war and the dictates of geography, continuity of treatment and supervision was very good, as is evident from the Medical Research Council's Special Report published in 1954.

The necessity for this segregation, this concentration of cases, is recognized increasingly. It is in the patients' interests; it also facilitates advances in understanding and technique, and encourages the co-operation of scientists. For example, during the decade that included the First World War two anatomists, Huber in the United States and Stopford in Britain, applied themselves to the study of nerve injuries with most fruitful results. During the Second World War the collaboration of clinicians and laboratory workers was extremely close. At Oxford I had the inestimable privilege of working

[1] Weir Mitchell wrote with unusual felicity. It is perhaps worth mentioning that he published eight slender volumes of verse. A selection from them was published in London by Macmillan in 1901; William Holmes gave me a copy, which I treasure.

[2] No attempt has been made to describe the many reconstructive operations that may be required, though a few are mentioned. There are two reasons for this. Reconstructive surgery is best dealt with in relation to all forms of peripheral paralysis; and to cover the subject adequately would involve making this book much too long.

with J. Z. Young, P. B. Medawar, William Holmes, F. K. Sanders, and Ernst Gutmann. And since then I have been blessed by equally close association with Hubert Sissons and his colleagues in the Department of Morbid Anatomy of the Institute of Orthopaedics.

There is one field of enquiry in which neither animal experiment nor access to a large number of patients is of much use; the study of disturbances of sensibility, more particularly cutaneous sensibility. It is no accident that the renowned investigations of Head, Trotter and Davies, Boring, Woollard and Weddell were done in times of peace. It is a leisurely occupation. Animal experiments, such as Sarah Tower's, have helped a little; but man alone, and an intelligent man at that, can describe the manifold sensations experienced after injury to a nerve and during regeneration. Moreover, the injuries themselves must be deliberately inflicted, with great precision, and the subject has to be a fully informed member of the experimental team. What is so astonishing is that in spite of the devoted efforts of many workers the riddle of sensibility is still not yet solved.

It may be said that this is rather the province of the physiologist and the anatomist. In methodology this is true enough, but the problem is intensely practical. In addition to the victims of nerve injury, there are some 15 million lepers in the world, most of whom suffer from disabling disorders of sensibility, the origin of which is in the peripheral nerves.

Causalgia is rare even in times of war, but what in Chapter 9 are described, for want of a better term, as irritative nerve lesions are always with us and there is as yet no rational basis for their treatment.

There are grounds for disquiet in this small, but absorbing and often rewarding field of surgery. We live in an age of unparalleled technological advance. A surgeon selects such new weapons as may help him to help his patients. But in some centres of endeavour established, proven and reliable techniques are being jettisoned in favour of what is novel. 'For all the Athenians . . . spent their time in nothing else, but either to tell, or to hear some new thing' (*Acts*, 17.21). And the old is sometimes abandoned when it is palpably better for the patient. This is noticeable in some of the recent work on nerve homografts.

There is a way of disciplining this ardour, this enthusiasm, which is too valuable to be censured. It is by using one of the most weighty weapons of contemporary research, the controlled clinical trial. Surgeons, by nature inventive, by temperament emotionally attached to their brain-children, find this more rigorous than do almost all other clinical experimenters. Yet the clinical trial is necessary. Its morality has been questioned. Today it is the other way round; it is often immoral not to embark on a trial. But the cost to the investigator must be counted. In many fields of work the duration of the trial may be 10 years; surgery of the peripheral nervous system is one of them. There are three reasons for this protracted ordeal. The first is that the inflow of patients is usually slow, though this can be remedied by a number of centres joining in a common investigation. The second is that the necessary period of observation after the performance of this or that operation is measured by years rather than months. The third is that comparisons are being made not between life and death, as was the case with tuberculous meningitis before and after the advent of streptomycin, but between methods of treatment that are more or less efficacious. It is a matter of finding out which is the better. In this I am obliged to confess negligence; opportunities that lay within our grasp have been missed. Now, in what seems to be a belated penitential exercise, I am involved in a clinical trial, in a field unrelated to the peripheral nervous system. From first to last it requires 10 years of unremitting effort on the part of a considerable number of people who are prepared to work to a common programme. It is costly too. The reward is unspectacular, but peculiarly satisfying: at the finish, certainty of knowledge that can be translated with complete assurance into action that benefits patients. This should be good enough. The technique of the clinical trial has been perfected. The problem is finding the people with sufficient self-discipline to use it.

For the management of damaged peripheral nerves the surgeon must arm himself with three weapons: detailed knowledge of the anatomy of the limbs; the special skills —and the patience—of the neurologist; and, in operative surgery, a delicacy of touch that lies between those of the neurosurgeon and of the otologist. I learned the second from George Riddoch and the third from Hugh Cairns. This book is dedicated to their memory; they were the best friends a man could wish for.

I am indebted to other friends. P. K. Thomas read the first, second and fourth chapters, and he supplied the best of the illustrations they contain. D. Lloyd Griffiths read the chapter on neurovascular injuries, and Hubert Sissons the one on nerve tumours. I am deeply grateful to all three for criticisms and suggestions—which I hastened to accept. My greatest debt is to John Crawford Adams who read all the other chapters; he brought to them the erudition and the superb command of our language which, over many years, have contributed so largely to the eminence of the British edition of the *Journal of Bone and Joint Surgery*. I cannot thank him adequately.

For over 20 years my partner in this work has been D. M. Brooks. He brought to it an innate wisdom which for me has been indispensable; and the elegance of his operative technique is of an order that I have never been able to achieve.

The most time-consuming labour was studying the records of some 2,000 patients. Under the guidance of Dr Ian Sutherland I designed an analysis card. The soul-destroying job of completing them was undertaken by Miss Ingrid Schoeberl, with endless patience and great accuracy. I scanned every dossier and card myself. After the information had been transferred to standard punch cards the analyses were made with a counter sorter that Dr Sutherland placed at my disposal at the Medical Research Council's Statistical Research and Services Unit. This work was costly, and would hardly have been possible but for a grant from the Institute of Orthopaedics, which I gratefully acknowledge, as I do the constant help of Mrs Mary Glen Haig, Medical Records Officer at the Royal National Orthopaedic Hospital.

Someone with the mind of an accountant could ferret out some statistical discrepancies. Although our notes have always been good, not every dossier contained all the information one was seeking. The gaps are small. Every set of figures is accurate in relation to the topic under consideration; they show what happened.

It has been my good fortune to work with a succession of able and enthusiastic junior colleagues. The consequence has been a steady stream of published papers on various aspects of disorders of the peripheral nerves. All this work has been incorporated in this book. But this formal acknowledgment is as nothing compared with what I owe them for constant mental invigoration, for transfusion of ideas. In working through our records, which were necessarily more their work than mine, I could not but recall with gratitude some words of Weir Mitchell's. 'No labour has been spared in making these clinical histories as perfect and full as possible. Those only who have devoted themselves to similar studies will be able to appreciate the amount of time and care which has been thus expended. We indulge the hope that we shall leave on record a very faithful clinical study of nerve injuries, and that we shall have done something at least towards lessening the inevitable calamities of warfare.'

I take the liberty here of mentioning three by name. W. Bremner Highet joined us at the outbreak of the Second World War. This talented young New Zealander was awarded the Jacksonian Prize by the Royal College of Surgeons of England for an essay on nerve injuries. The closure of the Mediterranean Sea left only the Cape route for the evacuation of men injured in the fighting in the Desert War. As a result of the shortage of transport shipping many of them piled up in South Africa. Highet was chosen to look after those who had suffered nerve injury. He was sent by sea; the ship was torpedoed and there were no survivors.

Ludwig Guttmann had come to Oxford from Foerster. He placed his master's and his own profound knowledge of peripheral nerve injuries at our disposal. His research work was superb. Guttmann (now Sir Ludwig) was soon to achieve worldwide renown when he set about establishing a spinal injuries centre at Stoke Mandeville.

Graham Weddell was and is a versatile anatomist. As a pupil of Woollard's he applied himself particularly to the problems of cutaneous sensibility. He also developed electromyography as a clinical weapon, and thus we were able to exploit this diagnostic aid at a time when the machines that today are commonplace did not exist.

In wartime we took our own photographs; their quality was only passable. Later, at the Institute of Orthopaedics, I was to benefit from the skill of Robert Whitley, that great master of medical photography. I thank him most warmly. Almost all of the line drawings and histograms are the work of Robin Callander of the Department of Medical Illustration and Photography in the University of Glasgow. I pay tribute not only to his skill as a draughtsman, but to his uncanny grasp of exactly what is required.

A number of illustrations, many of them my own, but a fair number from the works of others, have been reproduced from books and published papers. The generosity of many friends has been a great encouragement. I am grateful to editors and publishers for so willingly according me permission to reproduce pictorial material of great value. I acknowledge my indebtedness to: The Controller of Her Majesty's Stationery Office: The Association of British Members of the Swiss Alpine Club: *Bibliotheca Anatomica: Brain: British Journal of Surgery: British Medical Journal: British Surgical Practice: Canadian Medical Association Journals: The Hand: Journal of the American Medical Association: Journal of Anatomy:* The American and British Editors of the *Journal of Bone and Joint Surgery: Journal of Neurology, Neurosurgery and Psychiatry: Journal of Neurosurgery: Journal of Physiology:* E. and S. Livingstone, Edinburgh: *Physiotherapy: Plastic and Reconstructive Surgery: Revue de Chirurgie Orthopédique:* W. B. Saunders and Company, Philadelphia and London: *Surgery Gynecology and Obstetrics:* The Williams and Wilkins Company, Baltimore.

I am deeply grateful to my wife, to Mrs Helen Bamber and to Mrs Valerie Webster for their arduous and painstaking labour in preparing the typescript. I am no less appreciative of Miss Una Grant's devotion in checking and listing the (perhaps too numerous) references and preparing the index of authors.

None of the imperfections found in this book can be laid at the door of the publishers, Churchill Livingstone; they took endless trouble with it, and for this, and for their patience, they have my warmest thanks.

Stanmore, 1972 H. J. SEDDON

Contents

1. The Structure of a Peripheral Nerve

NERVE FIBRES

THE ESSENTIAL ELEMENTS of a peripheral nerve—its conducting fibres—are extraordinary in being cell processes that are mostly of immense length. In man the volume of the axon, without its myelin sheath, may be more than 200 times that of the cell body. The axon necessarily depends almost entirely on a local blood supply; yet severed from the cell body it degenerates, and robbed of its proper peripheral connection it fails to attain its proper size (Aitken, Sharman and Young, 1947).

An average cutaneous nerve may contain 10,000 fibres. The largest unmyelinated fibres, which predominate, may be about 1 μ in diameter, whereas the largest myelinated fibres are 20 times the size. There is an even greater range, about 1:100, of conduction velocities, the rate being greatest in the largest fibres. Nerve fibres in the periphery of a limb are smaller than those supplying the proximal parts; and it is possible that the longest fibres taper towards the end of their course (Young, 1950). It has been suggested (Sunderland and Ray, 1947) that the size of fibres in a nerve may have a bearing on its suitability for employment as a graft. There is no doubt that a large fibre growing into a very small Schwann tube cannot inflate it more than a little (Simpson and Young, 1945); but in the conditions that obtain clinically this is unlikely to be significant, because the differences in diameter are far less than those in the reported experiments, in which the proximal part of a somatic nerve was joined to the distal end of an autonomic nerve composed entirely of unmyelinated fibres.

Although we speak of fibres and although the axon appears fibrillar in stained preparations, the axoplasm behaves like a viscous liquid. The giant nerve fibres of some invertebrates show this property to a remarkable degree. When the worm *Myxicola* contracts the diameter of a cylinder of axoplasm trebles, and its length is reduced accordingly (Nicol and Young, 1946; Nicol, 1948). For surgeons this property of fluidity is of some interest. There is as yet nothing to indicate that when regeneration begins the outflow of axoplasm is any more purposive than a stream of molten lava making its way down the gullies on the slope of a volcano: with one proviso, that the streams of axoplasm have a particular affinity for the surfaces of Schwann cells, to which they adhere (Abercrombie, Johnson and Thomas, 1949).

All peripheral nerve fibres are enclosed by *Schwann cells*. There is one for each segment—the part between two nodes of Ranvier—in a myelinated fibre. In man the Schwann cells of unmyelinated fibres are remarkable. Whereas in some other species a number of nerve fibres are invaginated into the cytoplasm of the Schwann cell, in man the Schwann cell has pseudopodia—almost tentacles—which reach out to embrace neighbouring unmyelinated fibres. Thus one may find a number of fibres, each with its investment of Schwann cytoplasm (Fig. **1**, 1), but without any apparent connection with the main body of the relevant Schwann cell. Yet this is no more than a crude simplification of a remarkably complex arrangement (Eames and Gamble, 1970).

Both types of axon are invaginated into the cytoplasm of the Schwann cell and this gives rise to the formation of the *mesaxon*, which is clearly demonstrable electron-microscopically (Fig. **1**, 1).

Outside the Schwann cells is the *basement membrane* (Figs **1**, 1; **2**, 4 and **2**, 6, pp. 2, 11 and 13). In the case of unmyelinated fibres it encloses all that are embedded in the cytoplasm of one Schwann cell, in myelinated fibres it encloses only one with its investing Schwann cells. Thus a Schwann tube, to which reference will frequently be made, consists of a column of Schwann cells contained in a basement membrane. The membrane is continuous; the cells, however intimate their ramifications, are not—they do not form a syncytium.

The *myelin sheath* is the distinctive feature of

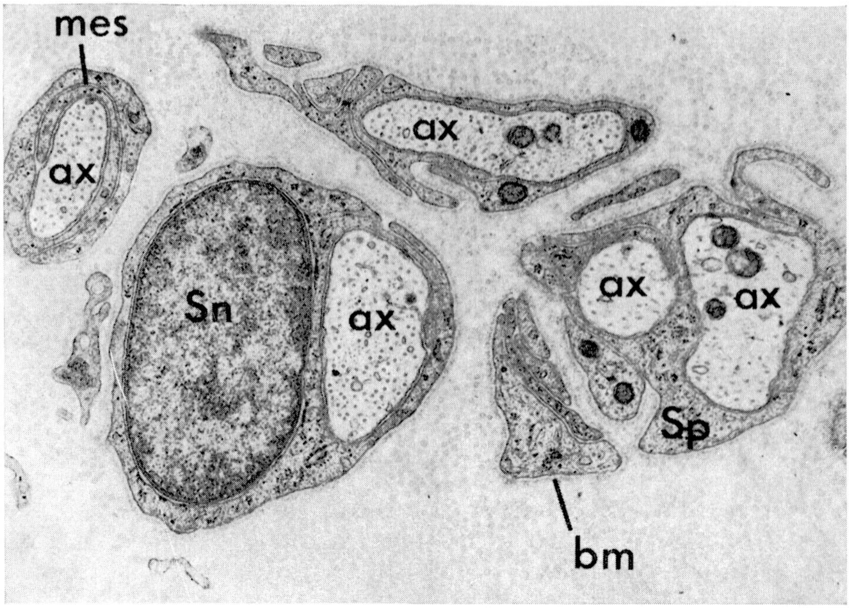

FIG. 1, 1. Electron-micrograph (×19,000) of a group of unmyelinated axons: human sural nerve.

ax	axon	bm	basement membrane
Sn	Schwann-cell nucleus	mes	mesaxon
Sp	Schwann-cell process		

(Courtesy of Dr A. J. Aguayo)

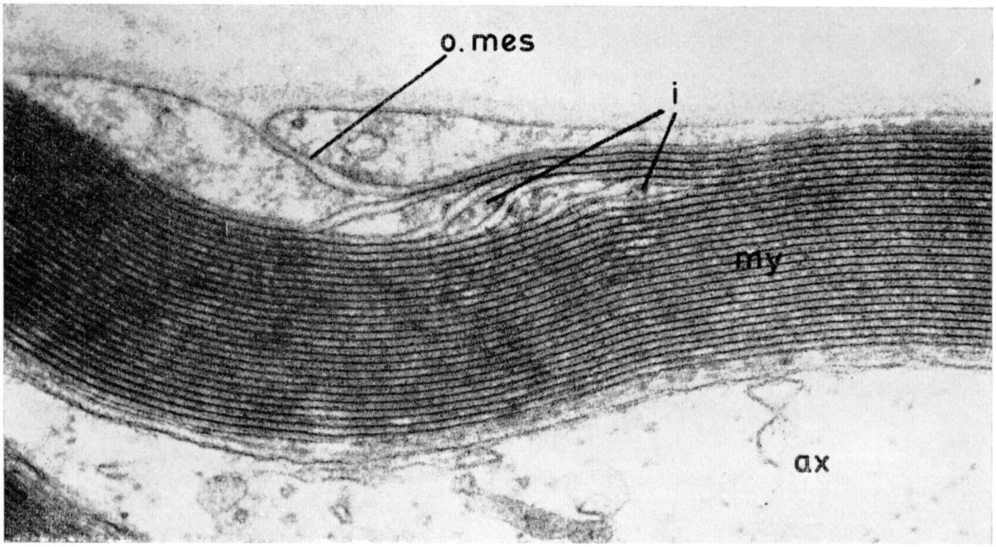

FIG. 1, 2. Electron-micrograph (×84,000) of a portion of a transverse section through a small myelinated nerve fibre. The myelin sheath displays a partial Schmidt-Lantermann incisure.

o. mes	outer mesaxon
my	myelin
i	Schmidt-Lantermann incisure
ax	axon

the large nerve fibres. Here the Schwann cells envelop only one axon. The myelin is derived from the mesaxon becoming wrapped spirally round the axon; obliteration of the intervening cytoplasmic layers producing the appearance of compact lamination (Fig. **1**, 2). There are also periodic funnel-shaped clefts in the myelin sheath, the incisures of Schmidt-Lantermann, where the lamellae are separated by cytoplasm (Figs **1**, 2 and **1**, 3).

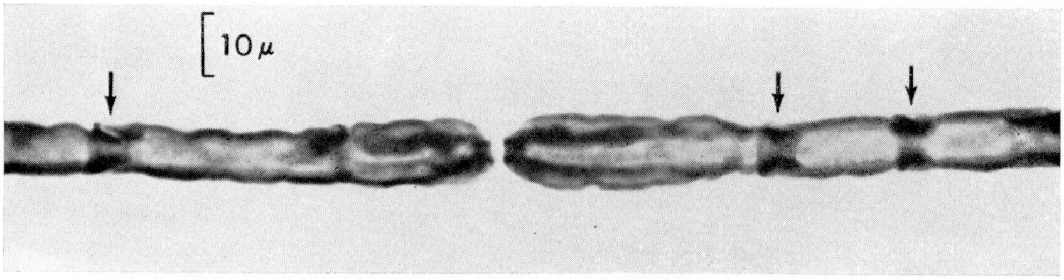

FIG. **1**, 3. Single myelinated nerve fibre showing one node of Ranvier and Schmidt-Lantermann incisures (arrows). Stain: osmium tetroxide. (Courtesy of Mr P. S. Spencer.)

The *nodes of Ranvier* (Fig. **1**, 3) demarcate the myelin segment. They represent the junctions between adjacent Schwann cells which have come into close contact with the axon membrane at the nodes. The basement membrane and collagenous ensheathment of the Schwann cell dip in at the nodes.

The distance between nodes is greater in the larger fibres, but the correlation is not strict. The internodal length is largely determined by the amount of longitudinal growth that has occurred after myelination. At birth the internodal length in large fibres is about 230 μ. In nerves supplying the forearm it increases fourfold by the eighteenth year: in nerves to the leg, the same; in nerves to the jaw only two-and-a-half times (Shepherd, Sholl and Vizoso, 1949; Vizoso, 1950). The jaw grows far less longitudinally than the distal segment of the upper or lower limb.

THE SUPPORTING TISSUES

The *endoneurium* is the supporting tissue of the individual fibre, a fibrocytic stroma composed of two layers of collagen. It forms the endoneurial tube, closely investing the Schwann basement membrane, but separating from it when degeneration occurs. The nerve fibres with their related endoneurium form aggregations variously called bundles, fasciculi or funiculi (the last is preferred) which are enclosed by a much larger, cellular and collagenous envelope, the *perineurium* (Fig. **1**, 4). This tube is composed of mesothelial cells in which are embedded 7 to 15 collagenous lamellae, the fibres being arranged longitudinally, circularly and obliquely (Sunderland, 1965). It has a smooth inner surface lined by flat polygonal mesothelial cells, and there are collagenous condensations dipping into the funiculus, so forming the intrafunicular septa. The nerve fibres are slack inside the perineurium; thus in longitudinal sections they present a wavy appearance.

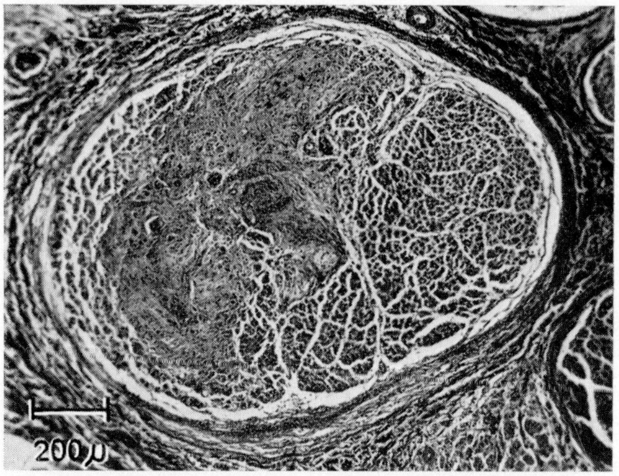

FIG. **1**, 4. The perineurium. The left half of its contents is abnormal, and this is referred to on page 272 (Fig. **15**, 26). On the right the pattern of the funiculus is normal, whereas on the left there is endoneurial fibrosis.

The funiculi are held together by a variable amount of collagenous connective tissue with a

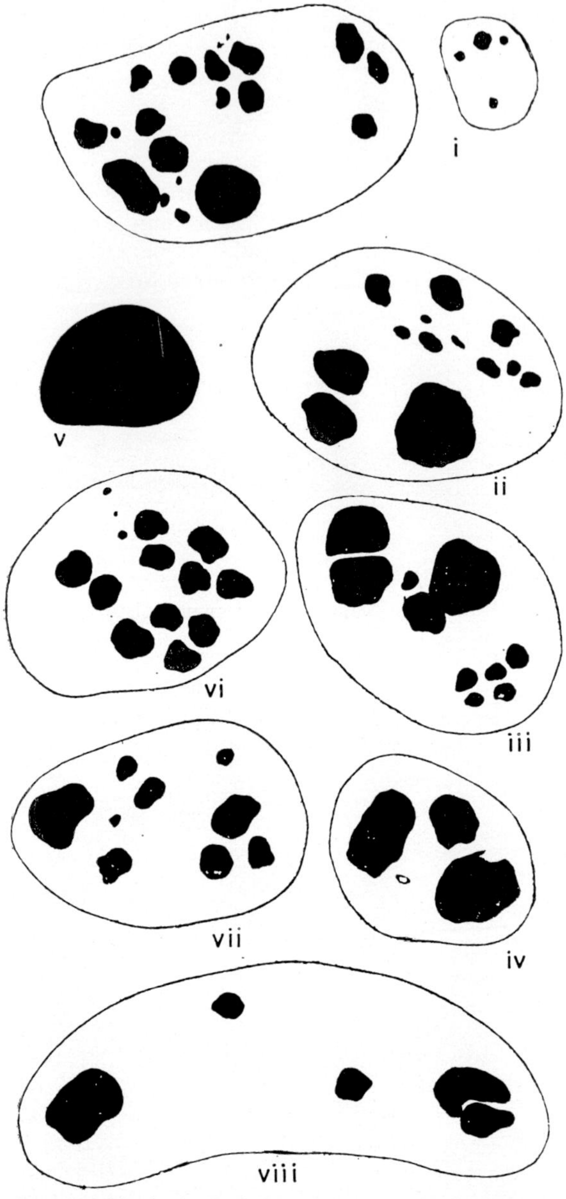

FIG. **1**, 5. The funiculi of the radial nerve at eight different levels. (Reproduced by kind permission from Sunderland, S., 1945, *Brain*, **68**, 243.)

little fat here and there; and enclosed by the outermost envelope, the *epineurium*, which is composed mainly of longitudinally disposed collagen fibres, fibrocytes and some elastin fibres (Thomas, 1963). Here again, the funiculi lie slack within the epineurium and, as surgeons are aware, they pout out when a nerve is transected. So there is double protection for the nerve fibres against stretching; inside the funiculi, and inside the nerve sheath, the epineurium.

Fluid injected beneath the epineurium passes easily proximally and distally and between the funiculi. Within a funiculus there is also fairly free passage. This is particularly significant in connection with the damage resulting from the intraneural injection of drugs (p. 135).

The amount of packing between the funiculi varies enormously as between one nerve and another, in different reaches of the same nerve (Fig. **1**, 5), and at corresponding levels in an individual on the two sides. The greater the number of funiculi the greater the quantity of interfunicular tissue; or, put another way, the greater the number of funiculi the smaller the proportion of the cross-sectional area they occupy. In most nerves the greatest area occupied by the funiculi is about 50 per cent—and the smallest can be as low as 16 per cent (Sunderland and Bradley, 1949).

The tensile strength and elasticity of a nerve are determined by the supporting stroma. The greater the number of funiculi and, therefore, the greater the amount of interfunicular tissue, the stronger the nerve (Sunderland and Bradley, 1961*a*). In spinal nerve roots the connective tissue is relatively scanty and poorly organized (Gamble, 1964), and in traction injuries of the brachial plexus (Chap. 11) the spinal roots are notoriously susceptible to damage. Sunderland and Bradley (1961*b*) found that in them it was the nerve fibres that ruptured first. That the nerve fibres and Schwann cells contribute little to the tensile strength of a nerve is suggested by the demonstration (Sunderland and Bradley, 1961*c*) that in this respect there is no difference between the proximal and the degenerated distal segment of a severed nerve.

The elasticity of nerve has recently acquired a new practical significance. It has long been known from experience of leg-lengthening operations that with care nerves can be elongated without suffering damage. Sunderland (1968, p. 63) gives precise details about the elasticity of human nerves, the important fact being its great variability which ranges from six to 22 per cent. The autologous grafting operation recommended by Millesi seems to be based on the supposition that in a sutured nerve the property of elasticity is best forgotten. This is discussed on p. 299.

INTRANEURAL PLEXUSES

From what has just been described it is evident that the internal topography of a peripheral nerve is plexiform; it changes from one level to another.

This subject has been studied since the early years of this century by a variety of methods:

1. Anatomical: dissection and histological examination (Bardeen, 1906; Stoffel, 1913, 1915; Langley and Hashimoto, 1917; Sunderland, 1945*a*; Sunderland and Ray, 1948).
2. Animal experiment: observing the distribution of Wallerian degeneration after partial section of a nerve (McKinley, 1921; Kilvington, 1940).
3. Very localized electrical stimulation (Langley and Hashimoto, 1917; McKinley, 1921).
4. Observation of the consequences of partial nerve injury (Sherren, 1908; Déjerine, Déjerine and Mouzon, 1915).

The most authoritative review, with an account of his own anatomical observations, is Sunderland's (1968).

The important practical conclusions are these:

1. The funicular pattern is inconstant, as between one subject and another, and as between right and left nerve trunks in the same subject.
2. The funicular pattern changes throughout the length of a nerve: the longest reach of any nerve showing a constant pattern is 15 mm, though individual funiculi may pursue considerably longer courses, especially where they are about to branch away from the main trunk. The average length of constant pattern is much less, only a few millimetres.
3. Not only is there communication between one funiculus and its neighbours but the number and size of the funiculi varies widely; and, as would be expected, the greater the number of them, the smaller their size.

The teleological explanation is simple enough. The grouping of neurons in the spinal cord and posterior root ganglia has to be translated into the appropriate innervation of muscles, skin and other tissues: for the limbs this is achieved first to some extent in the brachial and lumbosacral plexuses; but more delicate transpositions are required throughout the distribution of each nerve trunk. Yet there is an inescapable impression that this intermingling of nerve fibres and funiculi is rather overdone, and we are obliged to conclude that much of it is fortuitous, as is suggested by the inconstancies referred to above.

The clinical importance of the intraneural plexuses is considerable. In 1908 Sherren pointed out that one-third of a nerve trunk could be divided without producing any clinically detectable deficit. This is true enough—in certain situations, such as the ulnar nerve in the upper third of the arm. I have seen a patient with the ulnar nerve half severed at this level who showed no more than slight weakness of *all* the muscles of ulnar innervation and a trifling and *uniform* depression of cutaneous sensibility. The intermingling of the damaged fibres with the normal ones was just about complete by the time they reached the periphery. But because a branch of a nerve runs a well-defined course within it for some centimetres proximal to the point of separation, partial section of a nerve at this level and in the relevant sector has well-localized and easily recognizable consequences, that is, loss of function within the distribution of the branch.

The shifting funicular pattern makes it inevitable that any repair of a nerve in which the gap is considerable must be followed by confused re-innervation, however carefully the operation is done; the sizable cross-sectional area presented by the supporting connective tissue adds to the confusion and, worse, to wastage of axonal sprouts, some of which wander blindly in between the funiculi and lose themselves.

The separate course run by branches within a nerve, just above their points of departure, adds greatly to the effectiveness of surgical mobilization of a nerve; an indispensable feature of secondary suture. The distances over which important branches may be stripped from nerve trunks are given on page 269.

BLOOD VESSELS

That a peripheral nerve is less susceptible to ischaemia than voluntary muscle is proved by observations on patients with Volkmann's ischaemia in which sudden infarction, occurring in a previously healthy limb, deprives all tissues in the affected part of their blood supply. The nerves suffer less than the muscles (p. 94). Moreover, the apparent impunity with which nerves can be partially devascularized in the course of surgical mobilization has encouraged the notion that their blood supply is relatively unimportant. Yet this remarkable tolerance has a limit which, even if ill-defined, is entitled to some respect.

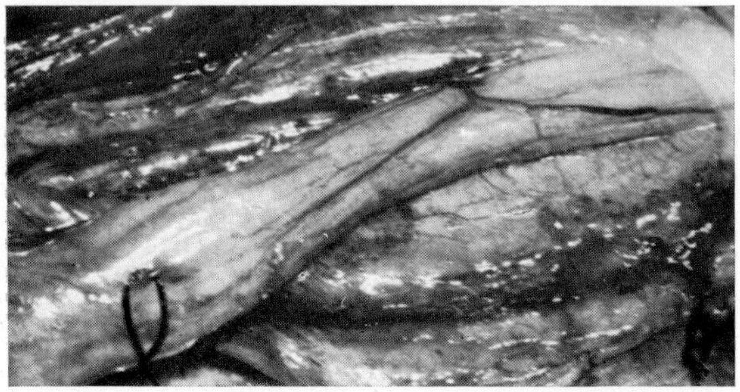

FIG. **1**, 6. Proximal stump of a severed nerve: guide suture, but not the end-bulb, visible on left. To show the ascending and descending branches of a collateral vessel.

Systematic studies of the blood supply of nerves, and of the effects of devascularization on regeneration have been carried out by a number of workers (see references in Sunderland, 1945*b*).

The blood vessels supplying a nerve always run in a web of connective tissue that Smith (1966) calls the *mesoneurium* because it resembles the mesentery. In certain situations arteriae nervorum join the nerve and may be up to 1 mm in diameter; the veins may run with the arteries or separately. Their length does not exceed 2·5 cm. Both arteries and veins exhibit some tortuosity, which helps to maintain the blood supply in situations where movement is often rapid, sudden and extensive. At some points, either in the mesoneurium or on the surface of the nerve (Fig. **1**, 6), there are longitudinal anastomoses, so ample that in certain sites—the median nerve in the upper arm, for example—hardly any collateral vessels join the nerve. Within the nerve, longitudinally disposed vessels are conspicuous beneath the epineurium and also between the funiculi (Fig. **1**, 7). Sometimes, when the proximal stump of a severed nerve is transected in preparation for secondary suture, a small artery within the substance of the nerve will spurt vigorously. Arterioles may be found even inside funiculi and, finally, there is a rectangular mesh of capillaries. It is doubtful whether there are any true end-arteries.

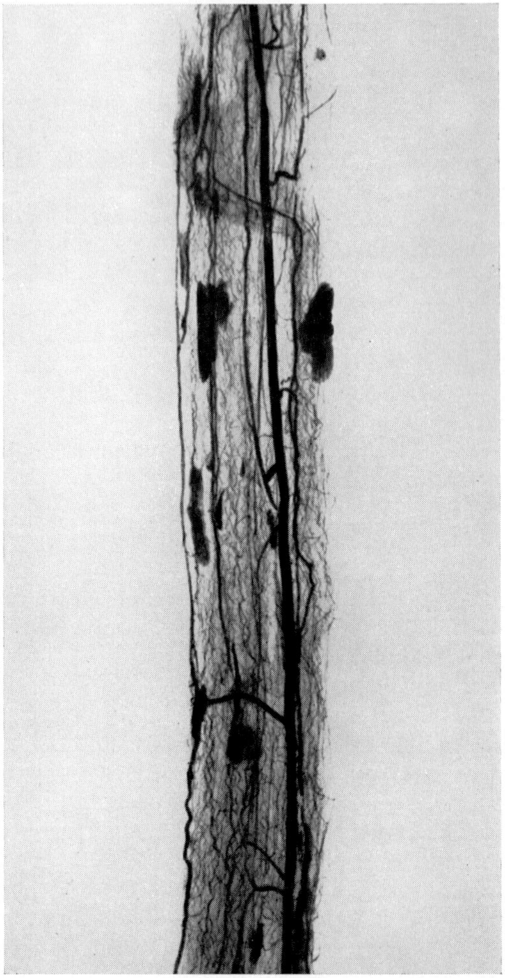

FIG. **1**, 7. Injected normal nerve. The large vessels anastomose freely. The significance of the large round or oval shadows is unknown. Dr Werner Nobel, who made these preparations and to whom I am indebted for this photograph, doubts whether they are extravasations. (Reproduced by kind permission from the proceedings of *5th Europ. Conf. Microcirculation, Gothenburg*, 1968. *Bibl. anat.*, **10**, 316.)

The result is that a nerve can be freed from its bed over a considerable length without jeopardizing its blood supply (Adams, 1943; Bentley and Schlapp, 1943). The longitudinally disposed blood vessels maintain it, although when the collaterals are severed they grow into the nerve again quite rapidly (Blunt and Stratton, 1956). A caveat is necessary here. Of the longitudinally disposed vessels those that descend are larger than those that ascend. Hence if both parts of a severed nerve are mobilized the nerve immediately distal to the point of transection may become ischaemic. Evidence of this, in the form of collagenization extending over perhaps a centimetre, has been found many times in sections of distal stumps resected at operation. Whatever the inferences from animal experiment (Bacsich and Wyburn, 1945*b*), mobilization of a severed human nerve retards regeneration (Nicholson and Seddon, 1957); and in the cases we reported the mobilization was largely confined to the proximal part of the nerve, that is to say, the part best able to withstand partial devascularization. There is an even greater risk of distal ischaemia if the injury has severed the accompanying main artery, because re-establishment of the circulation in the distal part of the nerve depends on the opening up of a roundabout collateral circulation. Striking examples of extensive peripheral ischaemia are shown in Figures **6**, 8B (p. 97), and **15**, 33 (p. 278).

The practical points emerging from these considerations are:

1. When mobilizing a nerve care should be taken to avoid, if possible, severance of major nutrient vessels, such as the one joining the sciatic nerve in the gluteal region, or the one running with the median nerve in the forearm.

2. Because some of the longitudinal anastomoses are situated in the mesoneurium, a millimetre or two wide of the epineurium, it is wise to conserve them by cutting the tissues surrounding the nerve so that a fringe of mesoneurium remains attached to it (Sunderland, 1945*d*). The mobilization should be no more than is essential.

3. If there is any choice the proximal rather than the distal stump of a severed nerve should be mobilized.

4. If the main artery as well as a nerve has been cut across there is a possibility of severe ischaemia of the stump of the distal segment. In such cases secondary rather than primary suture is preferable; after a few weeks the extent of the distal ischaemic changes will be easily recognizable as dense intraneural collagenization, and the resection can be planned accordingly.

MOTOR NERVES

At its termination a nerve fibre supplying voluntary muscle connects with a number of end-plates, and the ensemble is called a motor unit. In limb muscles there may be several hundred muscle fibres in one motor unit. An impulse causes simultaneous contraction of all the muscle fibres with which the one nerve fibre is connected, and this produces a characteristic electrical disturbance (Chap. 4). It is unlikely that the diameter of a motor nerve fibre is related to the number of end-plates it controls (Young, 1950). The muscle fibres comprising one motor unit interdigitate, an overlapping that explains why a number of motor-unit action-potentials can be picked up, on moderate contraction, by one concentric needle electrode (p. 61). This arrangement facilitates smooth muscle action.

The sudomotor, pilomotor and cutaneous vasomotor fibres are derived from the autonomic system; they are all unmyelinated, they run in the cutaneous sensory nerves and have much the same distribution. This permits an objective assessment to be made of the state of cutaneous innervation, particularly by observing sweat secretion (p. 45).

SENSORY NERVES

As was dramatically demonstrated at a Ciba Foundation Symposium (1966) the topics of tactile, heat, and pain sensibility, although the subject of intensive and continuing investigation by many distinguished physiologists and anatomists, still pose questions of bewildering complexity. There is no lack of elaborate receptors of which the Pacinian corpuscle is the most imposing, though some sensory nerve fibres appear to have none at all. The problem is deciding which does what, and also what happens when one modality such as the perception of heat merges into another, pain. Certain facts, besides the anatomically striking specialization of receptors, demand explanation on the basis of 'sensory units' comparable with motor units. The most obvious of these clinically is the almost constant pattern of sensory loss, as between one modality and another, after interruption of a cutaneous nerve. Tower (1940) went some way towards showing that in the admittedly unique surface of the cornea there are areas of innervation forming the peripheral expansions of 'sensory units'; the unit, somewhat like a motor unit, consisting of a central cell body, its axon and a considerable number of endings in a circumscribed but relatively large area, perhaps as much as 200 mm^2. The areas of contiguous sensory units overlap. On this hypothesis (Fig. **3**, 6, p. 40) the areas supplied by cutaneous pain units are much larger than the units subserving touch; and at the finger-tips, where two-point discrimination (p. 53) may be 4 mm or less, the tactile unit areas are smaller than, say, in the thigh, where two-point discrimination is far less accurate. Unfortunately, some consequences of interruption of a cutaneous nerve (p. 39) cannot be explained on a purely anatomical, specific sensory-unit basis, and indeed the whole concept of the specificity of the forms of cutaneous sensibility has been questioned (Weddell, 1961; Weddell and Miller, 1962).

But there is no getting round the fact that we perceived specific sensations and testing based on them is an important aspect of clinical examination. It will be considered in Chapter 3.

2. Degeneration and Regeneration

ONE OF THE great attractions of work on nerve injuries is the ease with which they can be studied experimentally in animals. But this has its pitfalls; it does not follow that the results of experiment can always be taken as a guide to clinical practice.

Kline, Hayes and Morse (1964) produced identical gaps in nerves—excision of a 1-cm segment, which left a gap of 2 to 3 cm—in dogs, rhesus monkeys, baboons and chimpanzees. The results were far from uniform both in the amount of connective tissue proliferation and the effectiveness of axonal regeneration. Bridging of the gap by outgrowing nerve fibres was poor in the baboon and still worse in the chimpanzee. In other experiments nerves were crushed, or divided and sutured. The chimpanzee's behaviour was poor in comparison with that of the other animals.

If the range of species were extended by putting the favourite animal for experiments of this sort, the rabbit, at one end and man at the other, the differences in capacity for regeneration would almost certainly be even more pronounced.

There are two other points: on the basis of experiments on small animals some workers, such as Gutmann and Holubar (1951), are so confident that the capacity for regeneration of spinal neurons is virtually unlimited that they boldly propose the clinical employment of operations designed to keep the cell bodies in a state of intense activity. Yet much clinical evidence (p. 312) suggests that in the human adult there is a limit to the quantity of axoplasm that, say, an anterior horn cell can synthesize. Differences in size of cell body (if this is relevant) as between a large and a small mammal are not great: they are less than the differences in size between cells of the same kind—for example, anterior horn cells—in one species. A human lumbar or upper sacral motor neuron is an astounding structure: it is very long, and the volume of axoplasm is 200 to 300 times that of the cytoplasm of the cell body. But a neuron with an exceptionally long axon does not have an outsize cell body. Recovery after repair of a proximal lesion of the sciatic nerve is always poor at the periphery. While it is true that retrogressive changes at the periphery—in the distal part of the nerve and in muscle—are fairly pronounced by the time regenerating fibres should arrive there, the picture, as will be explained later (p. 242), is rather that of axonal exhaustion. Nerve fibres capable of functioning do not reach the periphery. Hence, in considering the effectiveness of regeneration, the size of the animal can hardly be ignored. Another factor, as will appear later (pp. 296 and 305), is age. In a child—who has the added advantage of short limbs—recovery is far better than in the adult.

Thus, in the account that follows, the selection of evidence from animal experiment is influenced by its relevance to clinical practice.

It is not possible to make a sharp distinction between the process of degeneration and that of regeneration, because, almost from the first, the one is a preparation for the other.

DEGENERATION OF NERVE

When a nerve is cut across, its stumps separate more or less and the gap is filled with blood clot. The proximal end of the nerve swells because of the oedema and the non-specific cellular response that occurs in any recently damaged tissue. There is always retrograde degeneration, its extent depending on the kind of injury. It is slight after a cut with a sharp instrument, it may extend over 1 to 3 cm after the great commotion produced by a high-velocity projectile (p. 71). Thus the Wallerian degeneration that takes place throughout the whole length of the distal part of the nerve also occurs at the end of the proximal part (Fig. **2**, 1). As a result of the initial inflammatory reaction, collagen is deposited in the end-bulb or neuroma that forms (Fig **2**, 2), and the funiculi lose their mobility. The epineurium is fixed to them and it becomes much thicker than normal, this thickening extending some way proximal to the end-bulb. Scarring—collagenization—also occurs within the funiculi. The Schwann cells and fibrocytes in this degenerate part multiply but not to the same extent as in the distal end-bulb (Abercrombie and Johnson, 1942). That the neuroma is chiefly formed by regenerating fibres rather than collagen is suggested by the appearance of a nerve severely injured in two places: a large swelling forms only at the proximal site (Fig. **2**, 3).

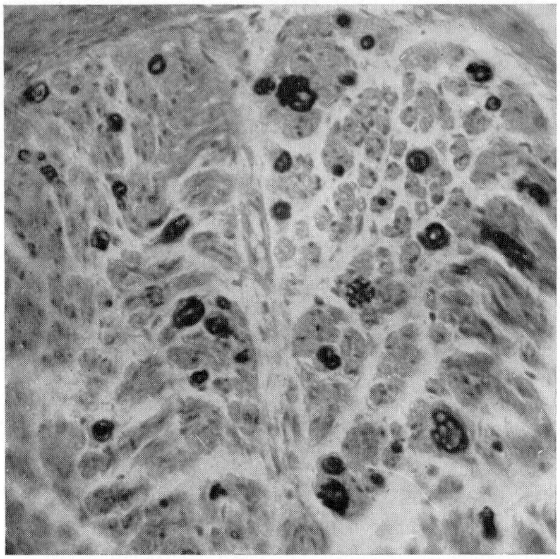

FIG. **2**, 1. A missile, accidentally discharged at close range, injured the median nerve. Six months later secondary suture was performed. The proximal resection was 2·5 cm above the lesion: it exposed good bundles, but, as is apparent in this section, there had been extensive retrograde degeneration. This picture is identical with what would normally be found in the distal part of the nerve. There are few myelinated fibres.

WALLERIAN DEGENERATION

Lively changes take place throughout the whole length of the nerve distal to the site of division. The mitochondria in the axoplasm swell and form clumps; the filamentous structure of the axoplasm is lost, it becomes a granular liquid of rapidly shrinking bulk, and this occurs before the myelin sheath begins to disintegrate (Vial, 1958). After 3 or 4 days all conductivity is lost because the axons and, if medullated, their myelin sheaths break up, the small fibres first. At about the fifth day macrophages move in (Doinikow, 1913) and begin to ingest the fragments; the Schwann cells also take up myelin remains. But macrophages account for only a fraction of the great cellular proliferation that takes place. In the rabbit the nuclear population of the degenerating sciatic nerve increases eightfold by the twenty-fifth day and is still fivefold at 225 days (Abercrombie and Johnson, 1946*a*).

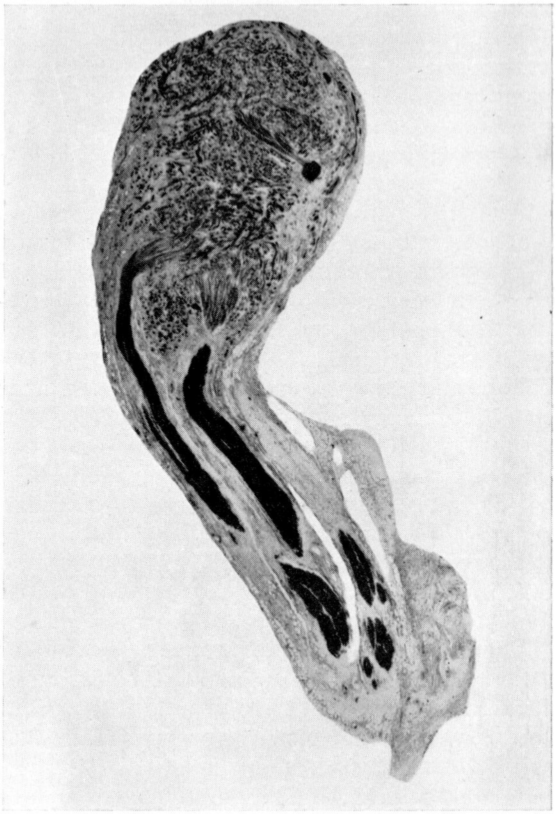

FIG. **2**, 2. A neuroma on a severed digital nerve. It is formed of collagen and a tangle of regenerating fibres, which in one place can be seen spreading out from the cut end of a funiculus. (Reproduced by kind permission of Professor William Blackwood.)

Schwann cells predominate, but the endoneurial fibrocytes are not far behind. It is suggested that the stimulus is the products of disintegration of the nerve fibres; but apart from the disappearance of the macrophages, when their scavenging is completed, it is not clear why the cell population gradually declines.

As the axoplasm and myelin disintegrate the basement membrane collapses into many folds (Fig. **2**, 4). Thus, where there had been a nerve

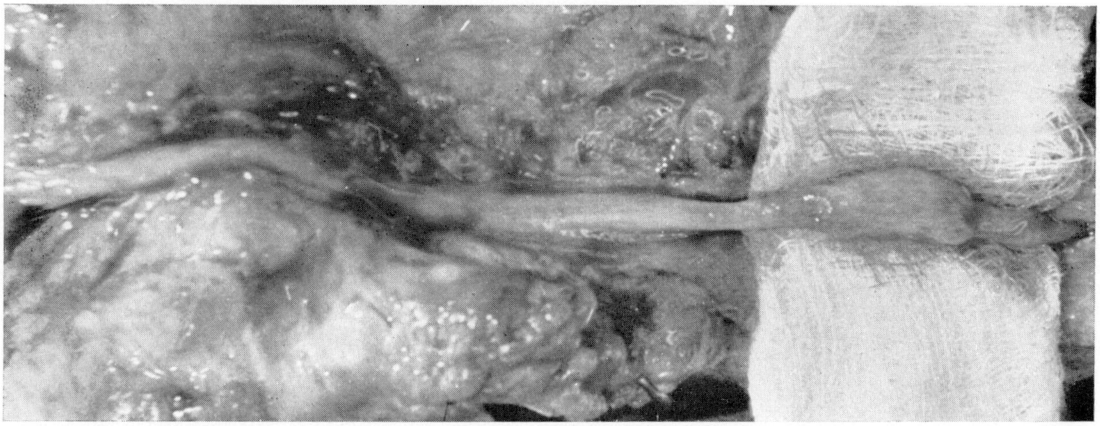

DISTAL PROXIMAL

FIG. **2**, 3. A nerve injured in two places: a neuroma formed only at the proximal site. Fortunately it was the ulnar nerve near the elbow, and after anterior transposition double repair was simple, the part between the two lesions becoming an autologous graft. (Reproduced by kind permission from M.R.C. Special Report Series, No. 282, 1954.)

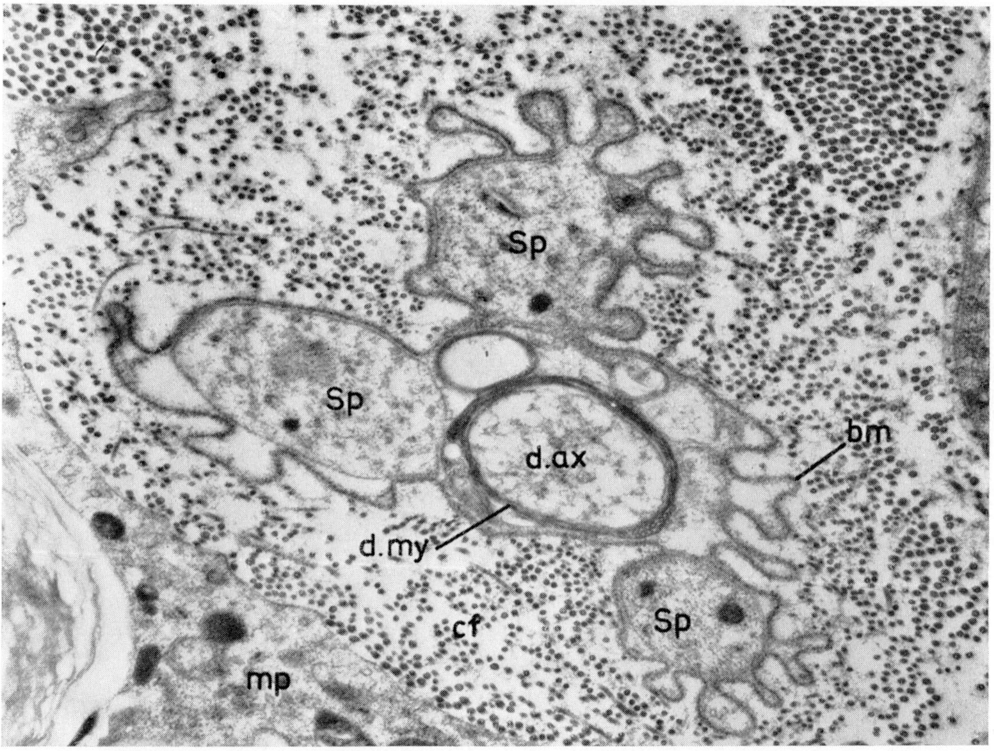

FIG. **2**, 4. Collapsed basement membrane enclosing Schwann cells, from the distal part of a rabbit's nerve severed 7 days previously. In addition to the Schwann-cell processes there are axon and myelin debris: ×23,000.

bm	basement membrane	d. ax	degenerating axon
Sp	Schwann-cell processes	mp	macrophage
d. my	degenerating myelin	cf	collagen fibrils

(The excellent photographs reproduced in Figs **2**, 4 to **2**, 6 and in Fig. **2**, 12 have been generously provided by Prof. P. K. Thomas.)

fibre the basement membrane alone indicates that there is a tubular structure, containing Schwann cells (Thomas, 1966). The Schwann nuclei are conspicuous (Figs **2**, 5 and **2**, 6), and their cytoplasmic processes interdigitate intricately (Fig. **2**, 5).

When a nerve is sutured this outgrowth from the distal stump is the most essential feature in the union of the nerve (Young, Holmes and Sanders, 1940). And because the activity of the cells is greatest relatively soon after the nerve injury this is a strong argument in favour of early repair (Holmes and Young, 1942). However, Abercrombie and Johnson (1942) suggested that because there is an appreciable interval before the power of multiplication reaches its peak, early secondary may be better than primary suture.

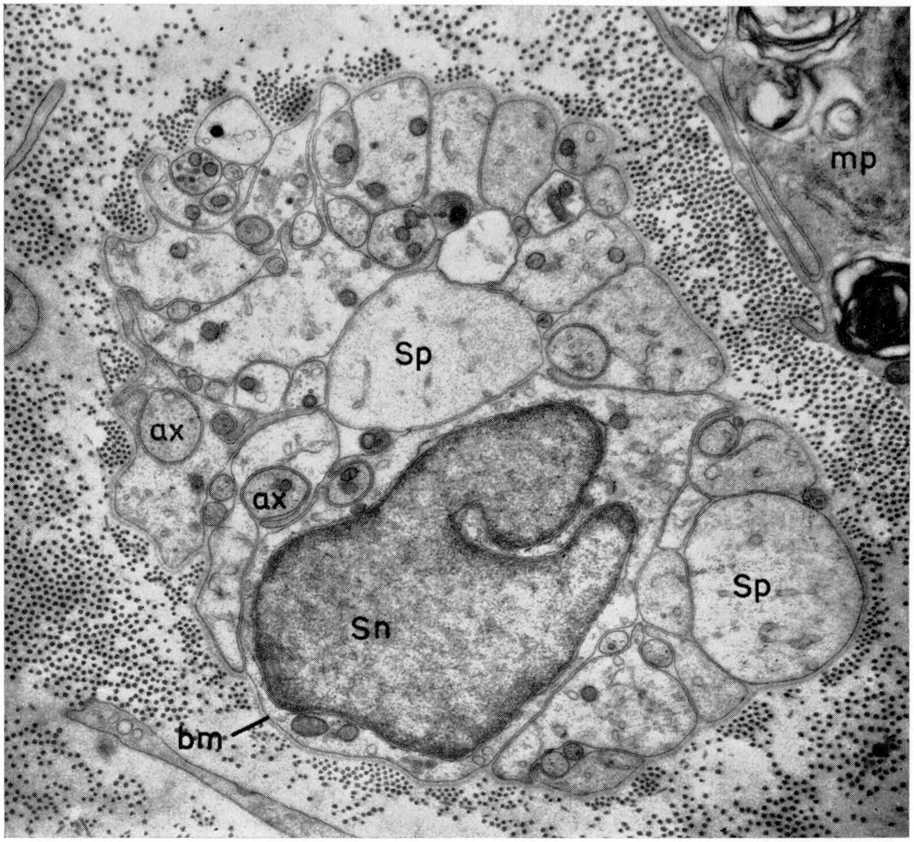

FIG. **2**, 5. Schwann tube from the distal part of a rabbit's nerve 3 weeks after nerve crushing, showing probable early re-innervation: ×15,000.

bm	basement membrane
Sn	Schwann-cell nucleus
Sp	Schwann-cell process
ax	probable axonal sprout
mp	macrophage

Particular interest attaches to the cellular proliferation in the distal end-bulb. Here, as in the proximal end-bulb, there is the usual response to injury, but the multiplication of Schwann cells and fibrocytes is so great that a visible swelling appears. The proliferation may even extend proximally, towards the proximal neuroma, forming what Young (1942) aptly called a 'ghost nerve'.

Masson (1932) and Denny-Brown (1946) took the view that the cellular outgrowth from the distal stump is mainly fibroblastic. Because of the difficulty in distinguishing proliferating Schwann cells (which are notoriously pleomorphic) from fibroblasts by light microscopy, the final answer could be given only by electron microscopy (Thomas, 1966). What happens is that Schwann cells grow out in columns invested by the same sort of basement membrane as exists in the distal part of the nerve, and these columns are surrounded by fibrocytes, blood vessels, leucocytes and macrophages. Furthermore, the perineurium participates, and thus in its cellular content this outgrowth is a proximal extension of the distal part of the nerve. But its structure is irregular, the Schwann-cell columns interlacing with each other. The fibroblasts contribute by laying down collagen; the collagen content of the degenerate nerve increases (Abercrombie and Johnson, 1946*b*), and it does not diminish when re-innervation takes place (Abercrombie and Johnson, 1947).

The endoneurial tubes shrink progressively (Holmes and Young, 1942), and there is an increase in the amount of collagen between them (Fig. **2**, 7). Collagen is deposited around the basement membrane surrounding a column of Schwann cells (Nathaniel and Pease, 1963; Thomas, 1964; Fig. **2**, 6). According to Nathaniel and Pease, collagen is laid down also between the basement membrane and the Schwann cells.

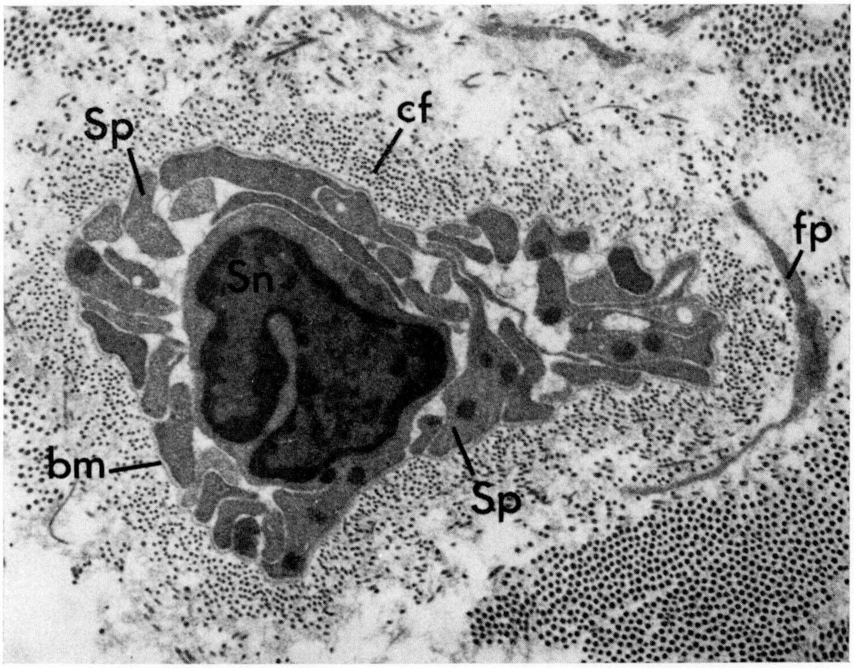

FIG. **2**, 6. Schwann tube from distal part of a rabbit's sural nerve 4 weeks after severance. Basement membrane surrounded by a dense zone of newly-formed collagen fibrils which are of smaller diameter than the more peripherally placed original endoneurial collagen fibrils: ×10,500.

bm	basement membrane
cf	collagen fibrils
Sn	Schwann-cell nucleus
Sp	Schwann-cell process
fp	fibroblast process

Sooner or later nerve fibres are to be found in the degenerate nerve. Some may have made their way across the site of injury; others (Holmes and Young, 1942) grow in along blood vessels.

After an initial increase in diameter the whole of the distal part of a nerve shrinks. Over a

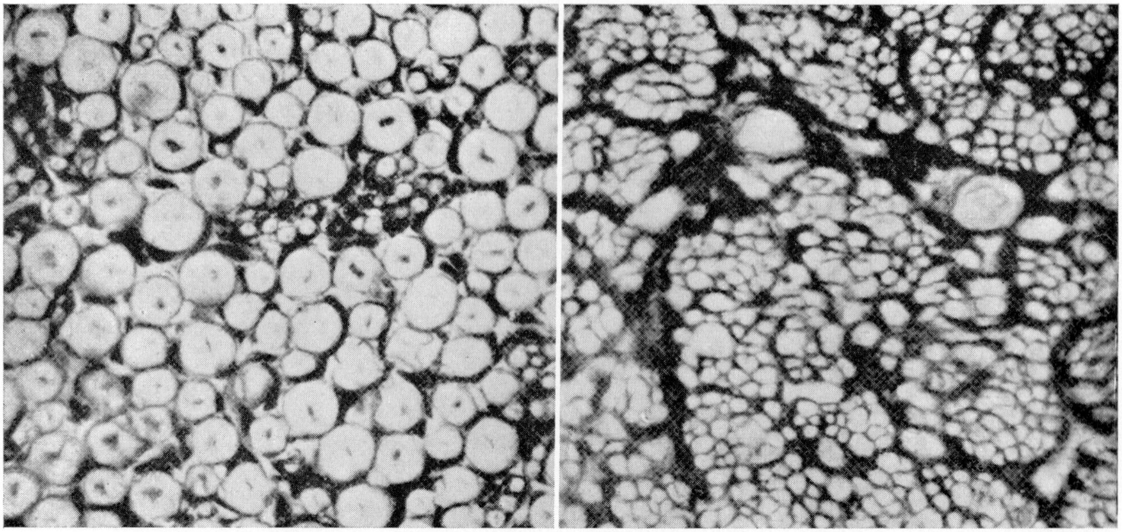

FIG. 2, 7. Transverse sections of the distal parts of the anterior tibial nerves in a boy of 9 years, who died from an unrelated condition 21 months after division of one common peroneal nerve about 5 cm above the head of the fibula. The sections were taken at the same level and the magnification is identical. (Reproduced by kind permission from *Br. J. Surg.*, War Surgery Supplement No. 2, 1948.)

number of years we have recorded both diameters (not all nerves are circular in section) of resected nerve stumps; we have found that after 6 months the shrinkage may be such as to make accurate suture impossible (Fig. **2**, 8). If, as is usual, epineurial stitches are used, there is bound to be some bunching of the proximal funiculi. This is an unfavourable factor.

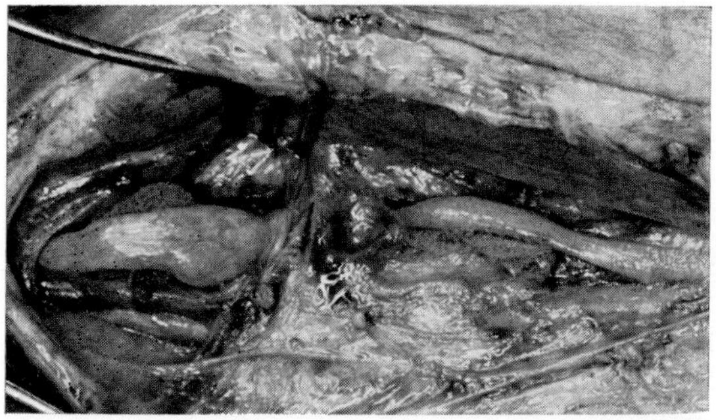

FIG. **2**, 8. The proximal neuroma is on the left. Shrinkage of the distal part of a severed nerve 27 months after injury. The diameters proximal to the neuroma—that is, at the far left—were 7 × 7 mm: distally 7 × 3 mm.

PERSISTENCE OF END-ORGANS

Of the more specialized end-organs Pacinian and Meissner corpuscles have been found in man 9 months after nerve injury (Lyons and Woodhall, 1949), and motor end-plates (Bowden and Gutmann, 1944) persist for at least a year.

CHANGES PROXIMAL TO THE SITE OF DAMAGE

There are changes in the nerve fibres proximal to the lesion. They become smaller and their conduction velocity is reduced (Gutmann and Holubar, 1951; Cragg and Thomas, 1957; Aitken and Thomas, 1962). That the shrinkage is not entirely due to the distal flow of axoplasm during regeneration is shown by the fact that shrinkage still occurs when the distal part of the nerve has been avulsed, so that regeneration is impossible. Furthermore, if a nerve has been severed and allowed to form a neuroma, the shrinkage is greater than after severance and suture. It appears to be a disuse atrophy.

The effect of nerve section on the cell bodies, the disappearance of the granules that bear his name, was described by Nissl towards the end of the last century. That centripetal atrophy occurs in the relevant parts of the central nervous system after amputation of a limb has been abundantly attested by many workers. There is even shrinkage of the spinal cord, and retrograde changes in the motor and sensory cortex corresponding to the absent limb (Campbell, 1905).

REGENERATION OF NERVE

This process, on which the effectiveness of repair of a damaged nerve ultimately depends, can be modified by local conditions. It is convenient to describe it in detail after ideal primary repair, that is to say, clean severance of a nerve with a very sharp instrument followed immediately by suture; and then to note more briefly what happens after early secondary suture, after late secondary suture, and after what is called unaided union in which regeneration of a sort occurs in the absence of operative intervention.

Ideal Primary Suture

The Junctional Tissue

The physical union of a severed nerve is the result of intense cellular activity mostly at the cut surface of the distal part. As has already been mentioned, the Schwann cells multiply vigorously and the fibroblasts of the distal endoneurium, perineurium and epineurium are equally active. The pattern of their growth towards the proximal cut surface and their ultimate union with it is not haphazard. Provided that there has been no distortion, such as is produced by tying the epineurial sutures too tightly, the orientation of the connective-tissue elements and of the Schwann cells is mainly longitudinal; the pattern of the Schwann tubes at the distal face of the severed nerve is extended proximally, but with interlacing between the columns of cells. The perineurium also participates in this bridge building (Thomas and Jones, 1967). However, when the columns of Schwann cells arrive at and join with the cut surface of the proximal part there is little chance of their uniting with the tubes to which they belonged. Nevertheless, the greater the pains taken to ensure correct orientation during suture of a nerve the less will be the resultant confusion. The cellular bridge that conducts the outgrowing axons to the periphery is now established.

Behaviour of the Axon

Some accounts of the behaviour of the regenerating axon are obscured by loose terminology. The individual outgrowing streams of axoplasm—even when confined, as they may sometimes be, within one Schwann tube (*see* axonotmesis, p. 21)—have been referred to as *fibres* or even *axons*. They are, in fact, only parts of *the* axon or nerve fibre. The Nile is still the Nile even when the body of water, diversified by rocks or islands, breaks up into many streams. The word branch is acceptable, provided it is not given a botanical gloss, and it is understood that the branches can coalesce.

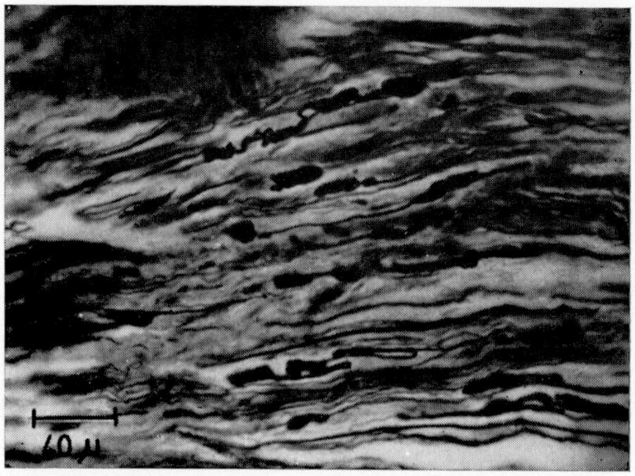

FIG. **2**, 9. The patient had great and persistent sensitivity of the left thumb after a metal splinter had entered it. The puncture wound was infected for a time. One year later a digital neuroma was excised.

A remarkable collection of Perroncito spirals was found where outgrowing axonal branches ran into a mass of scar tissue.

A regenerating axon always sends out a number of branches, the estimates given by various authors ranging from a few to dozens (Cajal, 1928). Whatever the nature of the injury this process begins some way proximal to the lesion, where the Schwann tubes are intact. When these axonal branches arrive at the cut surface of a nerve that has been severed they are free to wander anywhere. If obstructed some turn in their tracks and double back into the proximal part of the nerve forming the picturesque Perroncito spirals (Figs **2**, 9 and **2**, 10). Others turn laterally away from the line of the nerve, escaping into the tissues surrounding it. But if a suture has been well executed most of them go straight ahead, along the longitudinally disposed strands of Schwann cells that have bridged the gap. The branches—streams of axoplasm—have

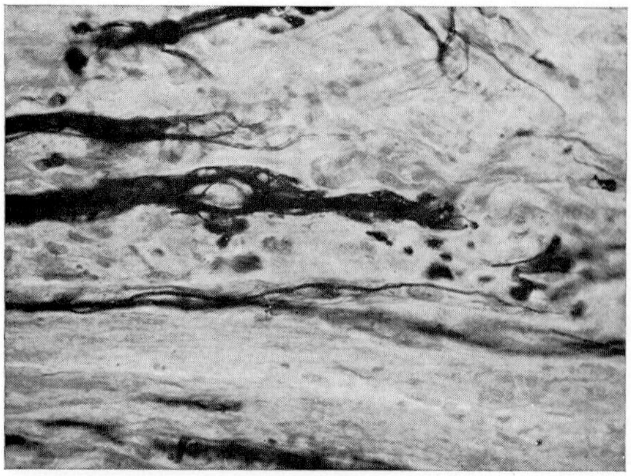

FIG. 2, 10. In the centre, advancing from the left, is a thick stream of axoplasm. It flows round a globule of degenerating myelin, then a little further on encounters some obstruction and doubles back on itself, thus forming a Perroncito spiral. Below this another finer stream of axoplasm is making its way uninterruptedly along the surface of long fusiform Schwann cells. (Reproduced by kind permission from Blackwood, W., 1954. M.R.C. Special Report Series, No. 282.)

an affinity for the surfaces of the Schwann cells and so reach the distal part of the nerve (Fig. **2**, 11). Here they come to the Schwann tubes, which have already extended in a proximal direction. Although the tubes are packed with

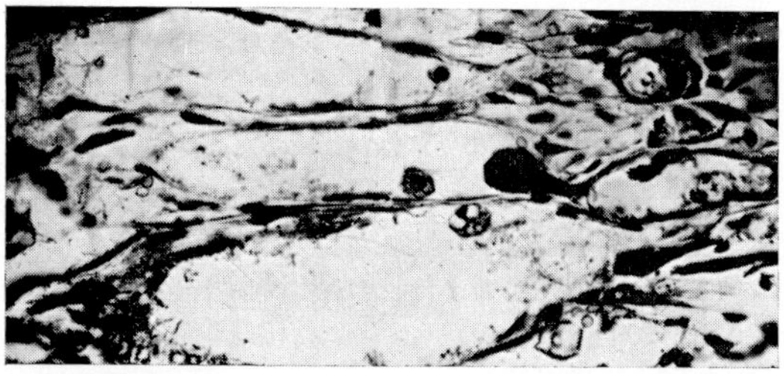

FIG. 2, 11. A blob of axoplasm, the advancing tip of a new fibre, about to cross a bridge formed by Schwann cells. Another small one, lower right.

Schwann cells and their processes, the streams of axoplasm squeeze their way in between them (Fig. **2**, 5); and up to 20 may be found in one tube (Holmes and Young, 1942). One branch may be centrally placed and rapidly develop a myelin sheath (Fig. **2**, 12); others are peripheral but still surrounded by Schwann cytoplasm, and several branches in one tube may become myelinated (Fig. **2**, 13). Secondary basement membranes may form within the original one (Fig. **2**, 12).

At this stage a transverse section of the distal part of the nerve presents the picture of great overpopulation; this has given rise to such statements as: 'The number of axons in the sutured region varied from 157 per cent to 440 per cent of the estimated normal number' (Shawe, 1955) which, if the term axon is interpreted in its strict sense, is a little misleading. Groups of these axonal branches must be derived from single axons above the level of the lesion. These branches continue distally and as they do so certain changes take place.

1. At any given time the number of branches is less in the most distal part of the nerve than in the part near the lesion. The further regeneration advances, the fewer the number of branches.

2. With the passage of time the number of demonstrable branches declines throughout the whole of the distal reach of the nerve, though as revealed by axon staining it remains well above normal.

3. A process of maturation takes place. Some of the branches that have penetrated Schwann tubes increase in diameter, a process that is greatly encouraged by the re-establishment of appropriate peripheral connections (Weiss, Edds and Cavanaugh, 1945; Aitken, Sharman and Young, 1947). These branches are on the way to becoming the new axons. Myelination also occurs around branches that have grown out from medullated fibres. Even if there are a number of branches within one Schwann tube several of them may become myelinated (Fig. **2**, 13).

4. But the final picture, even after ideal suture, is a population of mature fibres that is subnormal both numerically and in respect of diameter. Clearly there has been some elimination of the numerous branches that were present initially. It appears that some cease to grow; they may even atrophy and disappear, particularly those that lie outside the Schwann tubes. Those within the tubes may coalesce before or after myelination; or it may be that the one branch that makes an appropriate peripheral connection and becomes a mature axon squeezes the others out of existence.

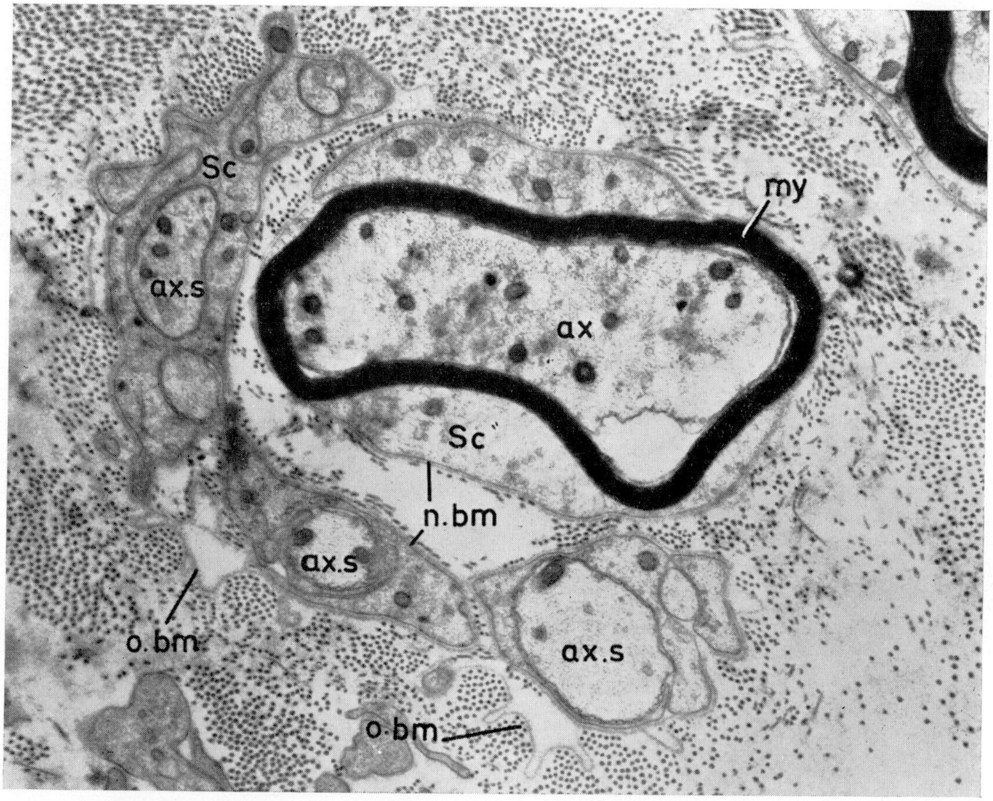

FIG. **2**, 12. Re-innervated Schwann tube from the distal part of a rabbit's nerve 3 weeks after a nerve crush: ×14,000.

o. bm	original basement membrane	ax. s	axonal sprout
n. bm	new basement membrane	my	myelin
ax	axon	Sc	Schwann-cell cytoplasm

The pattern of the regenerated nerve after suture is not restored to normal (Fig. **2**, 14), and there are functional as well as morphological deficiencies. Motor fibres, for example, become connected with muscles they did not formerly innervate. There is confusion too as between motor and sensory fibres. Thus there is inevitably a persistent impairment of function which even the crude methods of clinical examination will reveal if carefully applied. The conduction velocity of regenerated nerve fibres is reduced; even under the most favourable conditions, as when a nerve has been crushed instead of cut and sutured, and the pattern of re-innervation has been restored to normal, it is still about 25 per cent below normal at 12 to 16 months (Cragg and Thomas, 1964).

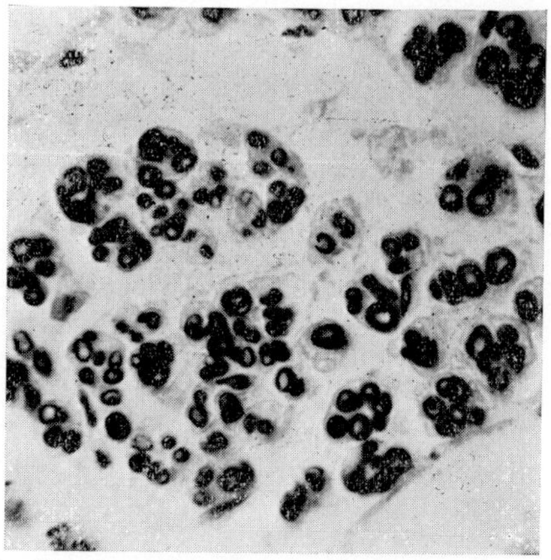

FIG. **2**, 13. Axonal sprouts, all myelinated, bunched together within single Schwann tubes (Reproduced by kind permission of Dr William Holmes.)

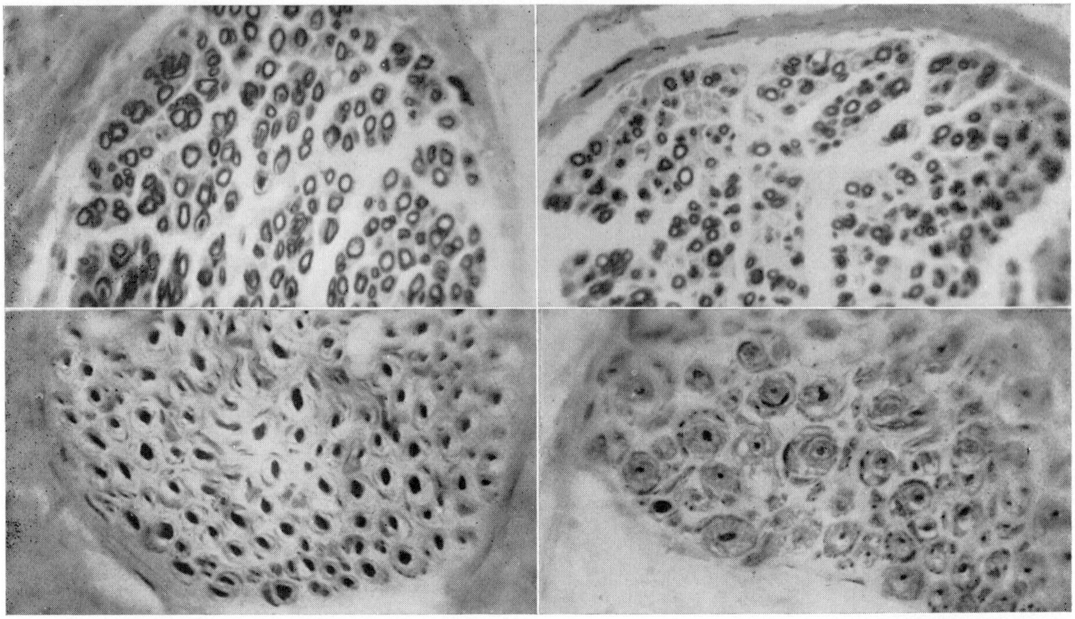

FIG. **2**, 14. The common peroneal nerve of a rabbit was crushed on one side (axonotmesis), on the other cut and re-united immediately by fibrin suture. At 107 days, re-innervation was apparently perfect on the crushed side (left). In the sutured nerve the distal part was well below normal, and in the lower right photomicrograph there are many small dots, possibly between the Schwann tubes, axonal branches that had gone astray. (Reproduced by kind permission from *Brain*, 1943, **66**, 237.)

Ambient temperature influences maturation (Jha, Goldby and Gamble, 1959). It seems likely that the most favourable temperature is slightly above that of the body; and also that the cooling of new nerve fibres when they reach a superficial position in a limb retards regeneration. This phenomenon has been observed in man (Haftek, 1967*a*) as well as in experimental animals.

Protection of the Suture Line

A recurrent penchant of surgeons interested in peripheral nerve repair is the employment of material that is wrapped round the suture line. The variety of wrappings used has been very great, and the search for what is considered the ideal still continues. Three reasons have been given for this practice.

1. It is supposed that the fibroblasts in the tissues surrounding the nerve invade the suture line and so give rise to harmful intraneural collagenization. It is overlooked that the nerve itself is richly endowed with fibrocytes, that they proliferate vigorously and lay down collagen and, as many observers have shown, rapidly re-establish something approaching the normal pattern of the stroma of the nerve. Indeed, after an improperly executed suture the impression conveyed (Fig. **2**, 15) is that collagenization *spreads out* from the nerve into the surrounding tissues. Even when a well-executed suture has come apart (Fig. **2**, 16) the epineurium may show perfect continuity. And on rare occasions when a suture line that is satisfactory has been inspected (as in a patient of mine who had violently extended the wrist soon after repair of the ulnar nerve, and separation seemed probable) the perineural adhesions were minimal. The invasive propensities of the extraneural fibroblasts are not established.

2. The second reason has substance; adhesions sometimes form between the suture line and the

surrounding tissues and it is conceivable that if the latter are highly mobile, tendons above all, there may be harmful traction on the nerve at the point of repair. In situations where this could happen an ideal wrapping material might be useful.

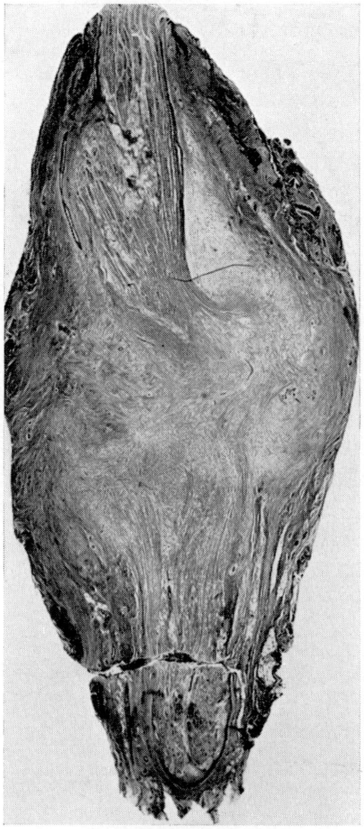

FIG. 2, 15. Forty-five days previously primary suture of the radial nerve had been performed, unwisely, after a missile injury. There was extensive interstitial damage of the nerve, and the subsequent collagenization presented the appearance of bursting out of it. There was little scarring of the surrounding tissues. (Reproduced by kind permission from Zachary, R. B. and Holmes, W., 1946. *Surgery Gynec. Obstet.*, **82**, 632.)

3. A third point, supported by experimental evidence, has been advanced by Campbell (Pinner-Poole, Tomasula and Campbell, 1967). However delicately a nerve suture is carried out and however favourable the conditions, the operation is undeniably an injury; and all injuries are followed by oedema, which involves the substance of the sutured nerve at least as much as the surrounding tissues. Campbell has shown that the swelling distorts the stroma of the nerve, and that this aggravates irregularity in the pattern of regeneration. If oedema can be prevented by appropriate wrapping of the suture line, then regeneration should be more regular, and Campbell has shown that this is possible. But this

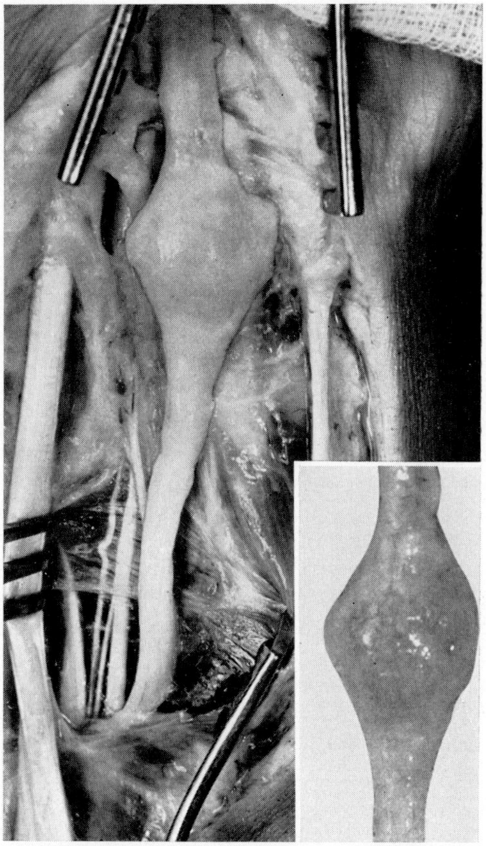

FIG. 2, 16. This was a well-executed secondary suture which unfortunately separated. Yet in spite of this mishap (successfully remedied later) the epineurium has remained intact. In the larger photograph there is no sign of invasion of the suture line from without; in the smaller one light is reflected from the intact epineurium which, undeterred by the separation, has sealed in the funiculi.

presupposes that the wrapping material itself produces no unfavourable reaction. Every material except the one currently in fashion has been found wanting, and it is noteworthy that most surgeons with considerable experience of surgery of peripheral nerves do not use these foreign bodies; they have seen too much of the damage, often irreparable, that has resulted from their employment. Campbell was the ardent advocate of Millipore, a porous cellulose acetate fabric (Campbell, Bassett, Giraldo *et al.*, 1956), but found that it became brittle and when fragmented provoked a brisk foreign body reaction. For this reason he favoured a silicone rubber (Silastic), said to be inert.

Early Secondary Suture

By this is meant repair within 3 months from the time of injury, and it suffices to note the features that differ from those obtaining in primary suture. Apart from entailing a second operation they are mostly advantageous. The epineurium is thickened over a short distance proximally and distally, and this gives the epineurial stitches a more secure hold. If there has been any disturbance of the circulation, such as damage to an adjoining main artery, any consequent ischaemia of the tip of the distal stump will have led to intraneural collagenization which is easily recognizable to the naked eye when the end-bulb is resected; the proper site for resection can be found without difficulty. Wallerian degeneration is well advanced and most of the remains of axon and myelin will have been removed from the Schwann tubes; though there is, however, no evidence that these fragments present any barrier to regeneration. The Schwann cells growing out from the distal end of the nerve are at about the peak of their activity and so rapidly form a good union with the proximal face of the nerve.

One disadvantage, in comparison with primary suture, is that instead of minimal trimming of the severed ends there is need to resect a fair slice from each: this entails some loss of congruity of the pattern of the funiculi.

Late Secondary Suture

The outgrowth of the Schwann cells across the gap is less vigorous. Although, as Blackwood and Holmes (M.R.C.R., 1954) have pointed out, the Schwann tubes may remain patent for up to 6 months after injury, the tendency is for them to become solid columns of small diameter, and the more advanced endoneurial collagenization may hinder the maturation of the regenerating nerve fibres.

Because fibre diameter and function are associated it is important to know whether, in the course of re-innervation, the shrunken tubes are capable of being distended by axons growing into them, or if the shrinkage can become so great and irreversible as to preclude satisfactory regeneration. The diameter of the largest tubes may decrease by up to 90 per cent (Sunderland and Bradley, 1950) and—in the Australian opossum—most of this occurs in the first 90 days. There is no doubt that axons artificially directed to grow into tubes that *never have been large* can distend them only to a small extent (Simpson and Young, 1945), but in simulating the clinical injury, in which shrinkage has occurred as a result of prolonged denervation, it is difficult to distinguish the harmful influence of the shrinkage of Schwann tubes from other noxious consequences of denervation. When we come to consider the practical implications of the shrinkage of the Schwann tubes and of kindred factors—that is to say, after what lapse of time it is futile to repair a severed nerve—it is best to rely on clinical evidence and, fortunately, it exists (pp. 242-249).

The distal part of the nerve as a whole will have shrunk and this makes tidy suture, and therefore orderly regeneration, impossible.

Unaided Union

The degree of separation of the nerve ends may be slight, particularly if the injury has left a strand of epineurium intact. I have seen recovery in a child following an unaided union of this sort which was, if anything, superior to that obtained after the most favourable suture (p. 252). The little bridge of epineurium not only prevented retraction of the severed funiculi but maintained them in the best possible apposition. This has a bearing on how exploration of a severed nerve should be conducted (p. 251).

But more often than not there is some separation. A neuroma forms and although regeneration occurs across the gap its quality is defective and better regeneration would have followed suture. In general, the presence of a neuroma, which in some situations is palpable or even visible, is an indication for formal repair.

Even when there is considerable separation some nerve fibres always jump the gap: thus, after a most destructive lesion one always finds a few nerve fibres, even myelinated ones, in the distal stump.

Axonotmesis

This term (Seddon, 1943; p. 32), is a convenient name for a type of damage that had long been recognized though not always clearly understood. If a nerve is crushed with smooth watchmaker's forceps (even if the nerve is small, firm pressure is necessary and it must be repeated several times at one spot) the axons and their myelin sheaths are broken, but the stroma of the nerve remains in continuity—the Schwann tubes, endoneurium, perineurium and epineurium. In their electron-microscopical study of this sort of damage Haftek and Thomas (1968) have shown that even the Schwann basement membranes persist. Within minutes of release of the pressure the translucent strand of crushed tissue is re-inflated. Yet the axonal damage and the consequent loss of function are as complete as after severance of the nerve. After a few days, a fusiform swelling appears and at its equator there is a transversely disposed patch of haemorrhage (Bacsich and Wyburn, 1945*a*). There is dilatation of blood vessels and proliferation of connective tissue elements. The degree of disorganization of the stroma depends on how the nerve has been crushed. Gutmann, Guttmann, Medawar and Young (1942), using smooth forceps, produced lesions in which the general architecture of the nerve was preserved, whereas Bacsich and Wyburn (1945*c*) inflicted 'a severe crush with artery forceps' and so produced tears in the supporting tissues. Either way both axoplasm and myelin are absent from the crushed segment. Yet even after a rough crush the initial disorganization is only temporary and by the fifteenth day (in rabbits) the crushed segment presents much the same architecture as the undamaged distal reach of the nerve. Wallerian degeneration occurs exactly as after severance of a nerve. The endoneurial tubes are in continuity throughout the whole length of the lesion and consequently there is no axonal confusion in the course of regeneration. This has a favourable effect on the rate and, still more, on the quality of regeneration.

One aspect of the restitution of the pattern of the nerve is shown in Figure **2**, 17. The intact, proximal axons shrink during regeneration and then—in axonotmesis, though not after suture—regain their original diameter as the new axons gradually mature and finally attain almost normal size (Gutmann and Sanders, 1943).

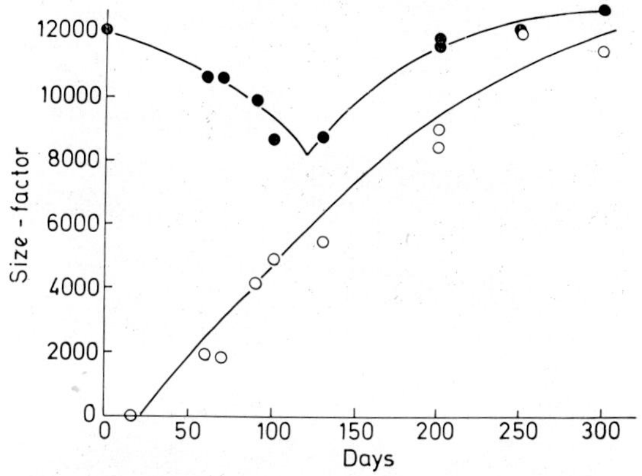

FIG. **2**, 17. Graph showing what Gutmann and Sanders (1943) call the size factor (of nerve fibres) in the proximal part of a nerve and in the distal part at various times after axonotmesis. Black circles: proximal. White circles: distal. (By kind permission of the authors and of *J. Physiol., Lond.*, **101**, 489.)

Although the lesions in continuity encountered in clinical practice include every degree of damage from pure axonotmesis to profound and irreversible intraneural disorganization, certain types of injury—for example, lesions of the radial nerve caused by fractures of the humerus—are often followed by the same kind of regeneration as is seen after experimentally produced axonotmesis. In such cases the term may properly be employed in diagnosis. And it is vitally important to recognize it, because restoration of function after axonotmesis is far superior to that seen after the most carefully executed nerve suture. It can be perfect.

Neurapraxia

At the time when this term (Seddon, 1943; p. 32) was introduced, it had no more morphological basis than its etymology suggests, and the word is best used to describe a clinical entity. A comparatively mild injury, moderate compression, slight stretching, or the passage of a missile near a nerve trunk produces a motor paralysis that is usually complete, but with only partial sensory loss and little or no disturbance of autonomic function. There is little or no evidence of

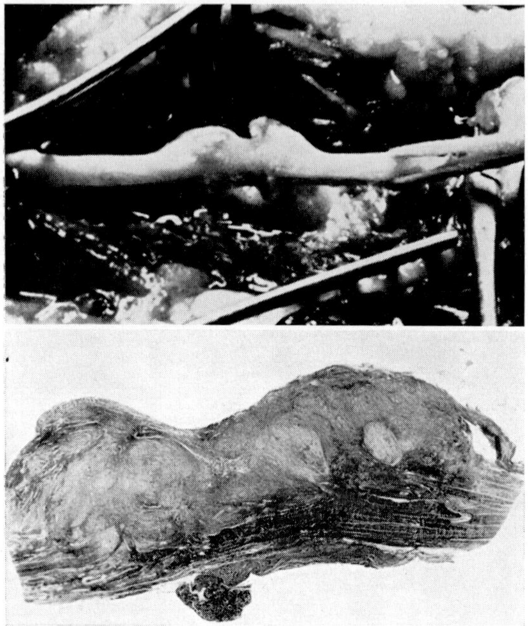

FIG. **2**, 18. A lateral neuroma with a double hump. Four months after the bullet wound that injured the radial nerve there was a little action in extensor carpi radialis longus. But no other muscles recovered and this is why the nerve was explored, resected and sutured. The serious damage involves at least five-sixths of the cross-section of the nerve. (Reproduced by kind permission from M.R.C. Special Report Series, No. 282, 1954.)

Wallerian degeneration; indeed, conduction in the nerve distal to the site of damage remains normal. Recovery may occur within hours, days, several weeks or a few months; and it does not follow a proximal-to-distal course, as is invariable during the ordinary course of regeneration.

Clinical evidence suggests a relationship between the vulnerability of nerve fibres and their diameter. The functions subserved by large fibres—motor and proprioceptive—are those chiefly disturbed.

Weir Mitchell (Mitchell, Morehouse and Keen, 1864) had noted this transient type of paralysis, and Erb (1876) remarked on the occasional persistence of faradic excitability in paralysed muscles, an indication that their nerve supply had not degenerated.

The experiments of Denny-Brown and Brenner (1944*a*, *b*) provided an explanation of the kind of neurapraxia that is more than fleeting. They showed that compression of a nerve by a tourniquet or a spring clip produced a dissociated paralysis, predominantly motor, exactly resembling the well-recognized clinical condition. The axons swelled and showed indentations, and their staining properties were altered. The myelin sheaths at the site of compression degenerated and there was oedema of the nerve above and below the compressed segment. These were the significant changes, though there were others. Conductivity returned well before there was restitution of the myelin sheaths, which occurred gradually over periods of up to 6 months. They describe the lesion as ischaemic demyelination.

PARTIAL DIVISION

Although nerve injuries can present any combination of the three kinds of damage that have just been described, with or without an admixture of normal elements, only one type need be considered here, namely partial division.

A sharp object—usually glass—may cut through part of a nerve, the remainder being little affected structurally or functionally; less commonly a missile damages the nerve in the same way. The severed part behaves like a nerve that has been completely transected. Proximally there is the usual swelling, a neuroma; and just below it the swelling arising from the distal cut surface, due to the proliferation of Schwann cells and fibroblasts. Thus, on one surface of the nerve, normal funiculi are distinguishable beneath the epineurium, whereas on the other there are humps like a Bactrian camel's (Fig. **2**, 18); the two swellings may be so close together as to form a single hump (Fig. **15**, 13; p. 263 and Fig. **15**, 17, p. 265). Either type of swelling is called a lateral neuroma.

If a high-velocity missile has nicked the nerve, exactly the same gross appearances result; but the part remaining in continuity is likely to suffer more severely. The damage of the part in continuity may approximate to an axonotmesis, or there can be such violent intraneural disruption that the ensuing collagenization precludes spontaneous regeneration. The total damage (Fig. **2**, 18) may be much greater than is suggested by the external appearance.

One of the most awkward problems facing the surgeon (pp. 262-266) is deciding whether to resect a lesion of this kind, in the hope of obtaining better regeneration by secondary suture. It has to be borne in mind that the severed funiculi can behave as an 'unaided union' (Fig. **2**, 19) and, as has been explained (p. 20), satisfactory regeneration can occur across a small gap without assistance from the surgeon.

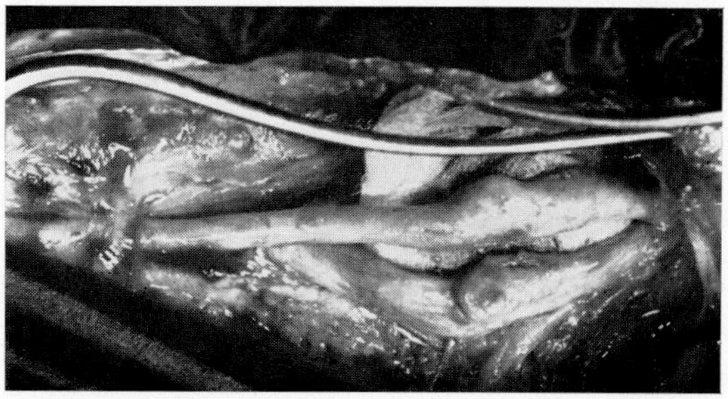

FIG. **2**, 19. Missile injuries of the common peroneal and tibial nerves; the upper (peroneal) shows a lateral neuroma with two humps; the lower (tibial) a single hump. There was complete motor paralysis of the peroneal nerve, but only partial sensory involvement. The tibial paralysis was incomplete. Exploration was performed because there was no clinical or electromyographic evidence of recovery in the muscles supplied by the peroneal nerve. It was decided that both nerves should be left alone and both recovered almost completely. (Reproduced by kind permission from *Br. J. Surg.*, War Surgery Supplement No. 2, 1948.)

SEPSIS

During the First World War it was found that a nerve could be damaged not only by a missile but by the infection that frequently supervened. In the Second World War no single instance of this was reported by British observers. It may therefore be concluded that this factor may now be disregarded so far as the nerve itself is concerned.

FOREIGN BODIES

Any missile may carry fragments of mineral matter or clothing into a nerve where they invariably set up the usual type of foreign-body reaction (Figs **2**, 20 to **2**, 22).

Two types of foreign body are introduced surgically; suture material, which will be considered in Chapter 15; and material used for wrapping round the suture line, on which some comment, mostly unfavourable, has already been made (pp. 18-20).

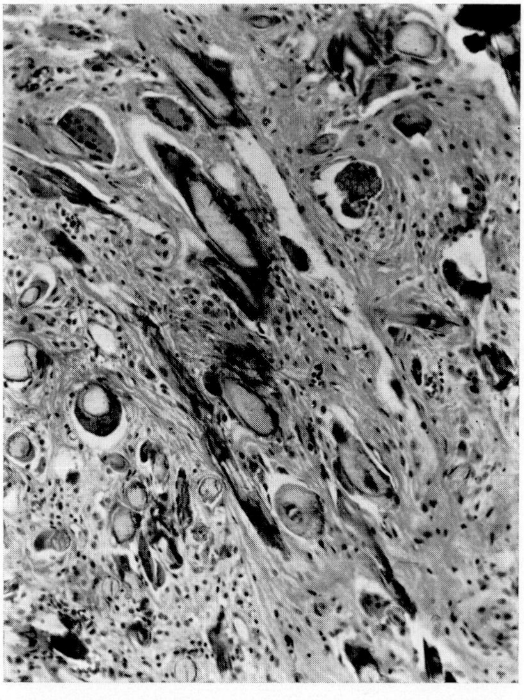

FIG. **2**, 20. Cotton fibres, not suture material and almost certainly from clothing, in the substance of a nerve, with some giant cells round them. (Figs **2**, 20–**2**, 22 reproduced by kind permission from Blackwood, W., 1954. M.R.C. Special Report Series, No. 282.)

MUSCLE

The consequences of denervation to be described are as follows: (1) atrophy; (2) fibrillation and (3) changes in motor end-plates.

Atrophy

Of all the consequences of denervation, muscle atrophy is the most striking. In poliomyelitis it may, after many years, go as far as complete disappearance of muscle and its replacement by fat. This atrophy far exceeds that due to disuse alone.

During the Second World War Bowden and Gutmann (1944) recorded the progressive changes that take place in man and so rounded off the large amount of information that had already been obtained experimentally.

Within the first few weeks the muscle fibres shrink rapidly. They are no longer compact and in longitudinal section present a wavy outline. Spaces also appear inside the individual fibres: the myofibrils become separated. The shrinkage is uneven (Fig. **2**, 23), some muscle fibres wasting more than others. The cross-striation persists; it has been observed for up to 23 years after denervation, but it shows up patchily in stained specimens and may be detectable only by polarized light.

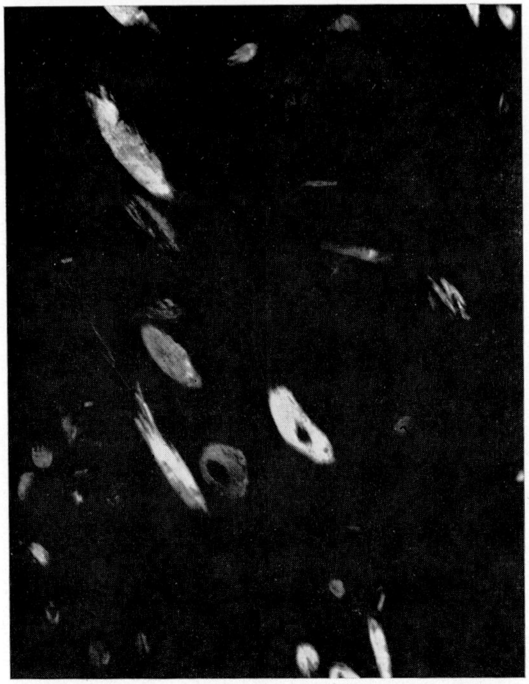

FIG. **2**, 21. The same as Fig. **2**, 20, except that the cotton fibres are picked out by polarized light.

With the passage of time there is a progressive increase in interstitial tissue, partly collagenous, partly fatty. As wasting of a muscle fibre continues, its nuclei become aggregated towards the centre of the fibre and, because of this crowding, give the appearance of being more numerous. Bowden and Gutmann found no evidence, such as Tower (1939) observed in animals, of transformation of muscle fibres into connective tissue. Nevertheless, after very long periods, even the minute atrophic fibres finally disappear and the muscle is replaced by a mixture of fat and fibrous tissue.

So long as muscle fibres persist they are capable of excitation by an electrical current of long duration and this property will be considered more fully in Chapter 4.

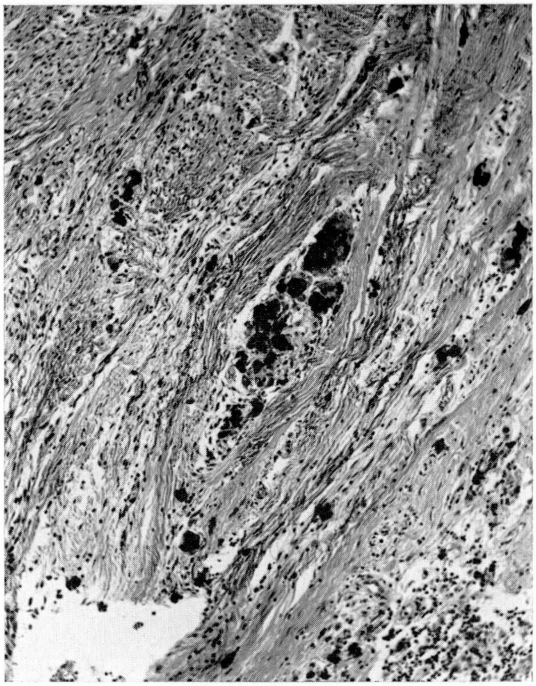

FIG. **2**, 22. Fragments of rock, the dark particles, embedded in a nerve and surrounded by fibrous tissue.

Fibrillation

This curious phenomenon, spontaneous contraction of individual denervated muscle fibres, was first described by Schiff in 1851. Within a week or less of interruption of the nerve, twitching can be seen in very superficial muscles such as those of the tongue, but not in those of the limbs. Schiff observed that after section of the facial nerve in the rabbit the vibrissae began to quiver about 4 days later. In other situations

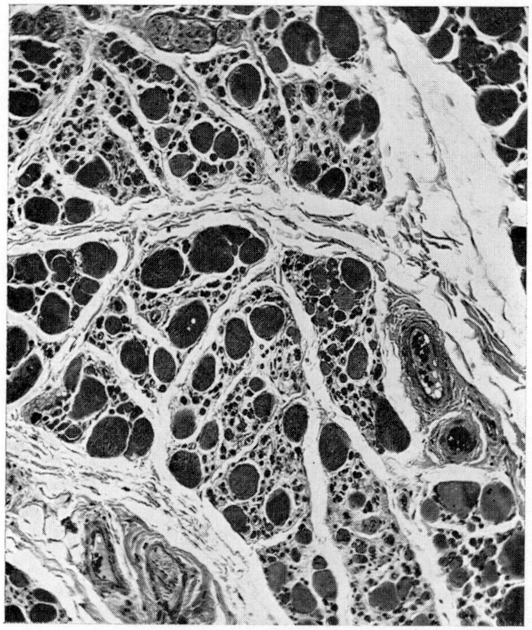

FIG. 2, 23. Uneven shrinkage of denervated muscle fibres.

fibrillation can be detected only in the exposed muscle. It continues for months but gradually decreases with progressive atrophy of the muscle. Fibrillation does not occur after transection of the spinal cord.

It is increased by warmth, decreased by cold; it varies from one species of animal to another, being greatest in the small mammals, and there is evidence to suggest that this is connected with the basal metabolic rate (Feinstein, Pattle and Weddell, 1945). Elaborate pharmacological studies have been carried out in attempts to elucidate the nature of fibrillation, and they are well summarized by these authors. It has been suggested that fibrillation is the chief cause of the atrophy, and that the increased oxygen consumption of fibrillating muscle is due to catabolic activity. But the atrophy begins before the fibrillation and it continues if the fibrillation is prevented by the administration of quinidine.

Minute action-potentials are produced by the fibrillating muscle; they are a sensitive index of motor denervation, but although they can be observed electromyographically (Chap. 4) it is sometimes difficult or impossible to detect them.

Motor end-plates

These elaborate end-organs are found where a motor nerve fibre makes contact with the surface of a muscle fibre. The structure of an end-plate is shown diagrammatically in Figure **2**, 24, and Figure **2**, 25 which have been drawn from good

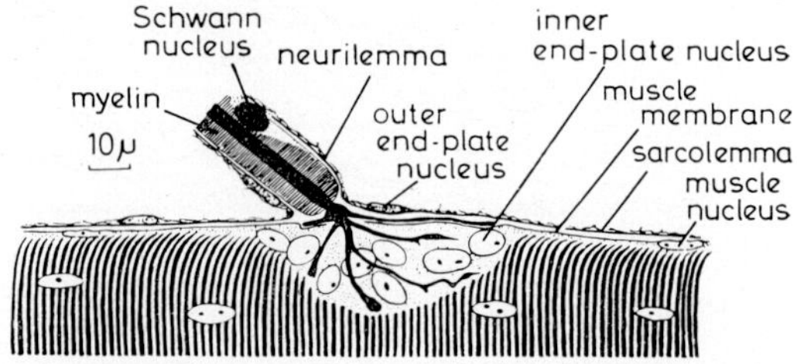

FIG. **2**, 24. Diagram of a motor end-plate. (Figs **2**, 24–**2**, 25 and **2**, 27–**2**, 30 reproduced by kind permission from Gutmann, E. and Young, J. Z., 1944, *J. Anat.*, **78**, 15.)

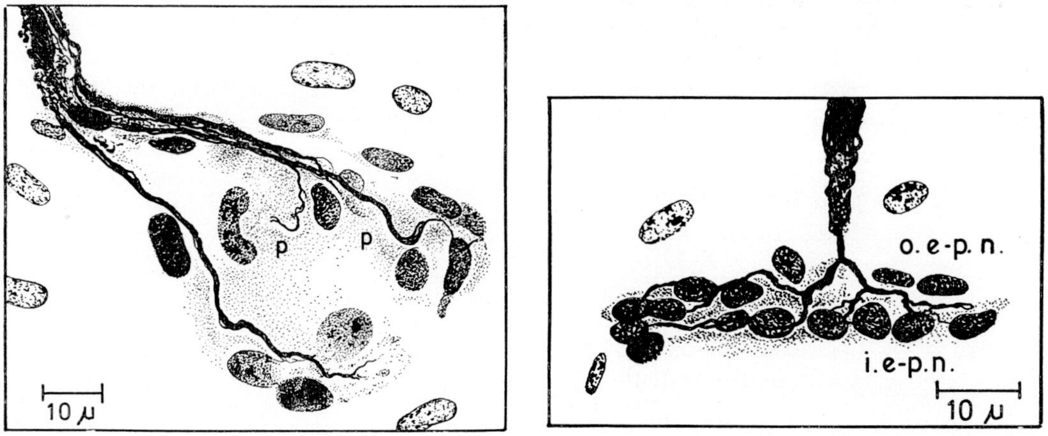

FIG. **2**, 25. *Left:* normal motor end-plate. *Right:* normal end-plate showing how the branches of the nerve fibre terminate between the outer and inner layers of end-plate nuclei. (After Gutmann and Young.)
p. protoplasm of end-plate o. e-p. n. outer end-plate nuclei i. e-p. n. inner end-plate nuclei

histological preparations. The electron microscope reveals much greater complexity of structure—see, for example, Engel and Santa (1973)—but none that need concern us here. After degeneration of the axon the fibrocytes become more numerous, and ultimately the collagen fibrils deposited round the termination of the Schwann tube and round the atrophying muscle fibre can obstruct re-innervation if and when it occurs (Fig. **2**, 26). The motor end-plates in denervated muscle persist for at least a year. If axonotmesis has occurred at a point not far removed from the muscle one nerve fibre grows down to its proper group of end-plates and rapidly re-establishes normal connection with them. If the period of denervation has been lengthy the down-growing fibre is obstructed, and it may extrude a stream of axoplasm running parallel with a muscle fibre; and at some more commodious point it may succeed in forming new end-plates (Figs **2**, 27 to **2**, 29). There is a profound change in the configuration of the motor units (Kugelberg, Edström and Abbruzzese, 1970). Instead of the muscle fibres being widely dispersed, mingling with those of other motor units (p. 7), they are bunched together and sometimes demarcated by perimysium. The prospects of satisfactory re-innervation are not so good after nerve suture because inappropriate fibres—sensory and autonomic—may find their way into the muscle (Fig. **2**, 30). They do not join up with the end-plates but ramify among the muscle fibres. Under favourable conditions, complete restoration of innervation of the end-plates may occur, as after distal axonotmesis, but otherwise, and more particularly after nerve suture, re-innervation remains subnormal. The longer the period of atrophy the less effective the re-innervation and many muscle fibres may never be re-innervated at all.

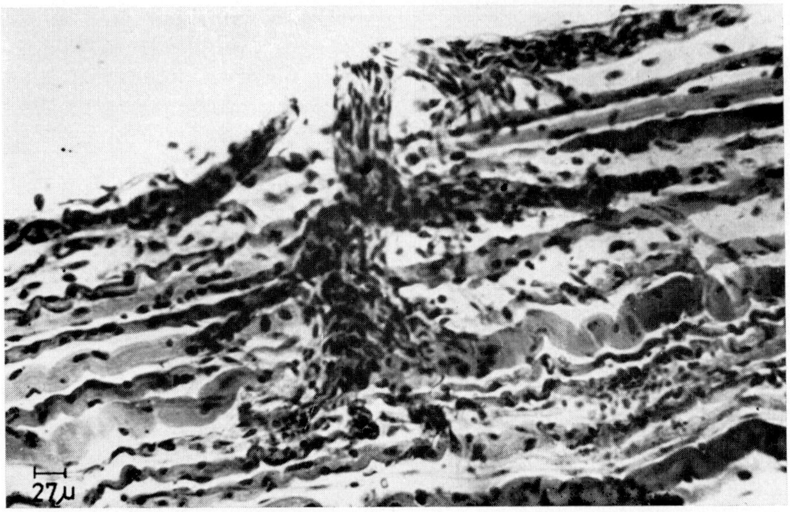

FIG. **2**, 26. Fibrocytic infiltration of the termination of a motor Schwann tube 250 days after the patient had suffered a nerve injury. (Reproduced by kind permission from Bowden, R. E. M. and Gutmann, E., 1944, *Brain*, **67**, 273.)

There is some delay between the arrival of regenerating fibres at their destinations and the return of functional activity, the duration of which again depends on whether re-innervation is early and complete or late and incomplete. Gutmann and Young found that after late suture of a nerve this delay could be as much as 55 days in the rabbit.

If a muscle has been partially denervated, so that there is an intermingling of normal and denervated motor units, the intact axons send out processes towards the denervated fibres which, on arrival, form new end-plates. This remarkable phenomenon, first described by Weiss and Edds (1946), occurs quite early; within a matter of weeks the partially denervated muscle begins to regain its weight and power and

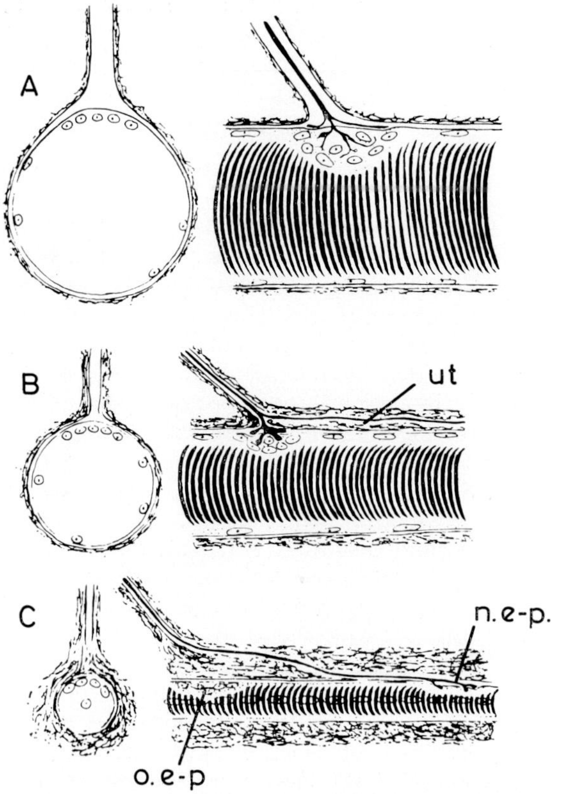

FIG. 2, 27. Diagrams showing how fibrosis round the terminations of motor Schwann tubes hinders re-innervation of muscle but does not necessarily prevent it.
A. Satisfactory re-innervation of a motor end-plate.
B. Fibrosis constricting the channel to the end-plate. Although the latter is re-innervated some of the axoplasm escapes laterally to form an ultraterminal fibre.
C. Channel obliterated by fibrosis. Old end-plate not re-innervated.

ut	ultra-terminal nerve fibre
n. e-p.	new end-plate
o. e-p.	old end-plate

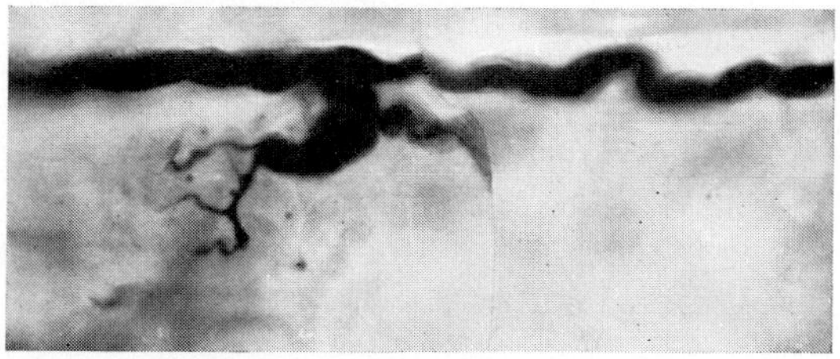

FIG. 2, 28. An ultraterminal nerve fibre that has formed an end-plate. The part of the fibre distal to the plate persists even 4 months after the fibre had arrived at the muscle.

in an increasing number of initially denervated fibres atrophy is reversed. Hoffman (1950) found evidence that the stimulus provoking this type of re-innervation is the local diffusion of a substance derived from the myelin of the

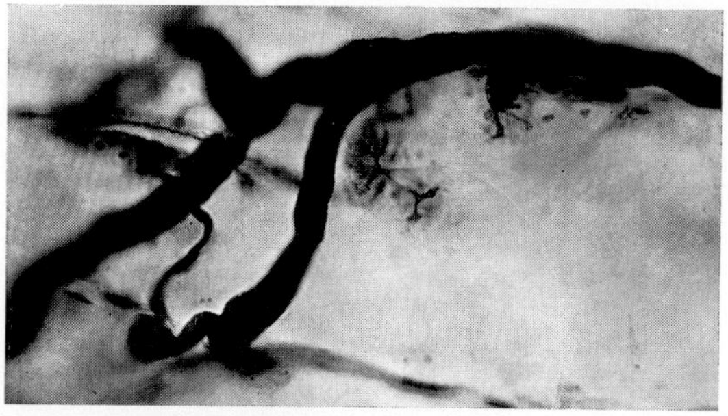

FIG. 2, 29. Fully formed new end-plates after a long period of atrophy and of recovery. It was 17 months before the nerve fibres arrived to form them.

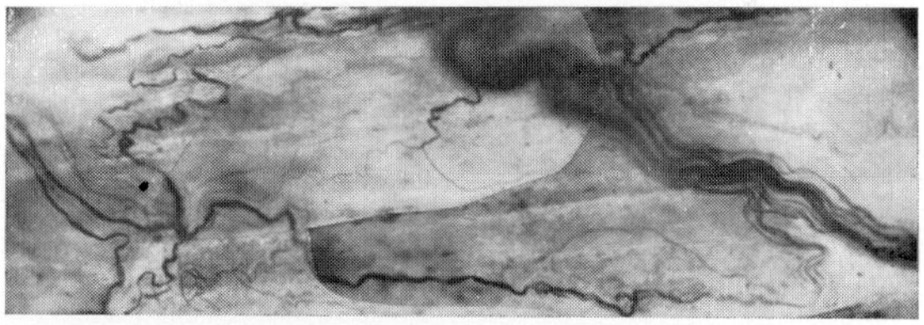

FIG. 2, 30. Sensory nerve fibres wandering aimlessly between muscle fibres.

degenerating nerve fibres. If the stump of a normal motor nerve is implanted into denervated muscle its fibres will ramify and form new end-plates (Hoffman, 1951); he also observed that a similar phenomenon could occur if the nerve was implanted into normal muscle—hyperneurotization—though to a lesser degree; and Sunderland (1952) found clinical evidence of this.

RATES OF REGENERATION

This has become a complicated topic, as Bowden and Sholl (M.R.C.R., 1954) have shown in their excellent review; only an abbreviated and simplified account of it will be given here. Two processes have to be considered, the advance of the axonal outgrowth and the advance of functional, that is to say motor and sensory, recovery.

The Advance of Regenerating Fibres

In animals, the first phenomenon can be studied by exposure of the distal part of the damaged nerve under light anaesthesia, and then pinching the nerve with fine forceps, beginning at the periphery and working proximally. The pinch that provokes a reflex response accurately indicates the point reached by the most rapidly advancing fibres (Young and Medawar, 1940). The advance of Tinel's sign in man, though it cannot be checked histologically, conveys much the same information. There is some delay before the new fibres enter the distal reach of the nerve; they are held up for a time at the site of damage. In rabbits the delay is about a week after suture, and 5 days after a crushing injury (axonotmesis); it is not possible to calculate the delay in man. The rate of advance is rapid, nearly 4 mm a day in the rabbit and about 3 mm in man.

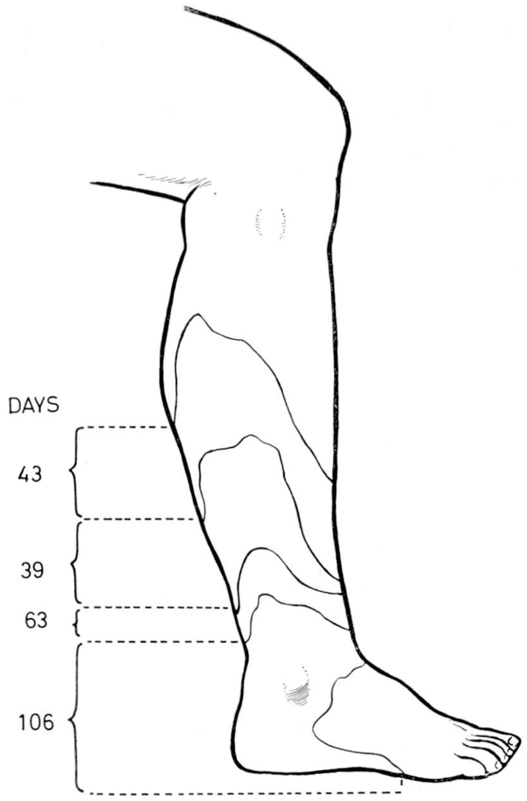

FIG. **2**, 31. The shifting boundary of sensory recovery can be followed conveniently in an extensive area of insensibility such as follows interruption of the sciatic nerve. (This figure, Figs **2**, 32 and **2**, 35 reproduced by courtesy of *J. Physiol., Lond.*, 1943, **102**, 191.)

The Advance of Functional Recovery

This process is much slower, because it requires maturation of an appreciable number of new nerve fibres, and their establishing appropriate motor or sensory connections. The rate of functional recovery can be studied in animals (Gutmann, Guttmann, Medawar and Young, 1942), but more easily in man. Sensory recovery can be plotted at intervals (Fig. **2**, 31). Motor recovery in patients requires knowledge of the levels at which motor branches enter the muscles under consideration, which are somewhat inconstant. Sunderland (1947) showed that even the order in which branches leave a nerve trunk is variable, and also that some attention ought, perhaps, to be paid to their intramuscular course. Armed with knowledge of the level of the lesion and with the levels of innervation of the various muscles, the observer then watches for the first appearance of activity in each muscle. This is difficult to organize; the patient must be seen at least weekly. The date of appearance of the first visible contraction is recorded (Fig. **2**, 32). Jasper (1946) very usefully recorded the rate electromyographically by the simple means of determining the interval between injury, or suture, and the time of the first appearance of motor-unit action-potentials 'subtracting 10 days for delay at the scar'. He measured the distance from the lesion to the site of insertion of the needle. He could obtain only an average rate but it is one that is valuable in clinical practice because electromyographic evidence of recovery precedes visible contractility. Bowden (Bowden and Scholl, M.R.C.R., 1954, pp. 277-283) went further and worked out rates of recovery based on electromyographic evidence of re-innervation. The times when motor-unit action-potentials first became detectable in each of the muscles supplied by a damaged nerve were utilized in exactly the same way as the first signs of voluntary contractility already referred to.

The Rates of Regeneration and the Latent Period

Because only a few points could be plotted on a graph, based on observations made on small animals, it was at first assumed, apparently with justification, that the rates of regeneration were linear. But evidence obtained clinically threw doubt on this. The points (Figs **2**, 33 and **2**, 34) seem to fit a straight line well enough, that is to say, the rates of regeneration are uniform, but

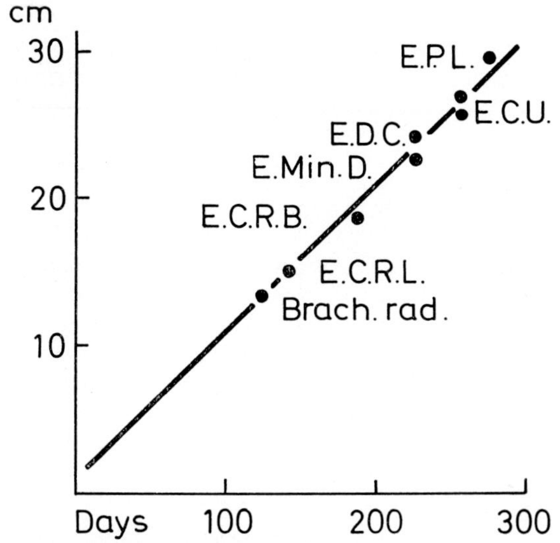

FIG. **2**, 32. Motor recovery after axonotmesis of the radial nerve. It will be noted that it appeared to begin a few days before the injury occurred: an absurdity.

Brach. rad.	brachioradialis
E.C.R.L.	extensor carpi radialis longus
E.C.R.B.	extensor carpi radialis brevis
E. Min. D.	extensor digiti minimi
E.D.C.	extensor digitorum communis
E.C.U.	extensor carpi ulnaris
E.P.L.	extensor pollicis longus

when these lines are extrapolated in order to determine the latent period before regeneration got under way it may be found, though not invariably (Fig. **2**, 36), that it is a negative quantity, which is absurd (Seddon, Medawar and Smith, 1943). It is evident that the rates cannot be uniform; the advance of the axonal outgrowth or of functional recovery is speedy at first, then settles down to what appears to be a uniform rate and, finally, as the process approaches completion, advances slowly. Occasionally (Fig. **2**, 35) the recordings can be fitted only to a curve.

Sunderland (1947, and in his earlier papers to which he makes reference) confirmed this discovery with a wealth of anatomical detail. To the biometrically minded it seems obligatory to make the curves smooth and expressible by mathematical formulae. The latter has been attempted by Seddon, Medawar and Smith (1943) and by Bowden and Sholl (1950).

The latent period before regeneration starts—that is, before the severed axons begin to send out

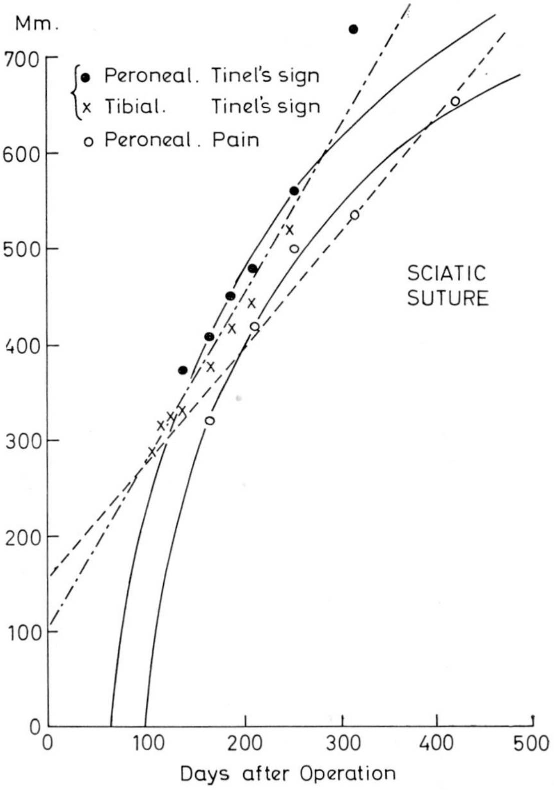

FIG. **2**, 33. Tinel's sign and return of pain sensibility after suture of the sciatic nerve. Although straight lines can be drawn quite convincingly, extrapolation of them gives a negative latent period.

branches—IS easily comprehensible; it is due solely to delay at the site of the lesion. But when the rate of functional recovery is being considered there are additional factors, maturation of the new axons, re-establishment of connections with motor end-plates, or in the case of sensory fibres their arrival in the skin in sufficient quantity to respond to appropriate stimuli. These all increase the latent periods, and if knowledge of rates of regeneration is to be applicable clinically we should know what they are; how many weeks or months.

A latent period can be determined only by extrapolation—this is where a formula should be useful—but when this is done a wide range of variation is revealed. Sunderland (1947) found

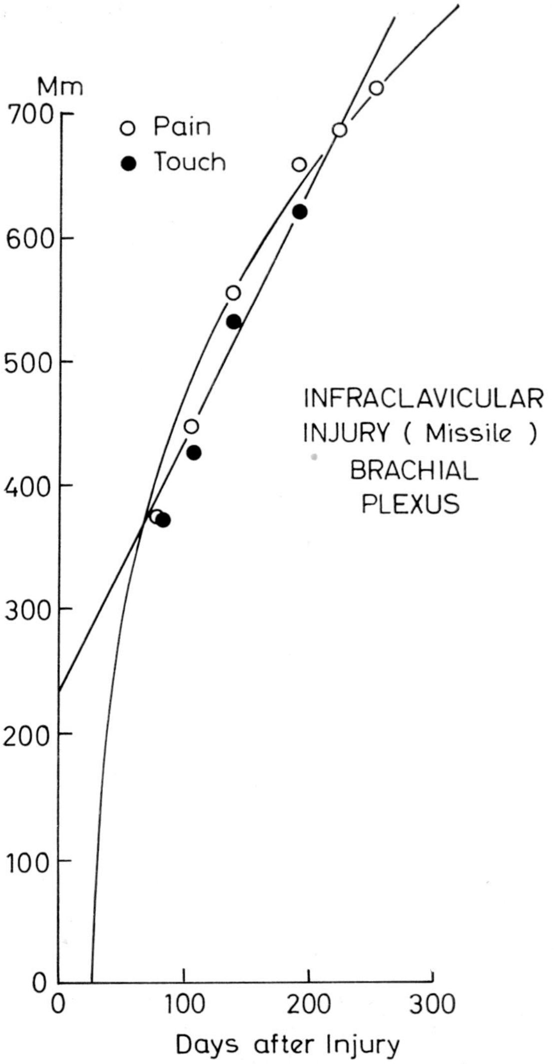

FIG. **2**, 34. Return of pain and tactile sensibility after an injury of the brachial plexus. The features are the same as those shown in Figure **2**, 33.

that it varied from 1 to 32 weeks, with a mean of 13 weeks after axonotmesis and 16 after suture. Figure **2**, 36 reveals a remarkable state of affairs; the patient was a man of 66 with a degenerative lesion of the radial nerve, presumably axonotmesis because the quality of recovery was ulti-

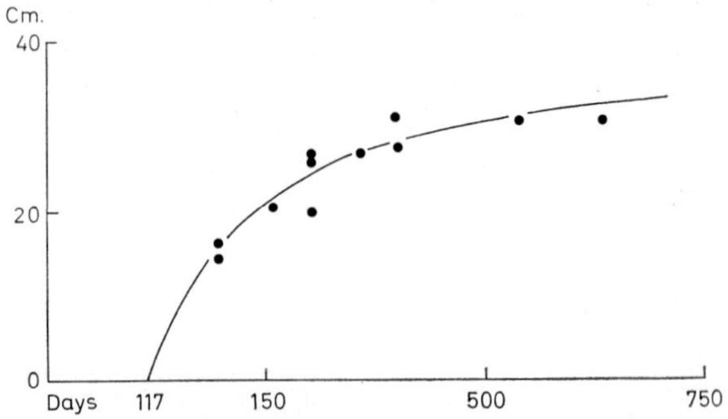

FIG. **2**, 35. These points, indicating the first appearance of motor recovery after an injury of the radial nerve, could be fitted only to a curve.

mately perfect. During the period of 200 days when motor recovery was occurring the rate was uniform and, at 2 mm a day, fairly rapid. If a straight line is drawn through the points the latent period must have been about 220 days—7 months. But because we know that the points lie on a curve the latent period must have been even

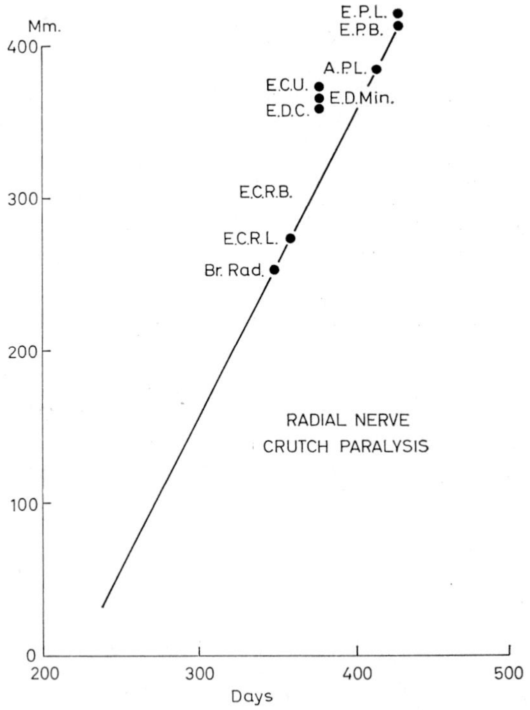

FIG. **2**, 36. Return of motor power in a man of 66 who had suffered a crutch paralysis of the radial nerve. Although the use of crutches was discontinued as soon as the paralysis started, a complete degenerative motor lesion developed.

longer, and the initial rate of advance much more than 2 mm a day. This very long latent period may have been partly due to the nature of the lesion; the paralysis was caused by pressure from a crutch, and the damage to the nerve probably extended over a reach of several centimetres. Recovery after traction lesions is slow, and here there is no doubt that the longitudinal extent of the damage is very considerable; it is sometimes the same with recovery after lesions in continuity caused by high-velocity missiles (Livingston, Davis and Livingston, 1945). If the process of motor recovery can behave in this odd fashion—and in this case (Fig. **2**, 36) much depended on it, whether or not tendon transplantation was required—it is clearly risky to base clinical decisions on any average latent period; or even on any average rate of regeneration, because the rate varies according to the level of the lesion (Fig. **2**, 37).

The burden of the discussion on indications for operation (Chap. 14) will be that, with the exception of nerve injuries in the upper limb due to fractures and dislocations, it is wise to base decisions on factors other than estimates of the time when signs of spontaneous recovery should appear.

The melancholy conclusion after all the work that has been done on rates of regeneration,

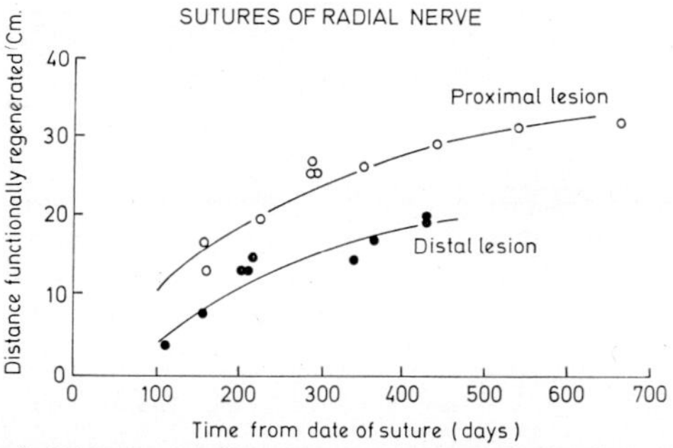

FIG. **2**, 37. Return of motor power after repair of proximal and distal lesions of the radial nerve (Reproduced by kind permission from Bowden, R. E. M. and Sholl, D. A., 1950, *Brain*, **73**, 251.)

although illuminating in itself, is that for practical purposes the old rule of a millimetre a day—ignoring all considerations of the latent period—is as good as any after nerve suture and a somewhat faster rate after lesions recovering without surgical repair.

3. Clinical Phenomena: Methods of Examination

CLASSIFICATION OF NERVE INJURIES

In a discussion of the clinical aspects of this subject some sort of classification is essential. A number of terms were used during the First World War (Medical Research Council, 1920) to describe the state of a nerve that had not been severed and was capable of more or less spontaneous recovery: contusion, compression, physiological interruption and injury of nerve fibres with intact nerve sheath. There was confusion between cause and effect and these ambiguous terms were employed with variable meanings.

During the Second World War a simple classification was introduced (Seddon, 1942, 1943). The original three terms used were quickly discarded in favour of rather startling neologisms suggested by Lord Cohen. It was the novelty of these words rather than what they were intended to signify that provoked a certain amount of opposition which, however, subsided fairly quickly.

A difficulty is that although there can be agreement between pathologist and clinician on the state of a nerve that has been so severely damaged that the interruption is complete and in the absence of surgical repair permanent, any injury less than total can produce grades of damage as numerous as the shades of colour in the spectrum. So any classification simple enough to be workable can be only a rough approximation. Nevertheless, it is remarkable how many nerve injuries can be fitted without difficulty into three classes or into certain fairly obvious combinations of them.

Neurotmesis (τμῆσις, a cutting which implies a separation of the related parts) is the word used to describe the state of a nerve that has either been completely severed or is so seriously disorganized by scar tissue that spontaneous regeneration is out of the question. This term is more inclusive than division because it embraces lesions in which the nerve preserves an appearance of continuity but is, in fact, totally destroyed over a longer or shorter distance. Traction injuries, the injection of noxious drugs and ischaemia can destroy a nerve in this way.

Axonotmesis, as has already been shown (p. 21), is a pathological entity, a lesion that can be produced experimentally. It is characterized by total interruption of the axons and their myelin sheaths, but the rest of the nerve—in short its stroma—is preserved. There is total peripheral degeneration, but regeneration occurs spontaneously and is of excellent quality because the intact endoneurial tubes guide the outgoing streams of axoplasm to their proper peripheral connections. It can only be inferred that a lesion of this sort occurs clinically, but the inference is extremely strong, particularly in one group of cases—that of nerve injuries caused by fractures (p. 78)—because well-nigh perfect spontaneous recovery occurs with considerable regularity. As will be evident from Table I, neurotmesis and axonotmesis are clinically indistinguishable except in their behaviour during the period when spontaneous recovery could occur. From the clinical standpoint this is of the utmost importance because it means that active steps must be taken to find out which of these lesions is the cause of a total paralysis.

The third term, **neurapraxia** (ἀπραξία, non-action), was perhaps unfortunate. It implied—correctly—that the nerve was out of action for a time, but gave no hint of the nature of the essential damage because, at the time of its introduction, this was not known. Two years later, Denny-Brown and Brenner (1944 *a*, *b*), showed experimentally that the main though not the only cause of this incomplete and comparatively short-lived paralysis was localized demyelination. However, it now appears that neurapraxia, like the other two terms, has come to stay and this does no harm provided that those who use the word understand what they mean by it, as indeed seems to be the case.

Because the clinical picture of neurapraxia is so strikingly different from that of the total paralysis—with peripheral degeneration—of neurotmesis and axonotmesis it will be described in some detail. This benign paralysis is seen fairly regularly in times of peace and frequently among the nerve injuries of warfare.

In 1864 Weir Mitchell described what we call neurapraxia with his habitual precision. 'This condition of local shock is very curious. A man is shot in the thigh, the ball passes near the sciatic nerve, and instantly the limb is paralysed; within a few minutes, or at the close of a day or a week the volitional control in part returns, but finally there may be left some single group of muscles permanently paralysed. . . .

'The most difficult fact to explain in this connection is the great frequency with which a gunshot injury of a nerve caused total loss of motion and very little of sensation. It would be natural to suppose that a ball striking a nerve, or passing near it, would equally damage its motor and sensory fibres. Practically, it is the motor filaments which suffer most severely, most often, and most extensively. Nor is this less true of the case in all stages, for we find that the lesions of motion are always the least readily relieved and the last to improve. As yet no plausible explanation of these facts has occurred to us. Nor can we conceive why, as sometimes happens, a ball should seem to have respected altogether the sensory fibres of a great nerve trunk. All of our anatomical views incline us to the belief that the two orders of nerves are intimately blended in the large nerves. Yet it appears scarcely possible that this could be, and one set escape the loss of function which the missile inflicts on the other. Is it possible that the fibres of motion and sensation may be grouped in bundles, and thus be liable to insulated disturbance, if we may so describe it? Or, if this view of the case be inadmissible, must we then concede to the two orders

TABLE I

	NEUROTMESIS	AXONOTMESIS	NEURAPRAXIA
Pathological			
Anatomical continuity	May be lost	Preserved	Preserved
Essential damage	Complete disorganization	Nerve fibres interrupted Schwann sheaths preserved	Selective demyelination of larger fibres: no degeneration of axons
Clinical			
Motor paralysis	Complete	Complete	Complete
Muscle atrophy	Progressive	Progressive	Very little
Sensory paralysis	Complete	Complete	Usually much sparing
Autonomic paralysis	Complete	Complete	Usually much sparing
E ectrical Phenomena			
Reaction of degeneration	Present	Present	Absent
Nerve conduction distal to the lesion	Absent	Absent	Preserved
Motor-unit action-potentials	Absent	Absent	Absent
Fibrillation	Present	Present	Occasionally detectable
Recovery			
Surgical repair	Essential	Not necessary	Not necessary
Rate of recovery	1-2 mm a day after repair	1-2 mm a day	Rapid; days or weeks
March of recovery	According to order of innervation	According to order of innervation	No order
Quality	Always imperfect	Perfect	Perfect

of nerves some difference in constitution or sensitiveness to foreign impressions, which makes one more liable to suffer than the other?—a conclusion which we should certainly hesitate to adopt.'

The conclusion that he was reluctant to adopt is one that has been forced on us by clinical observation, though it is not supported by the experimental work of Denny-Brown and Brenner. There is no doubt that the damage is selective and that it falls most heavily on nerve fibres of large diameter.

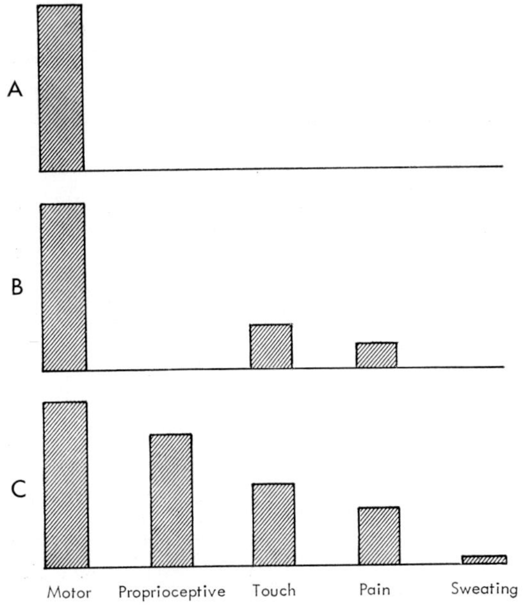

FIG. 3, 1. Relative involvement of the several modalities in neurapraxia. A and B are particularly characteristic of radial neurapraxia; as in degenerative lesions of this nerve there is no detectable impairment of proprioception, the median and ulnar nerves being chiefly concerned with this form of sensibility. (Reproduced by kind permission from *Brain*, 1943, **66**, 237.)

The widespread tissue commotion caused by the passage through a limb of a high-velocity missile is the most striking cause of neurapraxia. Weir Mitchell remarked: 'that a ball in thus passing may radiate effects, so to speak, upon tissues at a distance of an inch at least, is seen commonly enough, where a Minié, gliding over the sciatic nerve, palsies the limb as terribly as though the nerve had been in the very track of the ball.' Yet the paralysis is innocent enough and clears up more or less rapidly.

The very short-lived paralysis, lasting no more than hours or a few days, that Weir Mitchell described and that occurred in many of our own patients, can hardly have been due to so gross an organic change as localized demyelination.

A full account of the clinical findings was published long ago (Seddon, 1943) and it now suffices to recall (Fig. **3**, 1) how the various modalities are affected. The loss of proprioception is particularly striking. Spontaneous sensations are common and this is how they are described by patients: skin feels asleep or numb, with or without tingling or a sensation of heaviness; tingling or pins and needles, sometimes followed by loss of sensibility; aching which may be succeeded by tingling; wires pulling.

About two-thirds of the patients made one or other of these complaints, a considerably higher incidence of active sensory disturbance than is found after neurotmesis or axonotmesis. There is clearly an irritative element in this type of damage.

The time that elapses before recovery occurs varies widely. The paralysis may disappear within a few hours. In the cases that we have observed the duration ranged from 1 week to 6 months with an average of about 10 weeks. So however clear-cut neurapraxia may be as a clinical entity there must be more variations in its pathology than have yet been revealed by experimentally induced lesions. But there is nothing surprising in this because, as is apparent from Table II, there is a wide range of injuries capable of producing neurapraxia, some acting instantaneously, others such as pressure by crutches, slowly. On only one occasion have we had the opportunity of examining the site of damage, and the findings were bizarre:

A man, aged 22, was injured at 2.30 p.m. by a ·22 lead bullet which entered the antero-medial side of the right forearm and made its exit posteriorly near the olecranon. There was immediate burning pain at the site of injury and a little pain radiating down to the fourth and fifth digits; also immediate ulnar numbness and a feeling of weakness in the hand.

Two hours later he was admitted to hospital. Since the accident he had had acute 'pins and needles' in the fourth and fifth digits, which otherwise felt dead. There was a punctured wound of entry 10 cm below the medial epicondyle on the antero-medial side of the arm; the exit wound was between the olecranon and medial epicondyle. The diameter of both was 6 mm.

Neurological examination. Apart from slight power in flexor digitorum profundus (2: M.R.C. nomenclature) there was complete paralysis of all muscles of ulnar innervation. There was anaesthesia of the usual ulnar distribution on the palmar surface of the hand; on the dorsum a small area of anaesthesia medially and complete anaesthesia in the ulnar digital area. Analgesia was confined to the terminal phalanx of the fifth digit. In the rest of the area of anaesthesia, pin-prick was felt as a hot pain but there was no delay in appreciation nor was the pain persistent. Postural sensibility was normal, but the thresholds for deep pressure and deep pain were raised, the latter being felt as 'pins and needles'. There was a little sweating in the ulnar area of the palm but not noticeably less than in the median area.

Radiographic examination was normal.

It was evident that this was an incomplete lesion of some kind, because the motor disturbance was far greater than the sensory. A funicular division seemed unlikely because the dissociation could not be explained anatomically; the injury had evidently disturbed certain types of nerve fibres much more than others. A diagnosis of neurapraxia could not be made with certainty because, at this stage, it was impossible to know whether peripheral degeneration would ultimately develop.

The nerve was explored without delay and the findings were as follows:

1. Moderate bruising of the soft tissues and muscles from 4 cm above to 4 cm below the epicondyle.

2. The track of the bullet ran deep to the ulnar nerve.

3. There was haemorrhage round the nerve over a length of 8 cm but the nerve and its sheath were intact except at a point adjacent to the bullet track. Here, over a length of 14 mm, the sheath was torn and ragged but the bundles appeared intact (Fig. **3**, 2). The epineurium and perineurium were split to such an extent that it was possible to pass a small probe from one side of the nerve to the other between the bundles. The nerve was slightly thinner than normal and it was just possible that a few small bundles had been ruptured.

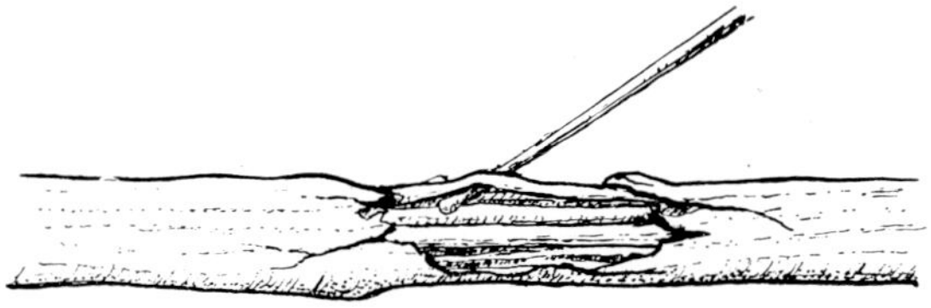

FIG. **3**, 2. The state of the nerve in a case of neurapraxia.

4. Proximal stimulation produced a powerful response in flexor carpi ulnaris and flexor digitorum profundus: a weaker response in adductor pollicis, and no response in other muscles of ulnar innervation.

TABLE II—Causes of the three main types of nerve injury

(Dominant causes are indicated by **bold type**)

NEUROTMESIS	AXONOTMESIS	NEURAPRAXIA
Cuts and Lacerations	Cuts and Lacerations	
Missiles	**Missiles**	**Missiles**
Fractures	**Fractures**	
Traction	**Traction**	**Traction**
	Compression: Prolonged	**Compression: momentary**
	Friction (a combination of traction and compression)	
Injections	**Injections**	
	Freezing	**Freezing**
Operation	Operation	Operation
Ischaemia	**Ischaemia**	**Ischaemia**

Subsequent progress. Sensory examinations were made at frequent intervals and recovery was rapid; some pain sensibility returned 2 days after the injury. Yet on the thirty-second day there was still some disturbance of sensibility. Light touch was not appreciated in the palmar distribution of the ulnar nerve; a slightly more powerful stimulus was felt and pinprick elicited a dull burning pain. It was a year before superficial sensibility had returned entirely to normal and this may mean that a few of the sensory fibres had, in fact, degenerated.

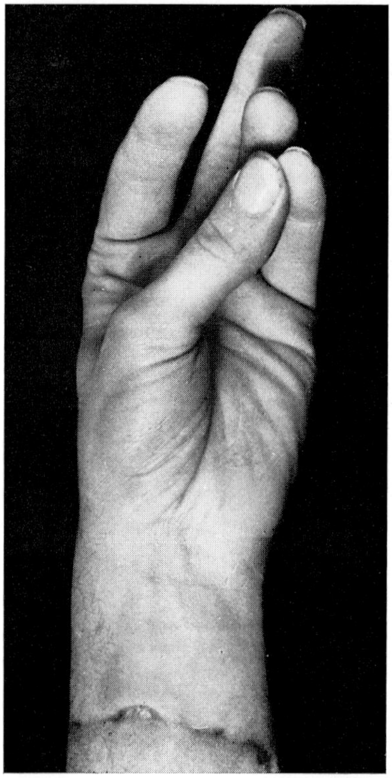

FIG. 3, 3. Action of the flexor pollicis brevis resembling though not exactly mimicking opposition in a patient with complete severance of the median nerve.

Twelve days after the injury, the first dorsal interosseous showed signs of activity and by the fourteenth day there was activity in all muscles of ulnar innervation. The electrical reactions were normal throughout and wasting was minimal. Progress to full recovery was rapid.

If appearances are anything to go by this was a violent injury and what was so astounding was the benignity of the paralysis. And as there was reason to believe that some of the sensory fibres degenerated so we may the more readily accept Bowden's finding (M.R.C.R., 1954) of fibrillation in cases that, clinically, could properly be described as neurapraxia: a certain indication that some motor fibres had degenerated. It is likely that 'pure' neurapraxia (like pure axonotmesis) is a lesion that can be produced only in the laboratory.

But in clinical practice this is unimportant; what matters is how to recognize the condition. The dissociated paralysis, predominantly motor, the persistence of normal excitability of the muscles after 18 days from the onset of the paralysis (the time required for the establishment of RD), and the conservation of nerve conduction distal to the lesion are pathognomonic.

MOTOR PARALYSIS

Paralysis of muscles is usually obvious enough though sometimes, after injury of the accessory nerve for example, it may escape detection at first.

After a few weeks the paralysed muscles become visibly wasted. When the onset is gradual, as when the median nerve is compressed in the carpal tunnel, the wasting may be the first feature of motor paralysis to attract attention.

DECEPTIVE MUSCLE ACTION

The extent of the nerve damage may be obscured by certain factors.

Anomalous Innervation

Paralysis of the thenar muscles may be overlooked, even when the median nerve is completely interrupted, because the flexor pollicis brevis is supplied by the ulnar nerve and its normal action masks the paralysis of the abductor brevis and opponens pollicis (Fig. **3**, 3). Anomalous innervation is therefore a pitfall and it will be described more fully in Chapter 11.

A striking example of anomalous insertion of a muscle is seen in some patients with complete radial paralysis. They are able to extend the interphalangeal joint of the thumb fairly powerfully against resistance though no movement of the tendon of extensor pollicis longus is detectable. Extension of the interphalangeal joint is brought about by the abductor pollicis brevis which occasionally sends a slip dorsally to be inserted into the terminal phalanx.

Supplementary Action

A muscle may have a secondary action that is not normally evident but becomes so when neighbouring muscles are paralysed. The most striking instance of this is the ability of the brachioradialis to flex the elbow. When the biceps and brachialis are paralysed, flexion of the elbow may remain strong.

Other examples of supplementary muscle action will be found on pages 200-201 and 219.

Trick Movements

These movements (Jones, 1919), which are all passive, trick the examiner. They are of three kinds:

1. If the strong contraction of normal muscles puts paralysed muscles on the stretch the latter become tense and so, like a tenodesis, produce a small movement through their normal range of action. In radial paralysis strong action of the wrist flexors sometimes causes the inert extensors of the digits to move them dorsally (Fig. **3**, 4).
2. When their antagonists relax, paralysed muscles, being elastic, produce a rebound movement. This is best seen in the extensors of the toes in common peroneal paralysis immediately after relaxation of the flexors of the toes.
3. The action of gravity can be deceptive, notably in extension of the elbow when the triceps is paralysed.

Deformity and Contractures

These can be the most devastating consequences of nerve injury (Fig. **13**, 2, p. 233), so much so that if recovery of the nerve occurs the affected part, usually the hand, may still be almost useless.

Deformity is not always synonymous with contracture. The claw hand of ulnar paralysis is at first a deformity without contracture; but the latter will develop if steps are not taken to deal with the deformity. By contrast, a moderate contracture may not cause deformity and the disturbance of function may be slight. A little shortening of the flexors of the wrist may be revealed by no more than slight limitation of extension of the joint.

Deformity without contracture is usually due to unbalanced muscle action, clawing of the fingers or toes being familiar examples. But it may be followed by true shortening of the active muscles and is then no longer correctable. It is then a contracture. Secondary changes occur

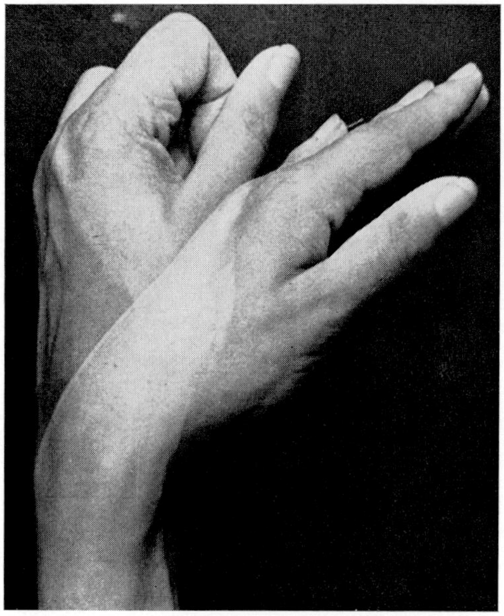

FIG. **3**, 4. In this case of radial paralysis there was moderate contracture of the (paralysed) extensors of the digits: consequently when the patient flexed the wrist the digits extended.

in the ligaments of the affected joints; in the claw hand the dorsal hoods of the proximal interphalangeal joints become stretched so that reconstructive tendon transplantation is then foredoomed to failure. Laxity of ligaments may lead to subluxation of joints, especially in children.

Shortening of ligaments may follow shortening of muscle, as in the case illustrated in Figure **13**, 2. But contractures can occur in denervated muscles, sometimes to a disabling degree, as in this same case. As Buchthal, Knapp and Lindhard (1936) and Tower (1939) have pointed out this is not entirely explicable in terms of shortening of the fibrous tissue that is deposited in denervated muscle; it appears that the contractile elements themselves are capable of shortening: they go into a state of continuous contracture. A curious feature, observed by Bowden (M.R.C.R. 1954), is that in the early stages of recovery and even before voluntary contraction is first observed some shortening of the affected muscles can occur quite suddenly.

Joint stiffness can be aggravated by oedema which, if prolonged, leads to deposition of collagen in all the swollen tissues and within the joint itself.

Cramp

Some patients with nerve injuries complain of painful cramp, always intermittent and sometimes temporarily disabling, confined to the affected muscles, but never those totally paralysed. It can occur during activity or at rest and is sometimes aggravated by cold.

With the passage of time it diminishes, although some patients observed for up to 18 years after nerve injury, complain of soreness in their weak muscles. Apart from kneading and stretching the affected muscles no remedy has been found; all drugs that might conceivably relieve the cramp have proved valueless.

Recovery

The essential feature of recovery, the re-establishment of axonal connections with motor end-plates, has already been described and it is followed by a steady increase in volume due to reversal of the shrinkage of the muscle fibres. The return of overt contractility lags behind re-innervation; and visible contraction cannot be detected until some time after motor-unit action-potentials make their appearance on electromyographic examination and until fibrillation, similarly observed, is waning (Chap. 4). Changes in the electrical excitability of muscle also precede clinical recovery.

Tenderness of the re-innervated muscles, distinct from the cramp referred to above, is common and it may be due to the ramification within the muscle of sensory fibres which, owing to axonal confusion at the site of injury, have lost their way.

The return of *independent movements* after a nerve lesion causing axonal degeneration depends entirely on the absence of axonal confusion at the site of damage. In axonotmesis the motor fibres regain their appropriate peripheral connections and so independent muscle action is restored. If, in spite of fairly good spontaneous regeneration, independent movements are defective (this is often seen after traction injuries of the brachial plexus) there has, presumably, been a good deal of intraneural disorganization. After the best possible repair of a nerve, independent movements are never fully restored, and we have not found that any process of relearning occurs subsequently.

SENSORY PARALYSIS

There is no mistaking the well-demarcated area of cutaneous sensory loss when a nerve has been completely interrupted. Although each nerve has its particular territory the boundaries are subject to variation, as will be shown in Chapters 11 and 12. The practical importance of this is that if the area is small, or even, in the case of the radial nerve, non-existent, there may still be complete interruption of the nerve.

The area of anaesthesia (loss of tactile sensibility) has particularly sharp boundaries which in a part where tactile discrimination is highly developed, above all the palmar surfaces of the fingers and thumb, can be delineated to within a few millimetres. There is a somewhat smaller area of analgesia, usually completely enclosed by the area of anaesthesia (Fig. **3**, 10, p. 45), though sometimes the area of analgesia has a promontory that transgresses the boundary of anaesthesia (Fig. **3**, 5). The area of total anaesthesia and analgesia is sometimes called (with slight misuse of the noun) the 'autonomous zone' of distribution of the nerve; that is to say, there is no overlap from any of the surrounding areas. The superficial radial nerve may have no autonomous area.

Between the boundaries of anaesthesia and analgesia are the limits of another area within which sensations of heat and cold are not appreciated. Like others we have found that in the investigation of peripheral nerve injuries nothing is gained by determining the area of thermanaesthesia.

Other forms of sensibility are affected too. Within an area even smaller than that of analgesia there is loss of pressure sensibility, postural and vibration sense. Yet even in a proximal sciatic nerve lesion the loss of deep sensibility does not lead to neuropathic joint changes such as occur in tabes dorsalis or in neural leprosy—though it is doubtful whether the joint destruction that occurs in the latter is purely neuropathic.

When we were permitted, even encouraged, to believe in the specificity of cutaneous nerve endings it was supposed that a 'pain fibre' had endings which covered a large area, a sensory unit in some ways not unlike a motor unit (p. 7). 'Touch fibres' came from smaller areas of skin, the higher the grade of tactile discrimination the smaller the area. The large pain sensory units overlapped considerably, the touch units far less (Fig. **3**, 6). This explained the difference between the boundaries for loss of pain and of touch. Unfortunately, as has already been mentioned on page 7, the whole subject of sensory perception has proved to be extraordinarily complex and, as yet, far from solved.

There is no denying that the comfortable anatomical explanation that we are being obliged to question is inadequate. In the marginal zone, between the boundaries of anaesthesia and of analgesia, there ought, according to the purely anatomical explanation, to be simply diminished appreciation of pain. In fact the sensations aroused in this area by a painful stimulus are extremely unpleasant, quite outside the range of normal experience. Immediately after the nerve injury the threshold is high; after a day or two it begins to fall, and then even gentle stimuli will evoke the most horrible sensations. There is a profound qualitative change. Fortunately, this dysaesthesia gradually diminishes, though stimulation of the marginal zone still provokes abnormal sensations.

PAIN

After even the most banal nerve injury the patient experiences spontaneous sensations which he refers to the area of sensory loss. From personal experience I can testify to the obtrusiveness of these hallucinations: mild pricking, itching, so that the subject finds himself rubbing or scratching the insensitive skin. These sensations are less noticeable if he is well occupied. They are aggravated by thinking about the affected part with the result that, during the first few weeks after the nerve injury, affirmative responses are given during sensory examination when, in fact, no stimulus has been applied to the skin. It is therefore wrong on this account to dismiss the subject as an unreliable witness.

A few patients, mostly those with incomplete paralysis but by no means all of them, suffer sharp pain on cutaneous stimulation. And still fewer suffer severe, even agonizing, spontaneous pain called *causalgia*. This topic is discussed in Chapter 9.

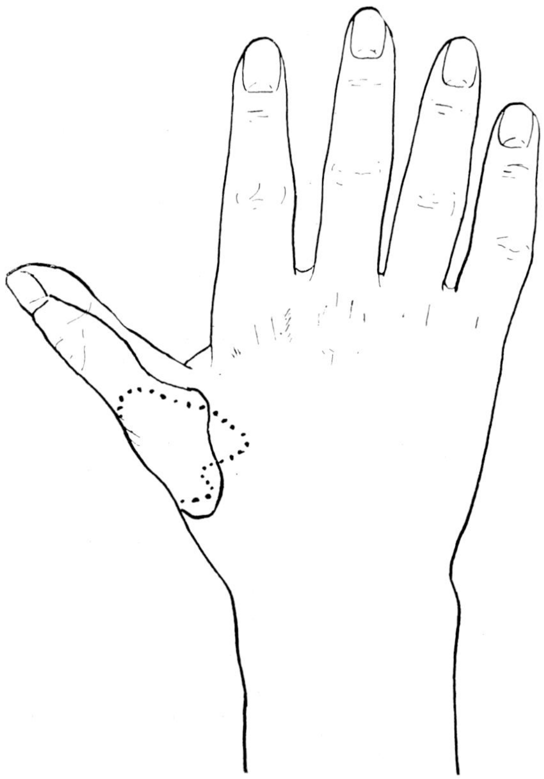

FIG. **3**, 5. An unusually small area of sensory loss in a case of radial paralysis. At one point the boundary of the analgesic area (dotted line) transgresses that of the larger anaesthetic area (continuous line).

Some patients with severe brachial plexus injuries experience *phantom sensations*, with or without spontaneous pain, and indistinguishable from the phantom hallucinations after amputation.

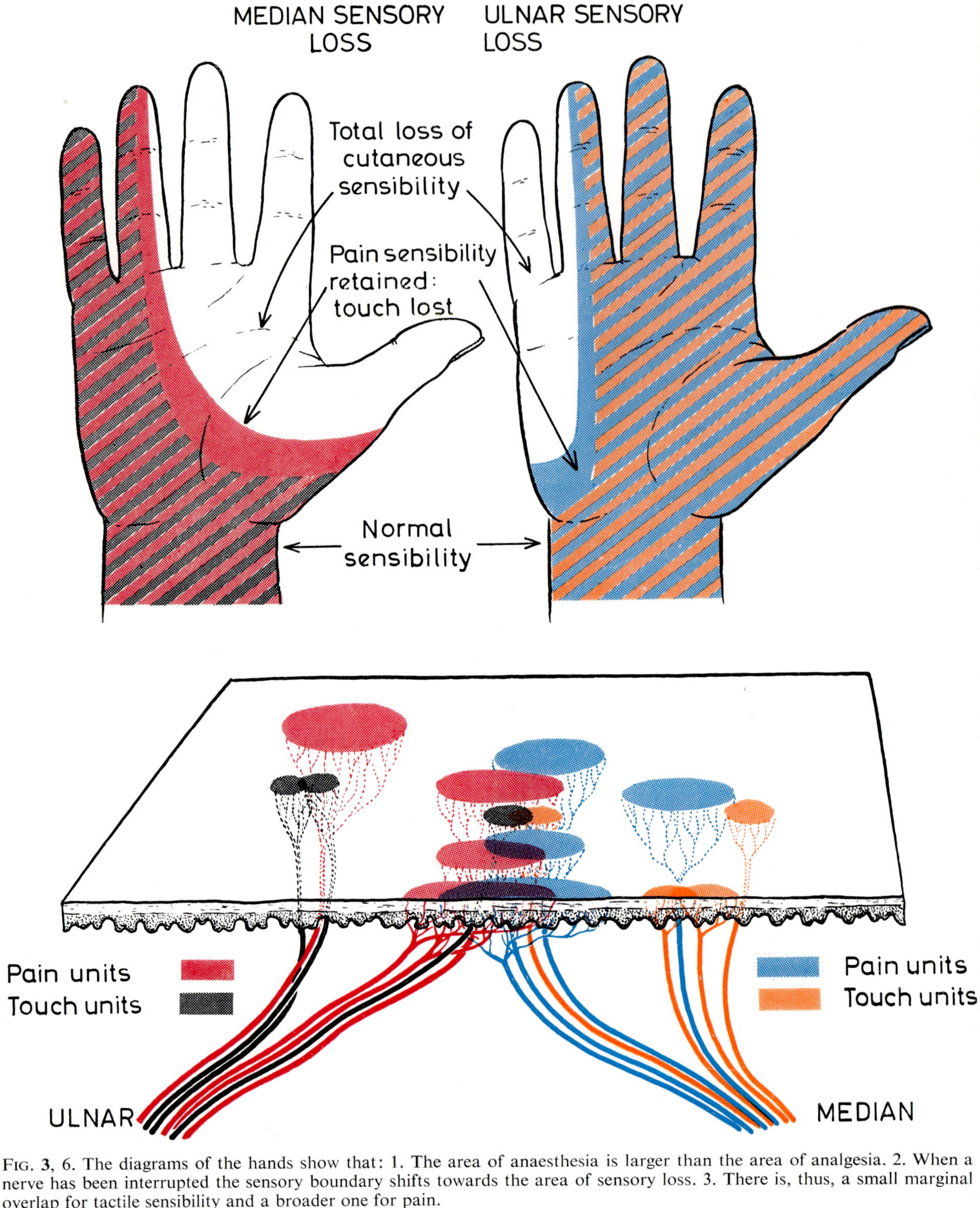

FIG. 3, 6. The diagrams of the hands show that: 1. The area of anaesthesia is larger than the area of analgesia. 2. When a nerve has been interrupted the sensory boundary shifts towards the area of sensory loss. 3. There is, thus, a small marginal overlap for tactile sensibility and a broader one for pain.

The lower diagram illustrates a plausible hypothesis, with some experimental support that sensory units exist. A comparatively large area of skin is innervated by a pain unit, a much smaller one (in the hand) by a touch unit. All these units overlap. Two-point discrimination, which in a finger may be 3 mm, is supposed to depend on the simultaneous stimulation of separate units. The smaller they are the more precise the discrimination.

Shrinkage of the Insensitive Area

Almost immediately after interruption of a nerve —within 3 days—the initial area of sensory loss shrinks. This very rapid return of circumferential sensibility (Figs **3**, 7 and **3**, 8) is thought to be due to the resumption of function in the terminal fibres of adjacent, normal cutaneous nerves which for some as yet unexplained reason were inhibited in their action by the sudden loss of sensibility in the area supplied by the damaged nerve. Then further, slower shrinkage of the area of sensory loss occurs and in a long narrow area (Fig. **3**, 7) anaesthesia and analgesia disappear completely, though the ultimate quality of sensibility is subnormal. This shrinkage has sometimes been mistaken for true recovery, but it takes place far earlier than could be accounted for by regeneration in the affected nerve; moreover it is strictly circumferential whereas true sensory recovery advances towards the periphery like a wave. This gradual encroachment into the insensitive area is the result of the ingrowth of fibres from the surrounding intact cutaneous nerves (Weddell, Guttmann and Gutmann, 1941; Livingston, 1947*a*; Fig. **3**, 9).

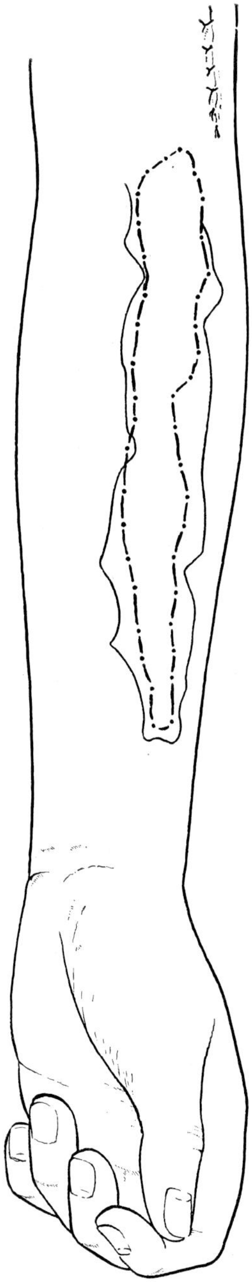

Fig. **3**, 7. This patient had persistent pain in the cutaneous distribution of the musculocutaneous nerve after an operation on a fractured humerus. There was little detectable abnormality of sensibility. When the nerve was exposed it was found to be caught up in the loop of wire that encircled the humerus and it was decided that the best remedy would be wide resection of the nerve.

On the day of the operation, when the patient was fully recovered from the anaesthetic, the area of sensory loss was outlined (continuous line). Forty-eight hours later the boundary (broken line) had moved in considerably.

Only the boundaries of anaesthesia are shown: the areas of analgesia were similar, but smaller.

Six months after the operation there was no detectable anaesthesia or analgesia, only diminished sensibility. There had been vigorous ingrowth of fibres from the surrounding intact nerves (cf. Fig. **3**, 9).

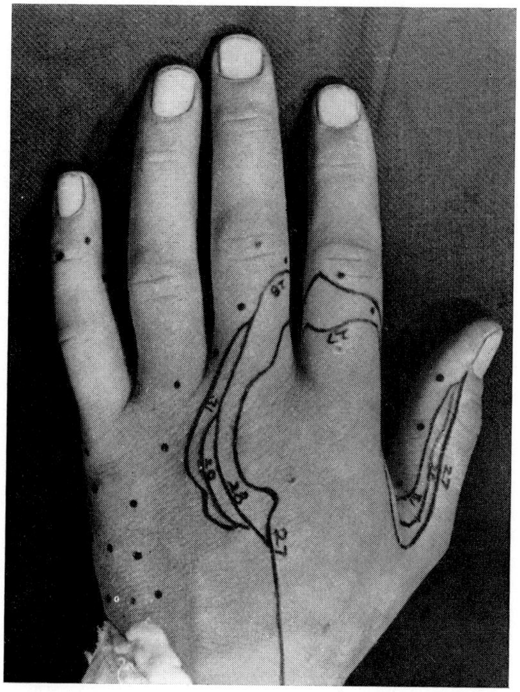

Fig. **3**, 8. This patient suffered a total median and ulnar paralysis on the 24th of a month. The increase in the area of supply of the superficial radial nerve between the 27th and 31st is shown.

Recovery

A curious legend arose during the First World War, almost comparable with the stories about Russian troops passing through Britain on their way to the Western Front, complete with snow on the roofs of the railway carriages. It was said that sometimes after nerve suture or nerve grafting—more particularly if the graft had been preserved in alcohol and not washed thoroughly—some sort of sensibility returned extremely early in the denervated area (Tinel, 1919). It was appreciated that this could not be accounted for by regeneration and various ingenious explanations were propounded. This phenomenon has never been observed in recent years.

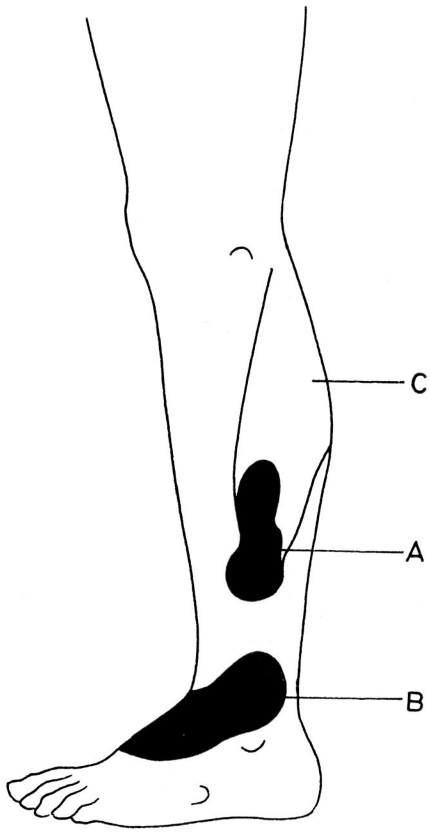

FIG. 3, 9. The common peroneal nerve was cut 6 years before the patient came for treatment. There was complete motor paralysis, but anaesthesia was confined to the areas A and B, and there was no analgesia. When he came into hospital for reconstructive surgery the opportunity was taken of inspecting the site of damage. The nerve was completely severed, the ends being joined by a narrow bridge of scar tissue. There was no response on electrical stimulation. The lesion was excised, after which there was anaesthesia and analgesia in the area C. It was then evident that ingrowth of sensory fibres accounted for the shrinkage of the distal part of the original area of sensory loss and that the proximal shrinkage was due to sensory fibres regenerating across the gap in the nerve.

Tinel's Sign

The earliest evidence of regeneration is Tinel's sign (1917). The examiner taps lightly over the affected nerve, starting at the periphery. At some point, as the examiner's finger moves towards the site of injury, the patient is suddenly aware of a curious sensation—an electric shock, pins and needles, or a stab of pain—both locally and radiating throughout the distribution of the nerve. (The test is not, of course, applicable where the nerve is deeply situated.) This phenomenon is the clinical manifestation of the advancing wave of regenerating sensory axons; but it has come to be regarded as unreliable because it is not quantitative. Suppose two-thirds of a nerve has been divided, a state of affairs that calls for operative repair: nerve fibres can still traverse the one-third that is in continuity and the positive Tinel's sign that develops may lull the observer into thinking that exploration is unnecessary. Yet Henderson (1948), more than anyone else, succeeded in making this sign informative. When he was a prisoner-of-war he made repeated observations in 400 cases of nerve injury and, because for a time he was unable to operate on those of his patients whose damaged nerves undoubtedly required exploration, he was well placed to assess the prognostic significance of his findings. Henderson found that Tinel's sign became important about 4 months after the time of injury. If it was strongly positive at the level of the lesion but persistently absent below, spontaneous regeneration could not be expected. If the sign was strongly positive at the site of damage and also appeared weakly distal to it, the quality of regeneration would be poor. But a strongly positive sign at the level of the lesion that gradually faded as the response moved peripherally and became stronger in the distal part of the nerve indicated that satisfactory regeneration was in progress. However, as Napier (1949) has pointed out, the absence of Tinel's sign is not always significant; there may be too much muscle over the nerve to allow adequate percussion of it.

As will be explained in Chapter 14, decisions for or against exploration can now be made on much firmer grounds than the behaviour of Tinel's sign, and its clinical significance is no longer great. Moreover, because delay is harmful it is unwise to take notice of a sign that does not become informative until, as Henderson said, 4 months have elapsed.

Return of Tactile Sensibility

Moberg (1958) has done more than anyone to emphasize the functional importance of restoration of what he calls tactile gnosis; this term, however lacking in euphony, does express what counts most in the hand, the ability to recognize what is being touched or grasped, the sum of sensations on which accurate performance depends.

In almost all areas, tactile sensibility advances towards the periphery. At first the threshold is high and in this phase the patient is bothered by the woolliness of the sensation; he feels as if he is wearing a thin glove. The advance of tactile sensibility lags only a little behind that of pain sensibility, though in order to demonstrate this a firm stimulus is necessary; this raises the possibility of the stimulus being transmitted by pressure to deeper structures and is one reason why Moberg has abandoned this type of examination in which one uses such implements as cotton-wool, a soft brush or a von Frey hair. He relies entirely on three methods: (1) two-point discrimination (p. 53); (2) the picking-up test (p. 53); and (3) the ninhydrin sweating test (p. 45), as an objective check on the other two.

These tests are valuable for assessing sensibility in the hand but are inapplicable elsewhere; reliance must be placed on the old-fashioned methods and there is not much to choose between them. My own preference is for the von Frey hair (Fig. **3**, 19. p. 52), though instead of being brought down perpendicular to the skin it is stroked across it. It is curious how the element of movement in tactile appreciation has been disregarded. A woman, even a man, selecting a fabric always examines its texture by feeling it between the fingers and thumb, which move over the material. The patina of old furniture, the softness of a fur are appreciated by stroking. The punctate tactile stimulus is unnatural, thrust on us by the devotees of punctate sensibility. If this gentle stroking evokes no response then the other, the blunt end of the bicycle-spoke holder is used instead. The usefulness of the ninhydrin test is that it is objective, but Önne's painstaking study of it (1962) leads one to doubt its value in the assessment of the finer grades of recovery which must, in the nature of things, be expressed subjectively. The chief value of sweat tests is diagnostic.

Return of Pain Sensibility

Pain sensibility returns in the same manner as touch and somewhat in advance of it. The most striking feature in the early stages of regeneration is its unpleasant quality, and having had personal experience of these sensations I understand why so many evocative terms have been used to describe it. The character of this abnormal pain seems to be the same as that of the pain felt in the intermediate zone soon after division of a nerve (p. 39).

Head's protopathic sensibility must be discarded because it embodies an erroneous theory. There is a free choice between what Boring called 'wicked' pain, hyperpathia (Foerster and Noordenbos) and what Riddoch and other British neurologists have called over-reaction, the term that we ourselves use. Over-reaction is a good description of the patient's response. It is astonishing to witness the behaviour of an intelligent subject who has submitted himself to an experimental nerve lesion and is as interested as his examiners in the findings. He braces himself to endure the stimulus, and however great his self-control he may withdraw the limb involuntarily as the needle approaches.

This over-reaction, the severity of which varies greatly from one patient to another, must be taken into account in the management of nerve injuries. As the time of recovery approaches it is wise to warn the patient that he must expect it, that it will have to be borne, and that the abnormal sensitivity may persist for several months before the return of something like normal feeling. I have known patients demoralized by bad management. The clinician may be unaware of this feature of nerve regeneration and in his anxiety to help the patient he resorts to sympathetic nerve block or even more drastic procedures. This is catastrophic because there is no known remedy for over-reaction and the failure to obtain relief convinces the patient that he is the victim of a distressing and incurable painful disorder. So he protects the hand, uses it as little as possible and finishes up with a good neurological recovery but a functionally bad one.

Sometimes, particularly after the repair of the sciatic nerve or its tibial division, recovery is imperfect and then over-reaction to pain may persist for a long time and can be mitigated only by supplying the patient with a soft and well-fitting insole. It is the risk of this persistent over-reaction that makes it doubtful whether repair of the posterior tibial nerve is worth while (p. 221), and in ischaemia of nerves below the knee the pain may be such that amputation is imperative (p. 108).

Proprioception

The proper performance of any movement is not possible if a patient is unable to appreciate the position of a limb and the sense of movement of joints. After a nerve injury, position and joint sense are lost, though not so extensively as cutaneous sensibility. However, the work of Halpern (1949), Brand (1964), and Moberg (1965) suggests that, at any rate in the hand, cutaneous sensibility is a most important factor in proprioception. In neurapraxia the nerve damage is always fairly proximal and, as has already been explained (p. 34), pronounced loss of proprioception may be found when there is only partial loss of feeling in the skin; and Bowden (M.R.C.R., 1954, p. 323) suspected that loss of proprioception could not be explained entirely on the basis of impairment of cutaneous sensibility. I agree with Moberg that nothing is gained by systematic recording of proprioception as an index of recovery.

Experiments performed by Barker and Young (1947) showed that the *stretch reflex* returns, though not to normal, after suture of a severed nerve; but Bowden found that even when fair power had returned in the calf muscle after suture of the sciatic nerve the ankle jerk was often still absent or feeble.

Grading of Recovery

For the systematic study of recovery after nerve injury and, more particularly, of the results of nerve repair, some sort of numerical grading is imperative. We have continued to use the scheme devised by Highet that was adopted by the Medical Research Council in 1941. Details of it will be found in Chapter 17.

AUTONOMIC PARALYSIS AND NUTRITIONAL DISTURBANCES

The autonomic nerve fibres supplying the skin run with and have much the same distribution as the sensory fibres. The pilomotor system may be ignored, but sweat secretion and vasomotor control are important.

SUDOMOTOR PARALYSIS

Guttmann (1933, 1940) was chiefly responsible for arousing interest in this subject.

When a nerve has been completely interrupted there is no sweating at all in the autonomous area, but in the intermediate area, in which there is some overlap of adjacent nerves, sweat secretion is present though greatly diminished. There is excessive sweating in the normally innervated zone surrounding the area of absent and diminished sensibility. The boundary of anidrosis corresponds most closely with that of anaesthesia though not infrequently it is nearer that of analgesia (Fig. **3**, 10).

Disturbances of sweat secretion can be demonstrated by staining techniques, by direct inspection of the skin, and by the measurement of skin resistance. The regular employment of one or other of these methods is unnecessary; we reached this conclusion after 10 years' routine use of the quinizarin method. Moberg (1958) has made a case for recording sweat secretion as an index of recovery after nerve lesions affecting sensibility in the hand; but there are occasions when the diagnostic value of estimating sweat secretion is very great.

Methods of Examination

1. The old *starch and iodine* method is so familiar as not to call for detailed description. Önne (1962) has an elegant way of using it.

2. The *quinizarin* method of Guttmann (1940) is the one of which I have most experience; it

gives very satisfactory results which are easily recorded photographically (Fig. 3, 10); but it can be trying for the patient, it is messy and it cannot be used if there is an open wound in the neighbourhood. The dye is the sodium salt of quinizarin 2-6-disulphonic acid. It makes a deep violet solution and because the powder is hygroscopic it must be kept dry. It is mixed with diluents in the following proportions:

quinizarin powder	35 g
powdered sodium carbonate	30 g
rice starch	60 g

This purplish-grey powder is dusted with some pressure over the area to be examined. A large radiant heat cradle is placed over the patient for a period of 15 to 45 minutes; sweating is accelerated if the patient has been given 0·3 to 0·6 g of aspirin and a cup of hot tea before the powder is applied.

During the heating the patient is observed from time to time; it is as important to ensure that sweating is not excessive as that it is adequate; rivulets of sweat will mar the result. When a satisfactory demonstration of sweating has been obtained the cradle is removed, the sweat must dry completely and then any remaining powder (there will be some on the anidrotic area) is dusted away. The result is photographed.

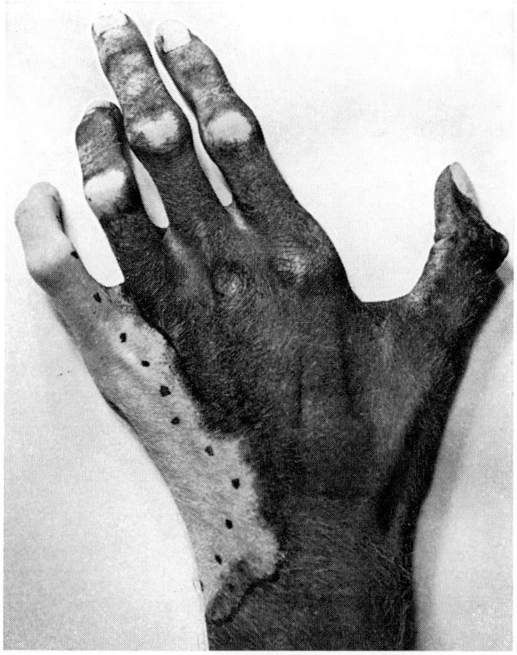

FIG. 3, 10. The area of anaesthesia (continuous line) is larger than the area of analgesia (dots) which it normally contains completely.

Sweat secretion, demonstrated by the quinizarin method—the dark staining—in ulnar paralysis.

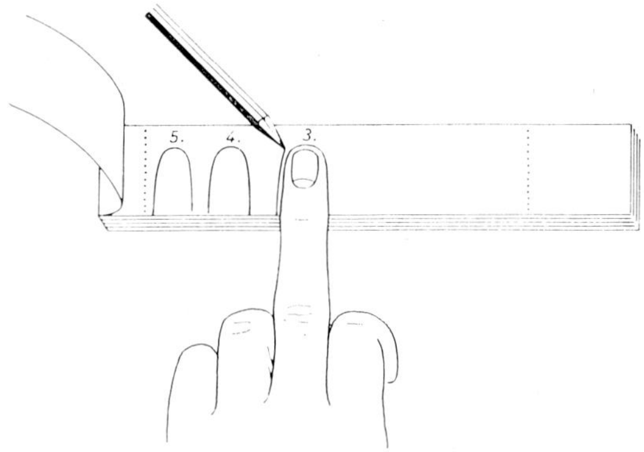

FIG. 3, 11. Tracing the outlines of the digits. (Figs 3, 11 and 3, 12 reproduced by kind permission of Professor E. Moberg.)

3. Moberg's (1958, 1964) *ninhydrin* method is suitable for the tips of the digits. This well-known colorimetric agent (indantrione hydrate) is colourless but becomes purple when exposed to very low concentrations of the organic components of sweat. Obtaining satisfactory prints requires great care. The pulps of the digits are pressed one by one against a strip of paper[1] about 3 × 15 cm in size and the outline of each digit is traced on the paper with a lead pencil that contains no soluble dye (Fig. 3, 11). Alternatively, and particularly with the thumb, the digit is rolled from one side to the other on the surface of the paper. If the digits are too moist they must be dried before the print is taken; if the patient's hand is dry, sweat secretion can be stimulated by a little exercise or by applying a blood pressure cuff inflated to 300 mm Hg. Both hands are examined. The prints are developed in a solution of 1 per cent ninhydrin in acetone, about 5 ml of which are mixed with a few drops

[1] Special paper produced by Gransholms AB, Gemla, and obtainable from AB Skandiadrog, Stockholm, Sweden (who also supply the ninhydrin spray and the ninhydrin fixing spray) may be used. It must be free from finger-prints.

of glacial acetic acid in a small dish. The stock solution will keep for a few months, the acidified solution for not more than 1 or 2 weeks. The paper can also be developed by spraying it with the acidified solution. After drying, which is rapid, the strips of paper are warmed in air at

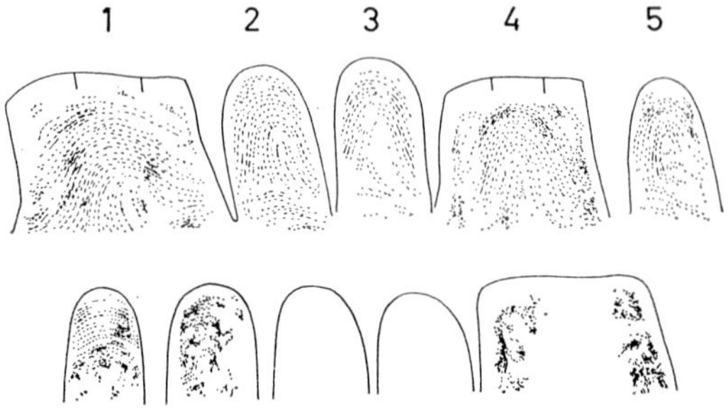

FIG. 3, 12. Ninhydrin prints. *Above:* normal. *Below:* median nerve lesion.

100° to 120°C for 5 to 10 minutes. Minute dots indicating beads of sweat then become visible (Fig. 3, 12). Moberg advises waiting for a few days before fixing the prints because by then the dots are more distinct. The strips of paper are dipped in a solution composed of:

copper nitrate	1 g
water	5 ml
methyl alcohol or acetone	95 ml
concentrated nitric acid	a few drops.

Prints can be kept as they are or photographed. The prints are said to be stable for a period of years.

4. A simpler method of which I have little knowledge is that described by Sakurai and Montagna (1964). The surface of the part to be examined is pressed on to a piece of medium-weight type-writing paper that has been previously immersed in 5 per cent *bromophenol blue* in acetone and dried. The sweat droplets leave bluish dots on a yellow background. The strip of paper is then dipped immediately into molten paraffin wax so as to avoid contamination and the colour will persist for a few months.

5. *Direct observation* of sweating. Kahn (1951) drew attention to the value of simply looking at the skin through the plus 20 lens of an ophthalmoscope which, if only qualitative, is quick and easy. It is possible, though unnecessary, to obtain elegant photographs (Fig. 3, 13); and permanent impressions can be made (Fig. 3, 14).

6. When the skin does not sweat its *resistance to the passage of an electric current* is greatly increased (Richter and Katz, 1943; Buratti, 1972).

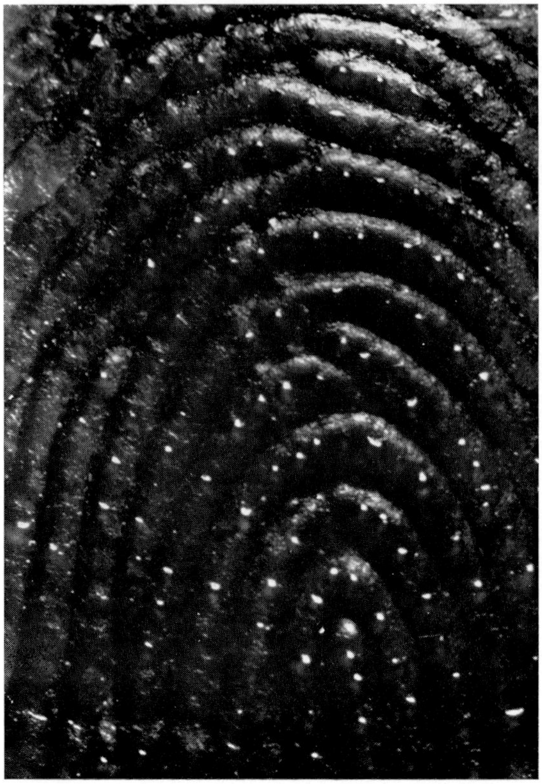

FIG. 3, 13. Sweating at the finger-tip of a healthy young (white) male: ×30.

Although this method of examination has never become popular it has the merit of being applicable in circumstances in which the dye tests would be inadmissible or difficult, but it lacks the simplicity of Kahn's method.

VASOMOTOR AND NUTRITIONAL DISTURBANCES

It is not certain that all the changes about to be described are due to interruption of the autonomic vasomotor nerve fibres. Our understanding of some of them is still incomplete. This account of them will be mainly descriptive and the reader who wishes to pursue the subject further cannot do better than consult Richards's excellent essay (M.R.C.R., 1954, p. 25).

These vasomotor and nutritional disturbances are noticeable after injuries of only four nerves: the median and ulnar nerves, the tibial division

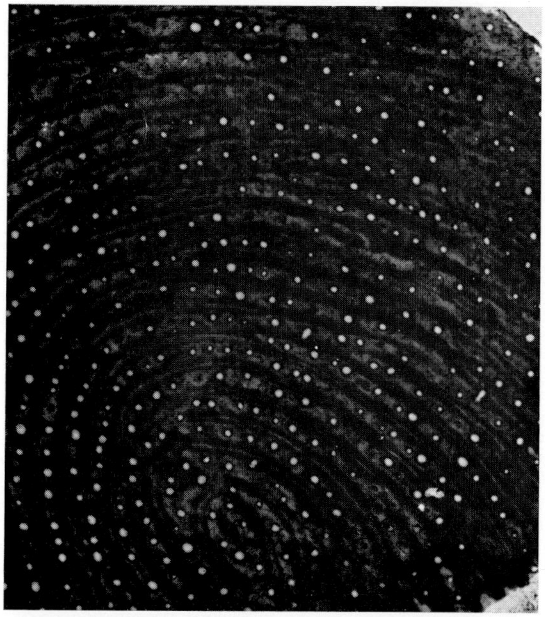

FIG. 3, 14. A plastic film taken from a finger-tip showing indentations produced by beads of sweat: ×20. This technique was devised by Sutarman and Thomson (1952). (Figs 3, 13 and 3, 14 reproduced by kind permission of Dr Pamela Mackinnon.)

of the sciatic nerve, and lesions of the brachial plexus causing paralysis below the elbow.

Temperature changes. Immediately after severance of one of these nerves, the autonomous area becomes hot, flushed and dry exactly as after sympathectomy. The affected area remains warm and its temperature is little affected by the environment. There are changes in the texture of the skin, which becomes smoother and may appear shiny. Then, after a few weeks, a cold phase supervenes, which in the absence of regeneration is permanent.

The time of transition to the cold phase may be 3 weeks or less in the hand, but in sciatic paralysis the foot may remain warm for several months after the injury. When the cold phase is established the patient usually has a good deal to say about it. Although the median or ulnar nerve alone may be affected the whole hand feels cold and the patient takes to wearing a thick glove. Objective evidence of coldness is not invariable but it is found more frequently when the nerve lesion is complete and it is commonest

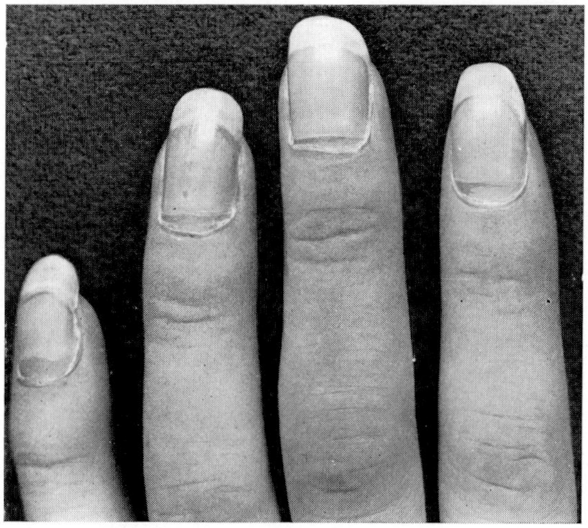

FIG. 3, 15. Transverse ridges on the nails in a case of median and ulnar paralysis.

after injuries of the median nerve. In cold weather the affected part is very cold; in warm weather the temperature may come up to that of the normal side.

Colour of the skin. In the area of analgesia there is usually redness, more commonly blotchy cyanosis. Pallor is rare.

Structure of the skin and its appendages. The sudomotor paralysis makes the skin dry; it becomes thin, scaly and peels readily, leaving a smooth often glossy surface though the ridges and papillae are preserved. Sometimes the skin is excessively keratinized, but in some cases this is due to the patient's having failed to wash and wipe the affected part with customary vigour.

The nails often become abnormal: in combined lesions of the median and ulnar nerves they may be long, curved and talon-like, but in ulnar paralysis there may be no more than a slight increase in curvature of the nail of the little finger. The nails become dry and brittle and often show pronounced transverse ridges (Fig. 3, 15); the cuticle disappears and the skin retracts from the base of the nail. The rate of growth is usually retarded. On account of the insensitivity of the part there is an increased risk of nailbed infections which may result in loss of the nail or great irregularity of growth (Fig. **3**, 16). Sunderland and Ray (1952) found this more

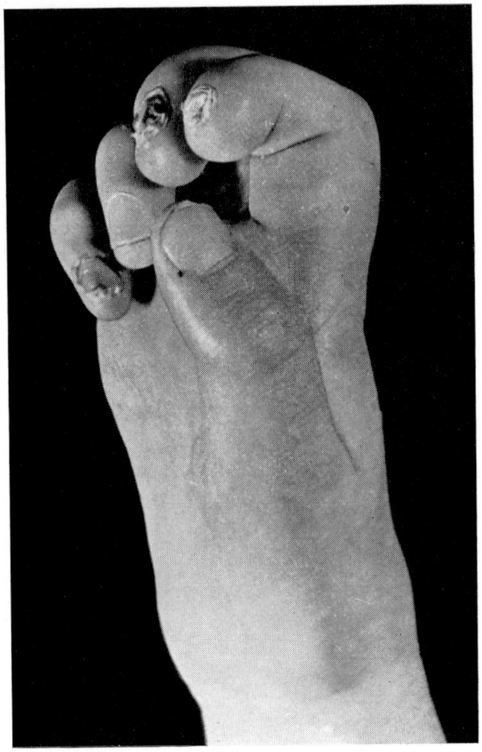

FIG. **3**, 16. Infected and deformed nails in a patient with median and ulnar paralysis. The hand was very stiff.

pronounced and regular when blood vessels as well as nerves were injured.

The apparent increase in the growth of hair on the forearm and leg is often due to shrinkage of the paralysed part.

Digital atrophy. Atrophy of one or more digits is invariable and in paralysis confined to the median nerve it catches the eye because it is limited to the index. A curious feature of the case illustrated in Figure **15**, 32 (p. 277), in which there was total median paralysis except for the index, was that at no stage did the index show any atrophy.

Ulcers, blisters, and other lesions. These are most commonly due to injury, the patient having burned the insensitive part; or, in sciatic paralysis, having been unaware of a nail or some other irregularity in the sole of the shoe. In the foot, exactly as in leprosy, ulceration may be secondary to deformity which causes excessive pressure on a prominent part (Fig. **3**, 17). Ulcers are usually

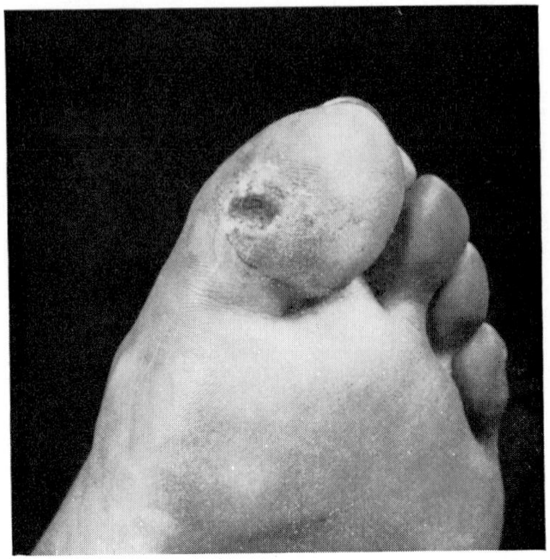

FIG. **3**, 17. A sore under a moderately clawed great toe. The patient had suffered transection of the sciatic nerve 6 years previously: recovery after repair was poor. (Reproduced by kind permission from Clawson, D. K. and Seddon, H. J., 1960, *J. Bone Jt Surg.*, **42B**, 213.)

superficial and, with reasonable care, heal rapidly. However, in the foot, neglect can cause an ulcer to go deep, with involvement of the underlying bones and joints.

Very occasionally there may be recurrent crops of small blisters that are not due to injury; they may appear in incomplete lesions in which sweating is excessive. Lesions that look like ordinary chilblains are sometimes seen, with the usual story of being worse in cold weather.

Oedema. In the upper limb swelling is seen only after extensive damage to the brachial plexus; in the lower limb it sometimes occurs after sciatic paralysis. In both, this is a serious matter because it can contribute to stiffness of the paralysed part which may develop rapidly.

Bone. The changes detectable radiographically are no more than could be attributed to disuse (Sprung, 1943), though in the case of extensive injuries, such as total paralysis of the brachial plexus, they can be extreme, particularly in cancellous bone. If paralysis occurs early in life there may be shortening and deformity due to unbalanced muscle action—as in poliomyelitis.

No matter how extensive the denervation, neuropathic disorders of joints never occur, nor even the type of arthropathy seen in neural leprosy, although the latter is a disorder of the peripheral nerves.

Observations on the Nature of the Vasomotor and Nutritional Disturbances

In the warm phase, exposure to cold does not cause cooling of the denervated part which behaves as after sympathectomy. In the cold phase, a cold environment produces an abnormally rapid fall in temperature of the denervated part and when the ambient temperature is brought back to normal the digit warms up very slowly, like an inert body.

Warming or cooling one normal limb produces reflex vasodilatation or vasoconstriction in the other three; but if one of these limbs is the site of a major nerve injury it responds differently. In the warm phase the part remains warm throughout; it does not respond whether another limb is heated or cooled. In the cold phase it is similarly unresponsive though it may warm up a little if there is great vasodilatation of the other three limbs.

If, however, the circulation is arrested with a pressure cuff the flushing that occurs on release is the same in normal and in denervated areas, which suggests that reactive hyperaemia is independent of the peripheral nervous system.

There is little doubt that the initial warm phase is due to vasoconstrictor paralysis but the cold phase is puzzling. It seems likely that the musculature of the blood vessels regains its tone and becomes hypersensitive to circulating adrenalin though this is not universally accepted (White, 1949).

The complaint of coldness has been attributed to the vasoconstrictor action of low temperature on denervated blood vessels (Lewis and Landis, 1930). It is less liable to be present where there has been good sensory recovery because the autonomic fibres run and regenerate with the sensory. However, this may not be the whole answer. In poliomyelitis coldness of a limb, although a direct result of increased peripheral vascular tone (Trott, Nesline and Green 1958), is associated with motor paralysis.

It is supposed that the reason why a sympathectomized limb behaves differently from one in which a main nerve has been interrupted is that in the former there is a general flushing, whereas in a limb in which one nerve has been injured the greater part of the limb is still responsive to vasomotor impulses and, as in a temperate climate these are mostly vasoconstrictor, the denervated area shares in the general coolness of the limb. Richards (M.R.C.R., 1954) pointed out that if the paralysis is extensive—involving the whole of the brachial plexus or the whole of the sciatic nerve—the general tendency of the paralysed part is to remain warmer than a small denervated area.

The nutritional disorders, from which ulcers ought perhaps to be excluded, are not confined to limbs in which a nerve has been injured. Changes in the skin (including chilblains) and nails and atrophy of the soft parts are seen in a variety of upper and lower neurone lesions of which poliomyelitis was formerly the best known example. Disuse is probably the chief common factor. If this is so then the more widespread the paralysis the more pronounced should be the nutritional disorder. Richards found the highest incidence of these changes in combined median and ulnar paralysis, which makes the hand almost completely useless, and he also noted that a proximal lesion of the median nerve, which innervates a considerable mass of the forearm flexor muscles, produced more severe nutritional changes than an injury of the same nerve at the wrist.

THE CLINICAL RECORD

A patient with a damaged nerve may present in one of several ways:

1. He is seen immediately after the injury; he may or may not be aware of paralysis and it is the clinician's business to search for evidence of it. If the patient is unconscious this is confined to noting the findings in any wound that has to be treated (p. 230), but there should be no hunting for possibly damaged nerves. The patient may be conscious, but shocked or in great pain or both; the tests must then be very simple.

They are described under individual nerves (Chaps 11 and 12).

2. The patient has suffered an injury and has recovered from its immediate effects. He may still be unaware of any paralysis and, as with the acutely injured patient, a search has to be made, but this time in detail if possible. However, the limb may be encased in plaster-of-Paris, or the skin may not be in satisfactory condition for thorough sensory examination.

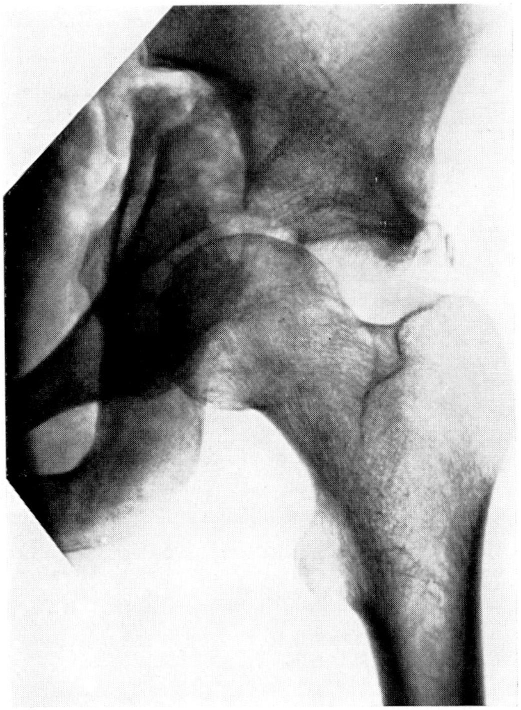

FIG. **3**, 18. A patient suffered a severe comminuted fracture of the lower end of the femur, and there was total sciatic paralysis thought to be caused by it. There were two reasons why this was unlikely: the fracture was hardly of a kind to damage both divisions of the sciatic nerve, especially as the popliteal vessels were intact. It was finally discovered that there was also a fracture of the acetabulum; this was the cause of the nerve injury.

3. The patient has suffered an injury and there is no doubt in anyone's mind that after it he had no disability attributable to nerve damage. Then paralysis supervened for some reason or other. Examples of this will be given later (pp. 81 and 91).

HISTORY

Among the details required in all records of patients *occupation* calls for particular attention. A nerve injury may oblige a patient to change his work; this is sometimes immediately evident and then there should be no delay in making plans for his rehabilitation and resettlement. If it is possible the *exact circumstances at the time of injury* should be recorded. If a man with an injured arm was dragged along the ground the nature of the nerve injury he has suffered may be entirely different from that in a case where this did not happen (p. 76). In missile injuries the position of the body when it was struck is sometimes relevant.

An external wound is or has been present. The time that elapsed before healing occurred should be noted and whether there was any sepsis. The wound may still be open. The patient may also have something useful to say about injuries to other structures such as bones, blood vessels or tendons.

No wound. Here it is particularly important to determine exactly what happened. If, for example, it emerges that the patient suffered a traction injury as well as a fracture the whole management of the case is influenced by this. There may have been two fractures and it is necessary to know which of them damaged the nerve (Fig. **3**, 18). The nerve may have been injured by an *injection*, and enquiry should be made about the site and about the pain the patient experienced at the time and subsequently.

Pain. Certain types of nerve injury are characterized by more or less severe pain and the following points should be noted:

1. Time of onset in relation to injury.
2. Distribution.
3. Site and direction of spread.
4. Quality and intensity.
5. Duration—continuous or intermittent.
6. Conditions that precipitate or aggravate it, e.g. posture, temperature, using the limb, emotion.
7. Conditions that give relief, e.g. posture, temperature, dampness, immobility, drugs.
8. Associated phenomena:
   Local, e.g. sweating, colour of skin.
   General, e.g. apprehension, insomnia, emotional state.

Evidence of recovery. Missile injuries are often followed by paralysis of the whole limb, but much of it turns out to be short-lived. If some considerable time has elapsed since the injury there may be further slowly progressive recovery due to spontaneous regeneration, entirely different from the early rapid recovery after neurapraxia.

The history is then summarized as follows:

1. Date of the injury.
2. Nature of the injury.
3. Date of healing if there has been a wound.
4. Sepsis.
5. Evidence of recovery.

LOCAL EXAMINATION

This should be leisurely and it requires the active interest of the patient. He should be seen in a quiet, warm room.

Wounds. All wounds are accurately described and, if healed, the dimensions and nature of the scars are noted. There may be local tenderness and sometimes a neuroma is palpable. If the track of the wound has been near a blood vessel particular attention is paid to evidence of an aneurysm or arterio-venous fistula. A stethoscope is essential.

If there have been several injuries in one limb it will be necessary, at some stage, to decide which is the one that damaged the nerve.

Joints. The passive range of movement in every joint of the affected limb should be recorded, and it is convenient to use the notation recommended by the American Academy of Orthopaedic Surgeons and the British Orthopaedic Association (1966). If a deformity is present it should be described or photographed and if the injury is in the lower limb the gait should be observed.

Joint stiffness is sometimes so severe as to present a more pressing problem than repair of a nerve, for however satisfactory regeneration of a nerve may be, the functional result will be marred if the joints of the paralysed part lack a full or at any rate a useful range of movement.

Motor function. The distribution of wasting is noted and the circumference of the limbs measured. In the adult a convenient level for measuring the thigh is 20 cm below the anterior superior iliac spine; the maximum diameter of the calf is measured. In the adult, arm measurements are made 10 cm above and 10 cm below the medial epicondyle of the humerus.

Voluntary power is charted in accordance with the following grading (specimen charts are shown on pp. 173-174 and 215):

0. No contraction.
1. Trace of contraction.
2. Active movement with gravity eliminated.
3. Active movement against gravity.
4. Active movement against gravity and resistance.

4+. Intermediate between 4 and 5.

5. Normal power.

Care must be taken not to be deceived by supplementary movements, rebound movements, and true trick movements.

When there is a possibility of ischaemia the affected muscles should be palpated and their consistence noted.

Sensory function. It has already been remarked (p. x) that the study of sensibility is a peacetime occupation. During the Second World War we were obliged to use simple methods of examination, to devise and adhere to a system of grading motor and sensory function that would at least give a rough idea of a patient's progress. It is notable that Highet's system of grading is still being used in countries other than the United Kingdom 30 years after it was invented. However, in view of the complexity of cutaneous sensibility it is not surprising that more elaborate methods of examination are being investigated; a good account of them is given by McQuillan *et al.* (1971).

If a limb has recently come out of plaster, if it is oedematous or cold, no response of any kind may be obtained. In such circumstances, examination should be postponed until the state of the part has been improved by massage, movement, and warmth.

This is the most exacting part of the examination. Both patient and examiner should be fresh and alert and the testing should be conducted with as few distractions as possible. First, the patient should be asked to outline with his finger what he considers to be the area of abnormality; he may indicate areas that might otherwise have escaped detection. Loss of *tactile sensibility* should be investigated first, because it imposes a strain on the patient's attention. It is not always possible for sensory examinations in a particular case to be made by the same person, but variations in technique can be considerably reduced if a constant stimulus is employed. The von Frey stimulator designed by Weddell is a simple and reliable piece of apparatus. A short length of nylon thread that bends when pressed on the pan of a balance against a weight of 1 g is mounted at the end of a bicycle spoke, with the part carrying the screw collar bent at a right angle (Fig. **3**, 19). The long handle enables the examiner to get round awkward corners without the risk of his hand or sleeve touching the patient's skin and so causing confusion. The area of skin under consideration is stroked with the hair from the anaesthetic towards the normal part, and a mark is made with black ink at the point where the hair is first felt. The areas examined should, in the first place, be about 4 cm apart. The ink dots will soon reveal the extent of the anaesthetic area. Stimuli are then applied to areas between those first examined, and the results will give some indication of the reliability of the patient's responses. In an intelligent subject it will be found that the second series of dots is roughly in line with the first. Indeed, the boundary of the anaesthetic area is usually so sharp that it is proper to mark it with a continuous line. The area outlined in this way is surrounded by one of hypoaesthesia, and in this outer belt a tactile stimulus, although readily appreciated, is less definite than normal—it feels 'woolly', as if something were interposed between the skin and the stimulator. However, the demarcation of this zone of hypoaesthesia is required only in partial or recovering lesions.

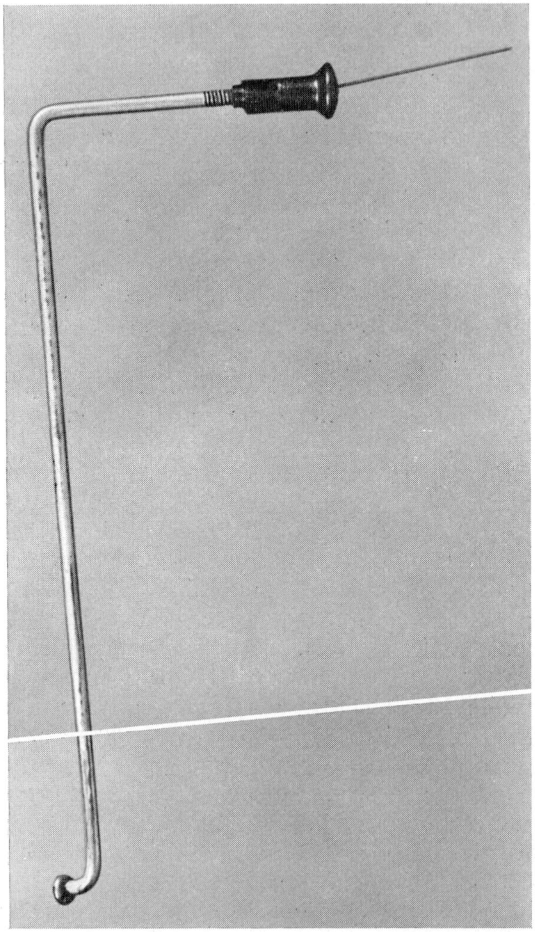

FIG. **3**, 19. Weddell's instrument for testing tactile sensibility. It is the full length of a bicycle spoke, but is shortened here to show the ends more conveniently.

Testing for *pain sensibility* is done with a needle such as is used for suturing skin, or a long hatpin. The difficulty is to know how deeply the skin should be penetrated, and the examiner should begin by determining the threshold in a normal area where the texture of the skin is similar to that of the part to be examined. Then, working from the analgesic towards normal skin, the needle is applied until a point is reached where pain is felt. This is indicated by a black dot. Any response other than one indicating pain should be ignored. Where the skin is thick the pressure necessary to puncture the skin may be felt as pressure even though the skin is completely analgesic. As in testing for touch, the areas first stimulated should be about 4 cm apart; then stimuli are applied in the gaps. It will not be found possible to mark a boundary as precise as that for anaesthesia; there is too much overlapping from contiguous sensory areas. Hence, it is best to indicate the analgesic area by a series of dots. As has already been mentioned (p. 38 and Fig. **3**, 10, p. 45) the analgesic area usually lies within the area of anaesthesia. The intervening area is hypoalgesic. It is here that one may find abnormal pain sensibility.

In partial or recovering lesions there may be nothing more than reduced sensibility in a part or the whole of the affected area. Here, the examiner can only indicate the boundary between normal and subnormal feeling, and this is conveniently indicated by a continuous serrated line (Fig. **3**, 20).

Two-point discrimination. This is valuable in the hand because it gives an index of tactile sensibility that can be expressed numerically. With the hand resting comfortably on a low table or pillow the blunted points of dividers are applied gently and simultaneously to the pulp of a digit (Fig. **3**, 21). At first the points are close together and the patient feels them as one; then the distance between them is increased until the patient —who must not see what is happening—gives fairly consistently correct answers when one and then two points of the compass are applied to the digit. The normal value in children may be as low as 2 mm, in adults 4 to 6 mm. We have come to regard anything above 15 mm as unsatisfactory; the patient always has appreciable sensory disability.

Picking-up test (Fig. **3**, 22). The patient is asked to pick up a number of small objects placed before him on a table and to put them as fast as he can into a small box, first with one hand and then with the other. He can then be blindfolded and asked to identify the objects. The difference between the behaviour of the hands is watched, though the result is difficult to quantify.

Coin test. Although I have used this test fairly regularly I did not—as has been stated—invent it; I learned it from Riddoch in 1940 and he made no claim to be the originator. This does not matter, but inaccurate descriptions of the test (Önne, 1964) have appeared. It has been said that the skin is stroked, first with a coin having a smooth edge and then with one having a milled edge. The test as used in Britain is in fact the precursor of the picking-up test. The patient, whose eyes must be closed, is given a coin and asked to identify it. If he has a median nerve lesion—and it is only in median or combined median and ulnar lesions that the test is applicable—he must not cheat by pushing the coin towards an area of normally sentient skin. A somewhat similar and quite elegant method has been devised by Porter (1966), who uses steel type letters, 1·0 by 0·8 cm. The letters must be identical in reverse and he has chosen H, O, U, V, and Y (Fig. **3**, 23). The patient scores no mark if he fails to identify the letter or takes more than 30 seconds to do so.

Tactile localization. This is the ability to indicate the location of a stimulus. On the abdominal wall or the thigh it is inexact: on the palmar surface of

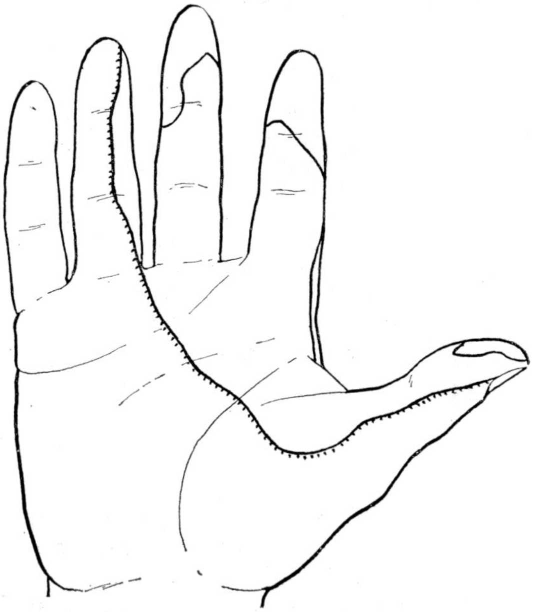

FIG. **3**, 20. Sensory chart during recovery.
—— boundary of anaesthesia: there is no analgesia.
⋯⋯ boundary of area of reduced sensibility.

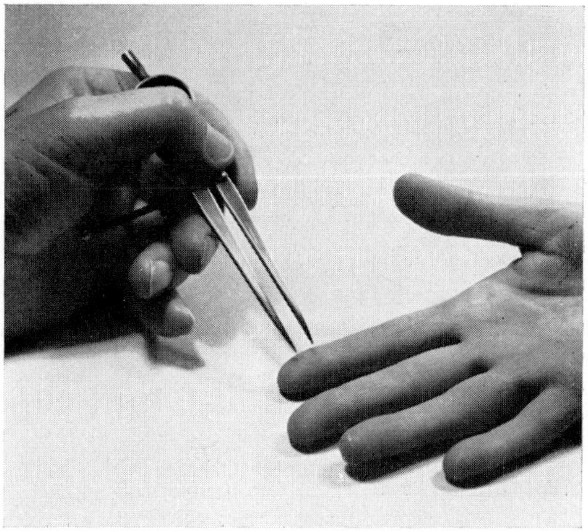

FIG. **3**, 21. Testing two-point discrimination: the points of the instrument must be blunt.

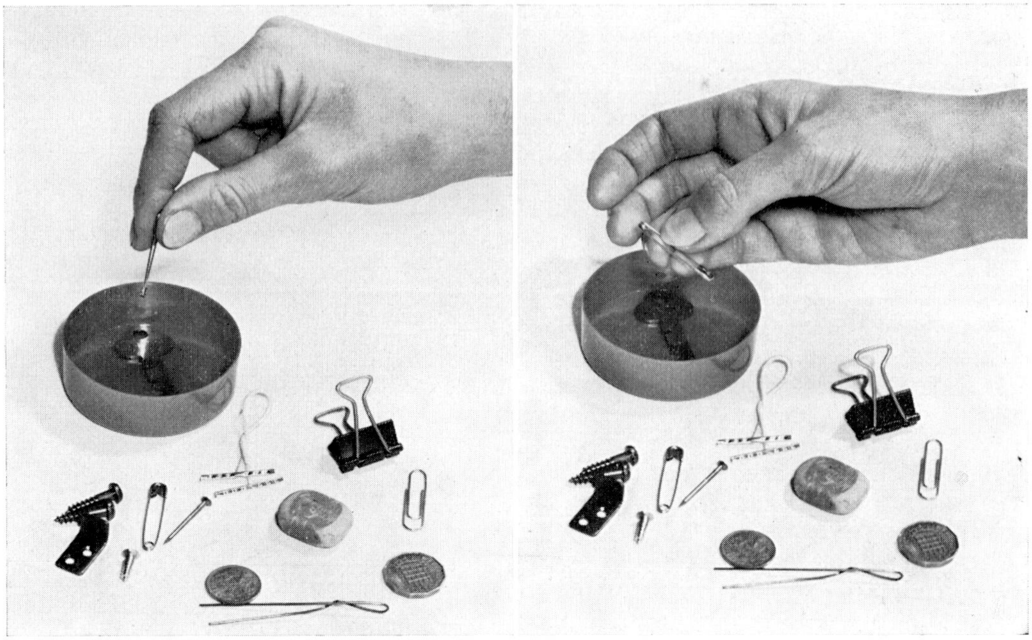

FIG. 3, 22. Moberg's picking-up test.

the hand it is normally most precise. During and often permanently after regeneration of a nerve it is faulty, particularly after nerve suture. A stimulus applied to the index finger may be

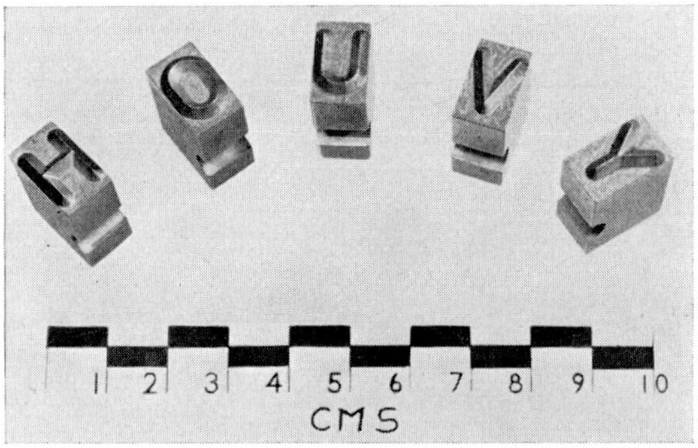

FIG. 3, 23. Tactile discrimination: Porter's steel type letters. (Reproduced by kind permission from Porter, R. W., 1966, *Br. med. J.*, **2**, 927.)

referred to a neighbouring digit or even to the palm; this is presumably due to axonal confusion at the site of the nerve lesion, as a result of which sensory axons arrive at destinations not their own. This is not a quality that can be graded and it is not used as an index of the completeness or otherwise of recovery, except that if tactile localization is normal then the degree of recovery is near normal too.

YOUNG PATIENTS. Tactile sensibility alone should be tested and this is not difficult if the child is first given the bicycle spoke and told to try it out on his own hand or his mother's. In infants the only satisfactory method, though it is crude, is testing pain sensibility under light narcosis.

The findings are recorded on the usual outline diagrams.

Tinel's sign. Percussion with the finger starts peripherally and the point at which a positive response is felt is noted. Tapping is then continued up to the level of the lesion.

Vascular and nutritional changes. Apart from the possibility of a vascular lesion at the site of nerve injury it is desirable to take note of the distal pulses and the colour and temperature of the skin. It is often possible by naked eye inspection or by using an ophthalmoscope to detect sweating. The texture of the skin, abnormalities of the nails and hair and the presence of blisters and ulcers are also recorded.

Ancillary Examinations

Radiography. Radiographic examination of the site of injury is at the discretion of the clinician, but it is always advisable when there has been a penetrating wound.

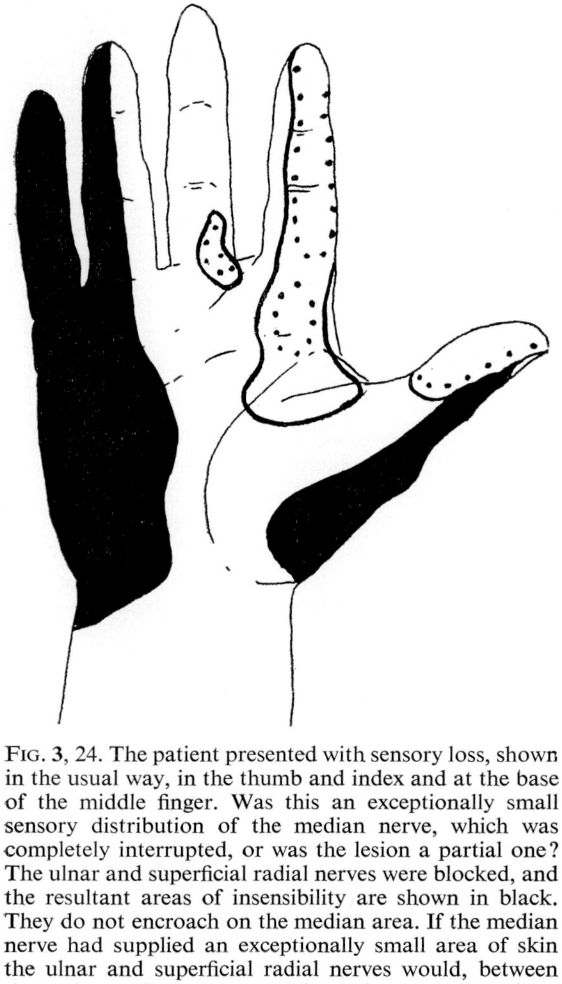

Fig. 3, 24. The patient presented with sensory loss, shown in the usual way, in the thumb and index and at the base of the middle finger. Was this an exceptionally small sensory distribution of the median nerve, which was completely interrupted, or was the lesion a partial one? The ulnar and superficial radial nerves were blocked, and the resultant areas of insensibility are shown in black. They do not encroach on the median area. If the median nerve had supplied an exceptionally small area of skin the ulnar and superficial radial nerves would, between them, have filled the gap. The lesion was, therefore, partial interruption of the median nerve.

Electrical examination. Unless the state of a nerve has already been established at operation one or more of the methods of examination described in the following chapter will usually be valuable. Even when it is known that, say, the median nerve has been severed electrical examination may be needed to elucidate some anomaly of innervation.

Nerve block. This method of examination was used extensively by Highet (1942) for the investigation of nerve injuries in which there was a possibility of some anomaly of motor or sensory innervation, and for indentifying partial injuries (Fig. 3, 24). It is not employed sufficiently, and

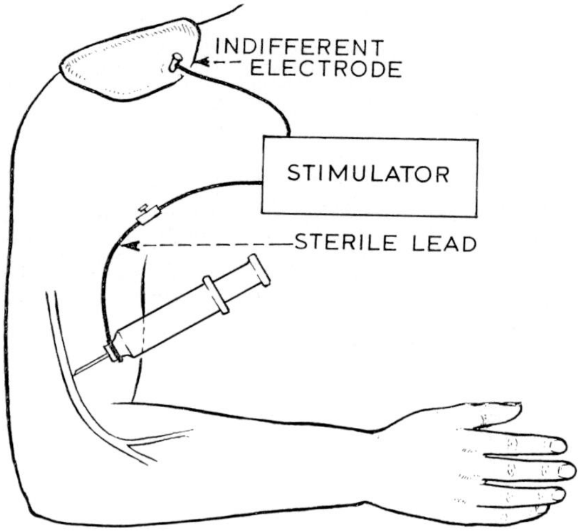

Fig. 3, 25. Highet's apparatus for nerve blocking. The needle is a stimulating electrode and is coated, except at its tip, with insulating resin.

because it is so valuable the technique will be described in detail. When a nerve can be easily localized by palpation—as, for example, the ulnar nerve at the elbow or the common peroneal at the neck of the fibula—there is no difficulty in making the injection which should be of a 2 per cent solution of procaine containing adrenalin at a strength of 1 in 50,000. Cutaneous nerves can be identified and their course followed by percutaneous unipolar electrical stimulation. But if a deeply placed nerve has to be blocked it is desirable to use Highet's apparatus (Fig. 3, 25), an electrical stimulator connected on the one hand to a large indifferent electrode and on the other to the metallic base of the injecting needle which must be coated with insulating resin except at its tip. The needle is inserted so that its point lies somewhere near the nerve and then, with a very small current flowing, it is moved until the patient feels tingling in the distribution of the nerve to be injected. It is then possible to anaesthetize the nerve with a small quantity of solution, so avoiding the risk of its diffusing widely and perhaps affecting a neighbouring nerve. This localizing needle-electrode can also be used to determine whether the block is complete, by increasing the stimulus and observing whether the patient feels anything in the distribution of the nerve.

The sweating test (p. 44). This is used as required but we have abandoned its routine employment.

Nerve and muscle biopsy. These two ancillary methods of investigation were used frequently during the Second World War, nerve biopsy by Holmes and Zachary (1946) and muscle biopsy by Bowden and Gutmann (1945). In cases of nerve injury the indications for the employment of either are now infrequent, though both are essential in the investigation of the more obscure disorders of peripheral nerve and muscle.

Neurography. Over many years there has been spasmodic interest (for example, Lohr and Jacobi, 1932; Saito, Kamizawa and Kato, 1933) in the radiographic investigation of peripheral nerve lesions. More recently (Cave, Fustec and Basset, 1965) it has been used in the study of the neuritis of leprosy, and for the localization of nerve tumours.

Now that the dangers of Thorotrast are appreciated we are assured that Lipiodol (Duroliopaque is specially commended) is harmless to human nerves although transient paresis has been noted in dogs (Karabarbounis, 1973). The usual technique has been to inject the nerve direct, but a most intriguing method has been used by this same author since 1957: the contrast medium is injected epidurally at an appropriate level, and after minutes or hours, depending on the region being examined, the peripheral nerves become radio-opaque.

Although I have never met anyone experienced in surgery of the peripheral nerves who employs neurography, and although it has been used unnecessarily in some cases (for example, Razemon, Petyt and Bonte, 1973) one can recall a few cases in which it would have been invaluable. This diagnostic aid does not deserve summary dismissal.

Progress Notes

The timing of subsequent examinations varies so much that generalization is impossible. If, for example, it is suspected that spontaneous recovery from radial paralysis caused by a fracture of the humerus will occur, weekly examination is necessary during the period when signs of recovery become due (p. 246).

4. Electrical Phenomena: Methods of Examination

IN THIS CHAPTER no more will be presented than the elements of a complex and expanding subject: the information that will enable a surgeon to assimilate what may be learned by electrodiagnosis into the observations on which decisions are based.

Well over a century has elapsed since the responses of normal and abnormal muscle to electrical stimulation began to arouse interest. The nerves too were stimulated through the skin and—after the advent of modern surgery—at operation. The old galvanic-faradic test gave way to the estimation of strength-duration curves. This in turn has now been largely eclipsed by more direct methods of recording the intrinsic electrical phenomena in muscle and nerve (see, for example, Desmedt, 1973). The recording of SD curves will therefore be described more briefly than in the first (1972) edition of this book. We shall then consider:

Percutaneous nerve stimulation.

Electromyography, that is the observation of electrical changes in muscle.

Nerve conduction and, what is intimately connected with it, nerve action potentials.

STRENGTH-DURATION CURVES

Certain tissues, nerve and muscle in particular, respond to electrical stimulation. The degree of excitability, which is much greater for nerve than for muscle, is the property that is being examined here.

The machine employed delivers stimuli of selected duration ranging from 0·3 second (300 milliseconds), which in this context is a current of unlimited duration and so corresponds to galvanism, down to 0·01 msec, which is much shorter than the stimulus from a faradic coil. Great attention is paid to ensuring that the potential is uniform throughout the stimulus which has, therefore, a square wave-form. The frequency of stimulation can be varied too. The strength of the stimulus depends either on amperage or on voltage. For technical reasons *constant voltage* is preferred; what this means is that the voltage is approximately constant at any chosen level throughout the circuit; thus the voltmeter reading indicates the voltage in the tissue stimulated. The curves given by a constant-current (amperage) machine cannot be compared with those given by a constant-voltage machine. Indeed, even when the same machine is used for repeated observations, strict precautions must be observed if comparable curves are to be obtained (Harris, 1952).

The conditions required are those that lower the resistance of the skin and subcutaneous tissues. It is useless to examine an oedematous limb. The limb, after brisk washing, should be well warmed by infra-red radiation. The indifferent electrode is placed at some convenient site and the stimulating electrode is placed over the muscle to be examined. The skin and electrode are kept well moistened with 1 per cent saline solution.

The duration-selector switch is set at 300 msec, the pulse repetition frequency at 0·5 second—that is two stimuli every second—and the strength of stimulus is gradually increased until the muscle contracts. By alternately increasing and decreasing the voltage the point is reached when contraction is minimal. If it is sluggish the muscle is likely to be denervated; if it is brisk, innervated; but no great attention should be paid to this.

The strength of current of infinite duration that produces a minimal response is called the *rheobase*. It has no absolute value but is indispensable as a quantity and term of reference.

Let us now suppose that normal muscle is being examined. Because the motor nerve fibres are more readily excitable than the muscle fibres the SD curve will in fact be that of nerve. For each duration of stimulus, there is a certain threshold response. The voltage required to evoke each response is plotted on a graph and the result is the SD curve for normal nerve. Figure **4**, 1 shows that with the shorter stimuli a higher voltage is required to elicit a response. The two curves mark the limits of normality. If a horizontal line is drawn at the level corresponding to twice the value of the rheobase it cuts the upturning curves. If from each point of intersection a

This is the nearest we can get to representing the excitability of a tissue by a single value, but as will shortly be apparent it is not invariably helpful.

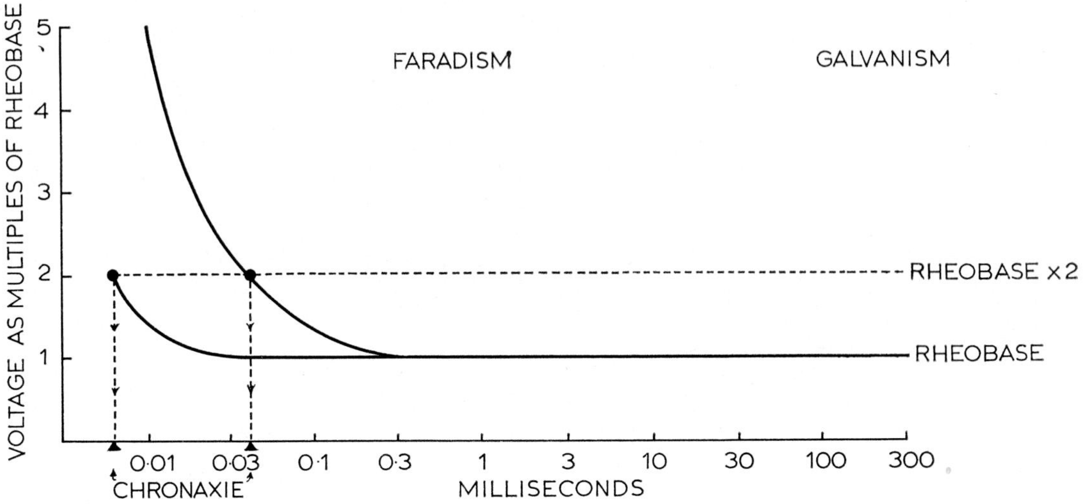

FIG. 4, 1. Normal strength-duration curves. (After Wynn Parry.)

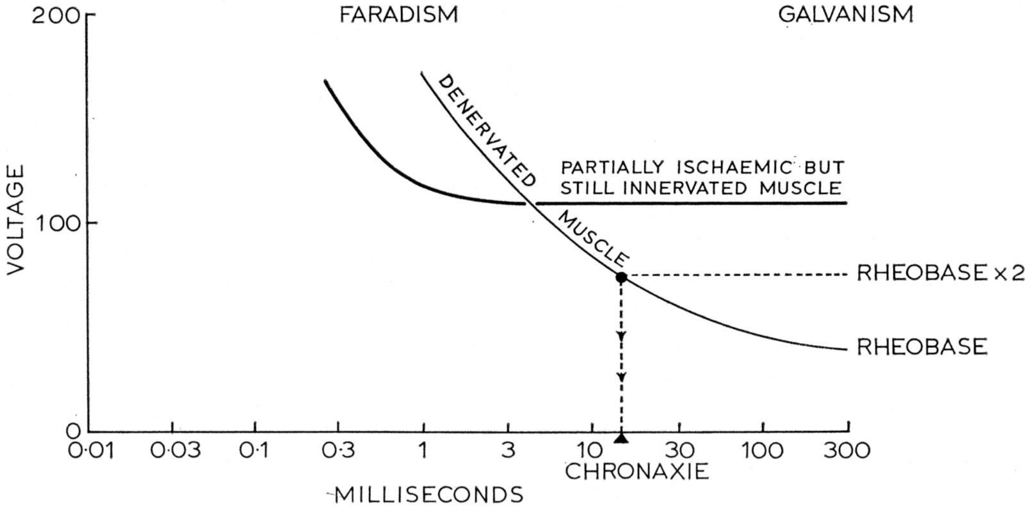

FIG. 4, 2. Strength-duration curves of denervated muscle and of muscle damaged by ischaemia.

perpendicular line is drawn it cuts the pulse-duration scale. The duration of the stimulus required to excite a response when the voltage is twice the value of the rheobase is the *chronaxie* (Bourguinon, 1923); in this diagram, with its two curves, a duration ranging from a little less than 0·01 msec to a little more than 0·03 msec.

If completely denervated muscle is examined the picture is very different (Fig. **4**, 2). The curve climbs quickly and the stimuli of short duration fail to evoke any response with a voltage that is tolerable. It will also be noted that the chronaxie of denervated muscle is long, about 15 msec, some hundreds of times the value for innervated muscle.

There is a third, the discontinuous, or more simply the kinked, type of curve (Fig. **4**, 3); and it is important. The more points there are on the graph the easier it is to demonstrate the kink; with 10 durations of stimulus it will certainly be apparent. This is the curve characteristic of muscle in process of re-innervation. It is, therefore, a sign of recovery, and the more the kink flattens out and shifts downwards towards normal (Fig. **4**, 4) the more certain is it that re-innervation is progressing satisfactorily.

Analysis of this kind of curve is instructive (Fig. **4**, 5). Consider first the chronaxie: it is almost identical with that shown in Figure **4**, 2. It is the chronaxie of denervated muscle and therefore gives no indication of the encouraging information conveyed by the whole curve. If the two parts of the curve are extrapolated it is apparent that there are two curves, one of denervated muscle (DN—dn) and one of nerve (N—n). But the rheobase for the latter (RN) is extremely high; it is commonplace that the threshold for excitation of regenerating nerve is elevated. So when the duration of the stimulus is long, denervated muscle is in fact more readily excitable than regenerating nerve.

Changes in the SD curve usually appear 2 to 3 weeks before there is clinical evidence of motor recovery.

Ischaemic muscle, if not totally destroyed, responds like normal muscle (M.R.C.R., 1954) in that currents of short duration can provoke contraction; but for all durations the threshold is very high (Fig. **4**, 2).

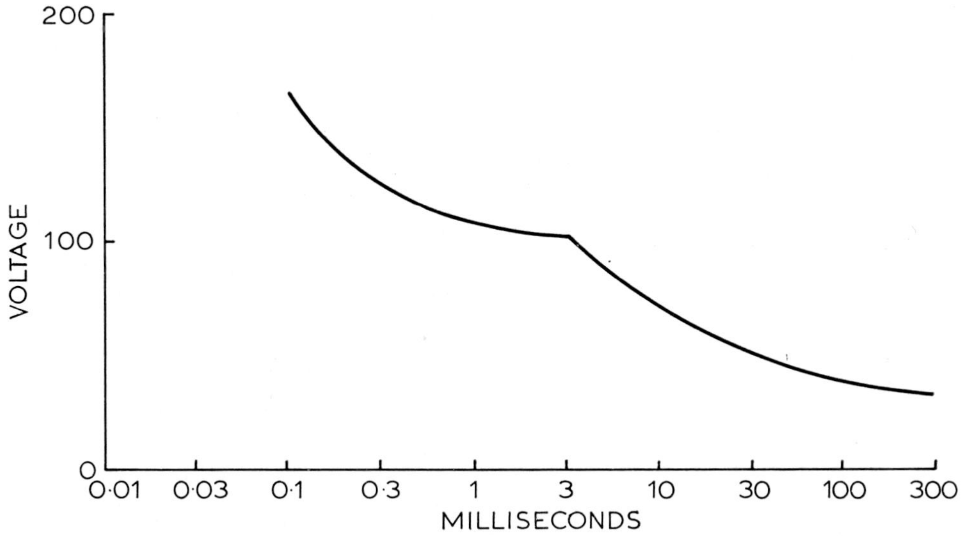

FIG. **4**, 3. The discontinuous curve found during re-innervation of muscle.

PERCUTANEOUS NERVE STIMULATION

This simple but valuable manoeuvre is applicable only to nerves that lie superficially. The stimulating electrode is placed over the nerve and the strength of the current is increased. If a positive response—that is, contraction of the muscles supplied by the nerve—is readily obtained on the contralateral side and not on the affected side then the damage has caused degeneration of the nerve. The test, whether positive or negative, becomes significant after the fourth day and herein lies its special value.

It is indispensable in the recognition of anomalous innervation, whereas electromyography is useless: and it is simpler than nerve blocking. If, in a case of median nerve injury with conservation of power in one or more of the thenar muscles (which is very common) stimulation of the ulnar nerve causes these muscles to contract, then it is certain that they are supplied wholly or to a considerable extent by the ulnar nerve. In such cases the median nerve injury is usually

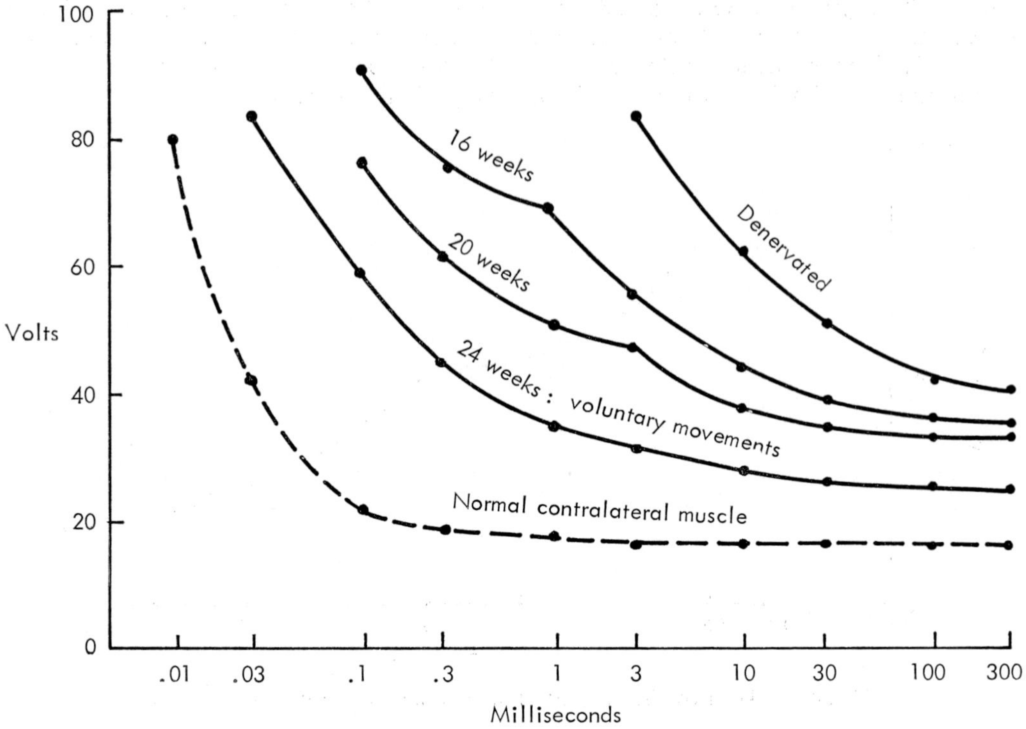

FIG. **4**, 4. The course of recovery as revealed by SD curves. (Reproduced by kind permission from Ritchie, A. E., 1954, M.R.C. Special Report Series No. 282.)

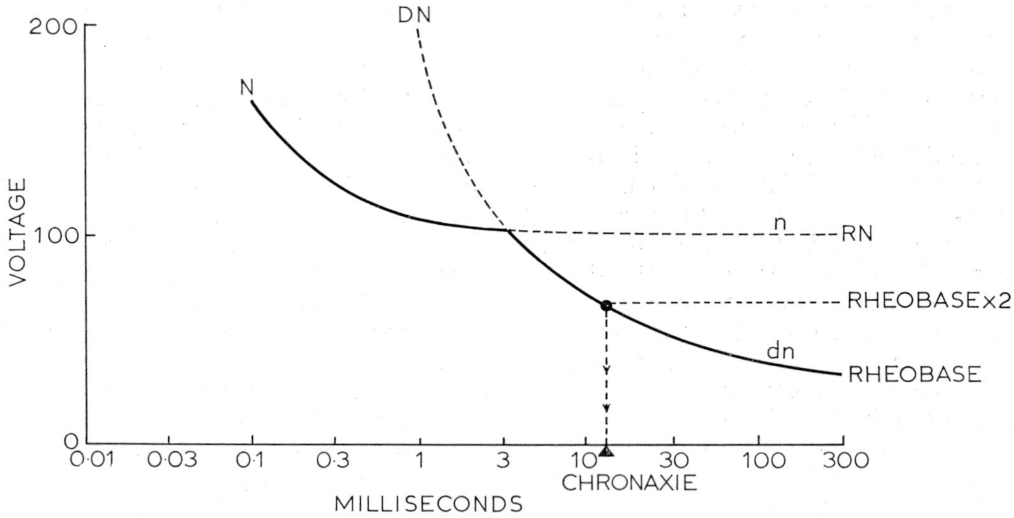

FIG. **4**, 5. Analysis of the discontinuous curve.

found to be complete and thus the indication for exploration is established.

Direct stimulation of the exposed nerve is also important in exploratory operations (p. 251).

ELECTROMYOGRAPHY

When muscle contracts there is a change in potential that can be recorded. For normal

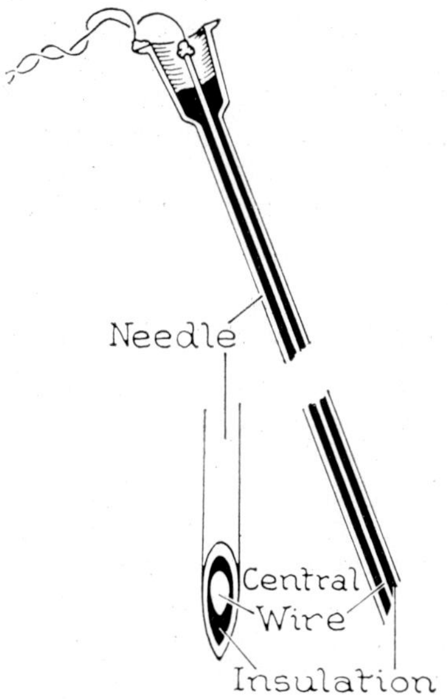

FIG. **4**, 6. The concentric needle electrode (Reproduced by kind permission of Dr J. V. Basmajian and the Williams and Wilkins Company.)

voluntary muscle, surface electrodes will suffice if the muscle is superficial; but in diagnostic work it is usual to employ the concentric needle electrode (Fig. **4**, 6) devised by Adrian and Bronk (1929) because it can be inserted into deep muscles, and because the small action-potentials produced by denervated muscle can be picked up only in this way.

Reference has already been made (p. 7) to the motor unit. On minimal contraction of a muscle it is the potential from this unit that appears on the cathode-ray screen (Fig. **4**, 7). Its amplitude is roughly proportionate to the number of fibres it contains. As the strength of contraction increases more and more motor units contract, and the needle picks up potentials from many in its immediate neighbourhood (Fig. **4**, 8). If a loudspeaker is connected to the apparatus the single AP sounds like the reverberation of one shot from a distant gun; the noise made by a strongly contracting muscle is like an artillery barrage.

The fibrillation of denervated muscle, which begins 14 to 28 days after a nerve injury, is due

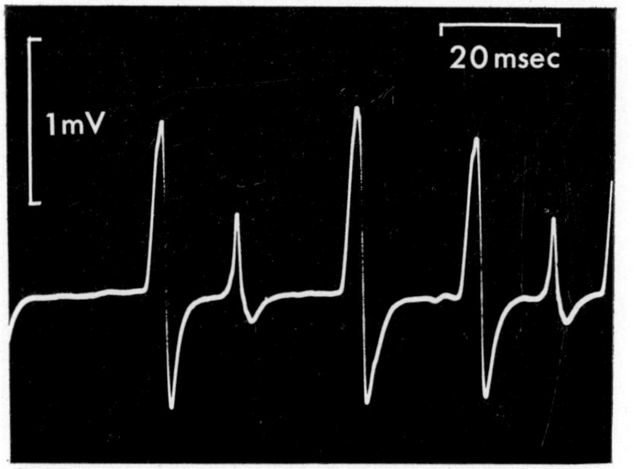

FIG. **4**, 7. Electromyogram recorded with a concentric needle electrode, showing normal motor-unit potentials. (The tracings in Figs **4**, 7 to **4**, 9 were kindly provided by Prof. P. K. Thomas.)

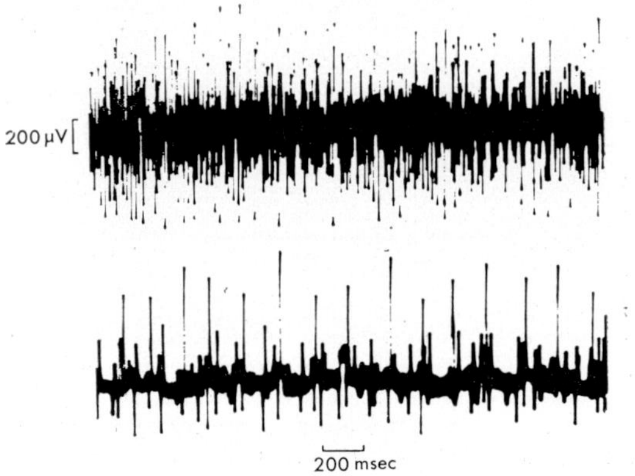

FIG. **4**, 8. Electromyograms recorded with a concentric needle electrode. *Upper tracing:* normal motor unit recruitment pattern on maximal voluntary effort. *Lower tracing:* reduced pattern in motor neurone disease.

to the regular contraction of individual muscle fibres. It is most easily detected by electromyography. The action-potentials have an amplitude of only 100 microvolts, compared with the 2 millivolts of a normal motor-unit AP. The duration of a fibrillation AP is shorter than that of a motor-unit AP (Fig. **4**, 9) which is why its amplification by a loudspeaker sounds like a sharp click. A curious feature of fibrillation APs is that a burst of them may be provoked when the needle electrode is inserted; it is called insertion activity. For some unknown reason some denervated muscles are electrically silent: so the absence of fibrillation APs cannot be relied on to exclude a degenerative nerve lesion.

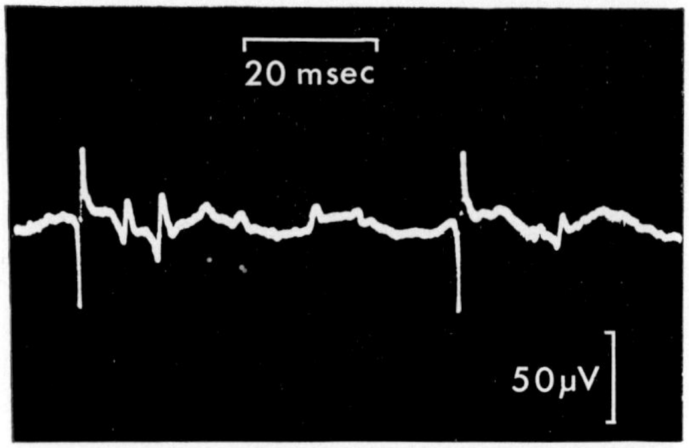

FIG. **4**, 9. Fibrillation potentials: recorded with a concentric needle electrode. Compare the voltage scale with that shown in Figure **4**, 7.

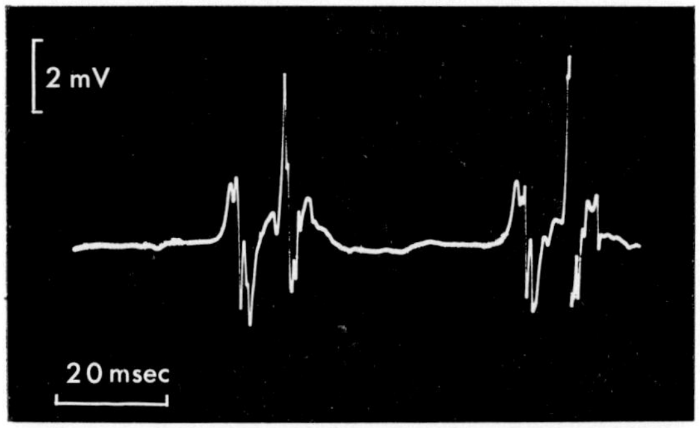

FIG. **4**, 10. Polyphasic motor-unit action-potential recorded by Prof. P. K. Thomas, who has kindly allowed this tracing to be reproduced: from a patient recovering from Guillain-Barré polyneuritis.

The re-innervation of muscle fibres from the nerve fibres supplying adjacent normal ones, a phenomenon that is independent of nerve regeneration (p. 26), is responsible for the appearance of giant motor-unit APs which differ from normal APs only in the voltage scale.

Whereas the normal motor-unit AP is usually triphasic the motor-unit APs that develop during true re-innervation of a muscle are often polyphasic (Fig. **4**, 10) and sound more like a troublesome motor cycle starting up than a gunshot.

A healthy muscle that is completely relaxed is electrically silent.

Motor-unit activity appears ahead of clinical evidence of recovery. As would be expected the interval is short after axonotmesis; there is no misdirection or wastage of the regenerating fibres. On the other hand, after suture of a mixed nerve, such as the ulnar, the axonal confusion is great and the first signs of motor recovery may not be detectable until 3 or 4 months after motor-unit APs have been detected.

This harbinger of recovery must be treated with caution; the detection of APs is no guarantee that useful recovery may confidently be expected. As Bowden showed (M.R.C.R., 1954 p. 282), what matters is electromyographic evidence of progressive re-innervation.

The possible Employment of Electromyography by the Clinician Primarily Responsible

Although electromyography has tended to become esoteric it is possible to assemble a simple and inexpensive instrument for use in the outpatient clinic with a great saving of the surgeon's and of the patient's time. All it will do is to indicate whether motor-unit APs (and, with luck, fibrillation APs) are present in a muscle. In peripheral nerve injuries as opposed to conditions such as carpal tunnel compression, this is often all the information that is required.

So anyone sufficiently interested may with advantage take a few lessons from an expert, with a simple mobile machine, and so enable himself to obtain possibly vital information with little effort and much expedition.

MOTOR NERVE CONDUCTION

In 1948 Hodes, Larrabee and German showed how the velocity of conduction in motor nerve fibres could be measured in man.

The arrangement of the various electrodes for examination of the ulnar nerve is shown in Figure **4**, 11. The rectangles A indicate indifferent (anodal) electrodes; only one is required, but the two sites are shown because these are the ones found to be the most convenient. S1, S2 and S3 are stimulating electrodes placed over the nerve just proximal to the wrist, a few centimetres proximal to the elbow, and in the axilla, respectively. The type of concentric needle electrode used in electromyographic examination is inserted into abductor digiti minimi at R1 and into the first dorsal interosseous at R2; these are the recording electrodes.

A stimulus—a brief condenser discharge—applied to the ulnar nerve through S1, S2 or S3 will be followed by contraction of all the muscles of ulnar innervation distal to the particular electrode, and the electromyographic responses picked up by R1 or R2 can be recorded in such a way as to indicate the lapse of time between the application of the stimulus to the nerve and the contraction of muscle, revealed by an action-potential, that indicates its arrival peripherally. Because the distances between the stimulating and recording electrodes are known, the velocity of conduction in the nerve can be measured.

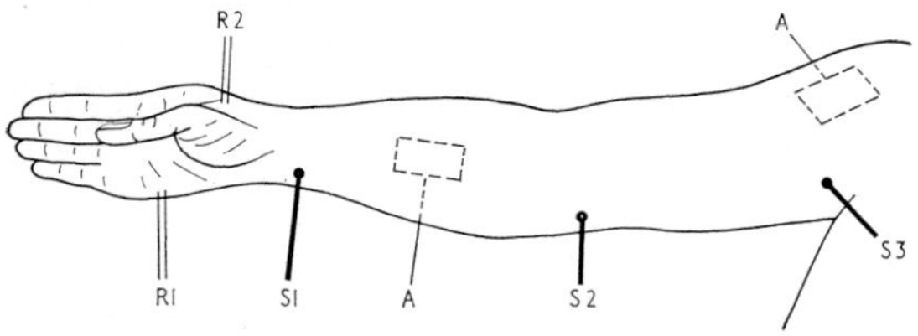

FIG. 4, 11. The arrangement of the electrodes for measuring motor conduction velocity in the ulnar nerve. (This figure and Fig 4, 12 reproduced by kind permission from Ebeling, P., Gilliatt, R. W. and Thomas, P. K., 1960, *J. Neurol. Neurosurg. Psychiat.*, **23**, 1.)

If recordings are taken at, say, R1 and the stimuli are applied at, say, S1 and then S3 the difference in the time intervals is due entirely to the time taken for the stimulus to travel along the nerve from S3 to S1. Thus it is possible to obtain values for normal motor-conduction velocity. It is normally about 55 metres a second, but allowance must be made for a reduction of up to 30 per cent *proximal* to the site of a conduction delay at the wrist (Thomas, 1960). In other words, there is an abnormality of conduction in a reach of supposedly normal nerve. Similarly if the level of stimulation is constant, say S1, and the responses at R1 and R2 are recorded simultaneously, the latency of the responses will differ because of the time taken for the stimulus to travel along the nerve between abductor minimi digiti and the first dorsal interosseous. Let us now suppose (Ebeling, Gilliatt and Thomas, 1960) that a lesion of the palmar branch of the ulnar nerve is suspected: not an injury, but some sort of compression that has not caused total paralysis. The conduction time between R1 and R2 will be increased, perhaps very greatly (Fig. **4**, 12). A simpler arrangement suffices for investigation of the median nerve at the wrist (Fig. **4**, 13). This method of investigation is invaluable not only in the early detection of

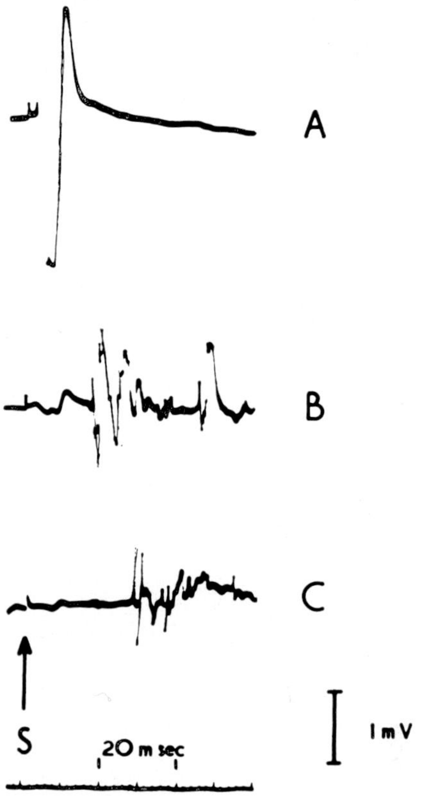

FIG. **4**, 12. Recordings from abductor minimi digiti, A, the fourth dorsal interosseous, B, and the first dorsal interosseous, C. The stimulus is indicated by S. The responses shown in B and C are delayed, thus indicating damage to the deep branch of the ulnar nerve close to its origin: the polyphasic action-potentials are also abnormal.

lesions such as compression of the median nerve in the carpal tunnel or of the deep branch of the ulnar nerve in the palm, but also, where there is doubt, for determining the level of damage.

The principles of motor nerve conduction are simple enough. The application of them is not and, unlike the three other methods of electrodiagnosis that have been described, this one is reliable only in the hands of an expert.

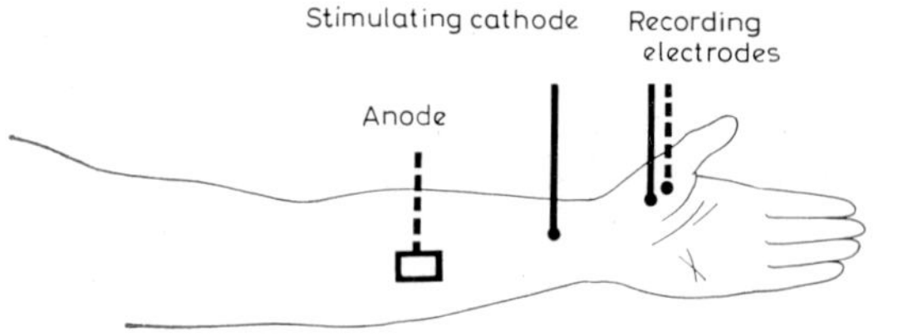

FIG. **4**, 13. The arrangement of the electrodes for measuring motor conduction in the median nerve. (Reproduced by kind permission from Gilliatt, R. W., 1962, *Br. med. J.*, **2**, 1073.)

RECORDING OF NERVE ACTION POTENTIALS

An even more sensitive method of examination—which in certain conditions, such as suspected ulnar nerve compression at the elbow, may be superior to motor nerve conduction—is the recording of nerve action-potentials (Dawson and Scott, 1949). It requires refined technique. In examining motor nerve conduction the amplitude of the evoked muscle action-potential is of the order of several millivolts, whereas nerve action-potentials are mostly in the range of 10 to 30 microvolts or less. For this reason complete muscular relaxation is required so that the recordings are not obscured by muscle action-potentials. If random artefact is troublesome a large number of responses are often recorded superimposed upon one another so that only a constant deviation from the base-line will be apparent. The response is picked up by surface electrodes and, because it is from the nerve itself, it does not matter whether the recording electrode is proximal or distal to the site of application of the stimulus. If the digital nerves in the hand are stimulated the action-potentials recorded at the wrist are purely sensory. A typical record is shown in Figure **4**, 14. If a mixed nerve is

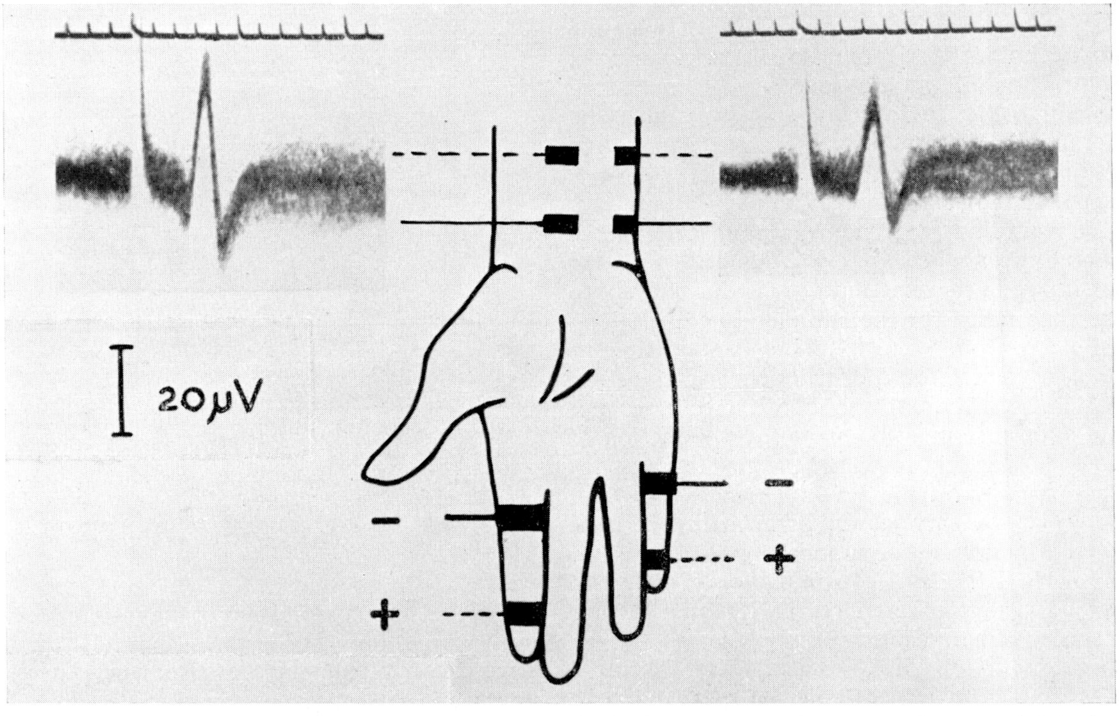

FIG. **4**, 14. In this arrangement the stimuli to the index and little fingers are electrical. The action-potentials in the median and ulnar nerves are picked up by the electrodes just proximal to the wrist. In each case 20 sweeps were superimposed. The first (left) spike in each of the recordings—both are normal—is produced by the stimulus. It is followed 2 to 3 milliseconds later by a triphasic action-potential. The time-scale is above the AP recording. (Reproduced by kind permission from Gilliatt, R. W. and Sears, T. A., 1958, *J. Neurol. Neurosurg. Psychiat.*, **21**, 109.)

TABLE III

QUESTIONS TO BE ANSWERED	SD CURVE	NERVE STIMULATION	EMG	MOTOR CONDUCTION	NERVE ACTION-POTENTIAL RECORDING
Is the paralysis due to a degenerative nerve lesion?	Examination usually conclusive after the 17th day	Invaluable in accessible nerves; reliable after the 4th day	Not very useful because fibrillation may not be detected	Not required	Not required
Is a brachial plexus injury proximal or distal to the posterior root ganglia?	Valueless	Valueless	Valueless	Valueless	Conduction present if lesion is proximal to the ganglia (see pp.191-192)
Is recovery (after, say, a supposed axonotmesis) impending?	Curve shows a kink	Not required and of doubtful value anyway	Motor APs present	Not required	Possibly a promising aid
Is recovery progressing satisfactorily?	Curve shifts down and to the left: kink flattens out	Valueless	Increasing APs, and spreading to the more distal muscles	Not required	Possibly a promising aid
Is an early compression lesion present: e.g. of the ulnar nerve at the elbow or in the palm, or of the median nerve in the carpal tunnel?	Valueless	Valueless	Valueless	Conduction rate retarded	Conduction rate retarded and amplitude of action-potentials reduced
If the site of the lesion is uncertain can it be localized?	Valueless	Valueless	Valueless	Conduction rates retarded at and distal to the lesion	Conduction rates retarded at and distal to the lesion

examined, such as with stimulation of the ulnar nerve at the wrist and recording at the elbow, the nerve action-potentials will be derived not only from sensory fibres but from antidromic impulses in motor fibres.

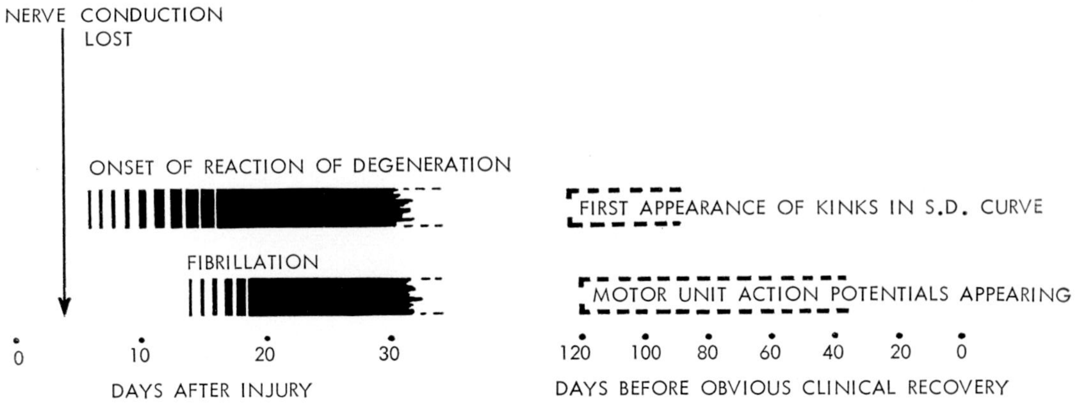

FIG. **4**, 15. The course of events after an ordinary nerve injury, showing how and when the various types of electrodiagnosis are applicable.

The important facts that have come to light from the application of these techniques are as follows:

In the course of Wallerian degeneration the conduction velocity (CV) changes little until it ceases completely on the third or fourth day (Gilliatt and Hjorth, 1972). Neuromuscular transmission fails rather earlier.

When a nerve is regenerating the CV is at first as low as 1 m/sec though it speeds up in the course of 12 to 18 months to about 75 per cent of normal in rabbits (Cragg and Thomas, 1964); but more slowly and incompletely in man, 50 to 60 per cent after 3 to 4 years. The threshold of regenerating fibres is at first so high that percutaneous stimulation is intolerable. This may sometimes be circumvented by stimulating the nerve proximal to the site of injury. The muscle APs evoked may have a latency of more than 10 times the normal.

In pressure and entrapment neuropathies (Chap. 7) the CV is reduced, and the localization of the lesion may indeed depend on CV studies.

Nerve action-potential recording can be valuable in investigating traction injuries of the brachial plexus, to determine whether the nerve roots have been damaged proximal or distal to the posterior root ganglia. If the damage is proximal there is no prospect of recovery (p. 186), because the nerve roots have almost certainly been torn out of the spinal cord. The recognition of the level of damage is necessary in order to establish the prognosis and plan the patient's treatment accordingly. If a nerve root is torn proximal to the posterior root ganglion the sensory fibres originating from its cells will not degenerate peripherally. There are several ways of demonstrating this (p. 191); the most recent and direct is by showing that these fibres are conducting although, maybe, the limb is totally paralysed and insensitive.

THE PRACTICAL APPLICATION OF ELECTRODIAGNOSIS

There are sins of omission and commission. Unless the clinician is aware of the potentialities of electrical methods of examination, both he and the patient may remain for a time, perhaps considerable, in a state of unnecessary uncertainty. Some of the questions that can arise are set out in Table III and it will be evident that the five available keys will unlock only certain doors. Ignorance of this accounts for an immense amount of wasted time and effort.

Of the five methods, determination of the strength-duration curve, direct nerve stimulation and simple electromyography are within the compass of any clinician with the inclination and time to employ them. Nerve conduction tests are best left to those with an occupational interest in them.

The course of events to be studied in an ordinary case of nerve injury is shown diagrammatically in Figure **4**, 15.

5. Common Causes of Nerve Injury: Open Wounds, Traction, Skeletal Damage

THE THREE CHIEF causes of nerve injury are open wounds, traction, and fractures and dislocations. Neurovascular injuries, though less common, have such remarkable features that they will be considered separately in Chapter 6.

There are also lesions mechanical in origin, not usually regarded as injuries and almost all slow in onset—the various entrapment neuropathies as exemplified by the ulnar at the elbow and compression of the median nerve in the carpal tunnel—which are described in Chapter 7. And in Chapter 8 we shall consider a miscellaneous collection of injuries that do not fit comfortably into the earlier chapters.

OPEN WOUNDS

Some sort of wound is by far the commonest cause of nerve injury though except in warfare this does not apply to certain nerves, notably the sciatic and the radial. Three types of wound have to be considered: incised, lacerated and those due to missiles, because there are differences in the resultant nerve damage.

In Table IV and Figure **5**, 1, the damage suffered by the median and ulnar nerves is shown in relation to the type of wound. The radial nerve and the sciatic and its terminal divisions are omitted because these nerves are so infrequently injured as a result of incised or lacerated wounds as to preclude any useful comparison. The state of each nerve was that revealed by operation: either obvious division, or partial division, or damage that could not be detected by the naked eye, that is, an injury in continuity which, if the subsequent spontaneous recovery was almost complete, was presumed to be predominantly an axonotmesis.

In each of the three groups a number of nerves were, for a variety of reasons, not explored. In the case of missile injuries, for example, the clinical evidence pointed to a neurapraxia or, at the other extreme, the damage was so extensive that no form of repair could be contemplated. But the proportion of unexplored nerves was not of an order that would invalidate the comparisons about to be made.

INCISED WOUNDS

There were 385 incised wounds of which 307 were caused by glass (79·7 per cent); but they were no different in their effects from the remainder. Table IV and Figure **5**, 1 show that in over 90 per cent of cases the nerve suffered complete or partial division. Thus, when a sharp object inflicts an incised wound that involves a nerve the likelihood that repair will be required

TABLE IV—Damage suffered by the median and ulnar nerves in relation to the type of open wound

TYPE OF WOUND	STATE OF NERVES						TOTALS
	Division		Partial division		No detectable division		
	Number	Per cent	Number	Per cent	Number	Per cent	
Incised	322	83·6	41	10·6	22	5·8	385
Lacerated	46	74·2	8	12·9	8	12·9	62
Missile	196	51·8	69	18·2	114	30·0	379

is so great (Fig. **5**, 2) that exploration of the nerve is usually necessary. The only exceptions to this are: (1) when there is *clinical* evidence of partial division, a condition in which good spontaneous recovery occurs fairly often (p. 263); (2) if the time at which the nerve injury first attracts attention is such that signs of recovery could appear within the succeeding 4 to 6 weeks, it being then justifiable to wait for that length of time; or (3) if there is already evidence of spontaneous recovery. There were 35 cases in which, for one of these reasons, exploration was withheld.

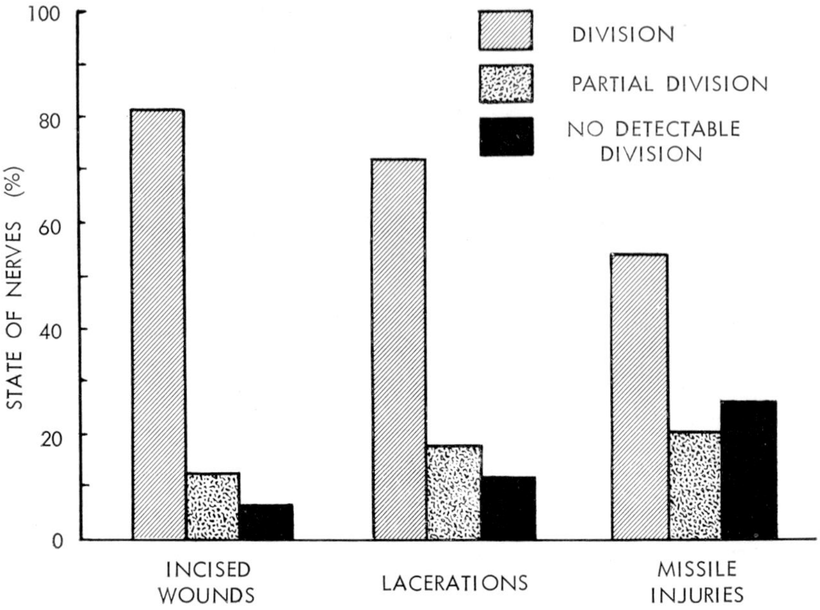

FIG. **5**, 1. The types of nerve damage encountered in the three kinds of open wounds.

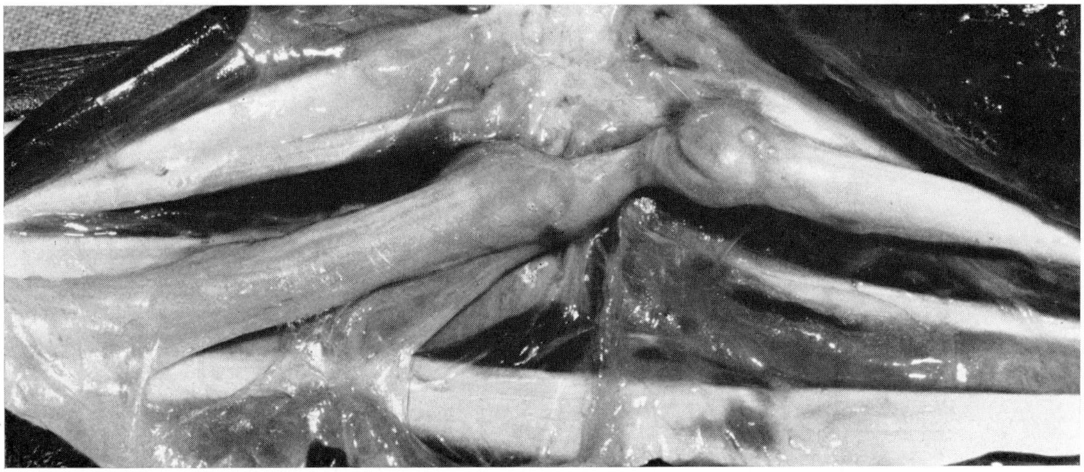

FIG. **5**, 2. A butcher nicked his forearm with a knife, causing a transverse wound 12 cm proximal to the wrist, 1·5 cm in extent. He cut the median nerve and three tendons. The proximal neuroma and the distal 'glioma' are about the same size. Interval between injury and operation 46 days.

The prime characteristic of a nerve injury

caused by some sharp object, which incises the tissues, is complete or incomplete division of the nerve. If exploration reveals no sign of either (the 22 cases of injury in continuity in Table IV) it is probable that the nerve was partially incised and that by the time the exploration was performed spontaneous reunion was well advanced. That this can happen is proved by the case reported on page 252. It is hard to conceive of axonotmesis or neurapraxia being produced by anything sharp; these injuries result either from a blunt blow, traction, or a near miss by a missile.

It is only in incised wounds of nerves, and not in all of them, that primary suture is permissible (p. 275).

LACERATED WOUNDS

Lacerated wounds involving nerves are less common. Anything can happen; a substantial segment of nerve may be torn away, or there may be a simple transection, complete or partial. If by chance the nerve is at the periphery of the laceration it may suffer axonotmesis or neurapraxia. However, the incidence of complete or partial division is so high (nearly 90 per cent) that, as with incised wounds, exploration is almost always called for as soon as sound healing of the laceration has occurred.

The laceration produced by a fracture has nothing to do with any injury that a nerve may have suffered. The broken bone is responsible and, as will be shown on page 79, a different plan of campaign is necessary.

MISSILE WOUNDS

Missiles produce the characteristic war injuries of nerves, though they are fairly common in civil practice. In warfare the missile may be anything from a small flake of metal to a mass several centimetres across; in civil practice pellets from a shotgun, flying glass or, particularly in industry, irregular metallic fragments.

The distinguishing feature of missile injuries is the pressure disturbance in the tissues caused by the passage through them of a mass travelling at high speed. The size of the missile and whether or not it is spinning are less important. There is no need to consider the ballistic details; what matters chiefly has been shown by experiments in which a bullet strikes a block of gelatin that has much the same physical characteristics as animal soft tissues. A mushroom of gelatin is blown out in the wake of the missile, a capacious tunnel opens in its pathway and a cone of gel is pushed out ahead of it (Fig. **5**, 3). The instantaneous photographs taken by Black, Burns and

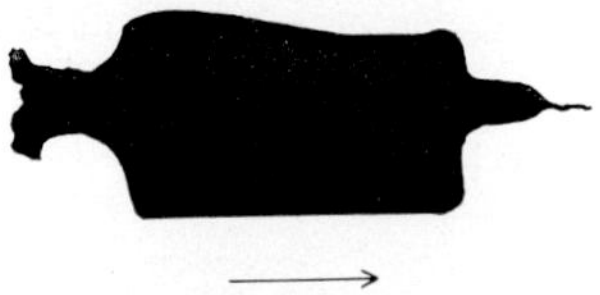

FIG. **5**, 3. Silhouette of a block of gelatin 207 microseconds after it had been pierced by a bullet in the direction shown. (Figs **5**, 3 and **5**, 4 reproduced by kind permission from Black, A. N., Burns, B. D. and Zuckerman, S., 1941, *Br. med. J.*, **2**, 872.)

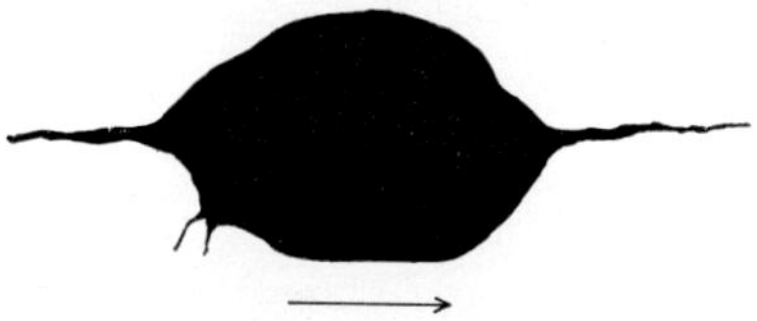

FIG. **5**, 4. The same at 840 microseconds. The distortion of the block must be due to the formation of a large cavity in the wake of the bullet.

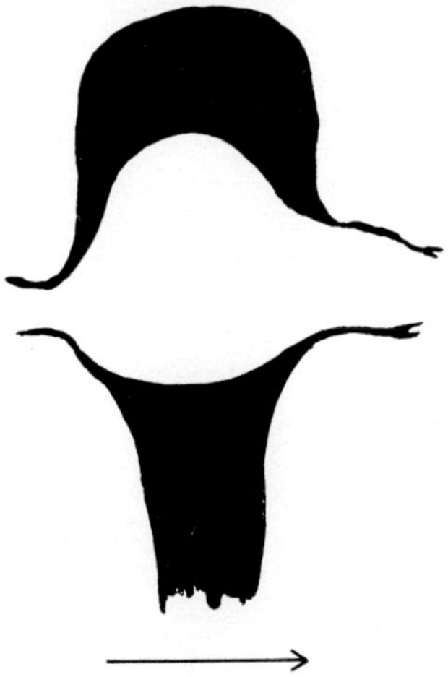

FIG. **5**, 5. Silhouette tracing from an X-ray taken just as a bullet had traversed a bag made from the skin of a cat's leg and filled with water. There is a large cavity. (Harvey, Butler, McMillen and Puckett.)

Zuckerman (1941) show this very well, and from Figure **5**, 4 it is evident that the great distortion of the gelatin block must be caused by cavitation. The cavity itself (Fig. **5**, 5) has been demonstrated by X-ray exposures of extremely short duration (Harvey, Butler, McMillen and Puckett, 1945).

The effect of the pressure wave specifically on nerve was investigated most elegantly by Puckett, Grundfest, McElroy and McMillen (1946). The sciatic nerve of a cat was rendered opaque to X-rays by injection of a contrast medium and the pressure cavity was photographed *axially* (Fig. **5**, 6). The resultant damage to the sciatic nerve varied considerably. It was impossible to ensure that the track of the missile was always at the same distance from the sciatic nerve; and, anyway, the nerves themselves were probably not all alike. In some cases there was no detectable disturbance of conduction. And here it is relevant to refer to a clinical record.

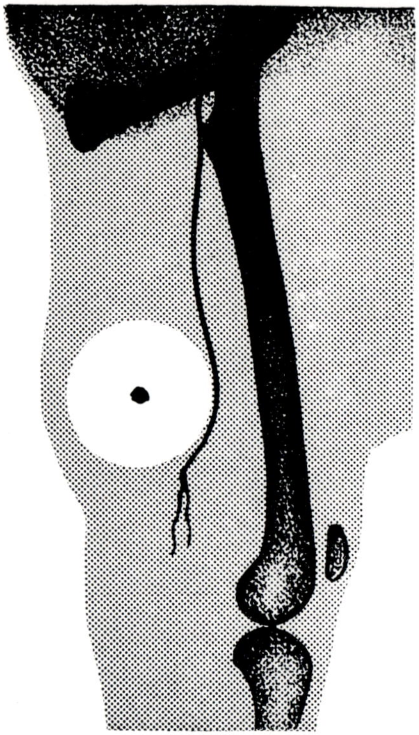

FIG. **5**, 6. Microsecond radiograph taken 200 microseconds after the cat's thigh was struck with a 3-mm pellet travelling at about 1,000 m/sec. The large cavity displaces the sciatic nerve: the black dot in the centre of it is the result of the missile making a hole in the X-ray film (Reproduced by kind permission from Puckett, W. O., Grundfest, H., McElroy, W. D., and McMillen, J. H., 1946, *J. Neurosurg.*, **3**, 294.)

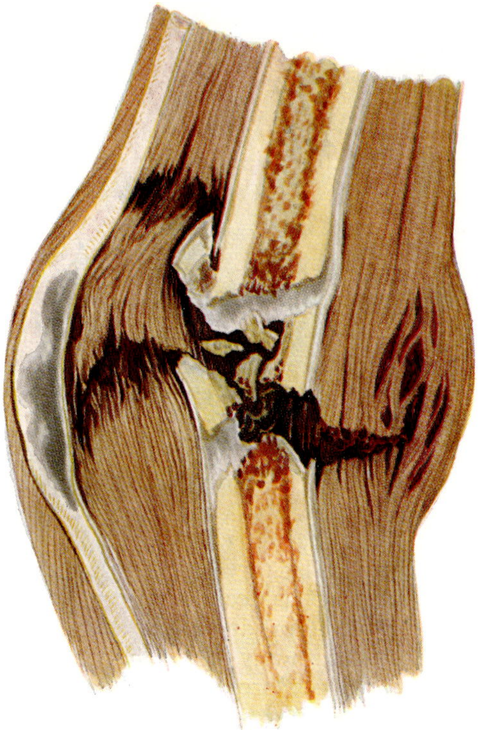

FIG. **5**, 7. How a nerve situated near the track of a missile is injured in continuity.

A man suffered a bullet wound that smashed the medial epicondyle of the humerus. There was paralysis of the median nerve but, oddly enough, ulnar function appeared to be normal. It was decided to remove the fragment; it was found to be rotated through 180 degrees so that its cortical surface was against the humerus, and the ulnar nerve lay on the anterior surface of the fragment. This nerve had no epineurium on one surface, the bundles were loose and separate and three of them had been severed. After the operation there was slight impairment of function for a time, but ultimately the only abnormality was slight diminution of two-point discrimination.

It is astonishing what disturbance a nerve can suffer without any serious consequences. But in a minority of the animals examined by Puckett and his colleagues the nerve showed obvious breaks in the funiculi, much kinking, separation and fragmentation of the fibres.

After a missile wound the elastic soft tissues spring back—though a bone may be shattered—leaving no more than a blood-filled track (Figs. **5**, 7 and **5**, 8), its diameter depending on how much tissue has been torn or blown away by the missile. But the shock wave has caused more or less disturbance of function and structure in the nerve, ranging from fleeting paralysis (many combatants remarked that the injured limb 'went completely dead' for a few minutes) to neurapraxia and axonotmesis and to internal disruption sufficient to cause moderate or severe intraneural fibrosis; all this short of actual severance of the nerve (Fig. **5**, 9). The longitudinal extent of the fibrosis is a reflection of the distortion that the nerve has suffered and in this there is probably an element akin to traction. If the nerve has been partially severed (Fig. **5**, 10) the paralysis is nevertheless likely to be complete because the part remaining in continuity has suffered severe interstitial damage. Complete resection and suture will be necessary. Similarly, if the nerve has been completely transected there is fairly extensive perturbation of both

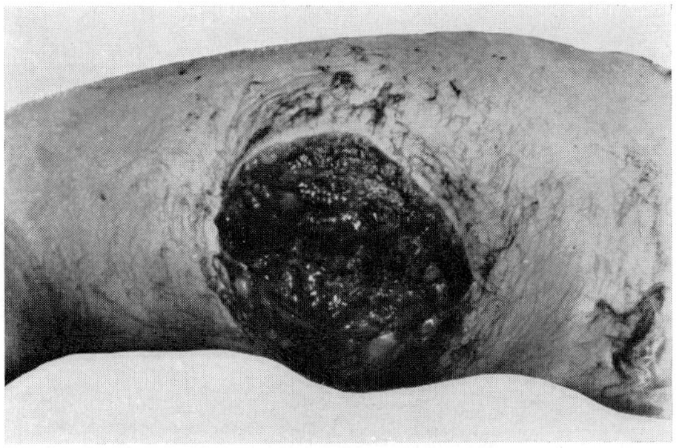

FIG. **5**, 8. A missile wound of the back of the thigh that shattered the femur and damaged but did not transect the sciatic nerve. Secondary suture of the wound was performed 24 days after the injury. The femur united well and the nerve recovered spontaneously.

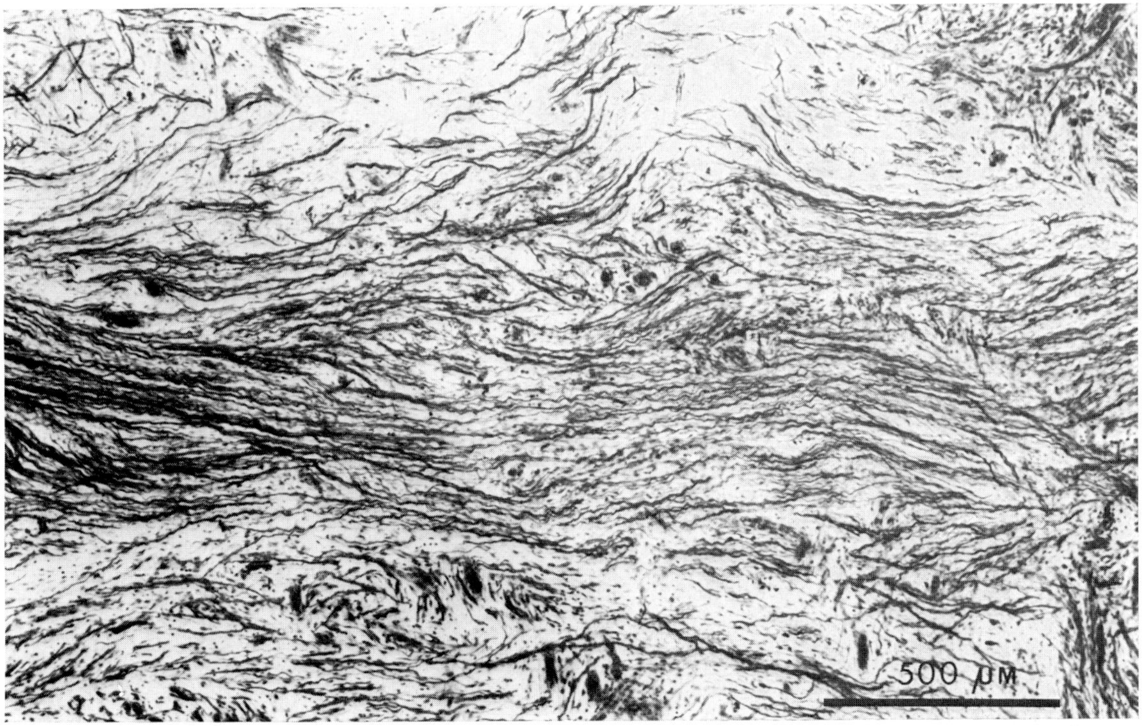

FIG. **5**, 9. Longitudinal section of the swelling on the ulnar nerve shown in Fig. **16**, 11, p. 249, stained to show nerve fibres. Regeneration of the latter is proceeding in spite of the gross disorientation caused by the near-miss of a high-velocity missile. But there is much intraneural fibrosis.

stumps. After a few weeks its extent is revealed by intraneural fibrosis and this is why secondary repair is obligatory; the proper level of resection of the stumps cannot be determined until the extent of the intraneural changes has become detectable by the naked eye.

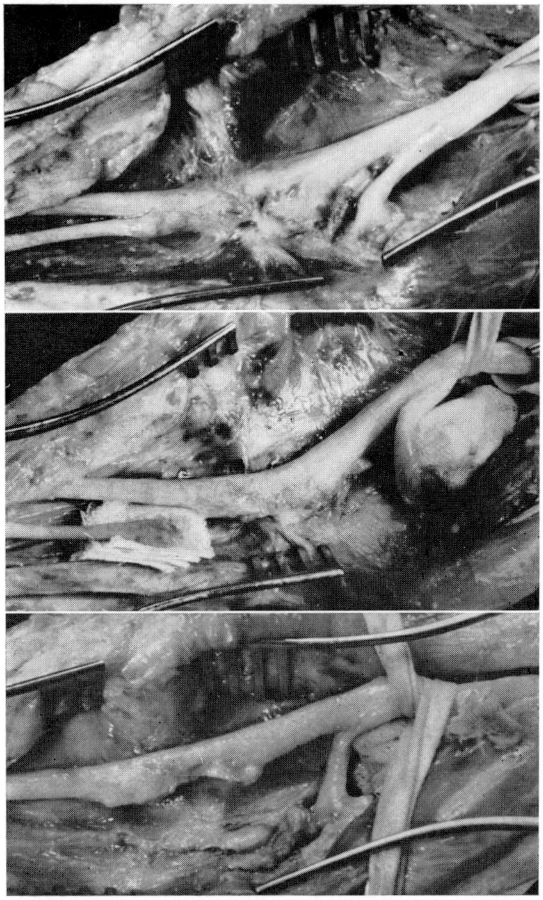

A

B

C

FIG. **5**, 10. A missile traversed the popliteal fossa transversely causing complete sciatic paralysis. At operation 8 months later the track is revealed by the scar tissue. The common peroneal nerve had been divided, (A), and after further dissection (B and C), partial division of the tibial nerve was found. But the internal disruption of the part remaining in continuity was so great that complete resection and suture were necessary. This is usual.

The pellets from a shotgun, provided it has not been fired at point-blank range, or larger missiles no longer travelling fast are much less harmful than the high-velocity projectile that causes a through-and-through wound.

It will be appreciated that for the reasons just given missile injuries are less likely than incised or lacerated wounds to sever a nerve, as is apparent from Table IV and Figure **5**, 1. Yet the frequency of complete or partial severance is high enough (70 per cent) to make exploration necessary. And indeed, as will be discussed in the chapter on operative treatment (p. 265), resection and suture are sometimes required even if the nerve shows no sign of division.

TRACTION INJURIES

If a nerve, or any other filamentous structure of limited extensibility, is violently stretched the severity and longitudinal extent of the internal damage is determined by the ultimate tensile strength of the material. A peripheral nerve has great tensile strength and, in man, very limited elasticity; so when it is stretched the intraneural damage may be most extensive. In a case of violent adduction of the knee I have found the common peroneal nerve damaged over a length of 30 cm. Traction lesions, therefore, present a very serious problem, not only because of the severity of the changes produced but because it is rarely possible to bridge the gap if the damaged segment of the nerve is excised.

It has already been pointed out (p. 4) that except in the nerve roots the toughest constituents of a nerve are the supporting structures. But there is no agreement about the order in which the various tissues give way. Denny-Brown and Doherty (1945) found experimentally that the first of them to break was the perineurium: the nerve fibres, lying slack within their collagenous envelopes, bulged out and formed a swelling. Liu, Benda and Lewey (1948) found that the nerve fibres broke before the perineurium; and Sunderland and Bradley (1961*a*), while allowing that the perineurium protects the nerve fibres, which are slack within it, against moderate stretching, described nerve fibres rupturing within funiculi before the funiculi themselves came asunder. According to Haftek (1970) these views are based on too limited examination of the specimens. He found (in rabbits) that the epineurium snapped first, often audibly. When this, the strongest structure, had yielded, the nerve fibres, being the weakest, could break anywhere at points remote from the site of epineural rupture; and within the perineurium which, being stronger, remained intact.

All observers are agreed that the vasa nervorum are damaged too and that this contributes to the changes suffered by the nerve fibres. Highet and Holmes (1943) found vessels in which there were gross abnormalities (Figs **5**, 11 to 13); Denny-Brown and Doherty (1945) noticed petechial haemorrhages; and recently Nobel (1966) found surprisingly large effusions that could produce a sub-epineurial haematoma 15 cm long in the human common peroneal nerve (Fig. **5**, 14).

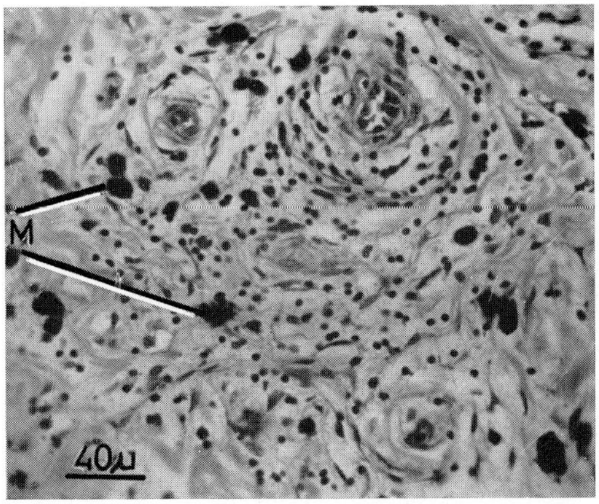

FIG. **5**, 11. Lymphocytes and macrophages (M), the latter stained with prussian blue to show that they contain iron pigment, surrounding the small blood vessels in the neuroma shown in Figure **5**, 16. (Figs **5**, 11 to **5**, 13, **5**, 16 to **5**, 19, **5**, 21 and **5**, 22 reproduced by kind permission from Highet, W. B. and Holmes, W., 1943, *Br. J. Surg.*, **30**, 212.

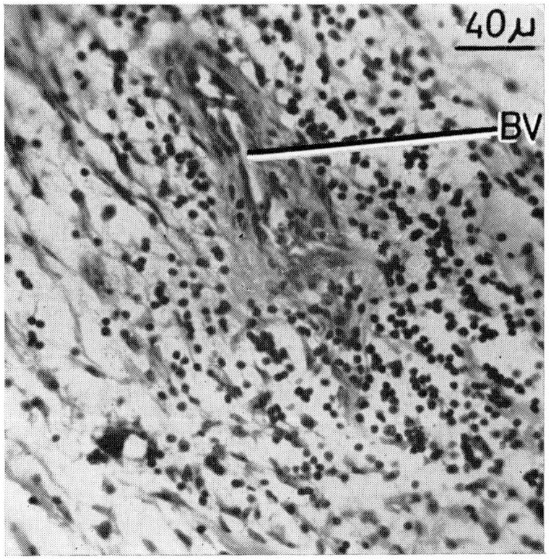

FIG. **5**, 12. Lymphocytes round an abnormal blood vessel (BV) in the same neuroma.

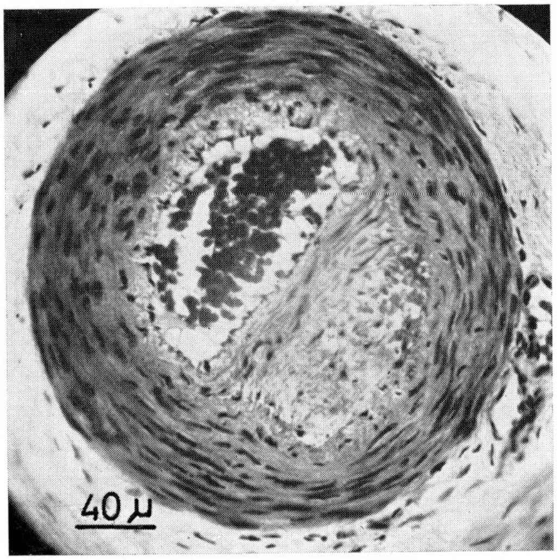

FIG. **5**, 13. Intimal proliferation in an arteriole in a traction neuroma.

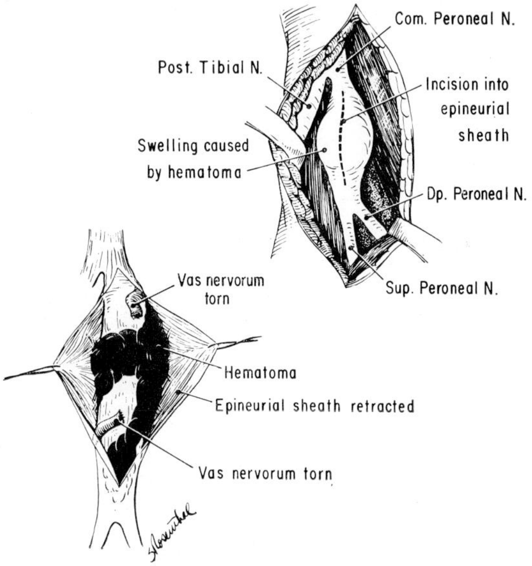

FIG. **5**, 14. Subepineural haematoma of the common peroneal nerve described by Nobel. (Reproduced by kind permission from *J. Bone Jt Surg.*, 1966, **48A**, 1484.)

The ischaemic changes in the nerve fibres, after moderate stretching, are segmental demyelination and beading of the axons; and there is more or less interstitial fibrosis. However, recovery is rapid, there being little or no axonal degeneration.

Mild distraction produces a lesion clinically indistinguishable from neurapraxia due to compression. The fibres are affected in order of their size; motor paralysis is complete, sensory disturbance minimal, and recovery occurs rapidly and completely.

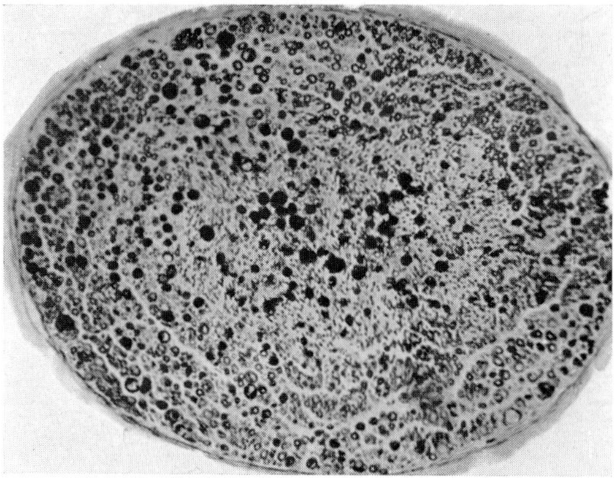

FIG. **5**, 15. Rabbit's sciatic nerve 50 days after a traction injury: almost all of the large, mainly motor fibres—shown as black dots (Weigert stain)—are degenerate. This selectivity of the damage was proved by examining the branches of the nerve; only the motor ones were degenerate. (Reproduced by kind permission from *Br. surg. Pract.* (*surg. Prog.*), 1948, **2**, 315.)

There may be more severe selective damage of the larger nerve fibres, causing Wallerian degeneration (Seddon, 1948; Fig. **5**, 15). This seems to explain a small group of cases in which there is extensive motor paralysis and little or no disturbance of sensibility. Recovery is slow but ultimately near normal.

Still greater violence causes such profound intraneural damage that the nerve is as completely disorganized as if it had been transected (Figs **5**, 16 and **5**, 17) and no recovery is possible. Finally the nerve may rupture (Fig. **5**, 18) and in addition to the solution of continuity

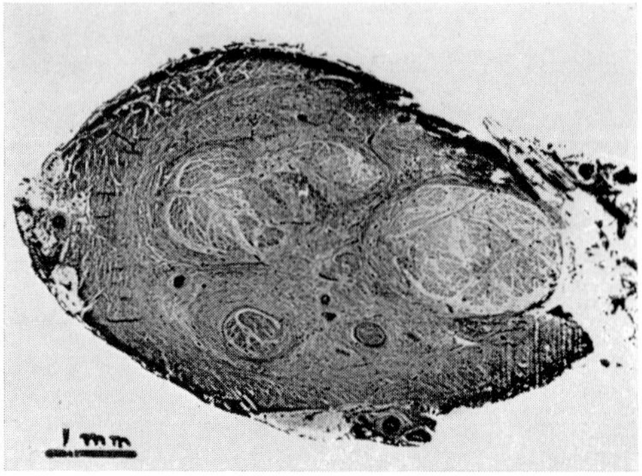

FIG. **5**, 17. Transverse section of the distal end of this fusiform neuroma. Five funiculi are visible, but there is gross scarring around them which replaces the other funiculi that should be present.

there are profound changes in both stumps of great longitudinal extent (Fig. **5**, 19). The force required to bring this about is enormous; it depends, of course, on the calibre of the nerve and, because the tensile strength of a nerve is largely determined by its connective tissue elements, on the abundance of the latter in relation to the nerve bundles. Detailed studies of human nerve have been made by Sunderland and Bradley (1961*a*) and the figures in Table V are taken from their paper. In the first column are given the range of loads, in kilograms, required to rupture each of the four main nerve trunks; in the second the range of loads per square millimetre of cross-sectional area. In both, the

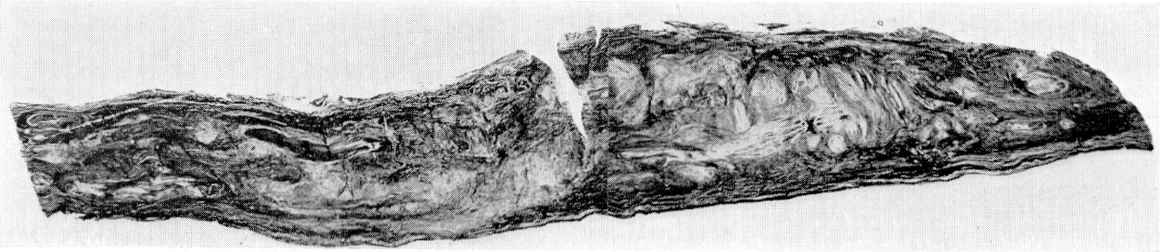

FIG. **5**, 16. A traction neuroma. Although the specimen—from the common peroneal nerve—was 7 cm long there are few nerve bundles at each end and the cross-sections showed a good deal of scar. Two-thirds of the length is nothing but irregular scar tissue.

scatter is very wide. However, it is doubtful whether anything like this order of violence is required to cause the commonest of all traction injuries, that of the brachial plexus. In nerve roots the supporting tissue has little tensile strength and it is the nerve fibres that take the strain. This is shown in Figure **5**, 20; and in Figure **11**, 20

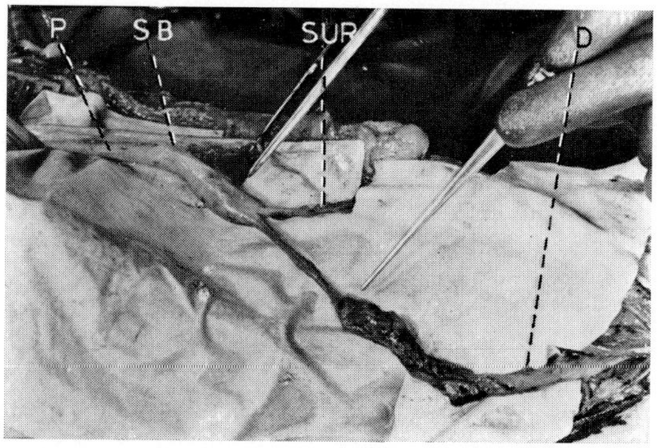

FIG. **5**, 18. Rupture of the common peroneal nerve due to an adduction injury of the knee. SB, sciatic bifurcation; P, proximal level of resection; SUR, lateral sural nerve; D, distal level of resection. The gap after resection was 15 cm. But after appropriate mobilization and pronounced flexion of the knee to 130 degrees (almost full flexion) the ends were brought together without difficulty. What happened subsequently will be shown in Figures **5**, 21 and **5**, 22.

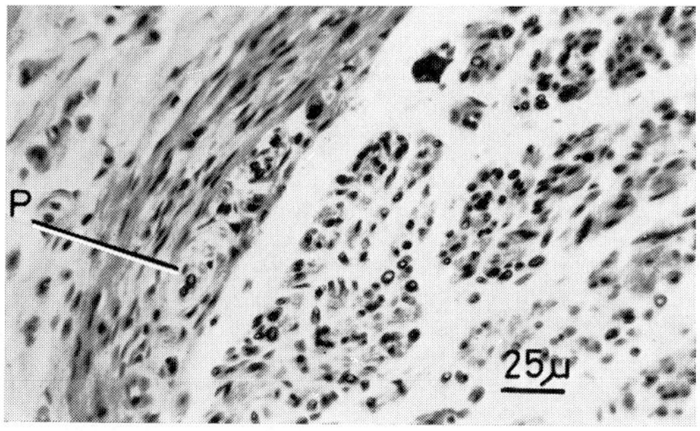

FIG. **5**, 19. Transverse section of a common peroneal nerve 9 cm above the point of greatest damage; 6 months after the injury. The nerve fibres are all small, indicating that there had been extensive retrograde degeneration. At the point **P** there are a few fibres within the perineurium, a certain indication that the latter had been ruptured.

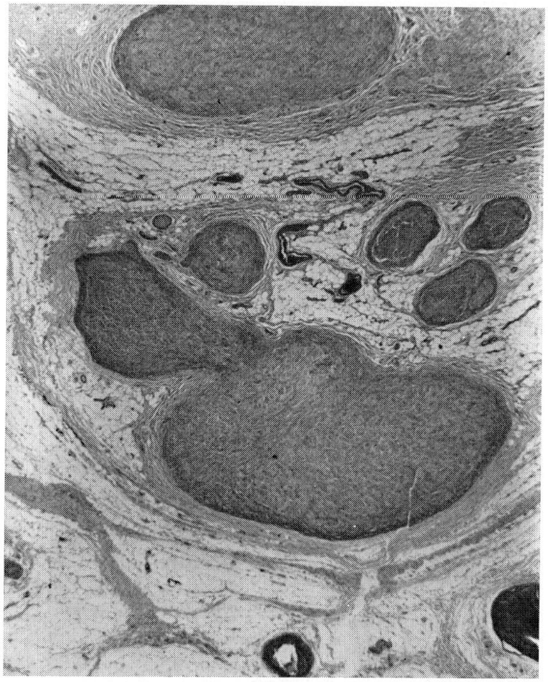

FIG. **5**, 20. Transverse section of part of the brachial plexus about 6 cm distal to the point of greatest damage. Every funiculus exhibits extreme endoneurial collagenization, though at this magnification (×25) it is not clearly distinguishable. What is even more striking, which is why this magnification was chosen, is the paucity of perineural changes. There is fairly dense collagenization around the uppermost funiculus, but hardly any around those in the centre of the field. This shows that in the brachial plexus it is the contents of the funiculi that break up first.

TABLE V—Loads required to rupture major nerves

	Load required to cause rupture (kg)	kg/mm^2
Median	7·3 to 22·3	1·0 to 3·1
Ulnar	6·5 to 15·5	1·0 to 2·2
Tibial	20·6 to 33·6	0·5 to 1·8
Common peroneal	11·8 to 21·4	0·8 to 1·9

(p. 188) it will be seen how the posterior root ganglia may be torn away from their connections with the spinal cord, remaining in continuity with the distal part of the plexus.

Our experience of the more severe traction injuries, the subject of papers by Highet and Holmes (1943), Bonney (1959) and Yeoman (1963) has been depressing. If recovery does not occur spontaneously the extent of the damage is usually such as to preclude suture; autologous grafting is rarely feasible (but see the case-history on this page) owing to the great difficulty or impossibility of finding enough material to bridge the gap. White (1968) has had some success with the common peroneal nerve; he has sutured two, with a good result in one patient and an excellent result in the other, whom I have seen. It may be that a nerve sometimes snaps with little interstitial damage in either stump (string and rope can be ruptured in this way); so perhaps one should approach these particular injuries less pessimistically.

THE MECHANICS OF TRACTION INJURIES

Some Structure Other than Nerve Must Give Way First

With the possible exception of the brachial plexus (and here rupture of the scalene muscles or avulsion fracture of the cervical transverse processes is often seen) no nerve can be damaged by traction unless some other structure is torn, broken, or dislocated. Nerves are normally well protected against this sort of injury.

The most familiar type of skeletal injury is the dislocated joint, such as the shoulder or hip, the nerve being stretched over the head of the humerus or femur. Less common, but well-recognized, is the tearing of important ligaments such as those that stabilize the knee; if they rupture, the common peroneal nerve may be stretched. What is insufficiently appreciated is that a traction injury may follow an ordinary fracture of a long bone.

This curious and often puzzling type of traction injury can occur when a limb has been broken and dragged on.

The first patient in whom I recognized this condition was a fighter pilot who was obliged to bale out of his aircraft. It was a windy day and as he landed his parachute dragged him violently along the ground; his arm was broken and, he discovered, totally paralysed. He came under my care four months after the injury and there was almost complete paralysis of the arm apart from the deltoid, pectoralis major and muscles proximal to them. It had been thought that he had a traction injury of the brachial plexus, but the neurological picture was explicable only in terms of injuries—presumably due to traction—of individual nerves at a level slightly higher than the fracture. I explored his arm and found that he had mild traction injuries of the musculocutaneous and ulnar nerves, and total disruption by traction of the median and of the radial nerves. This airman was fortunate in that the ulnar and musculocutaneous nerves recovered well, and the median moderately well after a gap of 14·3 cm had been repaired with a graft taken from the radial nerve distal to the site of injury (Fig. **16**, 12, p. 295).

I have since seen 13 similar cases. In four of them there were fractures of the humerus— the upper end, the shaft, or the lower end—with either supra- or infraclavicular traction injuries of the brachial plexus. In 1968 my colleague, J. N. Wilson, found paralysis of the musculocutaneous nerve and of the outer head of the median in a patient with a fracture of the upper third of the radius and dislocation of its head. This suggests that only moderate distraction (here the elbow may have been adducted) is required to produce these bizarre traction injuries remote from the site of skeletal damage.

Similar injuries can occur, though more rarely, in the lower limb, and Nobel (1966) has drawn attention to what may be traction injuries of the common peroneal nerve that can occur as a result of fractures of both bones of the leg, or even inversion sprains of the ankle. In the two cases that he described he operated early, on account of the pain the patients suffered rather than because of curiosity about the paralysis. In both he discovered an effusion of blood into the common peroneal nerve near its origin from the sciatic.

Missile Injuries

It has already been explained that a high-velocity missile blows out a sizable tunnel in its passage through soft tissues. Anything in the wall of this tunnel (except bone which may be shattered) is violently stretched. Thus a nerve that has escaped severance is subjected to a traction injury and this explains why the damage is fairly extensive, though less than when a nerve suffers longitudinal stress.

Stretching of a Nerve after Resection and Suture

By flexing a joint acutely it is possible to bring together the ends of a widely resected nerve without tension. Although the elasticity of human nerve can range from 6 to 22 per cent it has been found that its fibres may break, and at different levels, if stretched beyond 10 per cent of their length. That a normal nerve, given the opportunity, will shorten is certain; it happens in patients, adults as well as children, who develop contractures of the knee. That a nerve can grow longer—in a child or adolescent, longer than it would do naturally—is doubtful and, anyway, irrelevant because even the most long-suffering patient can hardly be expected to wait for this to happen after a nerve repair that has shortened a nerve appreciably. The flexed joint is straightened out within an arbitrary period of weeks. If the gap, in an adult, is of the order of more than 6 to 11 cm—depending on the nerve (p. 275)—gradual, unremitting post-operative stretching is likely to inflict a traction injury on the nerve which may be as devastating as any resulting from accidental injury. Bunnell (1964, p. 389) ascribed this to ischaemia: the vessels in the stretched nerve close down. For this reason he advocated intermittent stretching and this has influenced our technique of post-operative stretching (p. 275).

There is no doubt that fearful damage can result from continuous stretching (Figs. **5**, 21 and **5**, 22).

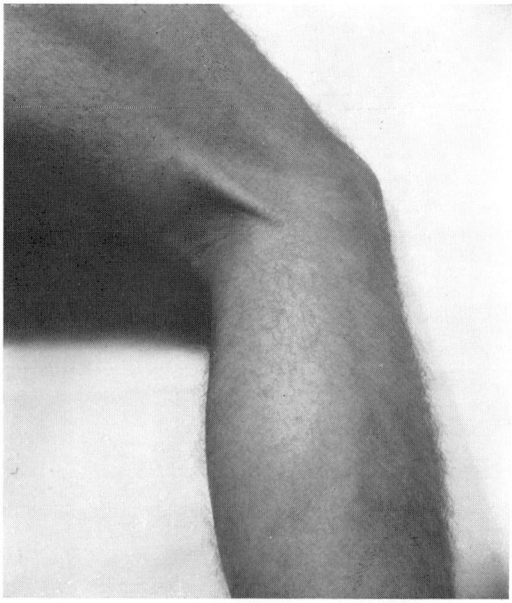

FIG **5**, 21. The common peroneal nerve shown in Figure **5**, 18 120 days after resection and suture. It is taut and stands out as if it were the tendon of the biceps.

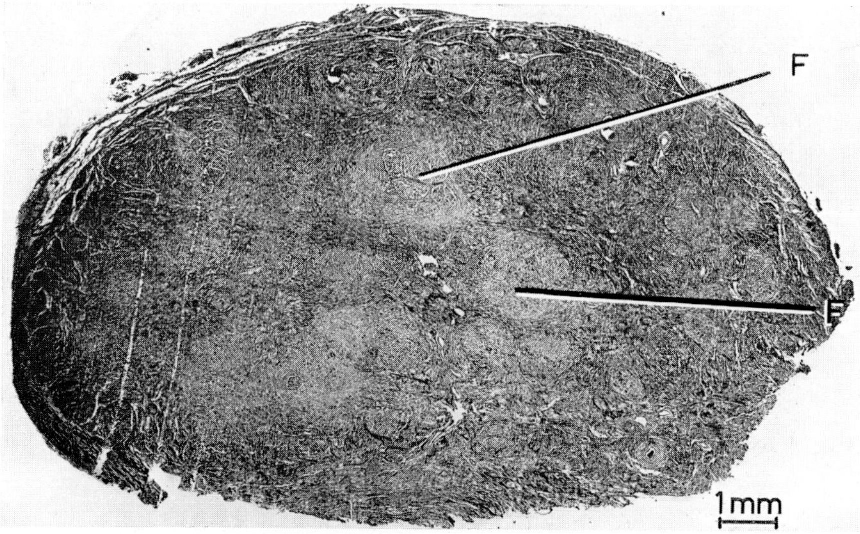

FIG. **5**, 22. The nerve was re-explored 245 days after suture. It is heavily collagenized, though funiculi are just distinguishable at F.

And now that autologous grafting is reliably established the surgical heroics of closing large gaps by end-to-end suture are no longer justifiable.

Accidental Stretching of Nerves during the Course of Operations

This is most likely to occur in exposure of the shaft of the humerus when the radial nerve is more or less tethered to it by scar tissue. A spike retractor forced between the bone and the soft parts does the damage.

Correction of Contractures, usually of the Knee

The hazard is much the same whatever technique is used unless it includes some shortening of the femur. The avoidance of traction injuries of the sciatic nerve—and in correcting severe flexion deformities of the hip, the femoral nerve—calls for considerable vigilance. It is the same after an operation for leg-lengthening.

THE COMMON FORMS OF TRACTION INJURY

Traction injuries of the *brachial plexus* head the list, with birth paralysis not inconspicuous in countries where obstetrics still lacks refinement. Dislocations of the shoulder may injure the *axillary nerve* (p. 81). Fractures of the shaft of the humerus or of both bones of the forearm, followed by violent dragging on the limb, may inflict a traction injury on *any nerve in the upper limb* below the level of the clavicle (p. 76).

In the lower limb posterior dislocation of the hip, with or without fracture of the acetabular rim, may stretch the *sciatic nerve*. It has also been seen after fracture of the shaft of the femur with extension of the knee and full flexion of the hip (p. 132). The *common peroneal nerve* is very vulnerable if the knee has suffered an adduction injury (p. 227). Dislocation of the knee may stretch both divisions of the *sciatic nerve*. An injury of this severity is liable to damage the popliteal artery as well, and then the picture may be complicated by concomitant ischaemic paralysis below the knee (p. 107). Fractures of the tibia and fibula and even inversion sprains of the ankle may disturb the *common peroneal nerve* near its origin (p. 76).

Detailed consideration of these injuries will be found in Chapters 11 and 12.

NERVE INJURIES CAUSED BY FRACTURES AND DISLOCATIONS

This topic has been the subject of more papers than it deserves. There is a recurrent theme: should the nerve or nerves be explored routinely, along with internal fixation of the fracture, or should exploration be limited to those cases in which spontaneous recovery has not occurred within the expected time?

The interventionists are of three kinds: those with limited experience who do not know what happens in the broad generality of cases; those who, while recognizing that the damaged nerve is usually in continuity, have an almost mystical faith in the virtues of neurolysis (p. 280); and those so addicted to the internal fixation of fractures that they regard the presence of a nerve injury that may possibly require surgical attention as reinforcing the desirability of intervention.

Here are some facts. Of 211 nerve injuries in the upper limb caused by skeletal damage, good or fair recovery occurred spontaneously in 91 per cent. If the shoulder injuries are excluded—with their particularly favourable prognosis—the percentage is 77. These patients were selected; they were referred to us because of their nerve injuries, not because of their fractures. There is therefore, a possibility that the true proportion of cases in which spontaneous recovery occurs is even higher than these figures indicate. Dr Jorg Böhler was good enough to supply me with information from accident services in Linz, Salzburg and Vienna in respect of fractures of the humerus, which are those most likely to cause nerve damage (Seddon, 1967):

Fracture of humerus	765
Radial paralysis	57

= 7·4 per cent

47 spontaneous recoveries = 82·4 per cent.

The conclusion to be drawn from these figures is the same as that reached over 25 years ago (Seddon, 1947*a*) and supported by many other observers; which is that, in general, nerve injuries caused by fractures are relatively benign. Yet, obviously, this is not to say that operative intervention is never indicated; one must look for the signs indicating that in a minority something is amiss and endeavour to secure recovery by timely intervention. Because the primary focus of interest is a skeletal injury rather than this or that nerve the whole subject will be covered in this chapter rather than in Chapters 11 and 12 which are devoted to lesions of individual nerves.

THE MECHANISM OF INJURY

The Irrelevant Fracture

In Figure **5**, 23 are shown the fractures commonly though not invariably seen in traction

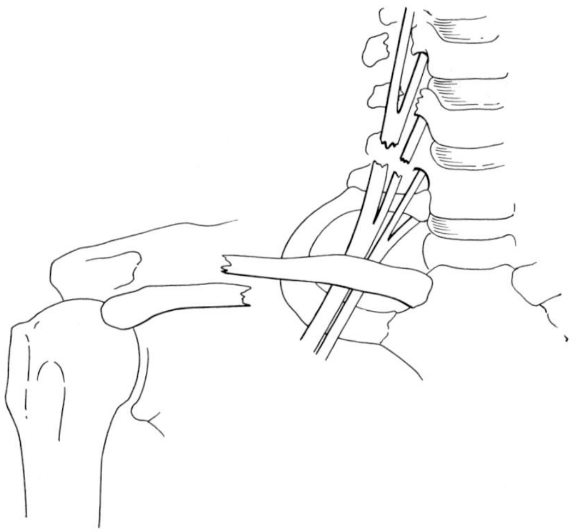

FIG. **5**, 23. The avulsion fractures of the transverse processes of the cervical vertebrae and fracture of the clavicle often found in association with brachial plexus injuries are no more than concomitant consequences of the traction force that damages the plexus.

injuries of the brachial plexus. They are produced by the violence that damages the plexus; the fractures are incidental though the break in the clavicle removes the last defence of the plexus against the distracting force.

The fracture produced by a penetrating wound (Fig. **5**, 7; p. 70) is again coincidental; it is the missile that smashes the bone and damages the nerve.

Fractures Injuring the Nerve Directly

Most of the nerve injuries we are considering are of the kind shown in Figure **5**, 24. When, as is usually the case, the nerve remains in continuity we can but speculate as to the exact

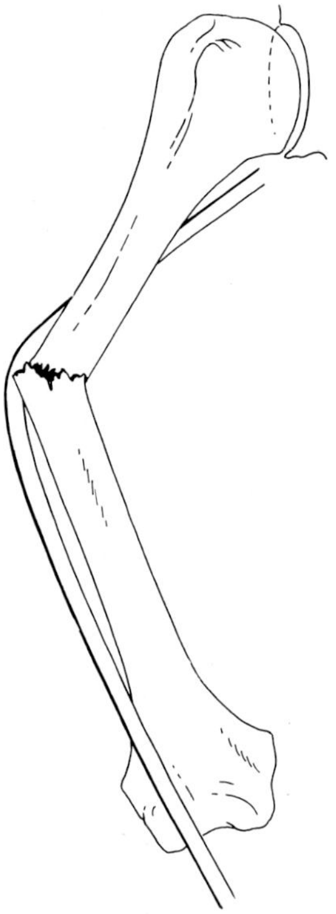

FIG. **5**, 24. The common sort of fracture that injures a nerve.

nature of the damage. However, the excellence of the recovery that so often occurs spontaneously even with a degenerative nerve lesion suggests that it is mainly an axonotmesis. But the sharp edge of one fragment may transect the nerve (Fig. **5**, 25) and the cardinal diagnostic problem is how to recognize these cases.

If there is an open fracture the prospects of spontaneous recovery are diminished, not because the breach in the soft tissues has any direct connection with the nerve injury but because the external wound may be an indication that the violence causing the fracture was very considerable, or it led to loss of muscle and skin with or without infection supervening. Either way the nerve is likely to be badly mauled.

If we consider the injuries in the upper limb, excluding those of the axillary nerve and the infraclavicular brachial plexus, in none of which was there an open wound, we find that spontaneous recovery occurred in 83·5 per cent of 109 cases in which there was a closed fracture

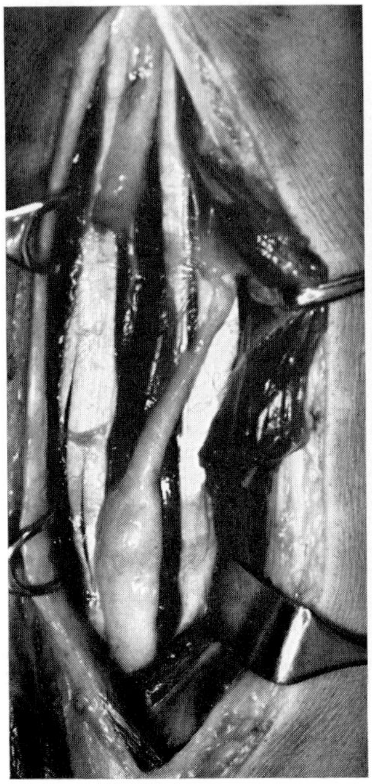

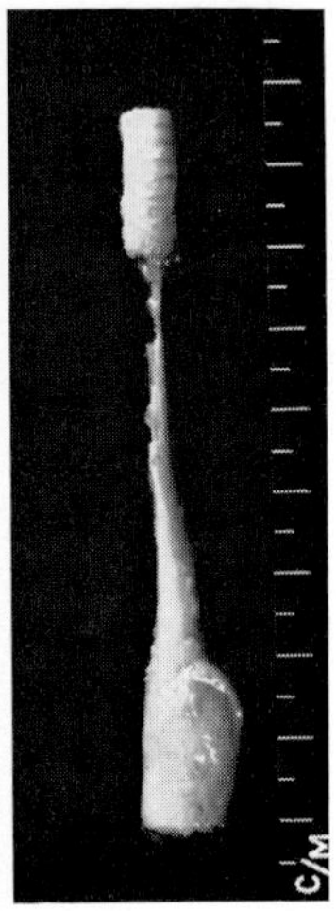

FIG. **5**, 25. An ordinary Colles's fracture transected the median nerve.

and in 65 per cent of the 37 in which there was an open fracture.

It is possible for a nerve to be trapped between the fragments, though not severed, and if this were at all a common event (Fig. **5**, 26) there would be a strong argument in favour of routine open intervention. However, as will be shown later, this hazard is limited to only a few skeletal injuries.

Dislocations

These can cause traction injuries of neighbouring nerves and the prognosis is therefore at best uncertain.

Fracture-dislocations

The damage that nerves may suffer as a result of these injuries is most varied. It may be comparatively benign, as is usual in fracture-dislocations of the shoulder. Rarely, the nerve may be trapped between bony fragments or even within the joint itself. In some situations exploration is required no more for the sake of the nerve than for restoration of the joint to something approaching normal.

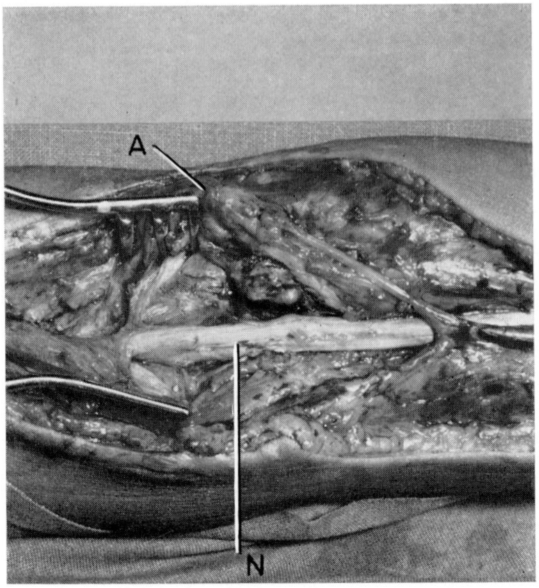

FIG. **5**, 26. A boy suffered a supracondylar fracture of the humerus. He was said to have developed partial median paralysis 2 months later, with complete sensory loss and paralysis of the abductor pollicis brevis. The nerve was explored 4 months after the injury and found to be trapped beneath the distal end of the proximal fragment of the (united) humerus, which projected anteriorly, A. The nerve is shown after liberation, and is slightly indented at N. The thenar muscles did not contract when the nerve was stimulated electrically, which proved that all except the short abductor were supplied by another, presumably the ulnar, nerve. Recovery was complete 2 months after the operation, which suggests that it was in progress before the nerve was freed.

Fractures allowing Nerves to be damaged by Traction

If a bone is broken in such a way that the limb is no longer protected against traction one or more nerves may suffer damage in this way; the characteristic neurological feature is that the level of paralysis is often proximal to the level of the fracture. This topic has already been discussed (p. 76).

Involvement of the Nerve in Callus

There are cases in which paralysis of a nerve appears at about the time when a fracture has united, and it is sometimes supposed that this is due to strangulation of the nerve by the new bone that forms during repair. I have never seen this. A more likely explanation of this paralysis of delayed onset is that the nerve is tethered by scar tissue at the site of fracture, more particularly if reduction has been imperfect, and when movement of the limb is resumed the nerve is damaged by stretching or compression. An example of this is shown in Figure **5**, 27.

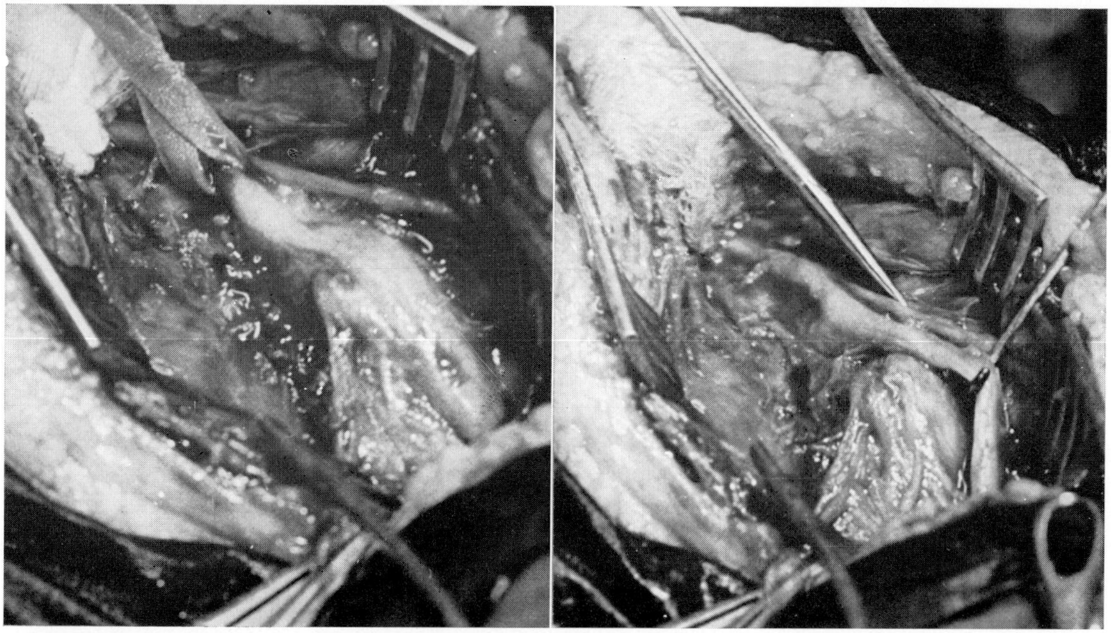

FIG. **5**, 27. Five months after a missile fracture of the humerus, which united satisfactorily though not in perfect alignment, the patient was troubled by weakness of the muscles supplied by the radial nerve and disordered sensibility in the superficial radial area. They began shortly after the time when he started to move the elbow. At operation the radial nerve was found spread out across a bony prominence, and adherent to it. After freeing of the nerve (right) the projecting mass of bone was removed.

NERVE INJURIES CAUSED BY FRACTURES AND DISLOCATIONS IN THE UPPER LIMB

The general distribution of these injuries is shown in Table VI.

Injuries in the Region of the Shoulder

DISLOCATION OF THE SHOULDER. The axillary nerve is sometimes injured and it may reasonably be inferred that the damage is by traction. As will be seen from Table VI the prognosis is uncertain. I have explored the nerve in two cases; in both, swelling and induration of the axillary nerve over a length of several centimetres strongly suggested a traction injury, and in one of them this was confirmed by histological examination of a minute biopsy specimen. Very occasionally a patient suffers paralysis of the deltoid after a heavy blow on the shoulder; there is no clear evidence of dislocation but it is reasonable to suppose, as Codman (1934) suggested, that there has been a momentary dislocation that reduced itself.

FRACTURES AND FRACTURE-DISLOCATIONS. This small but fascinating group, which includes minor injuries and some severe ones (Fig. **5**, 28), exhibits paralysis of the arm that ranges from involvement of one nerve to total paralysis below the level of the clavicle. The latter is hard to distinguish from a traction injury of the brachial plexus, and the presence of a severe skeletal injury makes it well-nigh impossible to examine the scapulo-humeral

TABLE VI—Nerve injuries caused by fractures and dislocations in the upper limb

NERVE	NUMBER OF CASES	GRADE OF SPONTANEOUS RECOVERY				
		Near normal	Impaired	Poor	Bad	Unknown
Infraclavicular brachial plexus lesions, partial or complete, due to shoulder injuries	45	33	10	1	1	—
Axillary nerve	15	6	4	1	2	2
Musculocutaneous nerve	1	1	—	—	—	—
Median nerve	18	14	2	—	1	1
Ulnar nerve	51	40	5	4	—	2
Radial nerve	74	46	8	—	19	1
Posterior interosseous nerve	8	6	1	—	1	—
TOTAL	212					

In 29 of the radial nerve injuries exploration was performed. In thirteen cases in which the nerve was in continuity satisfactory recovery occurred: in 12 of the remaining cases, in which the nerve had been severed, secondary suture was carried out with satisfactory results in eight.

muscles adequately. But the mere presence of the fracture-dislocation should put the clinician on his guard. In 1910 Delbet and Cauchoix pointed out that the distribution of the paralysis is usually infraclavicular, and Codman noted that the prospects of recovery were good. This is indeed the case as will be seen from Figure **5**, 29.

A series of 31 cases was studied by Leffert and Seddon (1965). We found nothing particularly significant in the mode of injury except that a fall from a moving vehicle was the

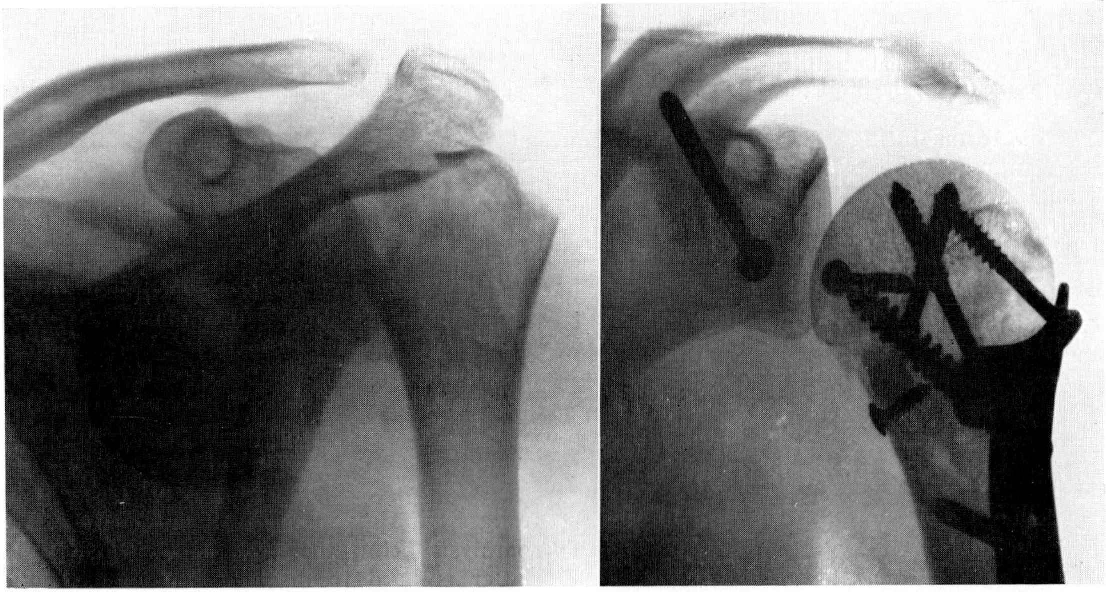

FIG. **5**, 28. Fracture-dislocation of the shoulder causing almost complete paralysis of the arm. A bold osteosynthesis was performed. The capital fragment of the humerus became ischaemic: the paralysis recovered apart from slight weakness of the intrinsic muscles of the hand.

cause in 12 cases and a fall while walking in seven.

Any combination of fractures with or without dislocation of the shoulder can occur, but dislocation of the shoulder with fracture of the greater tuberosity of the humerus is the commonest. An injury of the suprascapular nerve caused by fracture of the scapula has been reported to me by W. McKechnie; good spontaneous recovery occurred.

In such a heterogeneous collection the mechanism of injury must be extremely variable. When dislocation of the shoulder has occurred there is an element of traction. For the axillary nerve, running a short course, this may be noxious; but for the rest of the plexus—which is stretched at a point remote from both proximal and distal anchorage—the stretching is distributed over a wide reach of nerve and its effects are mitigated by the elasticity of the latter. In this respect infraclavicular brachial plexus lesions are much less harmful than the far commoner supraclavicular lesions which damage the plexus close to its proximal and structurally weak attachments.

Almost all of these injuries were in adults, some elderly. Treatment was for the most part conservative; the difficulty was preventing joint stiffness, especially in patients over 60 years of age. But assiduous mobilization of all joints, together with regular galvanic stimulation of the small muscles of the hand, the last to be re-innervated, was most rewarding.

But there are exceptions which the vigilant clinician will be quick to recognize. Two of our patients had traumatic aneurysms. One of them showed no more than a fracture of the greater tuberosity of the humerus, but he must have had a momentary displacement of the head of the bone. Operations were performed not for the nerve lesions but on account of the arterial damage. In one other case there was paralysis of three nerves which persisted for 16 months. Exploration ought to have been performed (we did not have the opportunity) as soon as it became evident that recovery in the proximal muscles—the biceps and the triceps—was overdue.

Humerus

FRACTURES OF THE SHAFT OF THE HUMERUS. These are the skeletal injuries that most commonly damage nerves, the radial nerve above all. Spontaneous recovery occurs in so large a majority that, so far as the nerve is concerned, the appropriate initial treatment is conservative. There is, however, no objection to inspecting the nerve if it is deemed expedient to treat the fracture by internal fixation; but the surgeon must beware lest the manipulation

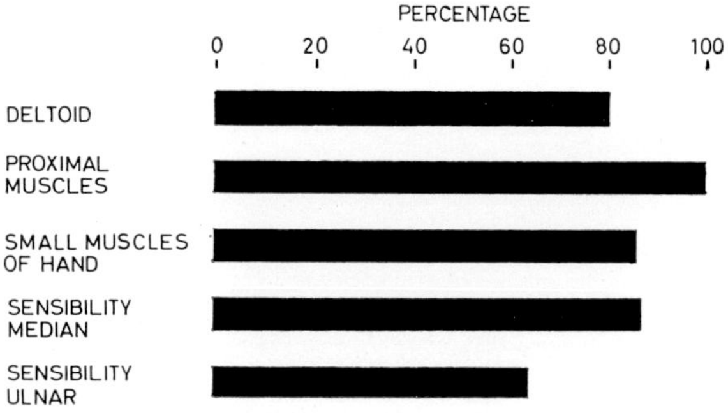

FIG. **5**, 29. Recovery after injuries in the region of the shoulder that damaged one or more nerves in the upper limb. In all cases the treatment was conservative (personal series of cases).

attendant on exposure of the fracture aggravates the nerve damage; a benign axonotmesis can be converted into a serious traction injury.

There is some significance in the type of fracture. It is usually displaced. One variety, that came to the notice of Holstein and Lewis (1963), is particularly liable to trap the radial nerve: an oblique fracture of the lower third of the humerus, running from below and medially upwards to the lower end of the spiral groove. If there is displacement the nerve may fall in between the fragments and it may well be, as these authors recommend, that open operation should always be performed (Fig. **5**, 30).

FRACTURES OF THE LOWER END OF THE HUMERUS. Sorrel and Sorrel-Déjerine (1938) reported 252 closed fractures of the lower end of the humerus in children (no schedule of ages is given, but they seem to have been mostly between the ages of 8 and 14 years); the ulnar nerve was damaged in 12, the median in four, both nerves in one, and the radial in four. Some nerves were explored, and although the reasons given are not always clear there is no doubt that in some cases the operation was necessary. I myself have found the radial nerve completely severed; and see also Fig. **5**, 26. Spitzer and Paterson (1973) in a somewhat similar study found spontaneous recovery in all; and they found nothing distinctive in the few cases in which median paralysis was accompanied by absence of the radial pulse. Lipscomb and Burleson (1955) have seen a number of supracondylar fractures in children in which the median nerve was caught up between the fragments. This can occur without, but more usually with, similar involvement of the brachial artery, the lesion that leads to ischaemic contracture of the forearm. They advised very early exploration.

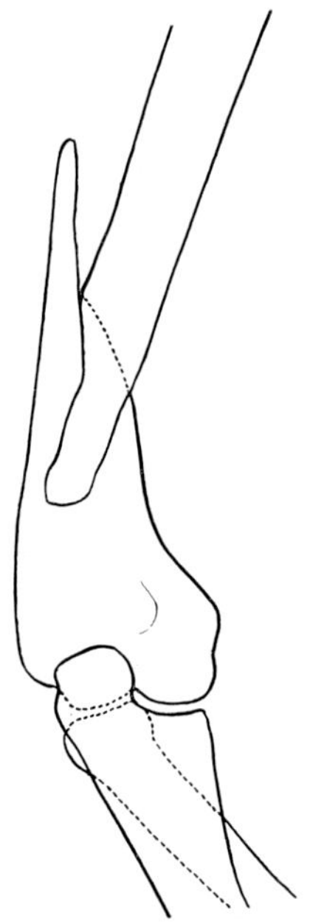

FIG. **5**, 30. Closed oblique fracture of the lower part of the shaft of the humerus. Radial paralysis. When the open reduction was performed the nerve, looking almost normal, was found lying between the fragments. The latter, after liberation of the nerve, were secured with two screws. Recovery uneventful.

This is rather confusing. However, on balance, it would seem proper to await spontaneous recovery of the nerve, provided that two conditions are satisfied. The first is reasonable apposition of the bony fragments, and the other *complete certainty that there is no threat of ischaemia of the forearm muscles.*

Elbow

Any dislocation or fracture-dislocation of the elbow may damage a nerve and it is usually the ulnar that suffers. Ulnar paralysis is particularly likely to accompany the fracture of the medial epicondyle in which the bony fragment is trapped in the joint, an injury that occurs more commonly in children than in adults. Operation is required primarily to free and replace the fragment; the ulnar nerve should always be transposed anteriorly.

But any fracture of the medial epicondyle can trouble the ulnar nerve; if not immediate ulnar paresis may develop several months, a few years, or many years later. The cause is always the same, an anatomical disturbance of the bed of the nerve.

A rare and most extraordinary injury is shown in Figure **5**, 31. There had been a fracture-dislocation of the elbow which must have opened up widely on the medial side. The ulnar nerve escaped damage but the median slipped into the joint and there was, naturally, complete paralysis of it. One similar case has been described by Mannerfelt (1968).

Radius and Ulna

Fractures of the upper ends of the forearm bones may damage the anterior or the posterior interosseous nerve. The prognosis is very favourable.

Fractures in the forearm may injure the median or ulnar nerve. Warren (1963) has described anterior interosseous paralysis caused by fracture of both bones. Spontaneous recovery occurs in all.

Wrist, Including Fractures of the Lower End of the Radius

A startling example of severance of the median nerve has already been given in Figure **5**, 25. But in most of these comparatively rare injuries the nerve is in continuity; spontaneous recovery may be expected with some confidence and exploration reserved for the case in which recovery has not taken place at the expected time.

Frykman (1967) found 14 cases of nerve injury (3·2 per cent) in a series of 430 fractures of the lower end of the radius, 10 affecting the median nerve, four the ulnar. He found no case of involvement of both nerves: I have never seen it, but it has been reported by Siegel and Weiden (1968).

Abbot and Saunders (1933) described four types of involvement of the median nerve:

1. Primary injuries, which are rare.

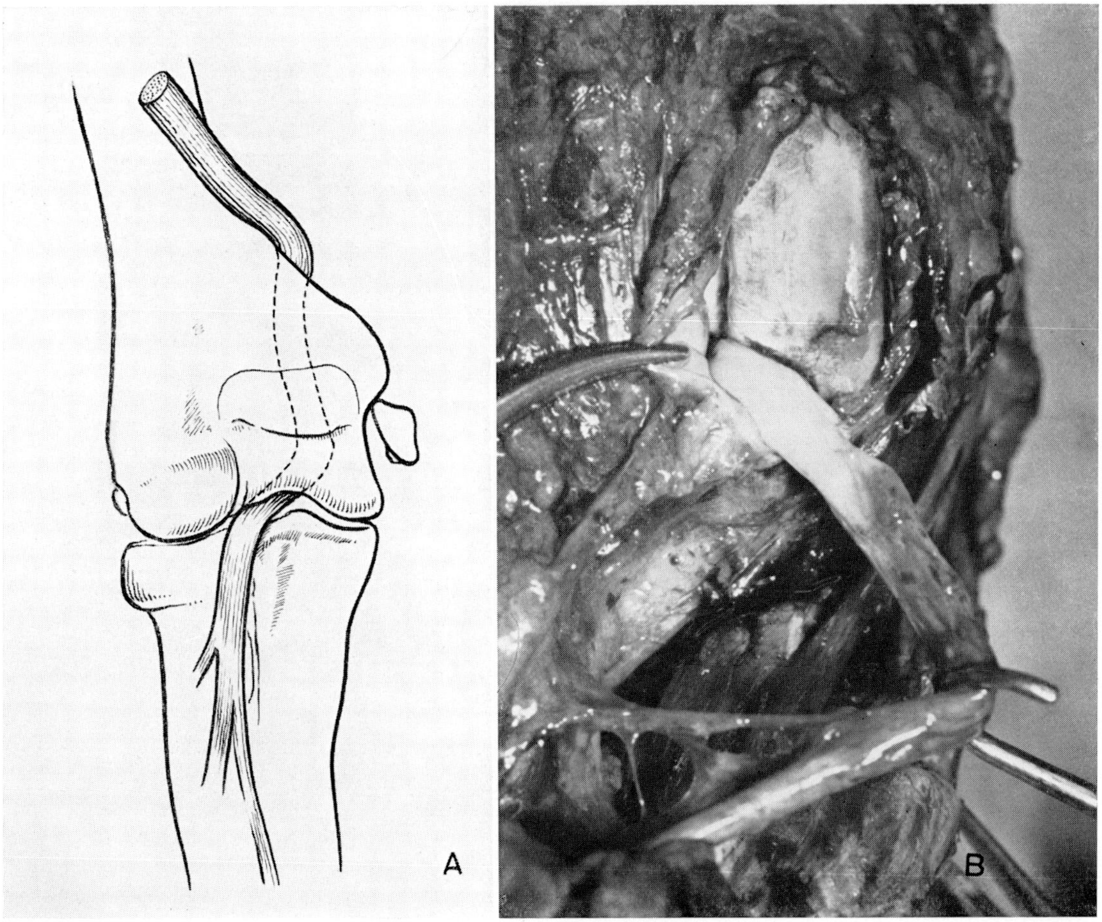

FIG. 5, 31. A, Diagram showing the median nerve trapped in the elbow joint when a fracture-dislocation occurred. B, The state of affairs revealed on exploration. The part of the nerve that had been caught in the joint is ivory white and completely collagenized. The ulnar nerve was, surprisingly, intact.

2. Secondary injuries due to pressure by an incompletely reduced fragment, the paresis appearing soon after movement of the wrist has been resumed.

3. Paralysis coming on very much later and due to bony abnormality in the bed of the nerve and to the rigidity of the anterior carpal ligament. I have seen what might be called traumatic median neuritis; there was malunion of a Colles's fracture (Zachary, 1945) with the result that the nerve followed a Z course, being caught between the lower end of the radius and the tight proximal rim of the carpal ligament.

4. Injuries associated with treatment in acute palmar flexion and ulnar deviation. This position undoubtedly narrows the opening into the carpal tunnel and Abbot and Saunders showed that it endangers the median nerve.

In the case of primary injuries, treatment should follow the usual line and be conservative in the first place; but operation is necessary when there is secondary involvement of the median nerve. I have only once found it necessary to deal with the ulnar.

Fractures of the Carpal Bones and the Bases of the Metacarpals

These fractures, particularly if the hamate is damaged, may injure the deep branch of the ulnar nerve (Howard, 1961). Howard suggested that if there is a haematoma round the nerve it should be evacuated and that if recovery is delayed the nerve should be explored.

Anterior dislocation of the lunate commonly injures the median nerve, but recovery follows appropriate treatment of the dislocation.

NERVE INJURIES CAUSED BY FRACTURES AND DISLOCATIONS IN THE LOWER LIMB

As is evident from Table VII these injuries are less common than in the upper limb: in this collection there were only 57 cases, compared with 212 in the upper limb.

Pelvis

Apart from fractures limited to the acetabulum, which are mentioned below under *hip*, there are the much more devastating injuries of the pelvis which may damage nerves. It happens that I have never encountered them. They are uncommon. A review of some 1,500 cases of fracture of the pelvis by Patterson and Morton (1973) revealed an incidence of 2·3 per cent. They remarked, however, that in the anxiety attendant on these grave injuries their less obvious neurological manifestations might be overlooked. As in nerves injured by fractures elsewhere the damage is usually at the site of fracture. But there are exceptions in which nerve roots are avulsed (as happens commonly in the brachial plexus) or compressed by a herniated intervertebral disc. Apart from the last the treatment is conservative.

TABLE VII—Nerve injuries caused by fractures and dislocations in the lower limb

NERVE	NUMBER OF CASES	GRADE OF SPONTANEOUS RECOVERY				
		Near normal	Impaired	Poor	Bad	Unknown
Sciatic: at the hip	20	8	7	3	1	1
femoral shaft*	11	5	5	1	—	—
Common peroneal: at the hip	2	1	—	1	—	—
femoral shaft	9	6	2	—	1	—
Both divisions of the sciatic at the knee	4	—	2	—	2	—
Deep peroneal (anterior tibial)	3	2	—	—	1	—
Posterior tibial	7	4	2	—	—	1
Saphenous	1	(irritative lesion treated by resection)				
TOTAL	57					

* In two cases the nerve was found to be severed and was sutured; one good and one poor result.

Hip

There are three kinds of injury that may damage the sciatic nerve: (1) dislocation; (2) dislocation with separation of a small or large fragment of the upper acetabular rim; and (3) central fracture of the acetabulum with more or less protrusion of the femoral head into the pelvis.

It is worth noting that in addition to the usual sciatic paralysis there may also be paralysis of the gluteus maximus.

DISLOCATION. This causes a traction injury of the sciatic nerve and, in our experience, nothing is gained by exploration.

FRACTURE-DISLOCATION. Here the mechanism is more complex. There may be an element of traction, but in addition the nerve may be trapped between the detached fragment and the body of the pelvis: it may also be caught up on the rim of the fragment. Because early

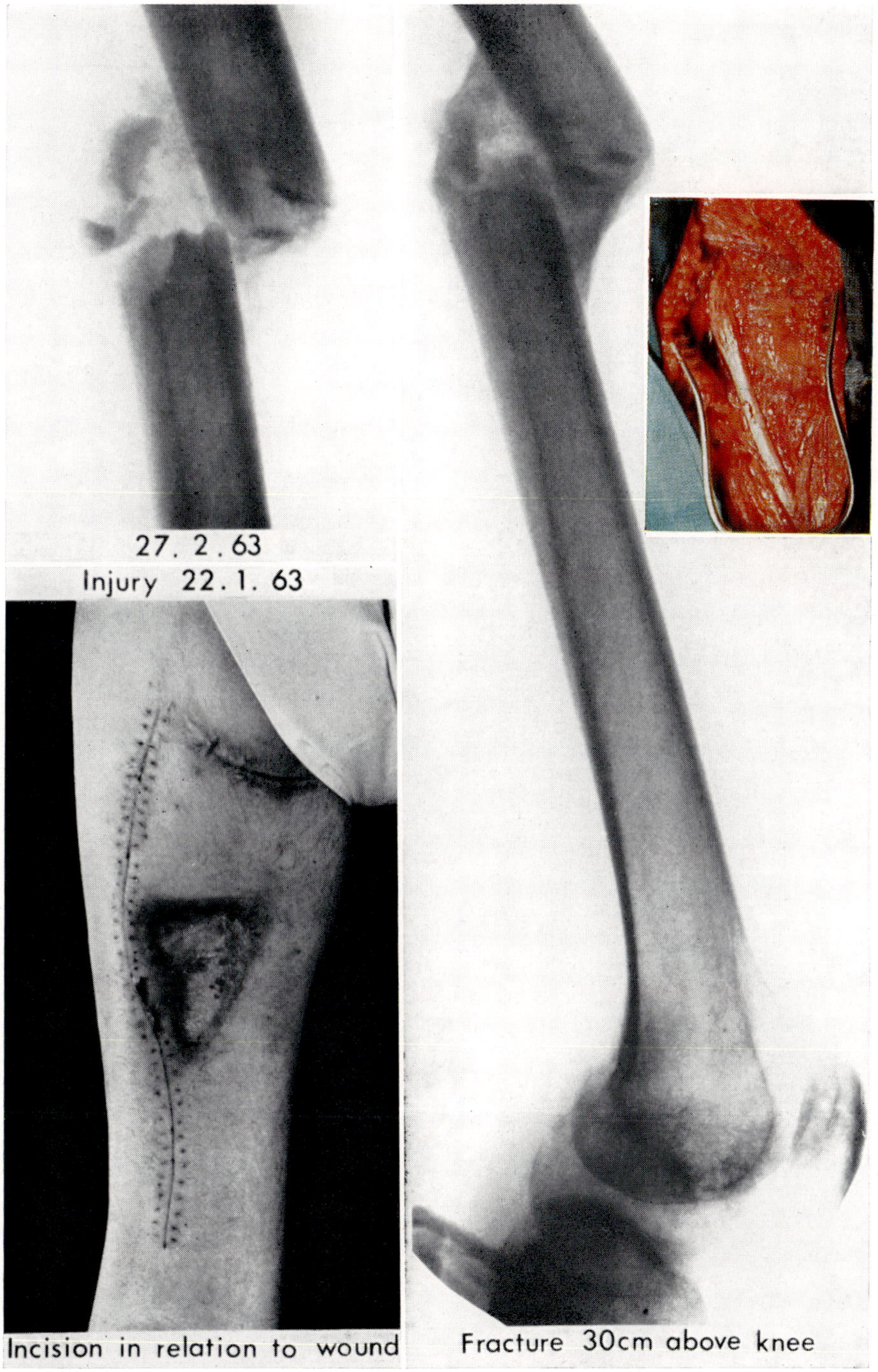

FIG. **5**, 32. When a fracture of the femur has injured the sciatic nerve it is wise to explore as soon as the fracture has united. In this case the nerve was found to be in continuity in spite of the severe open injury; and moderately satisfactory spontaneous recovery followed.

reposition of the acetabular fragment is always necessary, unless it is very small (in which case it could hardly involve the nerve), liberation of the nerve is carried out, so to speak, *en passant*.

CENTRAL FRACTURE OF THE ACETABULUM. Here the acetabulum is fragmented as if there had been a minor explosion inside it, the fragments flying centrifugally. Because the head of the femur is driven into the pelvis the sciatic nerve should be slacker than normal. But the postero-superior pieces of the acetabulum protrude towards the sciatic notch and here the nerve may be stretched over them. On four occasions I have removed the hump of bone: but this operation was carried out late and I was not convinced that it was beneficial. There is something to be said for early exploration when a central fracture of the acetabulum is accompanied by sciatic paralysis; I have never had the opportunity of doing it.

It will be noted from Table VII that the common peroneal division of the sciatic nerve alone may be damaged: not, it appears, the tibial division.

Femur

Very occasionally a fracture of the femoral shaft damages the sciatic nerve: it may even be transected. It is wise always to explore the nerve. The reason is that, as is shown in Figure **5**, 32, the time that must elapse before a benign lesion can declare itself by evidence of recovery in the proximally innervated muscles of the leg is so great—the femur being a very long bone—that if there is no recovery and repair is found to be necessary it is too late to obtain a satisfactory result.

The question, therefore, is whether to operate immediately or wait until the fracture has united. It so happens that my own experience is limited to the latter. However, I see no objection, in favourable circumstances, to internal fixation of the femur and exploration of the sciatic nerve at the same sitting.

Here again the common peroneal division alone may suffer injury.

Knee

Dislocation and fracture-dislocation of the knee can inflict fearful damage on the tibial and common peroneal nerves and all lesions I have seen were due to traction. Moreover, the popliteal vessels may be injured as well, with the result that there is ischaemia of the calf which in itself may damage the nerves at a lower level (for examples of this see p. 108).

Fracture of the Leg and Ankle

Nerve injuries due to these fractures (Bateman, 1962) are neither frequent nor serious. Either the posterior or the anterior tibial nerve may be affected (Table VII). In the one patient who showed little recovery there was most extensive muscle damage.

It is possible that nerve injuries due to fractures in the region of the ankle are not uncommon but escape recognition. I have seen only one (p. 280).

INDICATIONS FOR EXPLORATION

Although mention has been made of the indications for exploration in the three important types of nerve injury that form the subject of this chapter—those due to open wounds, to traction, and to skeletal damage—further reference to them will be found in Chapter 14, which precedes the discussion of operative intervention. The effective management of nerve injuries depends at least as much on deciding when to intervene as on technical skill.

6. Neurovascular Injuries

BROADLY SPEAKING, NEUROVASCULAR injuries, both open and closed, are of two kinds. There are those in which the vessels and nerve, or nerves, lying close together, are damaged at the same level; though it may be that the artery, or artery and vein alone are injured, the nerve becoming involved later as a result of the formation of a haematoma, aneurysm, or arterio-venous fistula. On the other hand, damage confined to an artery can cause ischaemia of the limb which is usually most pronounced some way distal to the site of damage; and one or more nerves may be affected where they traverse the ischaemic part. The pathological changes are very different: in the first group the nerve lesion is localized, in the second its longitudinal extent is considerable.

Both types of nerve damage can co-exist; the vessels and nerves are damaged, perhaps severed, at the site of injury; and ischaemia consequent on the arterial injury may cause ischaemic lesions of the same nerves more distally.

In this chapter there will be no detailed description of the treatment of arterial injuries, except of the spasm that so frequently accompanies the damage to the artery in Volkmann's ischaemia. Nor is it necessary to dilate on the treatment of a nerve injured at the same level as an artery because it differs in no way from the treatment of nerve injuries unaccompanied by arterial damage. It will, however, be necessary to describe the treatment of the damaged muscle, and of certain other structures, in Volkmann's ischaemia because the management of the ischaemic nerve cannot be considered in isolation.

Lastly, as a matter of convenience, certain related topics are considered in this chapter, namely, roller injuries, ischaemia due to anoxia caused by poisoning, and nerve damage caused by abnormal bleeding.

COMBINED OPEN INJURIES OF ARTERIES AND NERVES

These are predominantly war injuries.

Some idea of the frequency of nerve involvement may be gained from the following figures. Fromme (1917) reported 16 cases of aneurysm of the subclavian, axillary and brachial arteries with 13 nerve lesions, an incidence of 81 per cent; Maurer (1939): 71 aneurysms in the upper limb with nerve involvement in 25 per cent; Richards (M.R.C.R. 1954): 44 cases of aneurysm or arterio-venous fistula of the limb vessels with nerve involvement in 17—39 per cent. In Richards's collected records—from other centres—there were 31 injuries of the upper limb affecting arteries and nerves, and 52 nerves in all were involved. He found that apart from six cases of brachial plexus injury there were 12 in which more than one nerve was affected, the median nerve being the most vulnerable. There were 13 neurovascular lesions in the lower limb; the tibial nerve was not once affected alone, whereas in four the common peroneal nerve alone was affected.

There are three main types of injury, each with characteristic features.

SEVERANCE OF A MAJOR ARTERY WITH AN OPEN WOUND

These are the most alarming vascular injuries; the patient may quickly bleed to death. They were necessarily excluded from the reports that have just been referred to. DeBakey and Simeone (1946) showed how grave these injuries were during the Second World War, even apart from loss of life. The amputation rate was about 50 per cent if the artery was ligated or repaired by tube anastomosis. In their view ligation of the artery alone was inferior to ligation of the artery and vein. The loss of limbs was even higher: after repair by vein grafting, 57·5 per cent, but less, 36 per cent, after arterial suture.

The trouble about these wounds is that the great commotion caused by high-velocity missiles damages the neighbouring branches of the artery and, in consequence, the development of a collateral circulation is hindered or prevented. Thus the chief hope lies in re-establishment of the circulation through the main vessel, and some most encouraging experiences in the

Korean War were reported by Jahnke and Seeley (1953). Their first choice was suture of the vessel; if there had been such destruction that this was impossible they used direct suture after mobilization of the vessel, which might involve sacrificing some of its branches. Thirty-two repairs were carried out in the upper limb,

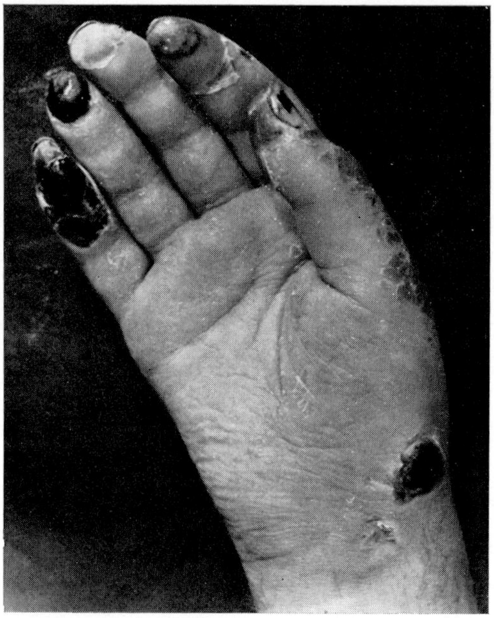

FIG. **6**, 1. A man aged 33 suffered a severe wound of the axilla that severed the axillary artery and vein and the ulnar nerve. The median and radial nerves were seen to be intact at the time when the vessels were ligated. Patchy gangrene occurred in the hand, but no certain evidence of ischaemia of muscle. The hand healed ultimately. The median and radial nerves recovered slowly and imperfectly.

with no subsequent amputations; and 45 in the lower limb with eight amputations. A curious finding was that ligation of the smaller blood vessels, those in the distal segment of a limb, led to amputation more frequently than did repair of a major vessel.

Any nerve injury that may be present is of no immediate consequence. What matters, however, is that when dealing with the artery, by whatever means, damage to adjacent nerves must be avoided. If the life-saving operation is carried out in a tranquil atmosphere, as is increasingly the case, the surgeon can spare time to take note of the state of the main nerve trunks in the neighbourhood, though if any of them are found to be severed it is best to postpone repair until the state of the limb is satisfactory and the tissues at the site of injury are supple. If the ends of a nerve can be tacked together this later operation will be facilitated. If the nerves are seen to be in continuity no further exploration will be required.

Saving the limb has as its objective a member that will be useful; an ischaemic appendage with, perhaps, peripheral gangrene (Fig. **6**, 1) is a poor affair. Richards (M.R.C.R., 1954) found that 16 per cent of missile wounds of major arteries in the upper limb were followed by ischaemia, and 45 per cent of such wounds in the lower limb. Makins (1919) noted that even in the absence of frank ischaemia a major arterial injury could cause a general depression of motor and sensory function in a limb. The case for arterial reconstruction rather than ligation is very strong.

OPEN WOUNDS LEADING TO THE FORMATION OF A HAEMATOMA, ANEURYSM OR ARTERIO-VENOUS FISTULA

Injuries of this kind are particularly liable to occur when the victim has been peppered by small high-velocity missiles, as from the explosion of a land mine, a common feature of modern warfare. The superficial wound may heal rapidly. There may be no sign of nerve involvement. What matters above all is observation of the patient during his recovery from the immediate effects of the injury. A watch has to be kept for:

1. The early appearance of a swelling, possibly pulsatile, which indicates that a haematoma is forming. A bruit may become audible.
2. The development of a swelling—usually pulsatile—at a later period, indicating the formation of a saccular aneurysm; here too a bruit may be heard.
3. The development of a bruit without any swelling, the noise being very loud, and there may be a palpable thrill. This indicates the formation of an arterio-venous fistula.
4. The onset of pain, a particularly significant symptom if a fleshy part, such as the buttock, has been injured. No swelling may be detectable but an aneurysm may be forming.
5. The state of the pulses. If a pulse diminishes

there is certain to be something amiss with the artery.

6. A change in the power of the limb. There may have been no paralysis; then some weakness of muscles and disturbance of sensibility appear, which strongly suggest that some abnormality of the blood vessels is beginning to involve neighbouring nerve trunks. There may have been some paralysis initially; its extent has to be accurately documented because it may be found that the paralysis spreads, indicating that something untoward is occurring.

Arteriography is particularly valuable if there have been injuries at more than one level, either penetrating wounds or fractures, especially closed fractures. The contrast medium will show where a block or leakage has occurred.

The timing of operative intervention is determined mainly by the nature of the vascular injury, though the presence of a nerve lesion may add some element of urgency. If there is increasing paralysis or severe pain or both, then there should be no delay. If there is a steadily enlarging haematoma the situation is urgent. If there is an aneurysm there should be no haste. With the passage of time the collateral circulation is likely to improve; the wall of the aneurysm will become consolidated and occasionally, as Richards recorded, the sac is obliterated spontaneously by thrombosis. He found little evidence to suggest that an aneurysm threatens the collateral circulation (Richards, M.R.C.R., 1954, p. 230), the incidence of ischaemia being lower in cases of aneurysm than in uncomplicated arterial injuries. There is usually no urgency in attacking an arterio-venous fistula, unless there is vascular insufficiency of the limb or evidence of systemic disturbance.

Combined Closed Injuries of Arteries and Nerves

These injuries are of two kinds. The patient always suffers some sort of an accident, usually a fall on the shoulder. Arterial damage may result from dislocation of a joint or a fracture, though it can occur in the absence of either (Gibson, 1962). The usual consequence is an enormous haematoma rather than a circumscribed aneurysm. These are dangerous injuries; of the 90 cases recorded by Calvet, Leroy and Lacroix (1941-42), 49 were fatal.

It is difficult to understand how a main artery such as the axillary can be torn without there having been any skeletal disturbance. It is possible that in some falls on the shoulder there was a dislocation that reduced itself; but in some of the elderly victims the artery may have given way because it was atherosclerotic, as in one of Gibson's elderly patients. Nerves may have been damaged by the original injury or paralysis may appear later. Typical examples are provided by the following case histories, one of which illustrates some of the mistakes that can be made.

A man of 42 fell off his bicycle on to the left shoulder. Paralysis of the arm came on *a few hours later* and within 48 hours there was total motor paralysis below the deltoid, and sensory loss in the distribution of the median and radial nerves. At this time the radial pulse was absent. There was no recognizable skeletal injury.

Four days after the accident there was complete sensory loss below the elbow and ecchymosis in the axilla.

He came under our observation 32 days after the accident on account of increasing pain in the arm and because a bruit was audible in the axilla. On the thirty-seventh day an arteriogram showed a saccular leak in the axilla, which was then explored after an arterial clamp had been applied to the third part of the subclavian artery. There was an enormous haematoma due to a small tear in the axillary artery. In the excitement of arresting the torrential haemorrhage, pressure forceps were applied above and below the rent, thus spoiling the chance of closing it by suture. The vessel was ligated. Subsequently he made a good recovery in all muscles except those of the hand, and the circulation was satisfactory; but the weakness of the hand was permanently disabling.

Two mistakes were made in the handling of this case. It was assumed that because there was paralysis of the arm after a fall on the shoulder he had suffered a traction injury of the brachial plexus, though the history of onset alone was sufficient to exclude this; the paralysis had not come on immediately and the sensory loss gradually increased. It was therefore thought that there was no element of urgency; this led to delay in recognizing the primary lesion—the tear of the axillary artery.

The second mistake was in using pressure forceps instead of arterial clamps on either side of the rent. Suture of the artery should not have been difficult.

A young man fell off a lorry; he suffered a number of injuries, including concussion, and the relevant one was a fracture of the left scapula with immediate and total paralysis distal to the shoulder. Accurate examination of the shoulder muscles was impossible.

By the twenty-sixth day, when he came under our care, he had fully recovered from his head injury but was complaining of severe intermittent pain in the left upper limb. There was an enormous haematoma filling the axilla, but it did not pulsate and no bruit was audible. The radial pulse was absent and no pulsation was detectable by oscillometry. On the twenty-seventh day the swelling was larger and had become pulsatile.

The axillary artery was explored on the following day. The approach was difficult on account of bleeding from many engorged small vessels. After a clamp had been applied to the third part of the subclavian artery (for details of technique see p. 93) the haematoma was evacuated. A longitudinal tear, 1·5 cm long, was found in the posterior wall of the axillary artery 5 cm distal to the clavicle, and two of the three cords of the brachial plexus were severed and very extensively damaged at the same level. The artery and two nerve trunks had been lacerated by a fragment of the fractured scapula.

Suture of the artery, though difficult, would have been possible, but at that time we knew nothing about repairing the plexus by autologous grafting. So the artery was ligated above and below the tear and cut across. The circulation was satisfactory. It later became evident that it was the outer cord of the plexus that had been spared. An appropriate amputation was advised.

Regional Distribution

Head and Neck

During the First World War, particularly in France, there was great interest in wounds of the upper part of the neck involving the last four cranial nerves, sometimes with damage to the neighbouring great vessels. As Pollock and Davis (1933) have pointed out, the clinical manifestations can be very varied; they call for searching clinical examination which should include laryngoscopy. We saw no cases of this kind during the Second World War, but Elkin and Woodhall (1944) described four, all with vascular injuries, and gave an excellent digest of the relevant literature. Treatment of the vascular lesions may prove most formidable.

Upper Limb

Combined open injuries are found predominantly in the upper limb (Richards's figure is 70 per cent) because of the contiguity of large blood vessels and nerves throughout their length.

The accident that most commonly causes a closed injury of the axillary artery is a fall on the shoulder. If there is a fracture there may be immediate paralysis which is indistinguishable from the infraclavicular brachial plexus injuries (with a favourable prognosis) that have been referred to on page 83. Then it becomes evident that something further is developing. The patient complains bitterly of pain in the arm, and a swelling of the shoulder gradually appears. The error here is delay in recognizing the vascular complication (Kirker, 1952). The treatment of this type of injury is the same as for a haematoma following a penetrating wound. When the paralysis comes on some time after the injury, hours or even a few days later, a potentially dangerous haematoma is certainly forming; falls on the shoulder, whether or not producing a fracture, are not ordinarily followed by paralysis of delayed onset. The lesion of the artery is greater than the sort that leads to formation of an aneurysm. When there has been no bony injury, and nothing to suggest a dislocation that has reduced itself, a diagnosis of rupture of the axillary artery is likely to be made quickly.

Lower Limb

Because the femoral artery is unaccompanied by any major nerve trunk, neurovascular injuries of the type we are considering occur at or below the knee. One exception must be mentioned though I have never seen it. Tönnis and Götze (1942) and others have described apparently minor wounds in the buttock that were followed after an interval by severe sciatica, which was found to be due to an aneurysm of the superior gluteal artery pressing on the sciatic nerve at its point of emergence from the pelvis.

The types of vascular injury are the same as in the upper limb though vascular damage due to closed injuries is very rare, its place being taken by aneurysms of the popliteal artery that arise spontaneously and may sooner or later involve the tibial or the common peroneal nerve.

Observations on Operative Technique

Injury of the Axillary Artery causing a Large Haematoma

The incision is made in the line of the axillary artery from the level of the clavicle down to just below the anterior axillary fold. If the haematoma is very large, or if it is high in the axilla, the incision should be continued over and above the clavicle (which should not be divided) so that the subclavian artery can be exposed and occluded temporarily with a rubber-covered arterial clamp. The incision is deepened through both pectoral muscles, but on no account should the fascia beneath them be incised until all the tissues down to this level have been cut through, and until all bleeding from the superficial tisues and from the muscle has been arrested. A roll of gauze, several layers thick, 6 to 7 cm wide and not less than 1·5 m long should be in readiness, unwound, in a heap. An incision about 7 cm long is then made through the fascia beneath the pectoralis major; blood clot and perhaps some bright blood well out instantly. The gauze is pushed through the hole very rapidly until it fills the axilla; a large quantity of clot is squeezed out. While the assistant presses on the mass of gauze the rest of the axillary fascia is cut from end to end. The assistant manipulates the gauze in such a way as to control bleeding from the artery but to give the surgeon sufficient room to expose the vessel as high up as possible, that is just distal to the subclavius. This muscle may be cut across to enlarge the exposure but it tends to bleed considerably and there are always troublesome distended veins. The artery is then freed and an appropriate clamp placed on it; there may already be one on the subclavian artery just proximal to the clavicle. Pressure on the ball of gauze is then shifted so as to expose the vessels in the lower part of the axilla or the upper part of the arm and here both the vein and the artery should be dissected out and occluded. Then it is safe to remove the gauze; yet in spite of the precautions that have been taken there may be disconcerting bleeding if the vessels, though damaged, are in continuity. Because the aim is restoration rather than ligation the surgeon should at all costs try to avoid the mistake described in the case already referred to, in which pressure forceps were applied to the torn artery.

When the bleeding is completely controlled, but before the arterial repair is carried out, the three cords of the brachial plexus are inspected; indeed a little dissection is permissible to facilitate this, provided that no branches of the artery or vein are disturbed. If the state of the nerves can be determined it is then possible to decide what, if anything, will be required later; if, for example, all three cords are found to be in continuity then no subsequent exploration of the nerves will be necessary.

Aneurysms

The formation of an aneurysm is a slower process resulting from a smaller leak. It will have been noted whether the paralysis has been present from the time of injury, or, if present, has deepened. If it is a recent development, there having been no paralysis initially, it can be positively affirmed (Fig. **6**, 2) that the aneurysm itself was responsible for the nerve involvement.

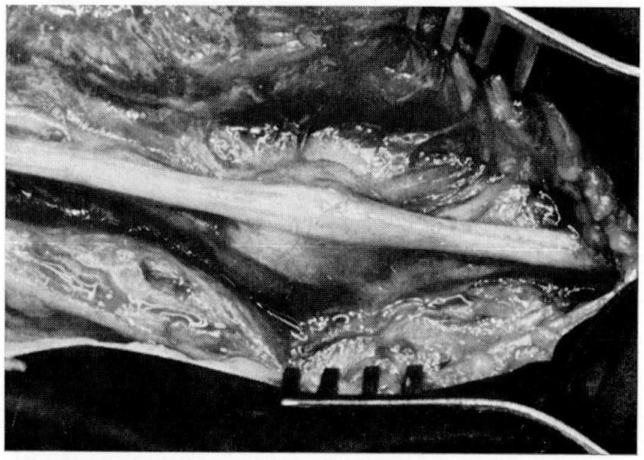

FIG. **6**, 2. Aneurysm of the brachial artery with the median nerve stretched over it. Treatment of the aneurysm sufficed.

All that need be said about the surgical approach to these aneurysms (and it is the same when there is no nerve lesion) is that the relationship of the nerve trunks to the sac should be clearly established. This calls for a long incision, exposure of the nerve trunks proximally and distally, where anatomical relationships are normal, and then they are traced towards the aneurysm. It may be found that one or more nerve trunks run into the sac (Fig. **6**, 3), in which case it is almost certain that there is serious damage, as in the case illustrated. After the aneurysm has been dealt with the nerve should be repaired. There are objections to a later operation; fresh adhesions will have formed between the repaired or obliterated vessel and the damaged nerve, and may make a secondary operation hazardous. The combined vascular and nerve repair can be time-consuming. In the axilla, even with an experienced vascular surgeon and another equally experienced in repairing nerves, the time from start to finish may be up to seven hours.

ISCHAEMIC NERVE LESIONS

Although it is the state of the muscle that has attracted most attention in Volkmann's and in kindred forms of ischaemia the characteristic infarction is no respecter of tissues; any of them—bone, tendon, and particularly nerve—can be involved though not necessarily to the same degree.

Pathology

There is no doubt that this condition can result from increased pressure within a fascial compartment (Parkes, 1945) as is sometimes seen in haemophilia, in fractures of the tibia and always in the anterior tibial syndrome; but the primary damage is usually arterial and there are three types. War wounds usually sever an artery; in civil practice the vessel commonly suffers injury in continuity as a result of a fracture; and, rarely, ischaemia is due to arterial embolism. The consequences, so far as the ischaemic damage is concerned, are much the same in all three but the mode of onset is rather different, as will be described later.

Changes in Muscle

Makins (1919), in his monograph *On Gunshot Injuries to the Blood Vessels*, observed that the

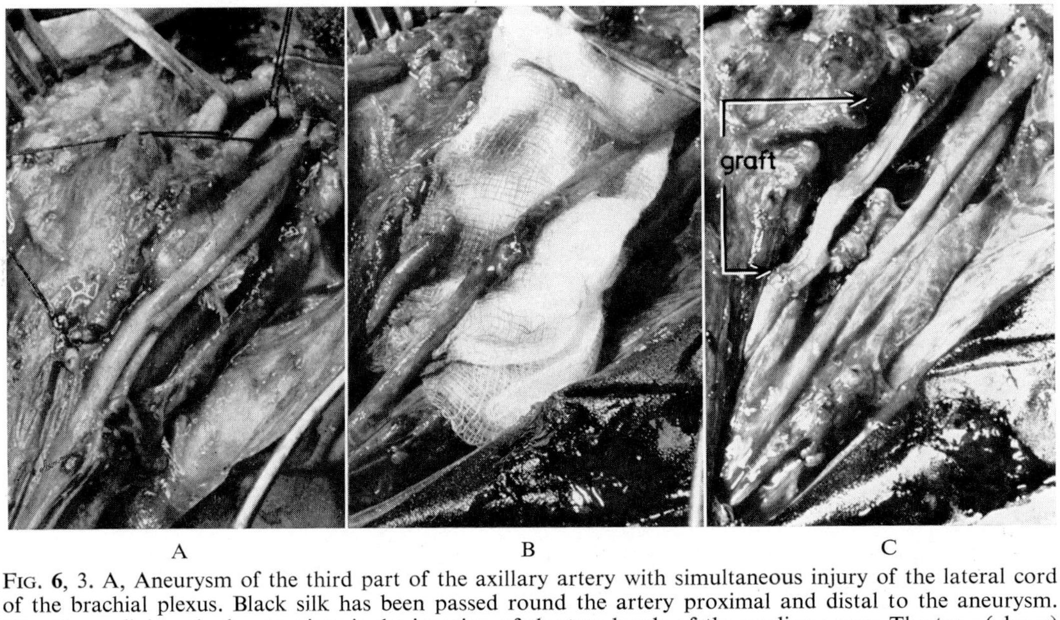

FIG. **6**, 3. A, Aneurysm of the third part of the axillary artery with simultaneous injury of the lateral cord of the brachial plexus. Black silk has been passed round the artery proximal and distal to the aneurysm. Directly medial to the lowest piece is the junction of the two heads of the median nerve. The tape (above) encircles the lateral cord of the plexus. B, The aneurysm has been ablated. The musculocutaneous nerve was found to be severed (proximal end turned upwards), and the lateral head of the median nerve, though in continuity, very badly damaged. C, Two strands from the medial cutaneous nerve of the forearm were used to repair the musculocutaneous nerve. Nothing was done to the outer head of the median nerve. The biceps recovered well: power 4 (M.R.C. grading): all the muscles supplied by the median nerve recovered to $4\frac{1}{2}$, but the terminal segment of the thumb remained insensitive.

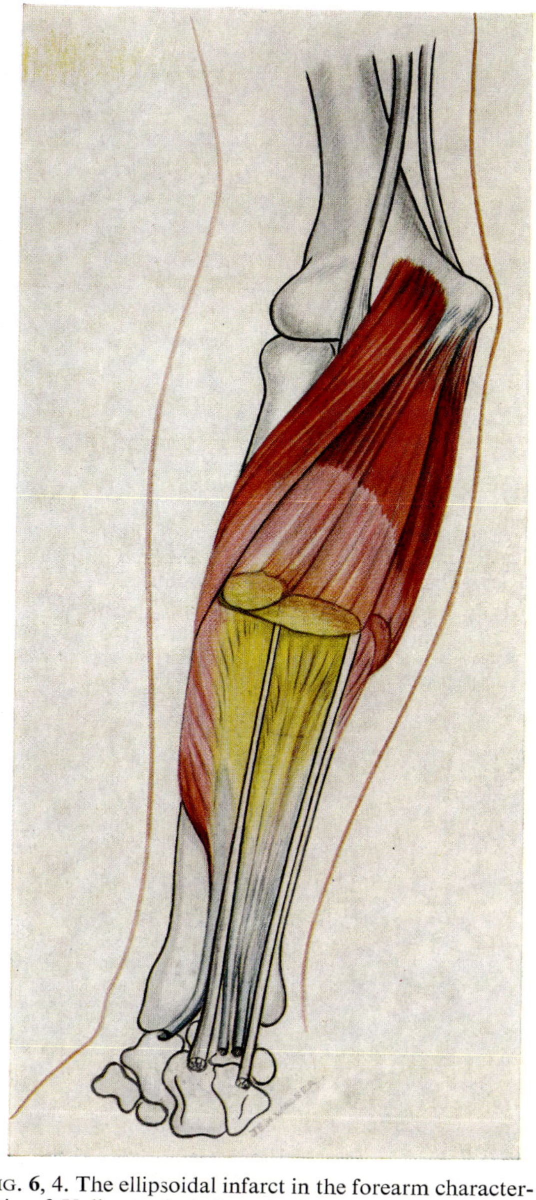

FIG. 6, 4. The ellipsoidal infarct in the forearm characteristic of Volkmann's ischaemia due to a supracondylar fracture of the humerus. The necrotic centre of the infarct is traversed by the median nerve; the ulnar nerve is at the periphery. (Figs **6**, 4 and **6**, 5 reproduced by kind permission from *J. Bone Jt Surg.*, 1956, **38B**, 152.)

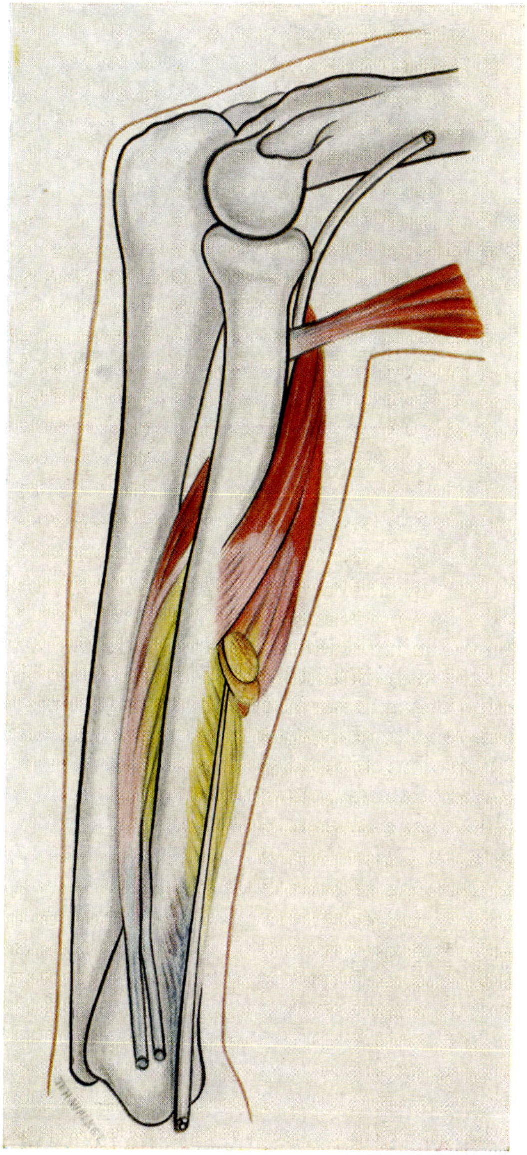

FIG. **6**, 5. A lateral view showing how the infarct may involve the deep extensor muscles.

state of the limb in a very unfavourable type of case can be just short of early massive gangrene. At the other extreme there is the case in which a patient recovers with no more than a moderate contracture of the forearm muscles. It might be supposed that in both cases and in all the intermediate grades of ischaemia the damage was diffuse, affecting all muscles (and other tissues) more or less uniformly. It was Tavernier (Tavernier, Dechaume and Pouzet, 1936) who showed that this was not so, that the lesion was in fact an infarct. This is so even in the worst type of case that Makins had in mind. The section

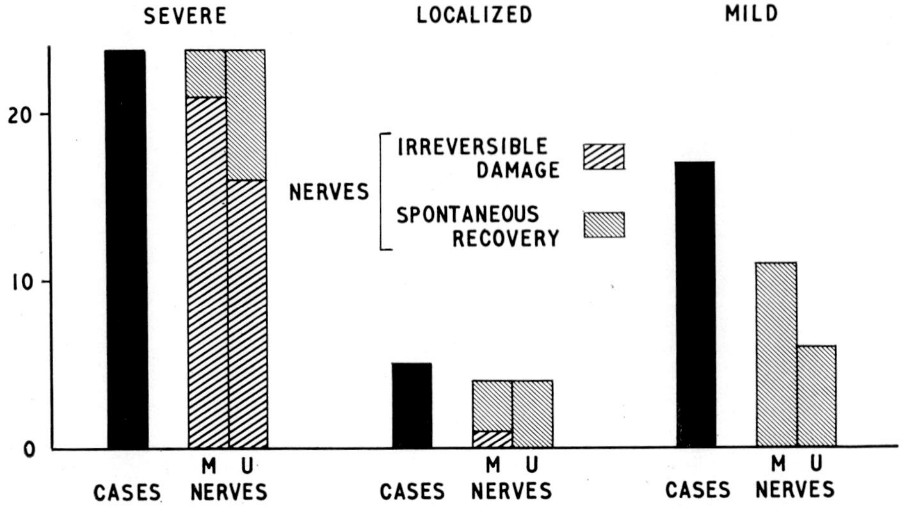

FIG. **6**, 6. Frequency of involvement of the median and ulnar nerves in ischaemia of the forearm. The ulnar nerve is not so severely affected as the median. The terms *severe, localized* and *mild* refer to the degree of ischaemia of the muscles. (This figure and Fig. **6**, 7 reproduced by kind permission from *Br. med. J.*, 1964, **1**, 1587.)

through the hand illustrated in Figure **6,** 7 was made through the distal part of an enormous infarction of the forearm, extending into the palm. Yet beyond the devascularized mass, which has the form of an ellipsoid (Seddon, 1956), as well as beyond its lateral boundaries, the vascularity of the tissues is near normal. The infarct is usually well distal to the site of the vascular lesion; a supracondylar fracture of the humerus damaging the brachial artery produces an ellipsoidal infarct in the forearm the centre of which is a little below its mid-point. The ischaemia may produce no more than a moderate fibrosis of the affected muscles which ultimately regain good contractility; at the other extreme most of the infarct is completely necrotic. But within the infarct itself there are differences (Figs **6**, 4 and **6**, 5) because the ischaemia is greater at the centre than at the periphery. If it happens that a nerve runs through the centre of an infarct, as does the median in the forearm, the nerve will suffer; if it lies more peripherally, as does the ulnar, it may escape altogether or be only slightly affected (Figs **6**, 4 and **6**, 6). The degree of nerve involvement is, as might be expected, a reflection of the severity of the muscle damage; thus the state of the muscle is a fairly reliable guide to the state of the nerve and hence to the appropriate treatment.

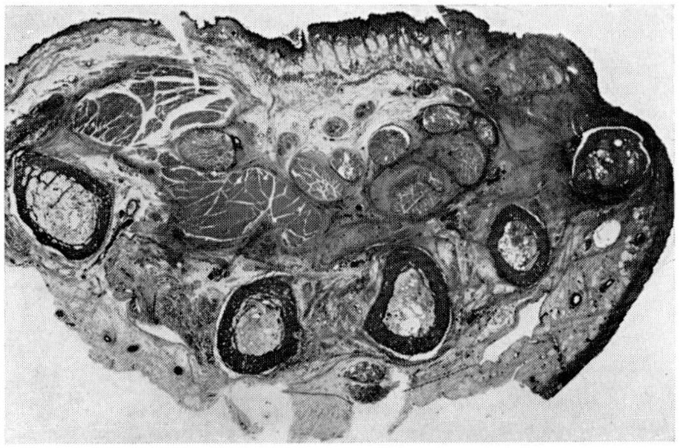

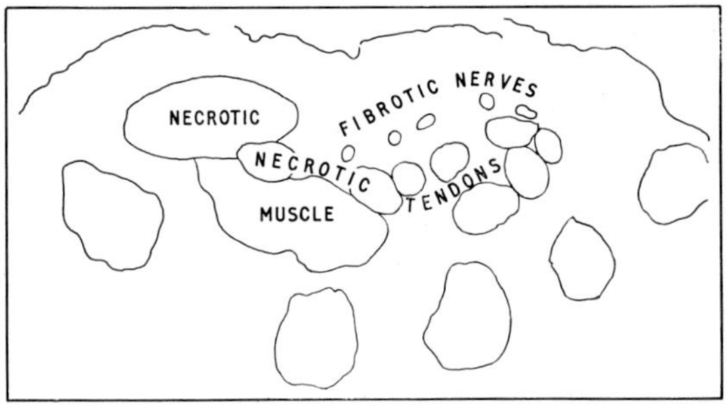

FIG. **6**, 7. In this case the infarction was so extensive that it involved the branches of the median and ulnar nerves in the palm and the intrinsic muscles of the hand. Amputation performed: no sort of reconstruction was possible.

Changes in Nerve

It was long believed that the nerve involvement was due to compression by the fibrotic muscle in the forearm. This, however, would cause paralysis of delayed onset, whereas the more carefully patients are examined the more certain it becomes that the nerve involvement is there from the beginning. Moreover, in mild degrees of ischaemia the nerves may recover spontaneously even while contracture of the muscle is developing. Nerves may show the changes of ischaemia where there is no overlying muscle to compress them (Fig. **6**, 7). Nevertheless, the progressive fibrosis of ischaemic muscle in the forearm can be an aggravating factor, as is well shown in a case of 'roller' injury described later in this

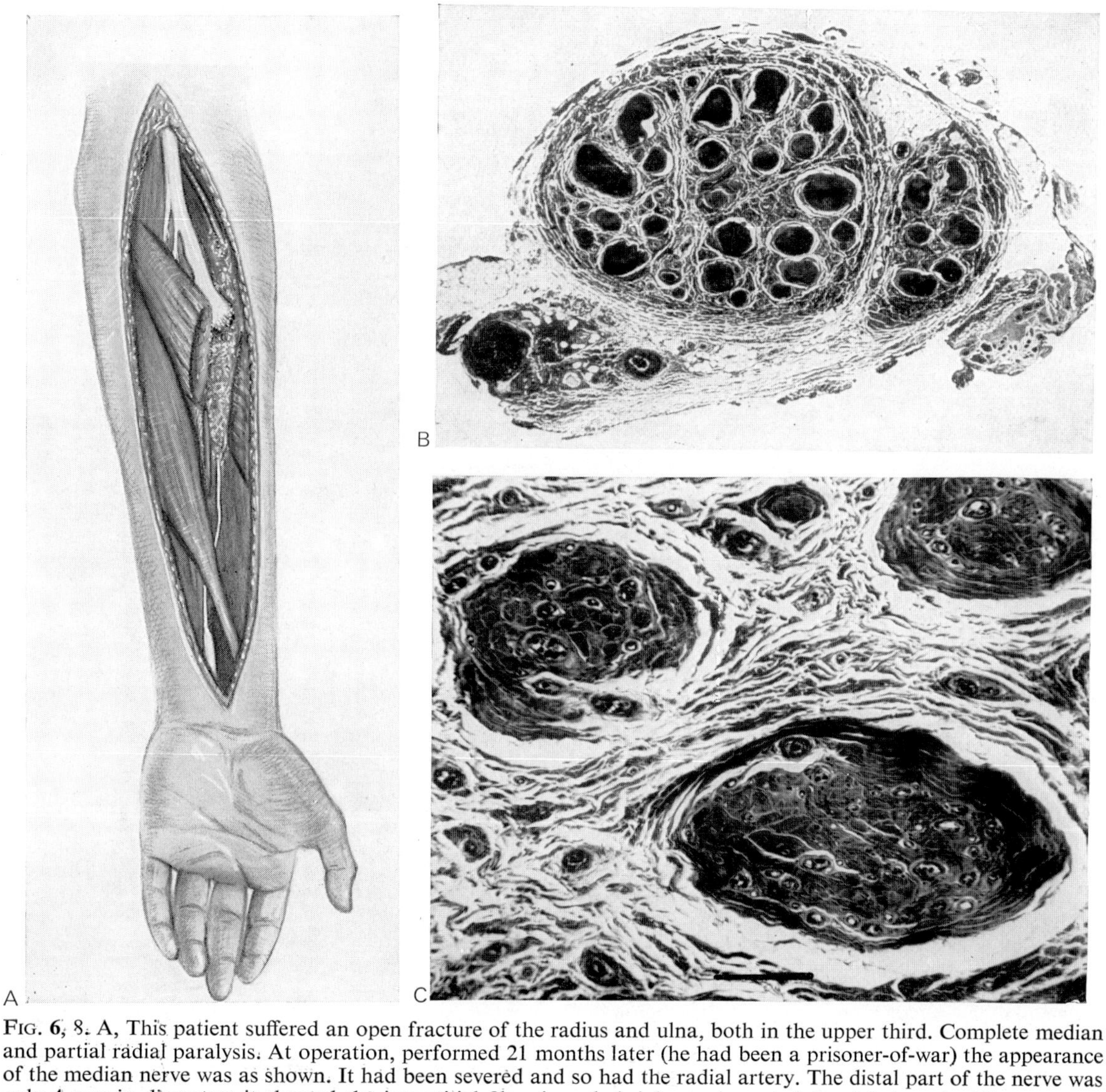

FIG. **6**, 8. A, This patient suffered an open fracture of the radius and ulna, both in the upper third. Complete median and partial radial paralysis. At operation, performed 21 months later (he had been a prisoner-of-war) the appearance of the median nerve was as shown. It had been severed and so had the radial artery. The distal part of the nerve was only 4 mm in diameter; it showed the interstitial fibrosis and shrinkage characteristic of ischaemia. There was no ischaemia of the surrounding muscles. The arteria comes nervi mediani had been destroyed. B and C, Almost total collagenization of the funiculi in isolated traumatic ischaemia of the median nerve. (Reproduced by kind permission from *Br. J. Surg.*, 1945, **32**, 389.)

chapter (p. 109). This fibrosis may hinder recovery that would otherwise have occurred spontaneously and justify an operation—neurolysis—for liberation of the nerve. Yet an operation done with this end in view may, if it is thorough enough, disclose that a short segment of the nerve is in fact totally ischaemic, that nothing short of excision and replacement of it by a graft will suffice and that the supposed compression by fibrotic muscle was inoperative. One final point in this venerable debate; an unusual injury (Seddon and Holmes, 1945; Fig. **6**, 8: Malt and McKhann, 1964; Fig. **6**, 9) may destroy the blood supply of a nerve without seriously upsetting that of the surrounding muscle. The nerve then exhibits the characteristic histological features of ischaemia (Fig. **6**, 8B) without there being any element whatever of compression by the surrounding muscles.

Mild ischaemia. Allbrook and Aitken (1951) have shown that in very mild ischaemia of muscle, the nerve fibres and motor end-plates within it degenerate and then, as the muscle

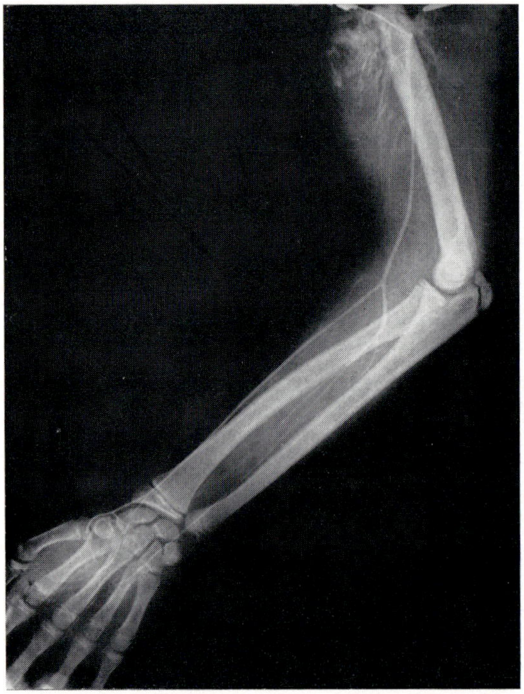

FIG. **6**, 9. An arteriogram of the first upper limb to be successfully re-attached. It will be observed that there is no filling of the profunda artery. It was subsequently found that the radial nerve had shrunk to one-fifth of its proper diameter. This must have been due to ischaemia consequent on the blockage of the profunda artery. The overlying muscle was not ischaemic. (Reproduced by kind permission from Malt, R. A. and McKhann, C. F., 1964, *J. Am. med. Ass.*, **189**, 716.)

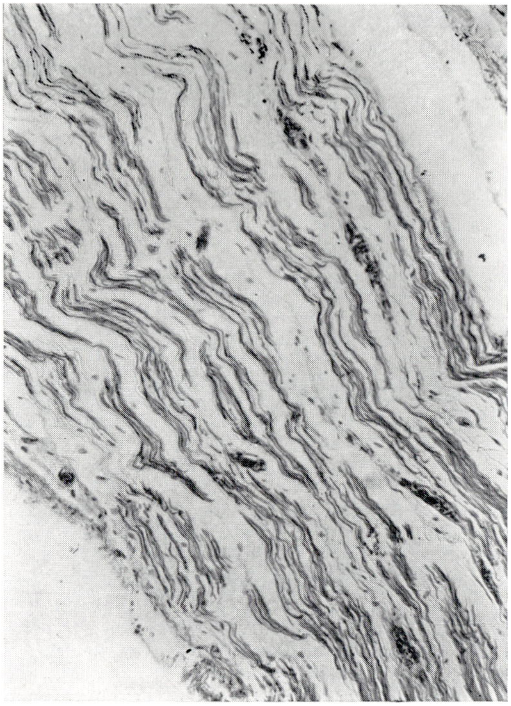

FIG. **6**, 10. Regenerating nerve fibres in an ischaemic branch of the ulnar nerve.

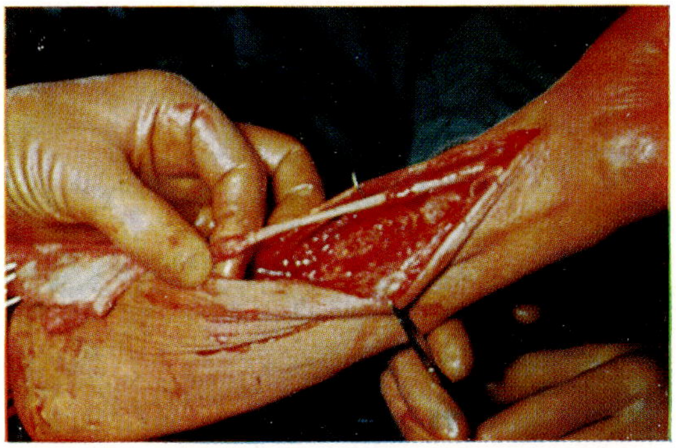

FIG. **6**, 11. A shrunken ischaemic segment of the median nerve.

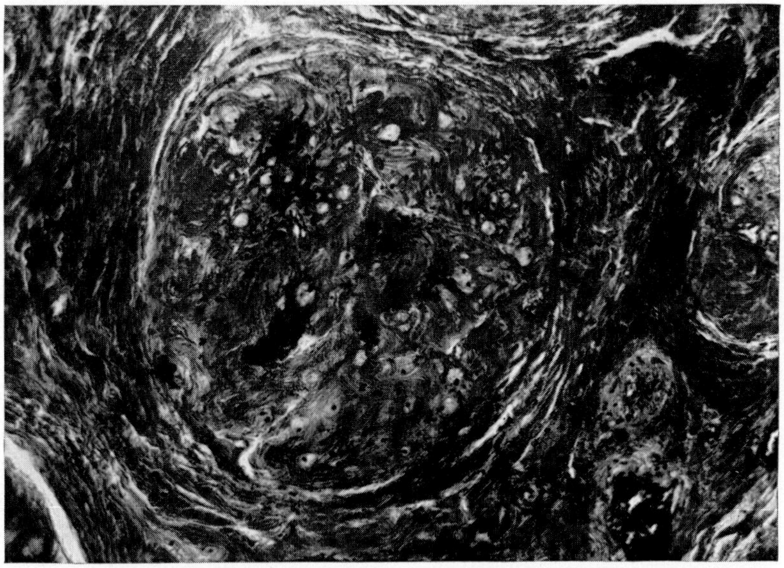

FIG. 6, 12. Section of an ischaemic nerve, not subject to compression, showing ubiquitous collagenization.

recovers, regenerate though not with entirely normal end-plates. Clark and Blomfield (1945) showed that devascularization sufficient to produce disintegration of the muscle fibres might be followed by regeneration of the muscle with the return of good contractility. The state of the nerves was not described, but in the course of similar experiments Allbrook and Aitken found new axons growing into the highly cellular tissue between the regenerating muscle fibres and, ultimately, regeneration of motor end-plates. They noticed that the pattern of innervation was abnormal, this being due, at least in part, to the deposits of collagen between the muscle fibres, the fibrous tissue that produces the contracture of an ischaemic muscle that has regained its contractility.

These experimental findings probably explain what happens in mild ischaemia in patients. I once had the opportunity (Seddon, 1956) of following recovery in a totally paralysed ischaemic forearm; the child ultimately regained almost full voluntary power, and sensibility that was apparently normal. Yet in spite of corrective splinting he developed a contracture that had to be corrected. Opportunities for carrying out biopsies are rare, but one example is shown in Figure **6**, 10 which illustrates the state of a nerve at the periphery of an infarct so ischaemic that it had to be excised.

On account of the capacity of ischaemic muscle and nerve to regenerate, time for this to take place must be allowed before any radical surgical treatment is carried out.

Severe ischaemia.[1] If the nerve runs through an infarct that has a small patch of necrosis at its centre the nerve is narrowed where it traverses the totally ischaemic part, its diameter being one-half of normal or even less. This attenuated reach of the nerve has a dirty yellow colour (Fig. **6,** 11); when examined with the aid of magnifying spectacles it is not possible to detect any epineurial blood vessels and if this abnormal part of the nerve is cut across no funiculi are detectable. Histological examination reveals intense collagenization of the funiculi and of the supporting tissues (Fig. **6,** 12). That this intense fibrosis can occur at all is an indication that some revascularization has occurred; but the barrier to regeneration is complete.

Extensive necrosis.[1] A nerve passing through the centre of a large necrotic infarct is as dead

[1] For a more detailed account see Holmes, Highet and Seddon, 1944.

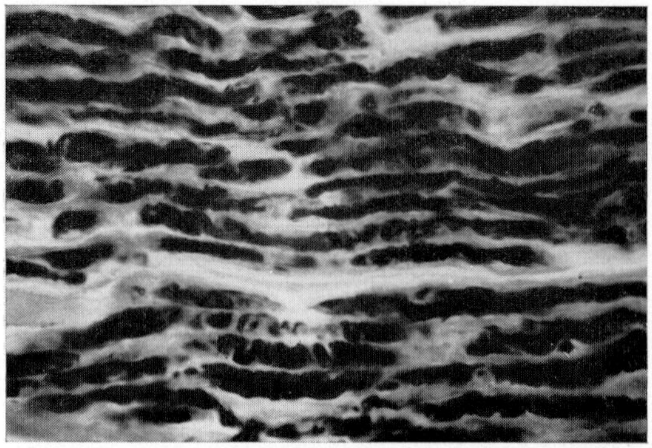

FIG. **6**, 13. Necrotic nerve in Volkmann's ischaemia. The myelin has broken up, but it is still present 6 months after the accident. All cellular elements have disappeared: no phagocytosis. This is death of a nerve, not degeneration. (By courtesy of Dr William Holmes.)

as the surrounding muscle. It does not shrink, there has not even been any reactive fibrosis, the myelin is still *in situ*, though fragmented, and only the Schwann nuclei have disappeared (Fig. **6**, 13).

Clinical Picture

When more or less acute ischaemia of a limb occurs, its paralytic manifestations are due to ischaemia of muscle and to ischaemia of nerve, which for a time cannot be differentiated. Even when nothing is done to relieve the ischaemia, regeneration of the nerves may occur, though sometimes imperfectly, in the absence of recovery in the ischaemic muscle. So if a patient is seen early there will be clear evidence of nerve involvement, whereas if he is seen for the first time many months after the event there may be no sign whatever of neurological abnormality. This is important in the management of established ischaemia (p. 103).

Arterial Embolism

Although this is a rare cause of acute ischaemia it is necessary to deal with it first because Jefferson's (1934) pain, pallor, paralysis and pulselessness have been too readily regarded as the characteristic signs of acute ischaemia, irrespective of the cause. What Jefferson described was the effect of the sudden complete blockage of main arteries, a sizable embolus being held up at a bifurcation. If these four signs were always present in the more common Volkmann's ischaemia due to a fracture it is hardly credible that it could ever escape recognition. The fact, attested by more than 50 cases, is that this unhappy accident occurs, though very rarely, in well-organized departments. Sometimes it is averted by prompt intervention; sometimes it is not, because the observer was not confronted with unequivocal evidence of vascular obstruction.

Severance of a Main Artery, With or Without Ligation

The consequences of this type of ischaemia were first described by Tinel (1917). There is severe pain, and with it a hypersensitivity to cutaneous stimuli which may change to total insensibility. In the upper limb the area of sensory disturbance is like a glove, and it may extend as high as the elbow; in the lower limb its upper limit may be anywhere between the ankle and the knee. There is no correspondence with the distribution of nerves, and the degree of sensory involvement is likely to be greatest peripherally. The ischaemic part is cold, bluish or reddish—not pallid—and all the soft parts are swollen. There may be partial or complete motor paralysis. The pulse cannot be felt. This is not a very different picture from that seen after arterial embolism but it is slightly less dramatic, perhaps because some circulation of blood has persisted through the collateral vessels, whereas in embolism (Griffiths, 1940) they are blocked. The signs of ischaemia may not come on until a few days after the injury (Richards, M.R.C.R., 1954), and in these cases it has been found that an aneurysm was developing or there was spreading arterial thrombosis.

Ischaemia associated with Fractures

This is the well-known and justly dreaded Volkmann's ischaemia of civilian practice. The distribution of fractures in 56 cases is shown in Table VIII. The supracondylar fracture of the humerus in a child, often with severe displacement (Fig. **6**, 14), is by far the commonest cause. In 38 of these cases the notes that accompanied the patient were very complete and from them a number of significant facts emerged.

TABLE VIII—Fractures causing Volkmann's ischaemia

Upper limb:	
Humerus, upper third	1
Humerus, supracondylar	25
Elbow, fracture-dislocation	4
Radius and ulna, including one post-operative case (plating)	13
Lower limb:	
Femur, mid-shaft	1
Femur, lower third	1
Knee, dislocation or fracture-dislocation	4
Tibia and fibula, including two cases of bone shortening and one osteotomy	7

Pain. In only a minority of cases was there a complaint of more pain than could reasonably be attributed to the fracture, though perhaps more care might have been taken in determining the site of the pain and whether there had been any change in its character.

Colour changes. There was pallor or cyanosis in only a minority.

Pulse. In only eight of the well-documented cases in the upper limb was the pulse recorded as having been absent. But it is probable that insufficient attention was paid to diminution of the pulse; Griffiths, with a wide experience of impending ischaemia, regards this as the only reliable warning sign and in itself a clear indication for exploration.

Paralysis. This was by far the most frequent manifestation of ischaemia, depression of sensibility (a certain indication of nerve involvement) and reduction or loss of voluntary power.

Another disturbing feature was that there might be no signs of ischaemia whatever until the third day. Thus the ischaemia associated with fractures—which, as Griffiths (1940) showed, is usually due to mural damage of the artery leading to spasm of the vessel which may extend over a considerable distance—can be considerably less dramatic than the ischaemia caused by a major arterial injury or by arterial embolism. The consequent infarction may be anything but massive and it is difficult to detect impending ischaemia in only two or three muscles. An indication of this is pain on passive extension of the digits. Griffiths thinks that this indicates that the damage is already done, and relies on observation of the pulse and on oscillometry. Yet this painful limitation of movement may be no more than a sign that the muscle is beginning to swell; and it is certainly not too late to save the situation by prompt operation.

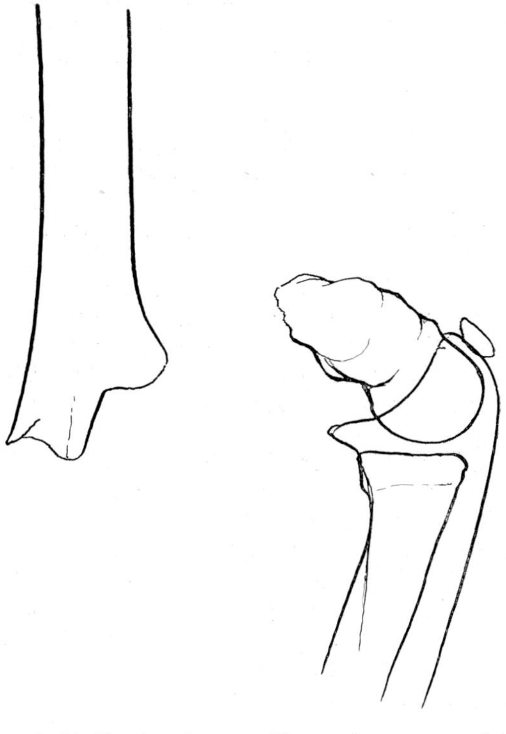

FIG. **6**, 14. Tracing from an X-ray of a supracondylar fracture with gross displacement. There is a great danger of injury to the brachial artery—present in this case—and also of *direct* injury to one or more nerves as well. Early open intervention is imperative.

Prevention

The chief cause of Volkmann's ischaemia in ordinary practice is fracture of a bone. Very few fractures threaten the circulation; even the notorious supracondylar fracture of the humerus in a child is only an occasional offender. But, if something does go wrong it may not be immediate; the onset of circulatory embarrassment can be delayed for as long as 72 hours and the signs of it are not always obvious. By contrast a wound of a major blood vessel, a war injury, is a matter of the utmost urgency. Saving a patient's life and saving his limb engage the surgeon's instant attention. If the circulation in the limb is embarrassed the signs of it are more immediate and more obvious. An emergency operation is imperative, nowadays repair of the vessel rather than simple ligation. The necessary degree of alertness is there from the start.

But in the treatment of a fracture, although the threat of vascular complications is there, it is in the background: attention is focussed on the fracture. Ischaemia can, so to speak, creep up from behind.

The question, still far from being settled, is: what are the early and reliable signs of impending ischaemia? Pallor and paralysis are undoubtedly late signs. Griffiths pins his faith on diminution of the pulse: others on painful resistance to stretching of the long flexors of the digits or, if the hand alone is threatened, of the intrinsic muscles.

In all well-ordered communities everyone now avoids tight external splints, or plaster-of-Paris that has not been split. Acute flexion of the elbow after reduction of a supracondylar fracture has gone too.

Unless some simple manoeuvre, namely a change of position or even abandonment of reduction of the fracture, quickly abolishes the signs of ischaemia, the site of fracture, which is the site of possible vascular damage, must be explored without delay. The characteristic lesion is a bruising of the artery; what cannot be seen is the intramural haematoma or rupture of the internal elastic lamina it produces. The artery is in spasm—contracted down and pulseless— over a greater or lesser distance. It is imperative to make an extensive incision through the deep fascia over the threatened muscles; impending ischaemia causes them to swell, often to such an extent that at the end of the operation it is found impossible to close the skin. Benjamin (1957) found that this decompression alone sometimes sufficed, though why this should be so is a mystery.

Kinmonth (1952), Kinmonth and Simeone (1952) and Kinmonth, Hadfield, Connolly, Lee and Amoroso (1956) have found that the only drug that may relieve arterial spasm—this is when the fascial incision has been unavailing— is papaverine, and wherever emergency surgery is performed a supply of it ought always to be available. Yet Kinmonth *et al.* (1956) reported only two cases of impending Volkmann's ischaemia in which the drug seemed to be valuable, and I have records of four in which it proved ineffective. Volkmann's ischaemia is different from embolic ischaemia in being due to an intrinsic—intimal—lesion of the artery. Whatever the mechanism that initiates the spasm of the vessel it is persistent. However, Kinmonth makes the point that because the spasm is myogenic, time must be allowed for the papaverine to soak into the artery; he has found that the thicker the wall of the vessel the longer the time required for the drug to act on it. Yet I cannot help wondering whether patience of the order of at least 20 minutes may be out of place when distal thrombosis can occur so easily and spread so rapidly.

Let us suppose that everything has failed: incision of the deep fascia, the application of warm normal saline solution to the artery, and bathing it with 2·5 per cent papaverine: what further steps can be taken? Sympathetic block is useless; it is worse than that, it is harmful because it wastes time. The contused segment of the artery should be excised. The effect may be dramatic; the spasm suddenly disappears proximally and the artery gushes blood. The distal end may do the same, but here a clot may be found in the mouth of the vessel; it may be possible to pull it out very gently with fine forceps or suck it out with a catheter. Then if there is another gush of bright blood the distal end may safely be tied. Finally, the neighbouring nerves are examined; the median in particular may have suffered direct damage.

With major vessels arterial repair is pretty well obligatory, but I have had the melancholy experience of assisting at an operation for rupture of the popliteal artery in the region of the knee, caused by a fracture, the diagnosis of ischaemia having been made very speedily, and at the end of it the circulation in the foot failed to return on account of distal thrombosis which had occurred with great rapidity.

Established Ischaemia

In the fully established condition there is nothing distinctive about the clinical features of the nerve involvement. The paralysis may be incomplete and transient; it may be complete, with total median and ulnar paralysis in the hand and perhaps even loss of sensibility in the superficial radial area too. The loss of sensibility in the forearm usually clears up rapidly, so that what remains corresponds with the distribution of one or more nerves. Although the damage to the nerves in the forearm is ischaemic, the parts distal to the ischaemic segments show ordinary Wallerian degeneration, and the muscles supplied by them the atrophy of denervation, not the fibrosis of ischaemia. They respond to electrical stimuli of long duration—the reaction of degeneration—whereas ischaemic muscle is inexcitable, unless there is only moderate fibrosis and the muscle fibres have not been destroyed. In the latter case, after some contractility of the muscle has returned, the strength-duration curve is of normal form but with a very high threshold (Fig. **4**, 2, p. 58).

If the ischaemic muscle is recovering, the nerve damage will not have been serious and spontaneous recovery is, in fact, likely to be ahead of that in the muscle. So in the category of muscle damage described as *mild* in Figure **6**, 6 (p. 96) there is no need for concern about the state of the nerves. The only condition that may require surgical treatment is the residual contracture which, in the forearm, is best dealt with by a muscle-slide operation (Seddon, 1964).

In the rare *localized* variety of ischaemia the infarction is none the less intense, and the appropriate treatment is excision of the affected muscle. In the forearm the distal parts of the deep muscles, flexor pollicis longus and flexor digitorum profundus (and perhaps the whole of the pronator quadratus) are destroyed. The operation affords an opportunity of inspecting the adjoining nerve trunk; but, as Fig. **6,** 6 shows, the need for repair is infrequent.

This raises the question of *how to decide that ischaemic nerve requires repair*.

If clinical examination reveals incomplete paralysis there is a strong probability that good recovery will follow. If it does not, if over a period of say 2 months there is no improvement, then it is probable that there is some hindrance and the nerve should be explored in the course of whatever operation may be needed for the damaged muscles. The need for this is rare; in the example of roller injury described on page 109 the median nerve was compressed by fibrotic muscle. In two other cases of mild ischaemia—one in the forearm, the other in the leg—the median and posterior tibial nerves respectively were found to be running through a small patch of necrosis affecting contiguous muscles; removal of the dead muscle was followed by recovery in the nerve.

If electromyographic examination of the muscles supplied by the affected nerve reveals motor-unit action-potentials it is safe to wait; the prospect of recovery is very good. If there is no response the nerve must be explored. This is likely to be necessary in all cases of *severe* ischaemia (Fig. **6**, 6); the proportion of cases in which spontaneous recovery occurs is small. When it has been decided that the flexor muscles in the forearm are so completely destroyed that they should be excised, exploration of the nerves, the median and the ulnar, is the first step in this operation.

Griffiths (personal communication) believes that in children the ischaemic nerves always recover sooner or later. In my series, in which there was a high proportion of cases of great severity, this was not so. In two patients, one 2 years old, the other 8, at the time of injury there was no recovery in the nerves 11 and 12 years later, respectively. In another child, aged 5, the median nerve had sloughed over a length of several centimetres. Repair of a nerve was carried out in patients in the following age-groups: 0 to 5 years—4; 6 to 10 years—4; 11 to 15 years—3; 20 to 35 years—2. In all cases histological examination of the excised segment showed irreparable damage.

Technique of Excision of the Infarct and Repair of the Nerves

A bloodless field. This operation should be undertaken at about 6 months from the time of injury, though as early as 4 months if it is certain that the forearm flexors are totally destroyed. Even in a bloodless field it is often difficult to trace the median nerve through the infarct; unless the circulation is arrested it is well-nigh impossible and most hazardous. So a compression bag must be used and the dissection of the nerves (the ulnar, lying on the periphery of the infarct, is easy to identify) can be completed in 40 minutes.

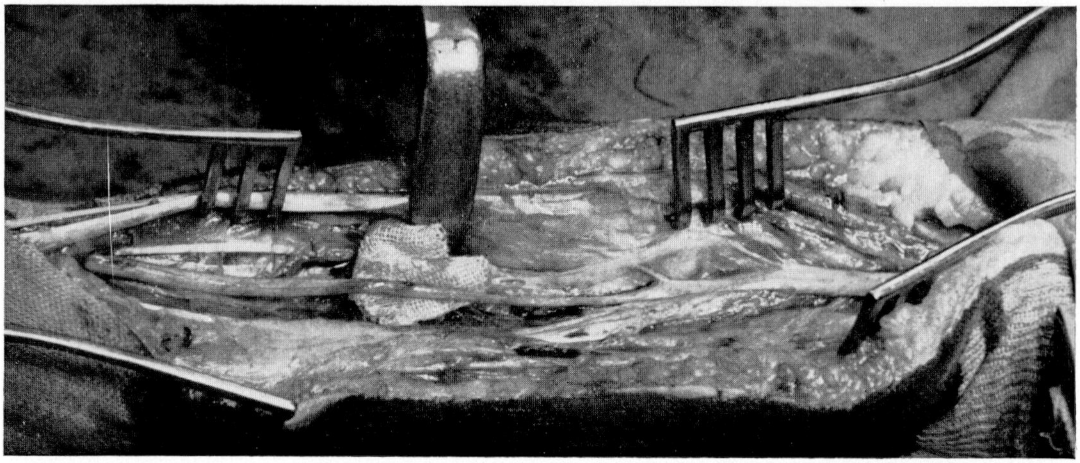

FIG. **6**, 15. The median nerve. The proximal part, on the right, gradually tapers to about a quarter of its proper diameter. Then, distal to the small swab, it enlarges. The narrow part is irreparably damaged. Treated successfully by nerve-pedicle grafting. (This figure and Figs **6**, 17, **6**, 18, **6**, 22 and **6**, 23 reproduced by kind permission from *J. Bone Jt Surg.*, 1956, **38B**, 152.)

The incision and exposure of the nerves. The longitudinal incision begins a little above the bend of the elbow and ends at the wrist. The two nerves are exposed proximally and distally in normal surroundings. They are stimulated electrically, even though the EMG may have been negative. If there is a positive response in the muscles of the hand the nerves will recover; dissecting out the nerves will then be necessary only to permit excision of the infarct. If some of the forearm muscles contract on excitation they will be conserved, and the excision will be limited to those muscles that are irresponsive. The nerves are traced towards the ischaemic region. This means cutting through the common flexor mass to expose the median nerve, and this should be done without hesitation if stimulation of the nerve has provoked no response in any of the forearm muscles it supplies. If, however, stimulation has provoked a moderate contraction in the superficial muscles, which are those likely to be the least affected, they should be elevated and retracted while the median nerve is being traced from above and from below into the fibrotic or necrotic deep muscles. Branches of the median nerve that enter muscles that are completely destroyed are severed but, for reasons that will be given in a moment, the leash of branches that includes the anterior interosseous nerve should be cut close to the muscle so that it forms a long tag. When the median nerve has been exposed from end to end it should be inspected (Fig. **6**, 15 and Fig. **6**, 11, p. 98). At this point the pressure bag is released so that the vascularity of the nerve can be observed. Distal to the ischaemic region it will have the greyish-pink colour of degenerate nerve. This appearance may be present throughout the ischaemic region with no reduction in the calibre of the nerve or change in its consistence. The nerve should then be left alone because, after removal of the ischaemic muscles, it will recover. On the other hand, if the nerve is narrowed, has the colour of ivory, is perhaps a little firmer than normal, and shows no blood vessels whatever when examined with magnifying spectacles it is so ischaemic that no recovery will be possible. The ischaemic reach of the nerve is always much

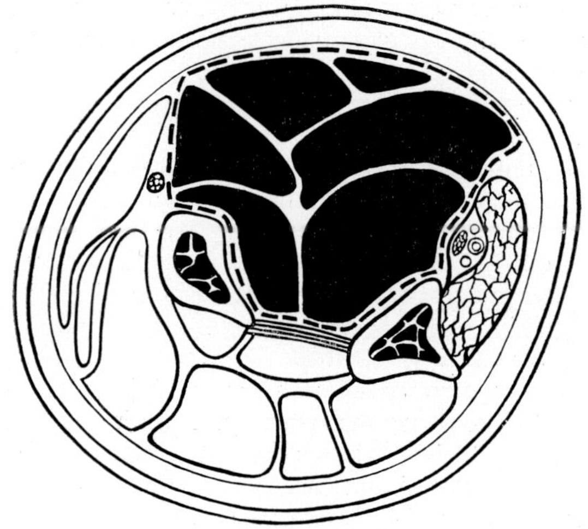

FIG. 6, 16. Excision of an infarct in the forearm with conservation of flexor carpi ulnaris, the ulnar vessels and, in this case, the ulnar nerve. (This figure and Fig. **6**, 19 reproduced by kind permission from *Rev. Orthop.*, 1960, **46**, 149.)

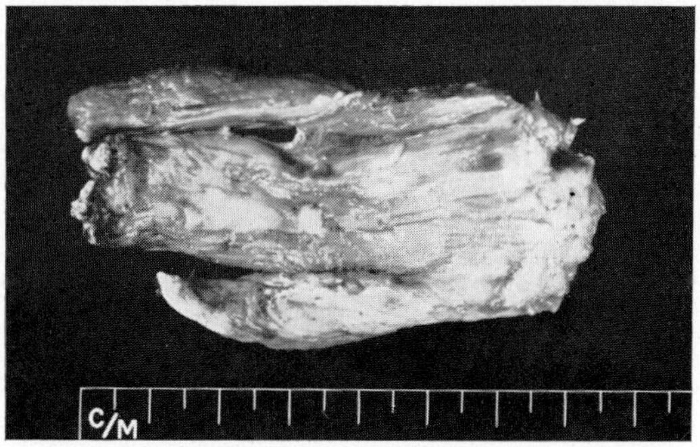

FIG. **6**, 17. An excised infarct.

less extensive that the ischaemia of the surrounding muscles; in the upper limb it has always been possible to repair the gap by grafting after resection of the nerve back to easily visible bundles with mobile epineurium around them. Total necrosis of a main nerve trunk without shrinkage is seen only when the necrosis of muscle is so extensive that the limb must be amputated.

The ulnar nerve is exposed by turning flexor carpi ulnaris medially, care being taken to conserve the ulnar vessels which may be patent. The vascularity of the hand may depend chiefly on them. The ulnar nerve is inspected in the same way as the median; if neither shows an ischaemic segment the ischaemic muscle may then be excised without further ado.

Excision of the infarct. The muscle mass is cut across transversely at the upper and lower limits of the ischaemia except for flexor carpi ulnaris which, whatever its state, is conserved (Fig. **6**, 16). Removal of this muscle carries too great a risk of injury to the ulnar vessels; if it is shortened its tendon can be severed just proximal to the pisiform bone, though if it is active a step-cut lengthening is performed. The state of pronator quadratus should be ascertained. If, as is likely, it is ischaemic it should be removed because it is chiefly responsible for the pronation component of the contracture. The muscle mass (Fig. **6**, 17) is gradually elevated from the radius, the interosseous membrane and the ulna, and at the finish the front of the forearm is left with no more than

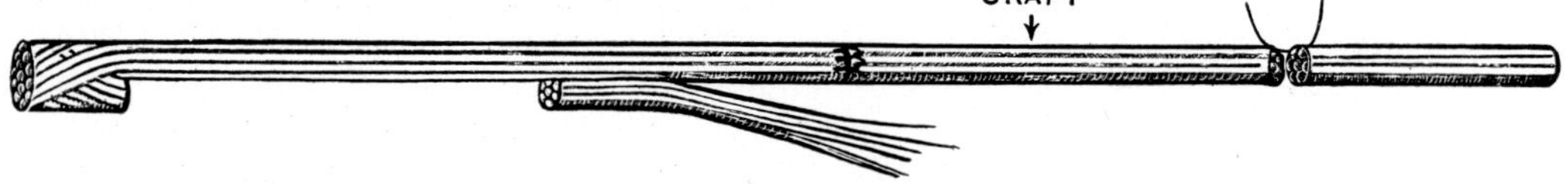

FIG. **6**, 18. A method of autologous grafting that can be used for repair of the ischaemic median nerve in the forearm. Because the flexor muscles have been destroyed by the ischaemia the motor division of the nerve is useless. It can therefore be stripped proximally until the intraneural plexus is encountered, and used as a graft.

the two nerve trunks, the flexor carpi ulnaris, the ulnar vessels and the stumps of the flexor tendons where they lie proximal to the wrist. If some of the superficial muscles have escaped damage they will have been conserved with their nerve supply; but their tendons will need lengthening.

Repair of the median nerve alone. The median nerve has been found ischaemic, but the ulnar presenting an appearance compatible with spontaneous recovery. The motor half of the median nerve is always proximal to the ischaemic segment; it is functionless because the muscles it supplies have been destroyed and have been removed. This leash of motor branches is dissected free from the part of the nerve supplying the hand, and this splitting of the nerve into two can be continued proximally above the bend of the elbow until an intraneural plexus arrests further progress. The free graft obtained in this way (Fig. **6**, 18) is long enough, after trimming of its distal end, to bridge the gap in the median nerve, though to avoid tension and to allow for shrinkage of the graft (p. 294) it may be necessary to bend the elbow to facilitate suture, which is carried out after all oozing from the large raw area has been arrested.

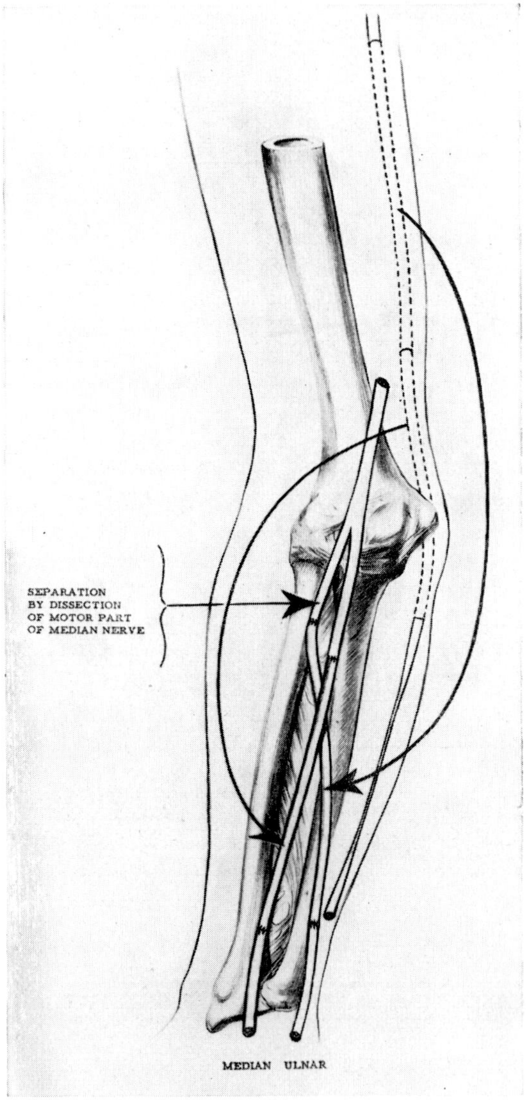

FIG. **6**, 19. A method for restoring innervation of all the intrinsic muscles of the hand in severe Volkmann's ischaemia.

Ischaemia of both median and ulnar nerves. The simplest remedy is to sacrifice the ulnar nerve for the sake of the median by means of Strange's (1947, 1950) nerve-pedicle operation (Fig. **16**, 9, p. 292). The ulnar paralysis is irremediable because such extensor muscles as are available for transplantation are required for the restoration of flexion in the digits. On two occasions, therefore, the operation illustrated in Figure **6**, 19 was employed. Two free grafts are taken from the ulnar nerve, which means exposing it almost up to the axilla; one is used to bridge the gap in the median nerve, the other to unite the useless motor division of the nerve (which lies above the ischaemic region) to the distal part of the ulnar nerve. It was gratifying to find that both children regained useful action in the ulnar intrinsic muscles sufficient to prevent clawing of the fingers, and to give a mass contraction of the interossei which enabled the patient to use the hand for coarse gripping.

Subsequent reconstruction. The extensor muscles will have been on the stretch as a result of the flexion contracture; time must be allowed for them to recover their normal length and greater power. After an interval of 2 or 3 months, when the forearm and hand are supple, one of the extensor muscles of the wrist, the short radial extensor for choice if it is powerful enough, is transplanted into flexor digitorum profundus, the tendons of flexor digitorum superficialis being pulled proximally and cut short. It may be possible to transplant an extensor muscle into flexor pollicis longus, but this has been abandoned because, after recovery of the thenar muscles, patients are well content with opposition without ability to flex the terminal joint of the thumb.

Instability of the wrist is sometimes a nuisance. It may be necessary to conclude the programme of operations with an arthrodesis of the joint.

Results. The results of the nerve operations (Seddon, 1964) are summarized in Table IX.

Volkmann's Ischaemia in the Lower Limb

Eighteen cases of Volkmann's ischaemia in the leg have come to my attention, and Table X shows that there was ischaemic nerve damage in 13 of them.

In four cases both divisions of the sciatic nerve had been damaged by traction, as a result of fracture of the lower end of the femur or dislocation of the knee (Figs **6**, 20 and **6**, 21). In one it was proved, and in the other three cases suspected, that there was ischaemia of the nerves at a lower level. It must be conceded that the patients were selected, but they were sent on account of the ischaemia, not because their nerves were affected. Even so, ischaemic nerve damage is a frequent, perhaps invariable, and extremely serious concomitant of ischaemia below the knee.

Another disturbing feature was the incidence of persistent pain; it was present in six of the 18 cases. This was not encountered in established ischaemia of the upper limb except in one case due to the hypoxia of barbiturate poisoning. The pain may be deep-seated, constant and burning, or it may be felt only when the foot is handled or comes in contact with the ground, then resembling the over-reaction sometimes seen after ordinary injuries of the sciatic nerve if they

TABLE IX—Nerve grafting in Volkmann's ischaemia of the forearm

	TOTAL	SENSORY RECOVERY	MOTOR RECOVERY
Median to median:			
children	5	4	4
adults	2	1	0
Ulnar to median nerve-pedicle graft			
children	6	6	4
adults	3	2	1
Ulnar to median and ulnar			
children	2	2	2

TABLE X—Ischaemic nerve involvement in the lower limb

NO INVOLVEMENT when first seen—1

ISCHAEMIA

	Common peroneal	Tibial	Both
Recovery	—	2	2
Partial recovery	—	1	1
No recovery	2	—	3
Too early to assess	—	—	1
Unknown	—	—	1

TRACTION INJURIES: all in severe damage to the knee—4

are partial, or in process of recovery after suture. One patient complained so bitterly that the pain was the chief factor determining amputation of the leg, after which it ceased completely.

Surgical exploration and dissection of amputation specimens shows that the extent of the damage is often considerably greater than in the upper limb. Moreover, the pattern of infarction is less regular (Seddon, 1966). After injury of the femoral or popliteal artery there is usually a clearly circumscribed ellipsoidal infarct situated distally rather than proximally in the leg. But when the injury is below the knee the distribution of the ischaemia is variable.

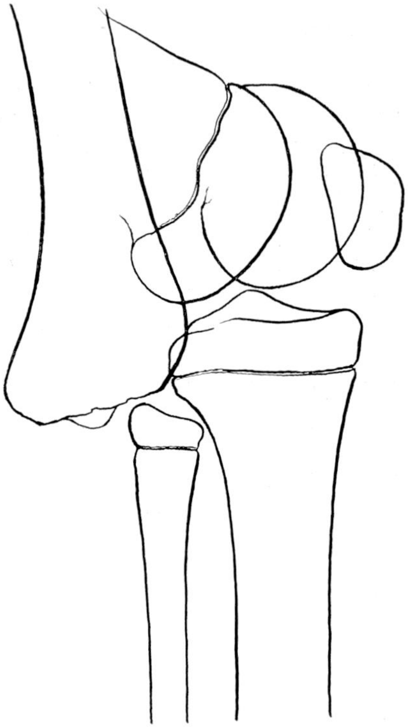

FIG. **6**, 20. A supracondylar fracture of the femur. Traction injuries of both divisions of the sciatic nerve: ischaemia of the calf and probably of the nerves.

It has not yet been possible to deal with the muscle and nerve damage systematically, as in the forearm. No nerve has been repaired by autologous grafting. It is doubtful whether such an operation would be worth while even if technically feasible; the results of ordinary suture of the posterior tibial nerve are discouraging (p. 227).

Treatment is usually limited to excision of the muscle that has been destroyed (Fig. **6**, 23), which permits correction of the contracture; though sometimes there must also be an extensive dissection at the back of the ankle to remove the scar tissue that may be the final hindrance to correction of the equino-varus deformity. In the course of this dissection the posterior tibial nerve is liberated and this may be followed by return of good sensibility in the sole of the foot. I am not convinced that the intrinsic muscles of the sole ever recover.

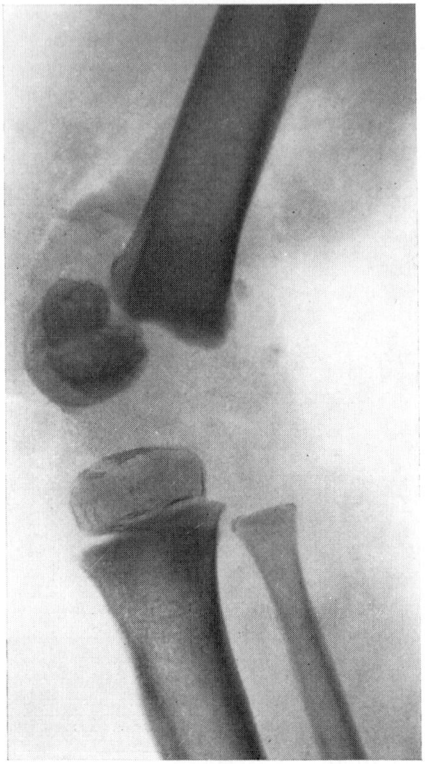

FIG. **6**, 21. Open separation of the lower femoral epiphysis. The popliteal artery was damaged; there was total ischaemic paralysis below the knee.

THE COMBINATION OF DIRECT NERVE INJURY AND ISCHAEMIC DAMAGE

An example of this has just been given; the cases of severe injury of the knee in which both divisions of the sciatic nerve were damaged by traction and there was ischaemia of the leg affecting the nerves more distally. Similar combinations are more common in the upper limb because the nerves, especially the median, run with the main blood vessels over a considerable distance.

In established ischaemia this state of affairs cannot be distinguished from an uncomplicated ischaemic lesion unless, in the course of electrical examination RD is discovered in the muscles *proximal to the ischaemic part*. Otherwise the only safe rule is to include the level of damage of the artery in any operative exposure that may be undertaken: this is pretty well obligatory anyway because the nerve or nerves must be identified proximally before they can be traced through the anatomically deranged ischaemic part.

From this it follows that the examination of any patient with an ischaemic upper limb in which there is involvement of peripheral nerves must be most searching and should invariably include electrical excitation of the muscles. Electromyography is unlikely to be helpful.

The best policy is to avoid these embarrassments by extremely early exploration. As Lipscomb and Burleson (1955) and Ottolenghi (1961) have pointed out, it is not uncommon, in supracondylar fractures in children that have caused vascular obstruction, to find that the median nerve as well as the brachial artery has been damaged, even trapped, by the broken bone.

Ischaemia due to Anoxia caused by Poisoning

It was known during the Napoleonic wars (Larrey, 1812) that in persons asphyxiated by carbon monoxide, tissue necrosis or something just short of it was liable to occur in parts of the body subjected to pressure. Several cases have been described more recently, notably by Gunther (1921, 1940) and I have encountered two. Very similar lesions have been described in other forms of intoxication that cause hypoxia: alcohol, alcohol and hypnotics, or hypnotics alone (Jasiński and Brütsch, 1952; Touzé and Thierry, 1952; Fahlgren, Hed and Lundmark, 1957) and I have seen two such cases myself. The stories of these four patients have been given together (Howse and Seddon, 1966). What happens is that the hypoxia resulting from these various forms of intoxication is such that, although the body as a whole may suffer no permanent damage, pressures that would be normal and tolerable in a healthy person—such as are sustained by the upper limb in someone lying on his side on the floor—tip the balance against the survival of the compressed tissues.

The relevant interest of this condition is that if (as in our four patients) the forearm is affected, the resultant damage is indistinguishable from ordinary Volkmann's ischaemia. The nerves may be involved in exactly the same way and exhibit the characteristic histological features. In none of our cases was the ischaemia of a degree sufficient to prevent spontaneous regeneration in the nerves; all that was required was appropriate treatment of the affected muscles.

Crush Injuries causing Ischaemia

If a limb is caught in machinery almost anything can happen; and injuries caused by short but intense, or by prolonged compression between hard objects such as pieces of masonry or, as in one of our cases, metal plates can seriously damage muscle and nerve. The damage may be direct, it may be ischaemic, or a combination of the two.

It is necessary to carry out an early and extremely thorough operation with exposure of the whole of the damaged area. This is best illustrated by reference to two such cases.

A man aged 33 years caught his right upper limb between the belt and roller of a machine. There was a wound 7·5 cm long on the medial side of the forearm near the elbow and a shorter one behind the olecranon. Pulsation was palpable in the brachial artery but not at the wrist. There was total loss of sensibility in the median area and diminished sensibility in the radial and ulnar areas. The hand was cool but its colour was normal; he complained of pain in the forearm which was swollen.

At operation the brachial artery was found ruptured at the elbow and its ends were ligated. The median and radial nerves were in continuity though the epineurium had been stripped from them over a length of about 5 cm. All soft tissues apart from the nerves had been severed down to the capsule of the elbow. A long incision was made through the skin and deep fascia from the cubital fossa to the middle of the forearm to relieve tension and 7 days later the gaping area was skin grafted.

Two months later the hand was swollen and there

was complete radial paralysis and paralysis of all muscles in the hand with total loss of sensibility in median, ulnar and radial areas.

Three months after the accident the oedema of the hand had almost gone but there was firmness of the forearm muscles both dorsally and ventrally.

Seven months after the accident, there being no further improvement, the forearm was explored. The pronator teres was shrunken to about a quarter of its normal size, consisting mostly of fibrous tissue with a few streaks of pale muscle. The other muscles looked fairly normal though a little pallid; there was no sign of necrosis. Pronator teres formed a tight band over the median nerve, liberation of which was a delicate affair. The nerve was found to be compressed over about 3 cm though there was little change in its consistence and its diameter was only slightly reduced; distally the nerve showed the grey appearance characteristic of Wallerian degeneration.

The patient made a complete recovery apart from an insignificant contracture of the forearm muscles.

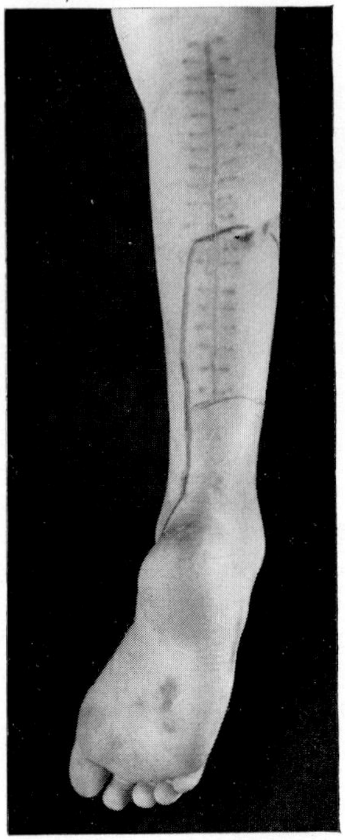

FIG. **6**, 22. The equino-varus deformity is characteristic. The line indicates the area of cutaneous sensory loss. The scar is of the incision made for evacuation of a very large haematoma.

There was a combination of causes of the paralysis in this case: (1) direct injury to the radial and median nerves; (2) almost certainly some degree of ischaemia affecting the median and ulnar nerves and (3) persistence of the median paralysis caused by compression of it by the tight pronator teres.

A boy aged 13 years was trapped beneath a block of concrete that fell on the back of his right calf and cut it. There was great swelling and immediate paralysis of the foot. Three days later and again 17 days later large haematomas were evacuated. When first seen by us 3 months after the accident he presented with an equino-varus deformity, paralysis of all muscles controlling the foot, loss of sensibility as shown in Figure 6, 22 and great induration of the

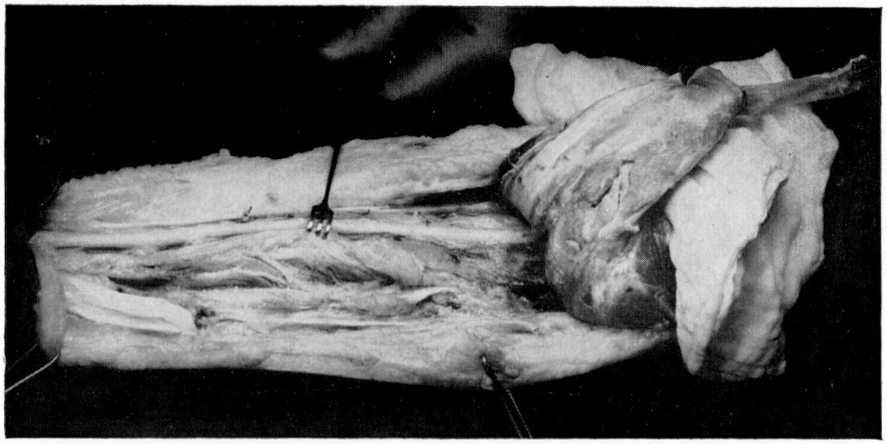

FIG. **6**, 23. The calf muscle was turned proximally and its deep part, the soleus, found to be necrotic, as was the flexor hallucis longus. The ischaemic posterior tibial nerve is beneath the rake retractor, the prongs of which are in the friable dead muscle.

muscles of the leg. At exploration (Fig. 6, 23) the soleus and flexor hallucis longus were found to be necrotic. The posterior tibial nerve may well have been damaged by the crushing blow, though it showed no sign of it; it was affected chiefly by the widespread ischaemia.

Nerve Damage caused by Abnormal Bleeding

In haemophilia and the much less common Christmas disease a large effusion of blood can occur anywhere in the body. If this happens in the neighbourhood of a nerve trunk the haematoma is very likely to cause paralysis. It has been seen a number of times in the iliacus muscle with involvement of the femoral nerve (Seddon, 1930; and see particularly Goodfellow, Fearn and Matthews, 1967) and in the forearm. The iliacus haematoma produces a striking syndrome; acute pain in the hip, restriction of extension of the joint, more or less complete femoral paralysis and, within a short time, an abdominal swelling.

If rest is enforced, which may include immobilization of the affected part, and if appropriate measures are taken to increase the coagulability of the blood (the administration of anti-haemophilic globulin, or of Christmas factor) the haematoma will shrink and the paralysis will usually clear up. But there is one situation—the forearm—in which the greatest vigilance is necessary. An effusion of blood into the flexor muscles of the forearm is very likely to cause median and ulnar paralysis; however, it may also interfere with the blood supply of the forearm muscles to such a degree as to cause ischaemia, which itself may damage the nerves. If there is the slightest suggestion of impending ischaemia the proper treatment is early evacuation of the haematoma, at a centre where facilities for controlling the bleeding are available.

7. Entrapment Neuropathies

WHERE NERVES pass near joints they are at risk not only on account of disorders arising in the joints or from deformity of the bony components but also because it is in these regions that nerves dive beneath tendinous arches from which muscles arise. In recent years the investigation of what are called entrapment neuropathies has become a minor industry (Kopell and Thompson, 1963; Staal, 1970).

The number of disorders seems to be limited only by the number of joints in the body, the nerves that course near them, and the pathological or anatomical disorders capable of upsetting nerves by compression and perhaps by stretching or friction. We are concerned here with a collection of neuropathies of insidious onset, and it is often most difficult to decide at what level an affected nerve is suffering damage. It is in this field particularly that the techniques of electrodiagnosis described in Chapter 4 are so valuable.

These entrapment neuropathies will be described on an anatomical basis, not in the order of their discovery or frequency.

- Pressure at cervico-brachial junction
- Elbow: Ulnar nerve
  - Median and anterior interosseous nerves
  - Radial and posterior interosseous nerves
- Wrist: Median nerve
  - Ulnar nerve
- Meralgia paraesthetica
- Sciatic nerve
- Common peroneal nerve
- Tarsal tunnel syndrome
- Morton's metatarsalgia (plantar digital neuroma)

PRESSURE AT THE CERVICO-BRACHIAL JUNCTION

Of all the disorders that form the subject of this chapter none is more controversial than that which I have followed Telford and Mottershead (1948) in calling pressure at the cervico-brachial junction. There is a variety of names for these conditions which it would be otiose to enumerate, and there is equal variety in the surgical remedies propounded. The heart of the problem is that the subclavian artery and the distal trunk of the brachial plexus emerge into the axilla through the lowest part of what may be a slit, or a triangle with a very small base, that is subject to any number of anatomical variations. The plexus itself may be at fault in being post-fixed.

A number of impressive series of cases have been reported, but none, to my mind, is so informative as Telford's. The conclusions he reached, based on some 40 years' observation, command great respect.

Anatomy. The slit, or triangle with a very narrow base, is bounded anteriorly by the scalenus anterior, posteriorly by scalenus medius and inferiorly by the first rib (Fig. **7**, 1). We will consider first the base of the triangle because it is the most important anatomically and historically the most notable. Above the first rib there may be a cervical rib with the artery and the lowest part of the plexus hitched up over it. Such a rib may be present without causing the patient the slightest trouble, and on the other hand an apparently normal first rib can compress the artery and the lowest trunk of the plexus (Falconer and Li, 1962). In this situation another possible offender appears, the clavicle. Costo-clavicular compression was first described by Eden in 1939 in relation to lesions of the artery; Falconer and Weddell (1943), who coined the actual term, invoked it to explain the nerve lesions. The observations of Telford and Mottershead (1948), both clinical and anatomical, do not support the clavicular component in compression of the plexus—unless there is a cervical rib—and the evidence in favour of it seems chiefly to be that during the course of a decompression operation at the cervico-brachial junction it is possible for the surgeon's index finger to be nipped between the clavicle and the first rib if the shoulder is pressed back hard enough, into an unnatural position which is exactly the reverse of the drooping posture commonly associated with cervico-brachial compression.

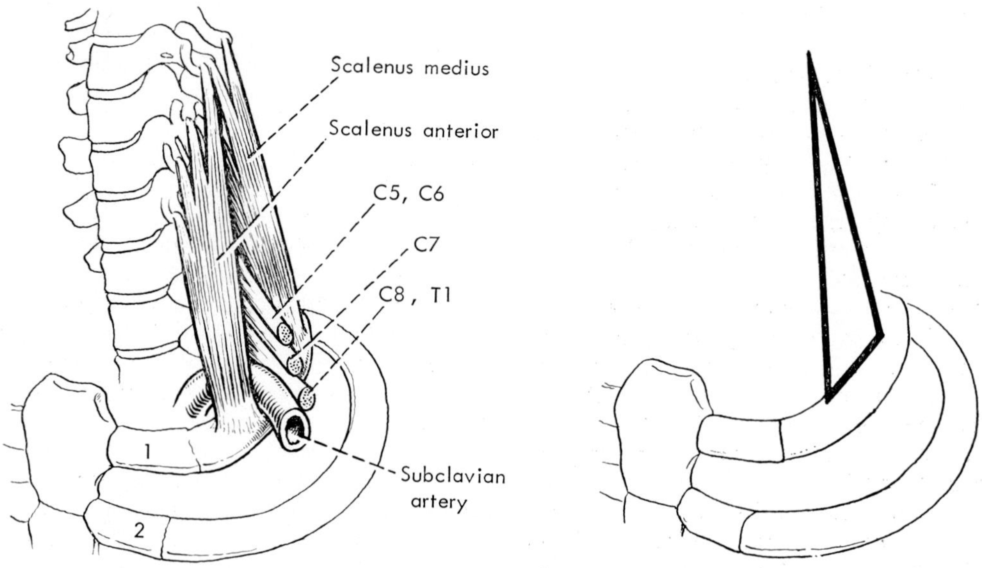

FIG. 7, 1. The cervico-brachial junction.

However, there is no doubt that a cervical rib can cause grave vascular trouble and neurological disturbances. Deformation of the thoracic outlet caused by fractures may affect the plexus (Mulder, Greenwood and Brooks, 1973). So may a tumour, such as a chondroma, but not (Manning, personal communication) cervico-thoracic scoliosis.

The anterior wall of the slit is of particular interest in that a scalenus anterior syndrome has been described. The idea is that either on account of some anatomical abnormality or because of completely unexplained spasm the scalenus anterior compresses the artery and the plexus; and division of its tendon was for a time the sovereign remedy. The spasm may be dismissed as imaginary but purely passive compression can occur occasionally. The scalenus anterior may be excessively tendinous at its lower end, with a falciform postero-lateral margin that kinks the artery and lowest nerve trunk. But the attractive notion that simple division of an anatomically normal scalenus anterior allows the neurovascular bundle to slide downwards and forwards along the first rib, thereby becoming relaxed, is incorrect and this operation is all too often futile. The subclavian artery may appear to pass through the scalenus anterior, the greater part of the muscle being in front of it; the posterior slip, in which there may be tendon, is the scalenus minimus which can compress the plexus but not, being behind it, the artery.

The posterior part of the slit or triangle is formed by scalenus medius. This muscle occasionally encroaches on the neurovascular channel if its insertion into the first rib is unduly broad and tendinous. If there is a cervical rib a sharp fibrous band running downwards and forwards from it to be inserted into the scalene tubercle is very liable to embarrass the plexus (Gilliatt, le Quesne, Logue and Sumner, 1970).

The patients' complaints. There are four kinds of complaint that direct attention to the cervico-brachial junction: pain in the arm, weakness of the hand, vascular symptoms and excessive sweating of the hand. The patients are mostly but by no means all middle-aged.

Pain. This is often continuous but varying in intensity, a grinding ache and sometimes a burning sensation. It may be worse at night; the patient then gets up, waves the arm about, shrugs her shoulders and feels better.

Neurological disturbances. These take the form of numbness and tingling, often predominantly in the ulnar half of the hand, with perhaps wasting and weakness of the intrinsic muscles, the thenar as well as those supplied by the ulnar nerve.

Vascular. Arterial thrombosis is a grave manifestation of cervical rib. There is gradually increasing pallor and coldness of the hand, which if of variable intensity may simulate Raynaud's syndrome. It is uncertain whether the arterial lesion, which may begin as an aneurysm situated distal to the rib, is entirely mechanical in origin or due to some sort of autonomic irritation which must certainly account for the last complaint in this list, namely, hyperidrosis. Whatever doubts there may be about the neural component of cervico-brachial compression there is none whatever about the arterial lesions.

Excessive sweating. As a presenting symptom excessive sweating is rare.

Differential diagnosis. It will be apparent from the above that there are many sources of confusion. At the present time, with the current disillusionment about cervico-brachial compression of the plexus and the equally widespread awareness of compression of the median nerve in the carpal tunnel, there is a tendency to decompress the nerve at the wrist when in fact the fault is in the neck. A complaint of pain in the arm, whether or not accompanied by muscle weakness or a demonstrable disturbance of sensibility, calls for an unusually searching examination of the patient; as does a disorder that is primarily circulatory.

Treatment. Successes have been claimed by the advocates of every form of decompression. The one most widely discredited is tenotomy of the scalenus anterior; the one most generally acceptable is removal of a cervical rib when exposure of the root of the neck reveals the plexus and perhaps the artery too hitched up over it. Removal of the rib can be a most delicate operation.

It seems to me, from limited personal experience, that the only safe approach is to be open-minded. When it has been decided that operation is desirable it should take the form of a thorough exploration of the whole region; and if some obvious source of compression can be found it is dealt with appropriately. It is significant that Telford recorded that in five cases in which no obvious cause of compression was demonstrable the patients' complaints continued.

ENTRAPMENT AT THE ELBOW

Ulnar Nerve

Although this condition was first recognized about 100 years ago its essential features have only recently been elucidated.

The ulnar nerve runs behind the medial epicondyle of the humerus. On its deep surface it is in contact with the medial ligament of the elbow and the medial lip of the trochlear surface of the humerus. It enters a tunnel, the roof of which is formed by the triangular aponeurosis that bridges the two heads of the flexor carpi ulnaris, its base situated proximally being thickened. We may call this transverse thickening a ligament. It is slack in extension; it tightens on flexion, in which position the medial ligament of the elbow tends to bulge.

Anything that distorts the course of the ulnar nerve, subjecting it to compression, may interfere with its function. The simplest example of all is pronounced flexion of the elbow during sleep. Another is pressure on the nerve during the course of operations (Wadsworth and Williams, 1973), which may be avoided either by keeping the elbows moderately flexed over the trunk, or if an arm has to be extended on a board for intravenous infusion keeping it fully supinated so that the olecranon process protects the postcondylar groove from pressure.

Any pathological anomaly of the elbow may distort the bed of the nerve. One of the earliest to be recognized was a fracture in the region of the elbow during childhood resulting in a valgus deformity. The ulnar paresis was customarily described as 'tardy' because it came on many years later. A few patients show what has been described as congenital cubitus valgus with anterior dislocation of the head of the radius; a probable explanation is that these were cases of 'pulled elbow', that is, dislocation of the head of the radius caused by a violent tug on an infant's hand. Wadsworth (1972) has also described injury to the capitular epiphysis leading to deficient development of the trochlea. Other causes are osteoarthritis (Fig. 7, 2), a ganglionic protrusion from the joint (Fig. 7, 3), osteochondromatosis of the elbow or anomalous muscle attachments.

The nerve may be held so loosely in its groove that it slips forward over the medial epicondyle on flexion of the joint though only rarely anterior to it. This can be harmless, but Osborne (1970) considers that if the nerve is enlarged on account of some pathological condition it is further damaged, secondarily, by the tightening of the 'ligament' in flexion. Sometimes this undue mobility of the nerve seems to have been precipitated by a blow on the inner side of the elbow. There may be a much more definite association with an open but not serious wound, as described by Platt (1926). The patient's first complaint is usually local; pain on the inner side of the elbow, and he may even have noticed the abnormal mobility of the nerve. But sooner or later there are symptoms referable to the distribution of the nerve; though in general relief is sought before ulnar paralysis develops.

Injury. A heavy blow on the inner side of the elbow may be followed by ulnar paresis. It is mentioned here, rather than under acute

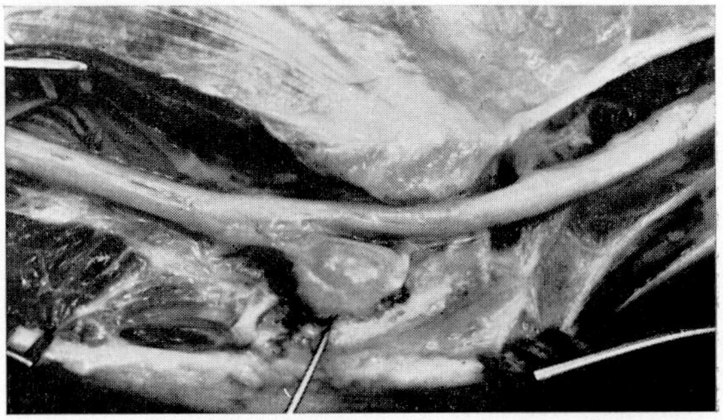

FIG. 7, 3. A man aged 44 years had suffered from ulnar paresis for 2 months. Twenty-seven years previously he had fallen off a bicycle on to the elbow, and an old fracture of the olecranon was discovered radiographically. No swelling was palpable. Exploration revealed a ganglion with no demonstrable connection with the joint. The ganglion was removed and the ulnar nerve transposed. (By kind permission of Professor J. I. P. James.)

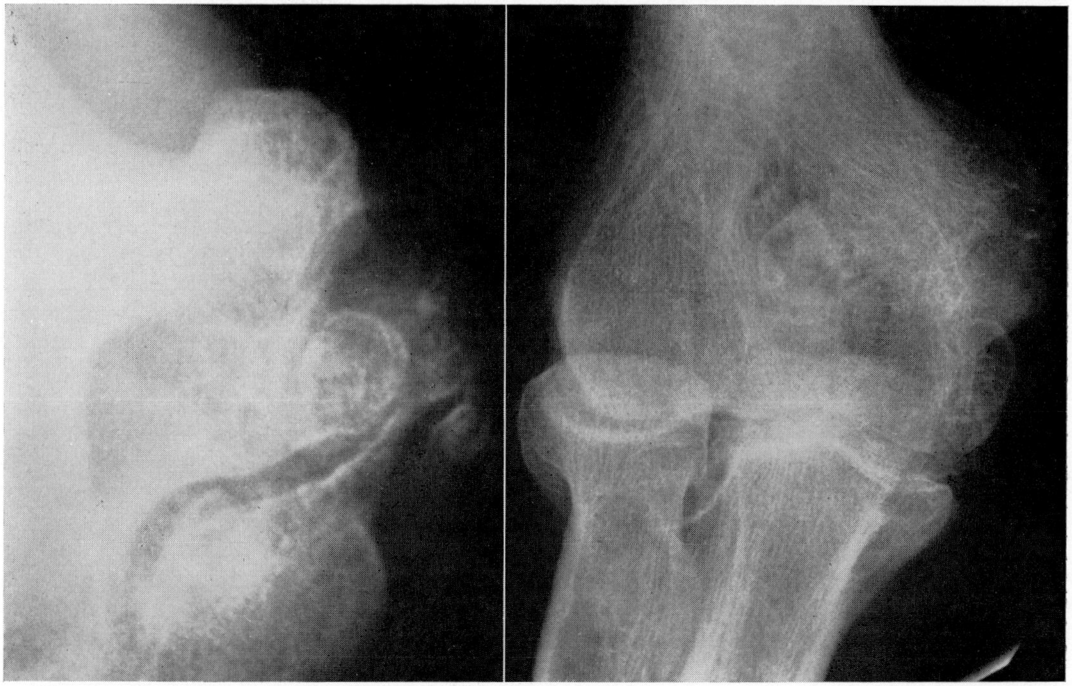

FIG. 7, 2. Osteoarthritis of the elbow causing traumatic ulnar neuritis. The ordinary antero-posterior view (R) shows a large osteophyte; an oblique view (L) shows a very irregular mass of bone in the track of the ulnar nerve.

injuries, because the patient may present with what seems to be the usual form of traumatic ulnar neuritis, and the history of the blow is elicited only in response to a leading question.

It is somewhat the same with the paralysis that comes on after an operation during which the patient lay on a hard surface with the elbows insufficiently protected against pressure. Lack of subcutaneous fat predisposes to this hazard.

The importance of these two varieties of traumatic ulnar neuritis is that spontaneous recovery can occur. But sometimes, for no apparent reason, it does not and all the relevant aids of electrodiagnosis may be required to determine if and when operative intervention is called for.

Idiopathic. Some patients present with the symptoms of ulnar irritation, perhaps even with demonstrable sensory and motor impairment, yet no abnormality can be found in the region of the elbow and there is no history of a blow or of compression. If the ulnar nerve is swollen and tender, or only tender, one is then obliged to label the disorder as idiopathic ulnar entrapment. Subcutaneous fat is usually sparse and close enquiry may reveal that the patient is in the habit of resting the inner side of the elbow on a hard surface. When tenderness of the nerve, with or without a palpable swelling, is present operation is advisable.

When a patient with symptoms referable to the ulnar nerve, perhaps with objective evidence too, has no tenderness or swelling of the nerve at the elbow a delicate diagnostic problem has to be solved. The lesion may be situated more proximally and in these circumstances the demonstration of changes in nerve conduction may be helpful (Gilliatt and Thomas, 1960; see also p. 63).

Prognosis. Most clinicians with considerable experience of these disorders can recall at least one patient, without serious involvement of the nerve and without deformity, who recovered spontaneously, but this is so unusual and so unpredictable that it is generally best to advise operation. The standard procedure has been anterior transposition of the nerve.

The prognosis after operation depends largely on the degree of nerve involvement. In 1950 McGowan classified 46 patients who had been under my care (the total has since risen to 97) according to the severity of the disturbance of the nerve:

Grade 1: Minimal with no detectable motor weakness.
Grade 2: Intermediate.
Grade 3: Severe, with paresis or paralysis of the intrinsic muscles of the hand supplied by the ulnar nerve.

Transposition, if properly performed, leads to almost immediate relief of any local discomfort and of ulnar paraesthesia. In patients with moderate sensory and motor impairment the hand becomes stronger, but slight residual weakness persists in over half the cases and slight sensory impairment in a quarter. Even when there is advanced paralysis of the ulnar nerve the intrinsic muscles invariably show some recovery; sensory recovery is even better, but normal function is seldom regained. In no case is the operation futile.

Prognosis after secondary transposition. There is a small group of patients, obtrusive because of their misery, who are made worse by operation because it has been incorrectly performed. The nerve may be kinked as it comes forward over the medial intermuscular septum, which ought always to be resected. Distally, it may be kinked, even to a right angle, where it dips backward (dorsally) from its transposed position to resume its normal course deep to the muscles of the forearm. But neither of these is so harmful as the deformation that can occur when a groove for the nerve has been cut in the common flexor mass. Between the muscle bellies there are dense fibrous septa which, when healing occurs after the operation, become firmly adherent to the nerve and distort it so that it looks like the twisted ornamentation of a piece of Jacobean furniture. With every contraction of the muscles the septa pull on the nerve. One cannot roundly condemn this operation because it has been done many times with good results, but the hazard described (Fig. 7, 4) is such that it ought to be discarded.

Patients whose transpositions have gone wrong are not merely unrelieved, they are much worse and often complain of constant pain in the distribution of the ulnar nerve. The only remedy is further transposition of the nerve deep to the common flexor origin, but a guarded prognosis should always be given because the prospect of complete recovery, even of complete relief from pain, is uncertain.

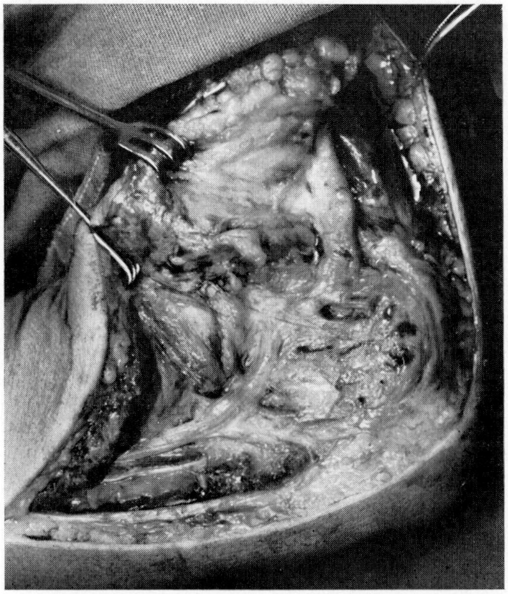

FIG. 7, 4. The distortion of the ulnar nerve found after transposition into a groove cut in the common flexor origin. The intermuscular septa became adherent to the nerve and this gives it a wavy appearance. The irritative symptoms that sometimes follow this type of transposition can be severe.

Treatment. The details of the operation of deep anterior transposition of the ulnar nerve are given in Chapter 15 (p. 258) but here it may be as well to mention an important feature in the immediate after-treatment.

When the nerve has been transposed deep to the common flexor mass the muscles are re-attached to the medial epicondyle with the fore-arm in pronation and the elbow flexed 90 degrees. This facilitates their approximation. It is essential that this position should be maintained for three weeks after the operation, which means that the arm must be put into plaster-of-Paris with the elbow at a right angle and the wrist fully pronated, a precaution that is unnecessary if the nerve is transposed superficially.

Osborne's operation. Osborne (1959) considered that the triangular aponeurosis that fills the gap between the two heads of origin of the flexor carpi ulnaris can compress the underlying ulnar nerve in much the same way that the anterior carpal ligament compresses the median. As at the wrist, a bony deformity or some other structural abnormality does not disturb the nerve directly; it is because the relationship between the aponeurosis and the nerve is upset. He observed that if there was any swelling of the ulnar nerve it was always proximal to the 'ligament'. So the appropriate treatment, as for the median nerve at the wrist, is simple longitudinal division of the offending structure. The operation is performed through a longitudinal incision, about 8 cm long, and the aponeurotic covering of the belly of flexor carpi ulnaris is divided as well as the ligament. The subcutaneous tissues and skin are brought together separately and the elbow is bandaged in extension for 10 days.

This operation has the merit of simplicity, whereas anterior transposition can cause trouble if not performed with some care. My experience of it is small, but satisfactory: though in some cases I have been so convinced that Osborne's ligament was not the operative cause of the damage to the ulnar nerve that I opted for transposition. Osborne has found that very occasionally the severed band regenerates and that compression of the nerve may recur. He therefore recommends that the constricted segment of the nerve should be mobilized over a distance of about 4 cm and the edges of the fibrous band are brought together with a few sutures beneath it. The nerve then lies superficial to what had been the roof of the tunnel in subcutaneous fatty tissue which is brought together separately before the skin is sutured.

Radial and Posterior Interosseous Nerves

Considering the anatomical awkwardness of the course of this nerve around the neck of the radius it is remarkable that compression paralysis of it is uncommon. It suffers much more frequently as a result of open wounds and fractures in the region of the elbow and in the course of operations on the head of the radius. A short distance above the lateral condyle of the humerus the radial nerve divides into its superficial and posterior interosseous branches. In an average adult the latter has a free course of only a few centimetres before its funiculi fan out to form a flat band that disappears into a slit-like tunnel in the supinator muscle. This muscle has an aponeurotic covering which means that the posterior interosseous nerve is firmly anchored.

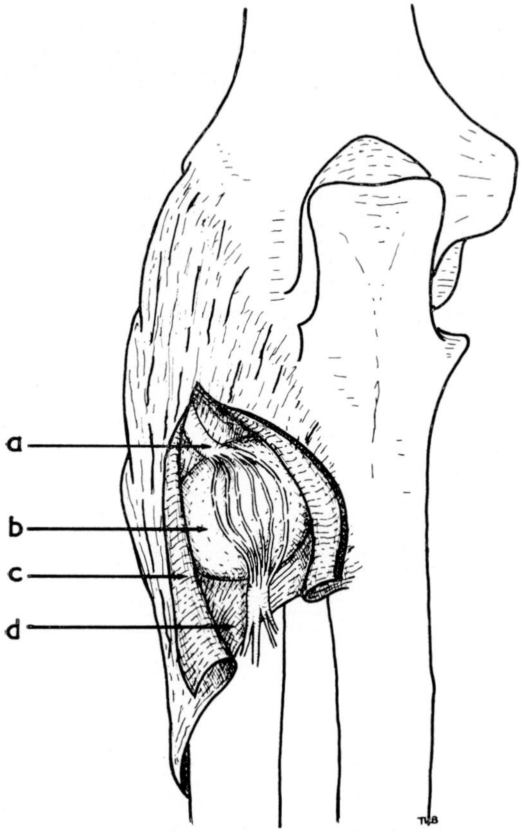

FIG. 7, 5. A ganglion pressing on the posterior interosseous nerve. *a*, the nerve: *b*, the ganglion: *c*, superficial fibres of the supinator: *d*, deep fibres. (Reproduced by kind permission from Bowen, T. L. and Stone, K. H., 1966, *J. Bone Jt Surg.*, **48B**, 774.)

The nerve emerges at the posterior border of the supinator to break up into its terminal branches. It is vulnerable in the proximal part of its course. Any swelling arising deep to it (Fig. 7, 5) can stretch the nerve and there are records of paralysis caused by lipomata, by ganglia and by other innocent swellings situated near the neck of the radius.

But posterior interosseous paralysis can develop in the absence of a swelling. The nerve may run entirely superficial to the supinator (Woltman and Learmonth, 1934); this could increase its vulnerability, the contracting supinator itself being the offending swelling. This is related to the cases in which occupation seems to be a significant cause of paralysis, though Mulholland (1966) found the evidence unconvincing. What is certain is that minor skeletal abnormalities can lead to traumatic neuritis of the posterior interosseous nerve not unlike that so commonly seen with the ulnar nerve at the elbow: cubitus varus, unreduced anterior dislocation of the head of the radius, anterior prominence of the capitulum and constricting fibrous bands such as Sharrard (1966) described. There is nothing unusual about the distribution of compression paralysis, but finding the cause of it may be difficult. A swelling is sometimes palpable but it may be concealed by the often considerable mass of overlying muscle. An abnormality of the elbow is readily recognizable: it may be an old fracture with or without osteoarthritis (the latter can produce a ganglionic type of swelling), an unreduced dislocation of the head of the radius or cubitus varus. Rheumatoid arthritis can be a snare because the nerve involvement may masquerade as rupture of extensor tendons at the wrist (Millender, Nalebuff and Holdsworth, 1973). Apart from bony changes, radiography is useful because it may reveal a circumscribed translucency suggestive of an innocent swelling; in one of Sharrard's cases there was a calcified lipoma.

There is no doubt that exploration is advisable: only by this means can one be certain of what is amiss, and more often than not the compression or stretching of the nerve can be relieved.

It is a different matter when entrapment of the posterior interosseous nerve is invoked as a cause of tennis elbow because it is a purely sensory disorder. However, resistant cases have been relieved by liberation of what was sometimes a definite constriction; see, for example, Roles and Maudsley (1972) who reported that in some of their cases there was delayed *motor* conduction.

MEDIAN AND ANTERIOR INTEROSSEOUS NERVE

In 1952 Kiloh and Nevin described an anterior interosseous paralysis that appeared for no obvious reason. Is it, as they suggested, a neuritis that should be treated conservatively? Fearn and Goodfellow (1965) thought not, because in a case that came under their care they found on exploration that the nerve was compressed beneath a crescentic fibrous band running obliquely proximally and laterally from the deep surface of pronator teres. It was proximal to and separate from the ulnar origin of pronator teres. Three months after division of the band recovery was complete. It is notable that although the main trunk of the median nerve also ran beneath the band it was unaffected.

The median nerve may suffer in a curious fashion if it runs deep to both heads of pronator teres. This 'pronator syndrome', well described—along with many other oddities—by Spinner (1972) is characterized by pain in the region of pronator teres, aggravated by resisted action of the muscle; paraesthesia in the median-innervated digits; some weakness of the corresponding intrinsic muscles; but normal action in the forearm muscles, though electromyography may reveal delayed conduction.

COMPRESSION OF THE MEDIAN NERVE IN THE CARPAL TUNNEL

Although this is by far the commonest cause of nerve compression, our understanding of it is comparatively recent. In 1909 Hunt described gradual atrophy of the thenar muscles, though the short flexor was often spared, with subjective sensory disturbance but little or no demonstrable diminution of sensibility. The patients were usually middle-aged or elderly. A few years later Marie and Foix (1913) performed an autopsy on a patient suffering from this condition and found the median nerve constricted in the carpal tunnel and swollen proximal to it. The frequent sparing of flexor pollicis brevis puzzled these and other observers; it was not known at that time that in three out of four patients, at any rate in Britain, the short flexor is supplied by the ulnar nerve (p. 206). Learmonth (1933) was the first to decompress the nerve by opening the carpal tunnel and in 1944 I operated on two patients, one of whom had old fractures of both scaphoid bones with osteoarthritis and the other a malunited Colles's fracture (Zachary, 1945). It was soon realized that compression of the nerve could occur in the absence of any skeletal abnormality (Cannon and Love, 1946; Brain, Wright and Wilkinson, 1947).

Clinical features. Women are affected more often than men in the ratio of about six to one. The symptoms are aggravated by pregnancy. The syndrome commonly occurs in middle life, in women at or just after the menopause, though the elderly may be affected. It can occur, though very rarely, in children who complain of severe intermittent pain in the hand (Martin and Masse, 1958), though in a patient of mine reported by Lettin (1965) there had been none at all. The disorder is often bilateral.

Stevenson (1966), in a series of 120 patients, found obvious causative factors in only 24. These are of the most varied kind and are as follows:

- old Colles's fracture, usually malunited;
- old fracture of the scaphoid bone, usually with osteoarthritis;
- old soft-tissue injury of the wrist, commonly called a sprain;
- tenosynovitis in rheumatoid arthritis;
- tuberculous tenosynovitis;
- non-specific tenosynovitis;
- simple ganglion (Brooks, 1952);
- Léri's pleonosteosis (Watson-Jones, 1949), which may cause paralysis even in children (Yeoman, 1961).
- Abnormal development of one of the long flexor muscles which cannot be detected until the wrist is opened (Fig. **7**, 6).

Most patients, however, show none of these things but, as Nissen (1959) has pointed out, there is often a great proliferation of the tendon sheaths which, if excised, are found to form a considerable mass.

An acute form of compression can follow bleeding into the carpal tunnel or acute infection of the hand.

It seems likely that in all cases the nerve damage is at first due to ischaemia (Fullerton, 1963), which if unrelieved goes on to progressive and finally severe structural changes (Fig. **7**, 7), the most striking histological feature of which is a reduction in fibre size (Thomas and Fullerton, 1963).

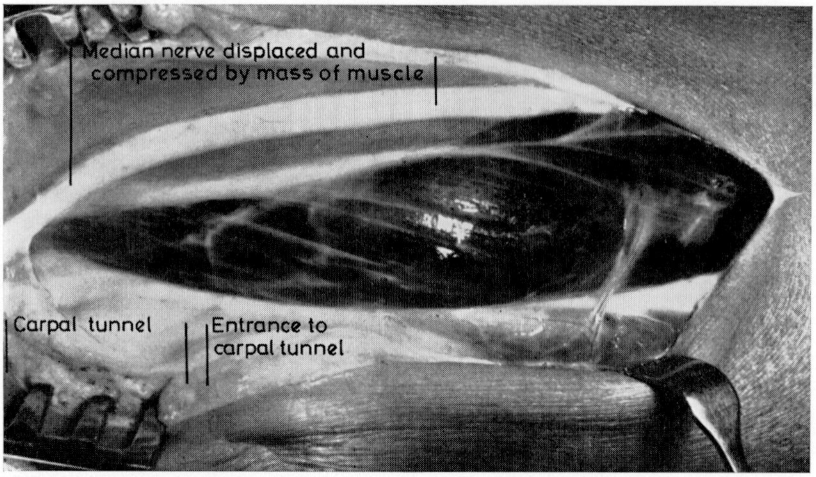

FIG. 7, 6. The radial half of the flexor digitorum superficialis formed a bulky muscular mass well into the carpal tunnel where it compressed the median nerve. The tunnel had been opened previously, but its contents were not inspected. The patient's symptoms persisted. Treatment: excision of the muscle but not of any tendon.

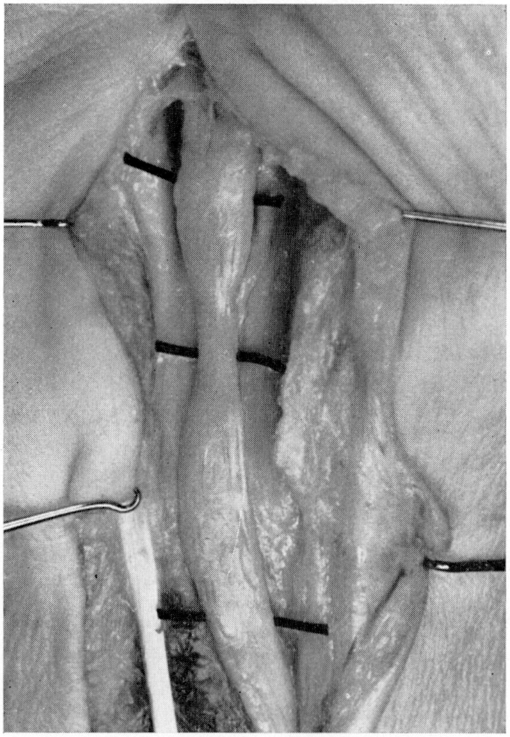

FIG. 7, 7. Compression of the median nerve in the carpal tunnel of a woman of 60. She had complained of pain for 20 years and had noticed wasting of the thenar muscles for two. Decompression relieved the pain, but not the paralysis. (By kind permission of Mr K. I. Nissen.)

The chief clinical features are well listed by Stevenson (1966); see Table XI.

Painful paraesthesia or numbness is the commonest complaint and nocturnal exacerbations are most characteristic. The patient wakes up with pain in the hand, which has been warm under the bed-clothes, and sometimes obtains relief by waving it about in the cool air of the room. The patient may say that all the digits are affected, but on close enquiry and examination it is found that the little finger is the least painful and that objective evidence of disordered sensibility is limited to the median area. When wasting of the thenar muscles appears it is first apparent in the short abductor, and at or before this time there is a feeling of stiffness of the fingers with, even, slight limitation of extension. This is due to limitation of action of the long tendons in the tunnel.

Patients usually put up with the complaint for months, even a year or two, before seeking relief. The objective signs of median nerve involvement become increasingly obvious: more or less weakness of the thenar muscles, the short flexor usually being spared, and diminution of sensibility within the median area. There may be slight fullness in the line of the nerve just proximal to the wrist, and pressure over it causes pain referred to the distribution of the nerve.

Diagnosis. When there are few or no physical signs the diagnosis may be difficult, particularly if there is co-existent cervical spondylosis. Several tests may be used and all are helpful. The application of a simple plaster splint will often relieve the symptoms; so will a local injection of hydrocortisone. Compression of the arm by a pneumatic cuff can aggravate the pain, though this may not happen until the cuff is deflated and the arm flushes. In a fair number of patients there is slowing of conduction in the nerve (Goodman and Gilliatt, 1961: see p. 64).

Treatment. *Palliative.* Resting the wrist in a light splint may give relief because it encourages shrinkage of the swelling inside the carpal tunnel. An injection of hydrocortisone may likewise decrease the turgidity of the tendon sheaths. These measures may suffice when the median nerve compression comes on during pregnancy because it clears up anyway after parturition.

Operative. This is the only satisfactory form of treatment, but the operation must be done properly. It is not sufficient to make a small incision and divide the carpal ligament blind. A transverse incision, however desirable cosmetically, is not recommended. The exposure of the carpal ligament and of the deeper tissues is inadequate and there is also a risk of damaging the small palmar branch of the median nerve with the result that the patient subsequently complains, often bitterly, of soreness of the scar or in the palm. The longitudinal incision should begin 4 cm proximal to the distal wrist crease and go as far into the palm as is required to expose the whole of the anterior carpal ligament. Its superficial surface must be exposed with caution and a watch kept for an anomalous motor branch (there may be two) that pierces it before entering the thenar muscles. It is equally necessary to obtain an adequate exposure of the main nerve after the carpal ligament has been severed or resected. There may be something unusual compressing the nerve. One of my two patients with compression of the nerve by an abnormal muscle mass (Fig. **7**, 6) had previously been operated on through an incision of adequate length.

Because this small operation must be done thoroughly, general anaesthesia and a pressure cuff to give a bloodless field are far superior to local anaesthesia.

Results of operation. About four out of five patients are restored to normal. The minority have some persistent though minor sensory disturbance, and if thenar paralysis has been present for a long time there may be little or no return of power. Curtis, dissatisfied with this, found that his results were better if he opened the epineurium and freed the funiculi from any fibrous adhesions that might be constricting them (Curtis and Eversmann, 1973). In some cases this endoneurolysis was promptly followed by a readily demonstrable improvement in motor conduction. More important still, the clinical results were better. Very rarely the elderly patient develops an irritative disorder that has most of the features of causalgia (p. 140), with constant pain though not of a degree to be demoralizing. The hand is puffy and there is likely to be stiffness of the wrist and digits. In the two cases that I

TABLE XI—Carpal tunnel syndrome: chief clinical features in 120 cases

	No. of cases	%
Paraesthesiae or pain in the hand	110	92
Nocturnal incidence of symptoms	98	82
Pain in arm and/or neck	29	24
Subjective numbness of fingers	72	60
Subjective stiffness or clumsiness of fingers	52	43
Sensation of swelling of fingers	12	10
Thenar wasting	36	30
Objective hypoaesthesia of fingertips	15*	12·5
Fullness of front of wrist or lower forearm	6	5

* Low, perhaps because not specifically tested in all cases.

have seen this complication resolved in about six months. It is imperative to maintain mobility of the hand, and considerable relief of pain may follow injection of the stellate ganglion—repeated two or three times if necessary—with a long-acting local anaesthetic (p. 149).

ENTRAPMENT OF THE ULNAR NERVE AT THE WRIST

Here again, as with compression of the median nerve in the carpal tunnel, the pioneer was J. Ramsay Hunt (1908, 1909, 1911, 1914). The disorder takes two forms. In the first, the paralysis

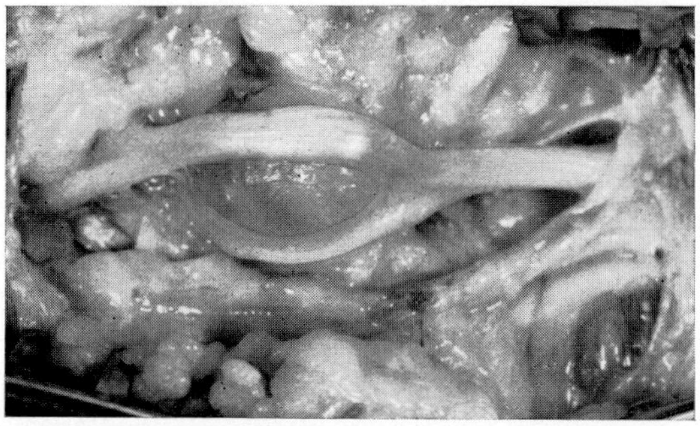

FIG. 7, 8. A ganglion protruding from a carpal joint with the terminal divisions of the ulnar nerve stretched over it. The deep motor branch is below.

is restricted to the deep branch of the ulnar nerve, with no sensory disturbance, no involvement of the hypothenar muscles and paralysis of all the interossei and of the two medial lumbricals unless, by chance, it happens that the first dorsal interosseous muscle is supplied by the median nerve. The other form of paralysis is much less common; there is usually complete paralysis of the deep branch of the ulnar nerve, some sensory disturbance and perhaps weakness of the hypothenar muscles.

Although the conditions can arise apparently spontaneously there is almost always a clear history of injury, often of a repetitive kind. Most of the patients are men. Some are ardent motorcyclists; others are engaged in significant occupations such as bootmaking, the leather-cutting knife pressing into the palm; telephone-cable splicing, wire-cutting shears being used hundreds of times a day; and gardeners are not exempt. Among the single injuries are heavy blows on the hand and, what amounts to the same thing, falls onto the outstretched hand. The interval between the injury and the onset of paralysis may be anything from a few weeks to many years and it is weakness of the hand that attracts the patient's attention.

If the offending occupation is abandoned and if the hand is rested, recovery may occur (Russell and Whitty, 1947; Ebeling, Gilliatt and Thomas, 1960).

It was supposed that the nerve was somehow compressed. But the deep branch of the ulnar nerve is uncommonly well protected by the hook of the hamate bone, the overlying hypothenar muscles and the long flexor tendons of the digits; this explanation was unconvincing. Certain local signs—slight swelling, crepitus on pressure over the pisiform bone and tenderness medial to the hook of the hamate—led me (Seddon, 1952) to carry out five explorations, four of which revealed a ganglion with the deep branch of the ulnar nerve stretched over it (Fig. 7, 8). This seemed to be the chief cause of the paralysis, which cleared up after removal of the swelling, though admittedly little faster than in cases treated conservatively.

Whether or not the deep branch of the nerve alone is involved, this is the commonest cause of compression of the ulnar nerve in the hand; many other surgeons have since found these ganglia. But I am no longer certain that exploration should always be carried out. In one of my patients there was almost complete motor paralysis when she was first seen, but two weeks later the muscles were much stronger. Exploration was performed (we were still groping in the dark at that time) and a ganglion was found though I doubted whether it was large enough to compress the nerve. It may have been doing so earlier and had shrunk as a result of relative inactivity while the patient was awaiting admission to hospital. The cases reported by Ebeling *et al.* support a conservative approach in the first place. Four of their nine patients made a good recovery without operation and a fifth, in whom exploration was negative, also recovered. On the other hand there may be compression by an innocent tumour or an aberrant muscle for which operative relief is essential.

We may well ask how the cases that need

decompression can be recognized. The answer is given by Ebeling and his colleagues (1960). They were particularly interested in nerve conduction and found pronounced slowing over the affected segment. In some of their cases the time taken for an impulse to pass from the wrist to the interossei was increased to five or six times the normal figure (see Chap. 4). This, of course, depended on the deep branch of the ulnar nerve conducting to some extent; in two of their cases the first dorsal interosseous muscle was inexcitable. It may therefore be suggested that exploration should always be performed if there is total paralysis of the interossei; this is uncommon but it indicates severe compression. When there is only paresis and when nerve conduction studies show improvement during the course of conservative treatment, i.e. rest, it is safe and indeed wise to wait. Unfortunately, facilities for carrying out these delicate tests are not universally available; the clinician must then rely on accurate clinical assessment of the power of the interossei; if it diminishes or if it fails to improve with two months' rest the hypothenar eminence should be explored.

MERALGIA PARAESTHETICA

This disorder, described by Roth and separately by Bernhardt in 1895, is due to an abnormality of the lateral femoral cutaneous nerve at the point where it leaves the pelvis. It emerges beneath the inguinal ligament, passes through the origin of the sartorius and enters a canal in the fascia lata before continuing distally into the subcutaneous tissues.

The patient, usually adult, complains of abnormal sensations in the area of distribution of the nerve, which is the whole of the outer side of the thigh; the symptoms are described as burning, scalding or tingling, aggravated by standing or walking and relieved by lying down, particularly if the hip is flexed. There is diminution rather than total loss of sensibility, the skin may be hyperalgesic and there may be loss of hair.

The exact nature of the lesion is uncertain. There is no doubt that the nerve is angulated at the anterior superior iliac spine and it also seems to be sensitive to pressure at this point because I have seen a number of patients complaining of meralgia when wearing a plaster spica or corset. It may be that the essential anatomical abnormality is that instead of passing beneath the lateral attachment of the inguinal ligament the nerve emerges through a slit in it (Fig. **7**, 9; Ghent, 1959). The nerve can be injured, presumably by pressure or stretching, during the enforced immobility of a patient undergoing an operation, usually abdominal.

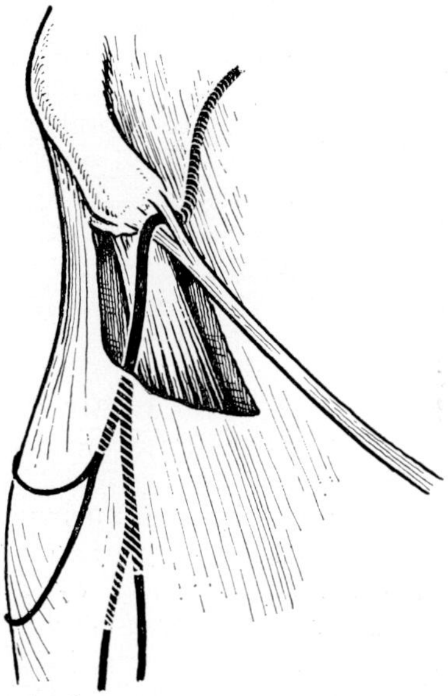

FIG. **7**, 9. This is probably the commonest anatomical anomaly predisposing to meralgia paraesthetica. (Reproduced by kind permission from Ghent, W. R., 1959, *Can. med. Ass. J.*, **81**, 631.)

An important warning is given in Stevens's (1957) classical paper. The lateral femoral cutaneous nerve has a long intra-abdominal course. Thus, in addition to being vulnerable to all the disorders that can involve peripheral nerves where they leave the spinal cord, this nerve may be affected by a great variety of abdominal conditions. Pregnancy is the commonest and the most benign. But Stevens lists more sinister causes, such as multiple sclerosis and deep-seated malignant disease, and points out that in such cases the area of sensory disturbance may extend beyond the territory of the lateral femoral cutaneous nerve. So there are two kinds of meralgia: that due to a lesion at the outer attachment of the inguinal ligament;

and what may be called secondary or symptomatic meralgia, which is analogous to sciatica. Therefore, just as the clinician habitually examines the spine, belly, hip, thigh and nervous system in any patient complaining of sciatic pain he should range equally widely in the investigation of a patient presenting with a sensory disorder of the outer side of the thigh.

If there is any doubt about the differentiation a small quantity of a local anaesthetic should be injected medial to the anterior superior iliac spine; in the primary variety of meralgia this will relieve the symptoms temporarily.

There is no unanimity about what should be done for primary meralgia. Stevens is unreservedly conservative. Because remission of the symptoms often occurs spontaneously within two years (Ecker and Woltman, 1938) reassurance of the patient is the most important measure, together with the removal or modification of any offending harness such as a truss or corset. Others, no less eminent, favour operation if pain and paraesthesia are persistent. There are two types of intervention, both of which I have used. The nerve—which may be found swollen and injected—is decompressed by cutting the deep, the inferior fasciculus of the inguinal ligament (Fig. 7, 9). It may also be resected. Neither operation can be relied on to give lasting relief, and resection always leads to paraesthesia at the circumference of the insensitive area (p. 39) which the patient may find as troublesome as the meralgia. Operation should therefore be avoided if possible.

Sciatic Nerve

I have seen two patients who suffered almost complete sciatic paralysis from pressure on the nerve in the thigh: one had taken an overdose of a hypnotic, the other was unconscious for a long period on account of a cerebral disorder. Neither presented any sign of ischaemia of the thigh muscles (cf. p. 109) and both recovered satisfactorily.

COMMON PERONEAL NERVE

External compression. This nerve has the misfortune to wind round the neck of a bone which, unlike the neck of the radius and the posterior interosseous nerve, is very near the surface and unusually vulnerable to external pressure. Millions of people in India sit cross-legged for long periods, and although pressure paralysis of the common peroneal nerve as a result of this has been described (Marwah, 1964) it seems to be something of a rarity even in the subcontinent. However, Garland and Moorhouse (1952) collected 19 British cases, mostly in men. In some of their patients the paralysis came on as a result of sitting with one leg over the other; or after kneeling with the knees acutely flexed, or kneeling while wearing the knee-pads used by coal-miners which have straps going round the back of the joint. They also record cases of the kind with which most surgeons are unhappily familiar, peroneal paralysis resulting from lying in the lateral position on the operation table without adequate protection, and paralysis due to tight bandages or adhesive strapping used for traction on the limb. However, in some cases there was no clear evidence of external pressure and it may well be that in them we are obliged to invoke some undue susceptibility to pressure such as is well recognized as a familial affliction (Earl, Fullerton, Wakefield and Schutta, 1964).

Entrapment. Sidey (1969) describes an entrapment neuropathy in which the most notable feature is pain, sometimes cramp, in the distribution of the nerve, frank motor paralysis being uncommon. For this he recommends division of the tendinous arch of origin of the peroneus longus.

The prognosis is good and the only treatment that may be required is a toe-raising apparatus attached to the shoe.

A sinister form of paralysis, because it can so easily go unrecognized, is that due to compression in patients paralysed as a consequence of a more centrally placed lesion (Lewin, 1943). A splint, or simply the posture in bed may be responsible. The diagnosis may be suggested by clinical examination: loss of sensibility corresponding to the distribution of the common peroneal nerve; excessive wasting of the muscles it supplies; their failure to participate in reflex contraction; their failure to recover when muscles in other groups are doing so. However, the proof must rest, as Lewin says, on the electromyographic demonstration of fibrillation in the anterior and lateral muscles of the leg and the absence of sweating in the cutaneous distribution of the nerve. Today one might add loss of nerve conduction.

Cyst of the nerve near the head of the fibula. This disorder, although rare, has attracted much attention because of its curious, indeed unique, features. There is a sausage-shaped swelling in the line of the common peroneal nerve at the level of the knee. The patient complains of pain, there is paralysis or weakness of the muscles of the anterior compartment of the leg, but the peronei are usually unaffected. There may be sensory disturbance too.

It is an intraneural ganglion (Wadstein, 1931); it could be a cystic neurilemmoma though I am unaware that this has ever been authenticated. This in itself is odd enough but, in addition, it may be multilocular and it may have a connection with the superior tibio-fibular joint.

It is possible that what began as a ganglion arising from a joint or tendon sheath can lose its original connection. In 1968 I operated on a woman who presented with a cystic swelling situated on the lateral side of the wrist and complained of tingling in the distribution of the superficial radial nerve. Fifteen years previously an ordinary ganglion arising from a tendon sheath had been removed. The swelling recurred in 1962. It proved to be a ganglion, inside the superficial radial nerve, which after the cyst had been dissected out was like gossamer. There was no connection with any tendon sheath or joint. Thus this is an example of a simple ganglion which many years later recurred as a strictly intraneural structure.

Because a cyst in the peroneal nerve causes more or less paralysis something must be done, but the surgical attack is much more formidable than in the other types of ganglia that merely compress a nerve. Our aim has been excision

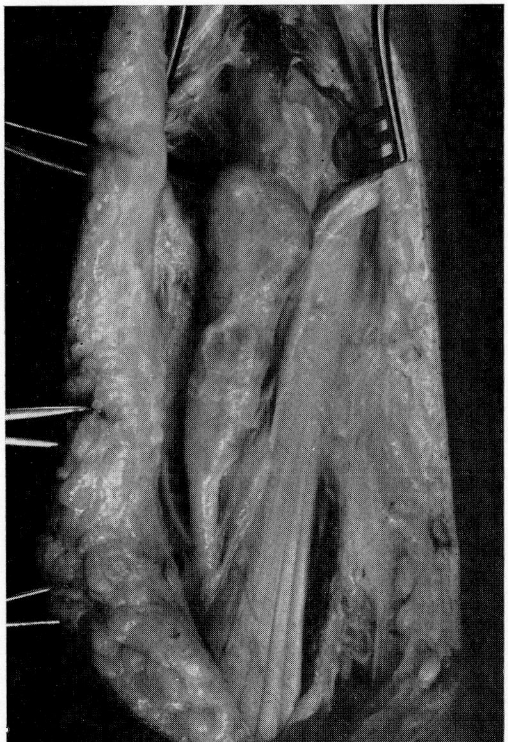

FIG. 7, 10. Multilocular cyst of the common peroneal nerve.

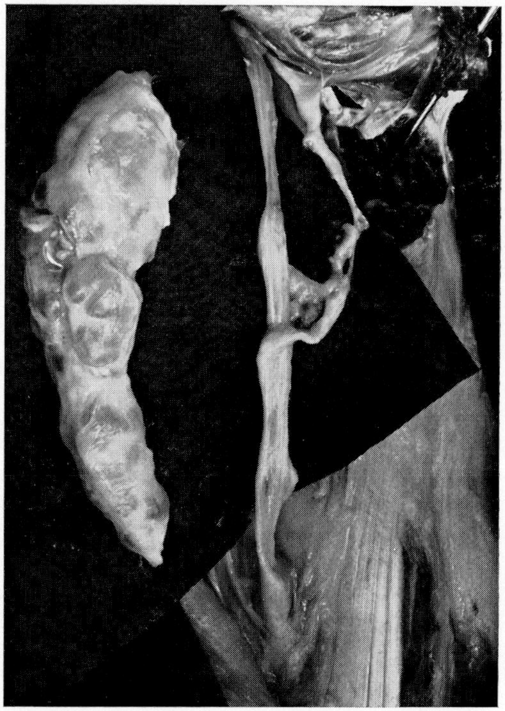

FIG. 7, 11. The ganglionic cysts after being dissected out of the nerve. (Figs 7, 10 and 7, 11 reproduced by kind permission from Brooks, D. M., 1952, *J. Bone Jt Surg.*, **34B**, 391.)

(Figs. **7**, 10 and **7**, 11), an operation of extreme delicacy involving risk of damage to some of the nerve bundles. It is clearly unsuitable for the multiple cysts described by Clark (1961) and he was probably right in resecting the nerve in his cases. Parkes (1961), who agrees with Brooks (1952) in thinking that there is invariably a connection between the ganglion and the superior tibio-fibular joint (Clark disagrees), advises extirpation of the pedicle of the ganglion and evacuation of its contents. This operation is the most conservative that has yet been devised. Parkes reports that it has not been followed by recurrence of the swelling and is therefore preferable to resection of the nerve, which may leave a gap too big to be closed, or dissecting out the cyst from inside the nerve.

Tarsal Tunnel Syndrome

This disorder was described in 1962 by Keck and by Lam and it bears a striking resemblance to the well-known compression of the median nerve in the carpal tunnel.

Men and women are affected alike and the complaint is of burning pain and disordered sensibility in the toes, in the sole of the foot and sometimes spreading up the leg. It may be particularly troublesome at night and, as in the hand, relief may be obtained by moving the limb or hanging it out of bed. There is tenderness over the course of the posterior tibial nerve at the ankle, a fusiform swelling may be palpable and there may be demonstrable impairment of sensibility in the sole of the foot. Pressure over the nerve can provoke the symptoms, as may the inflation of a sphygmomanometer cuff applied to the leg to produce venous congestion. The diagnosis is confirmed by observation of the conduction velocity in the nerve across the ankle.

As at the wrist the cause of the disorder is usually obscure. The tarsal tunnel differs from the carpal in that the flexor retinaculum is thin; but there are stout septa passing between the tendons and also enclosing the neurovascular bundle. The posterior tibial nerve is held fairly close to the medial side of the calcaneus. The only local causative factor that has been described is enlargement of the veins within the tunnel.

The appropriate treatment is thorough decompression through a medial incision in the line of the nerve.

It may well be, as Lam suggests, that a watch should be kept for this syndrome in patients suspected of having pain in the foot due to peripheral vascular disease.

MORTON'S METATARSALGIA: PLANTAR DIGITAL NEUROMA

In 1876 T. G. Morton described 'a peculiar and painful affection of the fourth metatarso-phalangeal articulation' that has been linked ever since with his name.

It is an affliction of adults, women more than men, though it can start in adolescence. It is not uncommonly bilateral. There is sharp pain somewhere near the head of the fourth metatarsal bone which comes on when the patient is walking, often quite suddenly, and is relieved by resting the foot with the shoe off. With the passage of time the attacks of pain, which can come like a stroke of lightning, may become so severe as to make the sufferer collapse; at the finish she is afraid to leave the house and walk on a hard pavement. Removal of the shoe and manipulation of the toes still helps but the foot remains painful and tender for some time afterwards.

Most patients have otherwise normal feet; if there is hallux valgus and loss of the metatarsal arch the sharp pain is felt distal to the callosities under the metatarsal heads. Footwear is important; high-heeled shoes aggravate the pain. It is felt not only in the sole but often in the fourth toe, or in the third, and there is sometimes diminished sensibility of the adjoining surfaces of these toes, the tips of which may be tender. A swelling may be palpable just proximal to the third web. Nissen (1948) found only one radiographic abnormality in his early series of 27 patients, in eight of whom the pain was bilateral. There was separation of the heads of the third and fourth metatarsals, which was caused by a mass of connective tissue; it was just visible and palpable.

Morton's metatarsalgia can occur in patients with rheumatoid arthritis (Vainio and Ritama, 1956) and it is suggested, though the evidence is thin, that the swelling in these cases may sometimes be a rheumatoid nodule.

The nature of the disorder. Although as long ago as 1893 Hoadley discovered and removed a neuroma on a digital branch of the lateral plantar nerve, which gave the patient complete relief; and although in 1935 Dott (personal communication), who never published his finding, performed an equally successful operation on his old teacher, Sir Harold Stiles, though without finding a neuroma; it was not until 1940 that Betts showed beyond peradventure that the pain was caused by a neuroma of the plantar nerve supplying the third digital cleft. There had previously been widespread fear that an incision in the sole would leave a painful scar, and various operations of a more mutilating kind had been done—not without success—such as removal of the head of the fourth metatarsal bone through a dorsal incision.

Betts's neurectomy cured the patient; but how did the neuroma come to be there? Figure 7, 12 shows that the nerve to the third cleft has two singular features. It runs obliquely across the tendons of the flexor digitorum brevis; then it is joined, though according to Nissen not constantly, by a communicating branch from the most medial branch of the lateral plantar nerve. The conjoint (or single) nerve then comes to lie on the plantar surface of the tough transverse metatarsal ligament (Fig. 7, 13). It lies alongside the digital artery. Then the nerve and artery divide to run on each side of the digital cleft; just before the artery divides it is joined by a small perforating vessel from the dorsum of the foot.

Betts took the view that 'when the foot is in action the flexor digitorum brevis contracts, fixing the origin of the nerve, while dorsiflexion of the toes in walking stretches it around the unyielding transverse ligament. The neuritis probably arises in the first place from minor trauma, the head of the fourth metatarsal taking most of the weight on the outer side and being the part of the tread most exposed to such injuries. . . . The origin by two roots anchoring the nerve at its base is probably the deciding factor. Each of the other digital nerves can slide easily longitudinally as the toes are dorsiflexed.' The neuroma is found on the nerve as it lies on the transverse ligament proximal to its bifurcation (Figs 7, 12 and 7, 14).

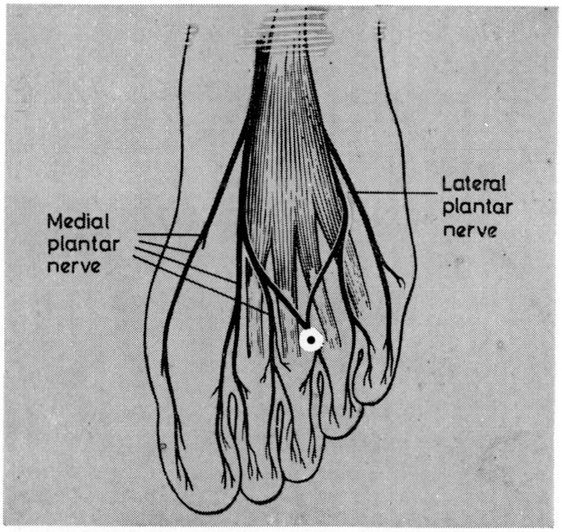

FIG. 7, 12. The site at which a plantar digital neuroma is most commonly found.

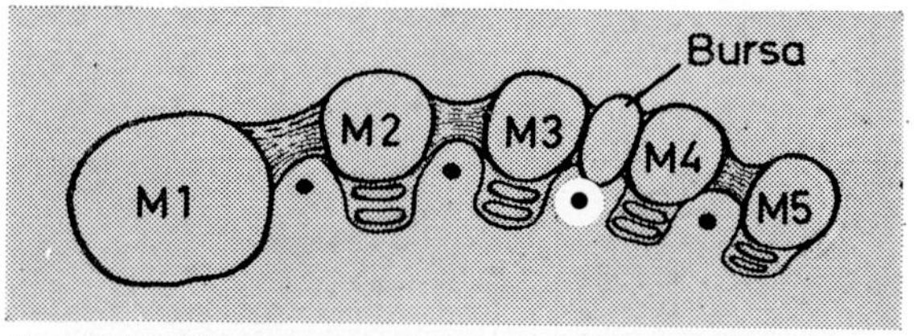

FIG. 7, 13. The common site for a plantar digital neuroma showing its relationship to the intermetatarsal bursa. (The bursae are not shown in the other spaces.)

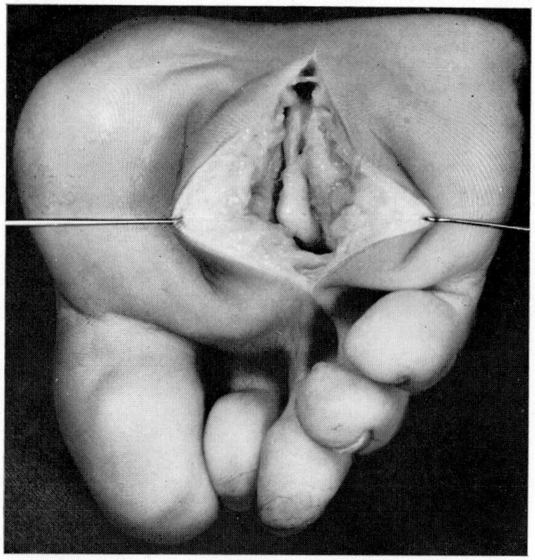

FIG. 7, 14. The usual finding at operation. (Reproduced by kind permission of Mr J. A. Cholmeley.)

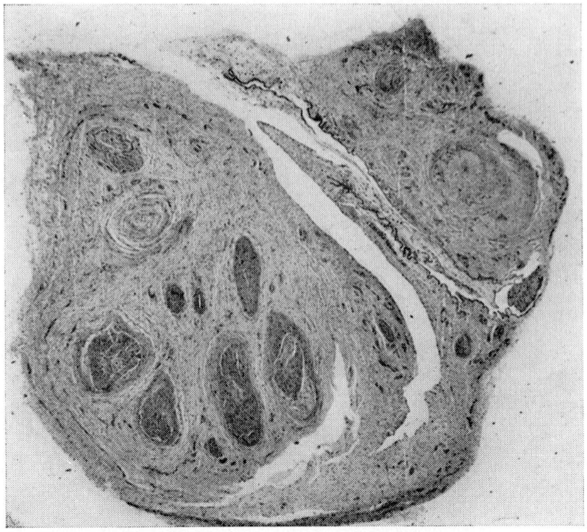

FIG. 7, 15. Transverse section of a plantar digital neuroma. The nerve bundles are separated by abundant connective tissue. The digital vessels, completely obliterated, are just distinguishable in the smaller part of the preparation, top right.

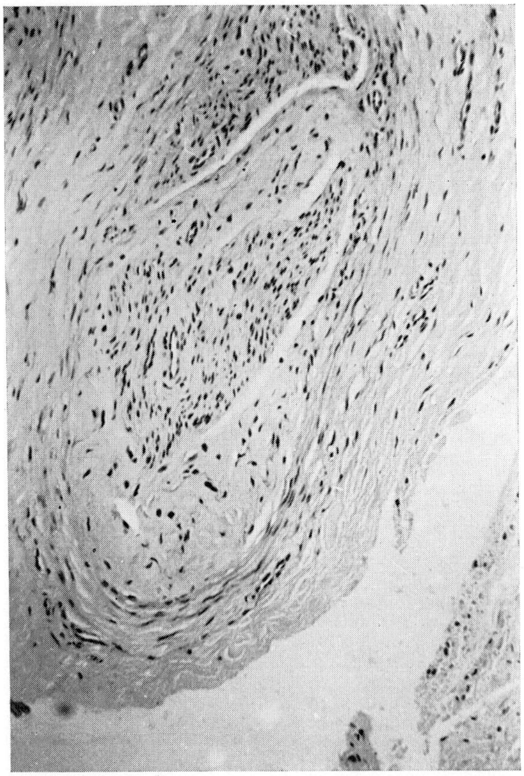

FIG. 7, 16. Section through a nerve bundle, showing collagenization within it.

A more recondite explanation was advanced by Nissen (1948). He observed that the digital artery was affected, showing changes ranging from thickening of the wall to complete obliteration of the lumen. He concluded that the nerve lesion was ischaemic in origin and in this he was supported by Holmes who examined his material histologically. It was said that according to Holmes, Highet and Seddon (1944) large nodules, like those found in Morton's disorder, may occur on the median and ulnar nerves in Volkmann's contracture with ischaemic nerve lesions. This is incorrect. Enlargement is not a feature of ischaemia of nerves, and the nodules referred to were neuromata produced by injuries, proximal to the zone of ischaemia. On the contrary, in every case they reported and in the many seen subsequently the ischaemic nerve was shrunken. For a nerve to be affected by ischaemia the longitudinal extent of deprivation of blood supply must be considerable (Chap. 1). Holmes pointed out that ischaemia can occur in injuries of the digital nerves (p. 278) when the adjacent artery is also severed, but he omitted to mention that this ischaemia is limited to the distal segment and is by no means an invariable finding; the distal part of the nerve is deprived of its important longitudinal blood supply. There is nothing to indicate that anything comparable happens in the plantar lesion. The site of damage in the latter is more proximal than a digital injury and in an area of fairly rich arterial anastomosis.

The histological changes (Figs 7, 15 and 7, 16) are unlike those of ischaemia in that there is immense interfunicular proliferation of connective tissue. The endoneural collagenization is similar to that found in ischaemia, but such changes are not specific; they can occur in traction injuries (see Chap. 5). It seems reasonable to conclude that the injuries to nerve and artery have a common cause.

Mulder (1951), dissatisfied with both Betts's and Nissen's explanations, has gone back to Morton's view that the plantar nerve is pinched between the metatarsal heads. He noticed that if the forefoot is grasped and if the thumb of the other hand presses firmly into the sole at the site of the suspected neuroma, alternate squeezing together of the metatarsals and pressure on the sole enables the observer to feel a small mass that jumps in and out of the space between the metatarsal heads. This can produce a palpable click and, if considerable force is used, the characteristic pain. This, he thought, might explain the sudden stabs of pain that some patients feel. He confirmed this observation at operation and it seemed to him that the digital artery might be damaged in the same way as the nerve. Mulder thought too that the intermetatarsal bursa played some part in the mechanism of injury.

Not one of these three theories is wholly satisfactory. Neither Nissen nor Mulder explains why the lesion is most frequently found at the third cleft, and Betts fails to explain why it is sometimes found in an adjoining one (Fig. 7, 17).

Treatment. Fortunately, there is no argument about this; Betts's neurectomy is most effective. The following description is taken from Nissen's (1948) excellent article. General anaesthesia is employed, a pressure bag is applied to the thigh, and the patient is placed in the prone position with the ankle resting over a sandbag at the end of the operation table. A generous longitudinal plantar incision is deepened down to the web between the toes. A longitudinal dorsal incision may be used, but it gives only a restricted exposure of the nerve. A transverse incision in the tread is permissible if the surgeon anticipates that more than one cleft must be explored. The incision is deepened between the common flexor tendon sheaths and the abundant subcutaneous tissue is held apart with a small self-retaining retractor. The digital nerve is sought where it crosses the transverse ligament, to which it is often adherent. It is traced proximally, and distally to the bifurcation. When symptoms have been present for only a short time no neuroma may be found. The extent of the resection should be not less than 2·5 cm and in some of Nissen's cases it was 4·5 cm. After removal of the compression cuff such slight bleeding as occurs should be arrested and the skin alone is closed with mattress sutures which are removed about 12 days later. If the patient insists on walking very soon, a generous dressing and a plaster shoe should be applied. Full weight-bearing ought not to begin in less than two weeks and exercises for the foot and leg are desirable for a further two weeks.

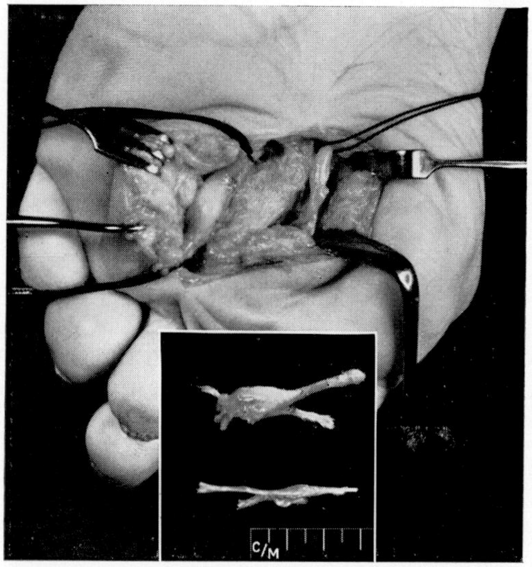

FIG. 7, 17. A double lesion. (Reproduced by kind permission of Mr K. I. Nissen.)

The results of this operation are extremely satisfactory, though patients sometimes complain for a time of the circumferential sensitivity that always follows resection of a nerve.

It must not be thought, however, that operation is imperative, though it is the treatment of choice. In some cases attention to footwear gives relief for long periods.

8. Miscellaneous Nerve Injuries

THIS CHAPTER IS devoted to a miscellany of causes of nerve injury. They are:

1. Birth injuries: traction affecting the upper limb, and the lower limb: compression injuries.
2. Maternal obstetrical paralysis.
3. Injuries arising during the course of surgical operations.
4. Crutch paralysis.
5. Nerve damage due to injections.
6. Injuries caused by physical agents: thermal burns, electrical burns, irradiation, and cold.

BIRTH INJURIES

These are of two kinds: traction injuries of the brachial plexus and, very rarely, of the lumbosacral plexus; and what for want of a better term may be called compression injuries, which are also uncommon.

BRACHIAL PLEXUS INJURIES

The decline in the incidence of these injuries during the past 40 years, which is not confined to what we are pleased to call advanced countries, is one indication of widespread improvement in the standard of obstetrics. Whereas Sever, an American, writing in 1925, could report 1,100 cases, my own experience is limited to under 50 cases over a period of nearly 40 years.

The paralysis is caused by dragging on an infant's arm during delivery and it takes one of three forms:

1. Proximal paralysis, associated with the name of Erb, caused by damage to the upper trunk of the brachial plexus with more or less involvement of the middle (C7) trunk and produced by forcible depression of the shoulder.
2. Distal paralysis (Klumpke) caused by damage to the lower trunk of the plexus (C8 and T1), the arm having been held up while traction was applied to the child's body during breech delivery.
3. Paralysis of the whole arm, a result of exceptional violence which may even damage the phrenic nerve (Grenet, Isaac and Ladet, 1937). Sever (1925) encountered bilateral paralysis in 63 of his 1,100 cases, and in the remainder the incidence of proximal paralysis compared with paralysis of the whole arm (distal paralysis was not mentioned) was four to one.

Proximal paralysis. This affects the muscles supplied by the fifth, sixth and, sometimes incompletely, the seventh cervical nerves; the most important are the deltoid, the proximal part of pectoralis major, the spinati, possibly the subscapularis, always the flexors of the elbow and, to a varying degree, the extensors of the elbow, wrist and digits. The posture of the limb is unmistakable, what has so aptly been described as the tip-hand position: the arm hangs by the side of the trunk, medially rotated; the forearm is pronated, the wrist slightly flexed, and the digits also flexed as if ready to receive a solatium. It is not always possible to demonstrate any sensory disturbance, and this is not due solely to the difficulty of examining a new-born child, who responds to pin-prick as briskly as does an adult. There may, indeed, be no sensory paralysis, which suggests that the damage is confined to the motor fibres (p. 74). It is rare, too, to find a neuromatous swelling in the posterior triangle of the neck.

A remarkable, a unique feature is that within a very short time, and even when splinting and passive movements have been started early, a contracture at the shoulder develops, abduction and lateral rotation being limited. It was this that led Thomas (1916: where references to his earlier papers may be found) to the conclusion that the primary damage was in the joint. But his view was not accepted by his contemporaries or immediate successors. Taylor (1920) could find no evidence of derangement of the shoulder in any infant under the age of 3 weeks. Moreover, in the limbs that he explored early, the damage was confined to the nerve roots; such extraneural scarring as was present did not involve the shoulder. Yet it must be conceded that no satisfactory alternative explanation of this curious tendency to contracture has been offered.

Taylor was not alone in favouring exploration and repair of the plexus in infants who failed to show satisfactory evidence of recovery within three months. But the results reported by him and by others were not encouraging, and the operation was abandoned. At that time the pathology of traction injuries was still obscure; the great longitudinal extent of the damage (p. 74) was not appreciated, though Taylor (1920) himself noted degenerative changes in the nerve trunk *proximal* as well as distal to the main site of damage. A birth injury of the brachial plexus is essentially the same as the now much more common traction injuries in older subjects, and in view of the extremely poor prospects of successful repair in the young adult there can hardly be justification for attempting the operation in the new-born child.

The proper treatment is conservative, and it can scarcely begin too soon. The chief aim is preventing, or at any rate minimizing, the contracture of the shoulder. The arm is splinted with the joint abducted 90 degrees and in full lateral rotation, the elbow being flexed 90 degrees and, when the infant is old enough to make it practicable, with the forearm supinated. All joints are put through the fullest possible range of movement twice a day. This regime is followed for one year. Any subsequent treatment is surgical; correction of residual contracture of the chief offender, the subscapularis; and muscle transplantation, moving the latissimus dorsi and teres major—so that they act as abductors of the shoulder—being the most useful (Brooks's operation: Roper, 1972).

Distal paralysis. A typical example is shown in Figure **8**, 1. The flexor group of forearm muscles is paralysed, as are the intrinsic muscles of the hand, and, as in the case illustrated, Horner's syndrome may be present. Loss of sensibility, at the least of the palmar surface of the hand, is easily demonstrable. No splinting is required, but passive movements must be carried out assiduously. When the child is older, reconstructive surgery may be useful.

Paralysis of the whole arm. This depressing condition is fortunately now very rare. In addition to the extensive motor and sensory paralysis there is likely to be swelling and cyanosis of the forearm and hand, a consequence of vasomotor paralysis. The treatment is the same as for distal paralysis.

Prognosis

Our own records are useless because most of the children with birth injuries of the brachial plexus were referred to us late, the paralysis being fairly severe. The best recent information comes from Wickstrom, Haslam and Hutchinson (1955; Table XII). They found that proximal paralysis is commonest and has the best prognosis, good muscle power returning within three to six months after birth. In the whole series of 54 patients, eight showed little or no recovery; in three of these Horner's syndrome was present, and in four paralysis of the levator scapulae, rhomboid and serratus anterior muscles indicated damage close to the spinal cord, possibly even avulsion of the nerve roots.

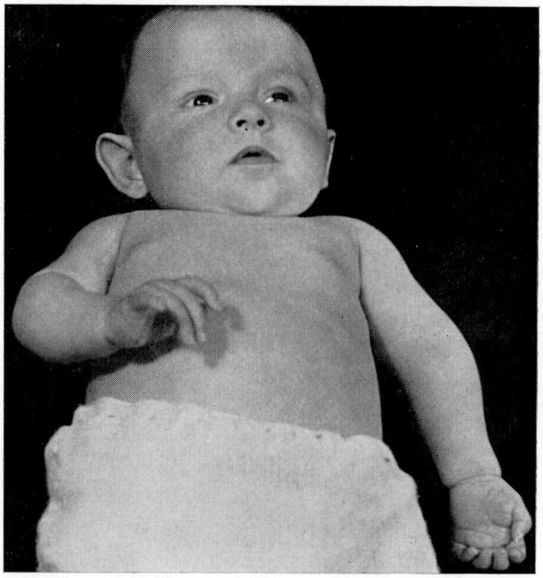

FIG. **8**, 1. Distal type of obstetrical paralysis. The narrowing of the palpebral fissure was constant and the left pupil was also smaller than the right.

LUMBO-SACRAL PLEXUS INJURIES

I have not encountered sciatic paralysis caused by traction on the lower limb with the knee extended and the hip flexed, but it is mentioned by Reuss (1920) and Ehrenfest (1931). It seems more likely that for the sciatic nerve to be injured the shaft of the femur must break first, so permitting hyperextension of the limb with the hip flexed, as in the following case.

A difficult breech delivery was accompanied by signs of foetal distress, and for this reason had to be hastened. When traction was applied to the flexure of the acutely flexed right hip there was an audible crack. It was found that the lower end of the femur had fractured: the knee must have been fully extended. The whole limb was paralysed and there was weakness of the right lower abdominal muscles. No detailed sensory examination was made until nine months after birth, by which time there was a little action in the gluteus maximus, the calf muscle and the flexors of the toes. Sensibility was present in the sole of the foot, absent in the leg and possibly impaired in the thigh. It was concluded that the infant had suffered a traction injury of the lumbo-sacral plexus. Myelography, which might have revealed traumatic meningoceles, was unfortunately unsuccessful. There was no spina bifida.

Lance (1937) described paralysis of both lower limbs following difficult breech delivery. There was no mention of spina bifida having been excluded though it could hardly have been overlooked. Ehrenfest (1931) and others have pointed out that bilateral paralysis may be due to intraspinal injury.

Craig and Clark (1958) reported what may have been a traction injury of the obturator nerve in an infant in the breech position delivered by Caesarean section.

Compression Injuries

The radial nerve is the most susceptible to this type of damage, which can occur before birth. It is possible that it can be compressed by amniotic bands (Langen, 1930), by the umbilical cord, or against the rim of the mother's pelvis (Ottow, 1932). Prolonged labour (Hauch and Ottsen, 1939) or a fracture of the humerus can injure the nerve, as can obstetrical forceps (Dunham, 1955).

A number of cases of prenatal radial paralysis have been reported by Craig and Clark (1958) and they also described three cases of posterior interosseous nerve paralysis which seemed to be caused by traction, the wrist having been actually flexed. There can be overt signs of compression, such as a groove on the outer side of the arm or a haematoma.

A new-born infant may suffer radial paralysis if an arm is gripped tightly (Craig and Clark, 1961). These injuries are benign affairs (neurapraxia) and recovery is rapid.

TABLE XII—Response to non-operative regimen in 54 patients

	EXCELLENT		SATISFACTORY		POOR		TOTAL	
	No.	Per cent	No.	Per cent	No.	Per cent	No.	Per cent
Minimal damage	7	12·9	21	38·8	—	—	28	51·8
Moderate damage	—	—	2	3·7	16	29·6	18	33·3
Severe damage	—	—	—	—	8	14·8	8	14·8
Total	7	12·9	23	42·6	24	44·5	54	99·9

MATERNAL OBSTETRICAL PARALYSIS

Although this is a rare condition—Tillman (1935) found only nine examples of it in 18,800 deliveries, and I myself have seen it only twice—it deserves more than passing reference because of a dispute about causation that has an important bearing on management.

It is commonly described as a paralysis in the distribution of the common peroneal nerve coming on during labour and persisting for several months afterwards, possibly permanently. Tillman found that it was most frequent in primiparae, also if there was a contracted pelvis, a difficult delivery, if forceps were employed, and if the baby was large. He accepted the popular view that the lumbo-sacral cord, which is the one part of the plexus that runs over the rim of the pelvis, was compressed by the foetal head. His views were shared by Whittaker (1958).

A critical appraisal of this disorder was made by O'Connell (1944). He noted some objections to the compression theory; in some cases the long diameter of the foetal head is away from the side of the paralysis; the paralysis sometimes comes on after delivery; labour may be easy, short, with no pelvic disproportion, and no application of forceps; the paralysis can be bilateral; and, lastly, femoral paralysis has been seen, which cannot possibly be explained on the basis of any sort of compression. O'Connell concluded that these patients suffer from prolapse of an intervertebral disc, precipitated by the general softening of pelvic ligaments that occurs towards the end of pregnancy. Moreover, there are three distinct syndromes: firstly, an unmistakable disc prolapse coming on at any time during or soon after delivery; secondly, paralysis, unaccompanied by pain, appearing during or after labour—this being rare; and, lastly, the same sort of paralysis, but accompanied by pain of sciatic distribution, this being the commonest type of maternal obstetrical paralysis.

Review of the records of the two patients who came under my care has convinced me that one certainly had a disc lesion and the other may have had. The implications of this are obvious; if compression of the lumbo-sacral cord is the cause of the paralysis no active steps can be taken to relieve it; the most that is possible is avoiding action in any later pregnancy. Prolapse of an intervertebral disc, on the other hand, may require intervention; a strictly conservative regime could amount to neglect.

The conclusion to be drawn from this conflict of views is that anyone faced with a case of maternal obstetrical paralysis should not accept the traditional explanation (which is shaky anatomically anyway) until he has satisfied himself that the patient is certainly not suffering from prolapse of an intervertebral disc.

NERVE INJURIES ARISING DURING THE COURSE OF SURGICAL OPERATIONS

Paralysis caused by the position of the patient on the operation table. These paralyses cause the patient great distress and the surgeon much anxiety, though fortunately the tendency is for them to clear up spontaneously (Ewing, 1950). They are particularly liable to occur in prolonged operations in which the upper limbs are fixed in abduction for the convenient measurement of blood pressure and the administration of intravenous fluid. The Trendelenburg position is particularly hazardous. It is unlikely that the shoulder-rests press on the brachial plexus above the clavicle. What happens is that, with the arms secured in abduction—the crucifix position—and the rest of the body tending to slide towards the head end of the table, the shoulder girdle is depressed in a patient whose muscles are totally relaxed. Moreover, the abduction of the shoulder causes the head of the humerus to protrude into the axilla, which increases tension on the brachial plexus. If the anaesthetist turns the patient's head to one side, as he often does, there is further tension on the brachial plexus on the other side. The greater the abduction of the arm the greater the risk, and tethering the patient's arm or arms above the head is particularly to be avoided. The risk of damaging the brachial plexus is not confined to patients in the Trendelenburg position; it can occur when the spine is extended, as when the bridge of the table is raised to facilitate operations on the gall bladder (Kiloh, 1950). The brachial plexus is safe only if the arms are folded across the chest or lying unsecured at the side of the trunk. The one comforting feature about this type of paralysis is that it is often a neurapraxia or, at worst, an axonotmesis; and complete recovery may be expected, though this may sometimes take some months.

The ulnar and common peroneal nerves are liable to be damaged by compression, particularly in thin subjects. Fortunately both can easily be protected by pads of plastic foam placed under the vulnerable sites, the hand being supinated if the extended arm is strapped to a board.

Tourniquet paralysis. This disappeared with the tourniquet, but the rubber bandage is still a hazard (Princeteau, Abadie and Desqueyroux, 1913; M.R.C.R., 1954, p. 218); yet the bandage cannot be altogether banished because, unlike the pressure cuff, it can be sterilized and in certain circumstances (p. 104) this is most advantageous. The bandage must be removed after one hour though it can be reapplied, if necessary, after a short interval. Pressure by a cuff, which is far safer, has been maintained for operations lasting three or four hours without harmful consequences, but to be on the safe side it is wise to deflate the cuff after an hour and a half. If the dissection, possibly intricate, has not been completed within this time the cuff can be reinflated after reapplication of a sterile rubber bandage.

This form of paralysis has been the subject of much experimental investigation, admirably summarized by Richards (M.R.C.R., 1954). It seems to be due to direct pressure rather than ischaemia (Ochoa, Danta, Fowler and Gilliatt, 1971).

There are three kinds of paralysis. The mildest clears up very rapidly. Next, there is paralysis without Wallerian degeneration, but with demyelination of the nerve fibres, which is greatest at the site of compression; this is neurapraxia and recovery may take several weeks. Lastly, there may be Wallerian degeneration, and recovery is then slow, being dependent on regeneration. This degeneration may be limited to the larger nerve fibres, the paralysis being predominantly motor. Permanent paralysis is fortunately rare, but cases have been recorded by Speigel and Lewin (1945), and I have seen one case. In no case has more than one nerve been affected, which is suggestive of compression rather than ischaemia. In the three explored by Speigel and Lewin obvious damage was detectable four to six months after the injury.

Injury of the nerves in the field of operation. The most vulnerable of all nerves are the accessory and the posterior interosseous. Of the 14 cases of accessory paralysis that we have seen eight were caused by operation. This nerve sometimes lies superficial to the sterno-cleido-mastoid and is then in a most exposed position. The mistake is always the same, making too short an incision. In any operation on the side of the neck, biopsy in particular, the field of vision should be wide enough and dry enough to permit the surgeon to see exactly what he is doing.

In a quarter of all cases of posterior interosseous paralysis the nerve was injured in the course of an operation on the head of the radius (p. 203).

The nature of the pathological disorder may aggravate the risk of nerve damage, and in this respect diaphyseal aclasia leads the field. Everyone with experience of excision of these protuberances is aware of the alarming fashion in which major nerve trunks pursue their course in the most intimate contact with these firm and sometimes large tumours. Here again extensive exposure is essential but the nerve trunks at risk must also be exposed early above and below the mass, and the dissection planned in such a way that it is always away from a nerve trunk, never towards it. Sometimes, and particularly at the upper end of the humerus, two or more nerve trunks traverse the field of operation and it may prove impossible to remove the mass without risk of damaging one of them. There should then be no hesitation in removing it piecemeal even though this means sacrificing a pathological trophy.

Nerves are sometimes damaged in endeavours to arrest bleeding. A pressure forceps applied hastily in the depths of a bloody wound may seriously damage a nerve. I have known the femoral nerve to be severed when a surgeon was dealing with a reactionary haemorrhage following repair of a simple femoral hernia.

The radial nerve is liable to injury when the shaft of the humerus is exposed, and especially if there is much fibrosis of the overlying muscles. The nerve may be cut, but it is more likely to be injured by a retractor passed around the shaft of the humerus subperiosteally, depression of the handle of the instrument stretching the tissues through which the nerve runs.

Three of the popular operations for osteoarthritis of the hip can endanger the sciatic nerve, and the paralysis is often permanent. In upper femoral (displacement) osteotomy the nerve may be injured if the posterior retractor is not subperiosteal. The nerve can then be compressed between the retractor and the back of the femur. In prosthetic replacement of the hip the acetabular component may be secured with a plastic cement that sets rapidly and in the process becomes hot. The sciatic nerve has been damaged by the hot cement coming into contact with it. The much older operation of ischio-femoral arthrodesis—which has a wide application—carries the risk of transfixion of the nerve by the bone graft that unites the femur to the pelvis. Adams (1964) has shown how this hazard may be avoided.

CRUTCH PARALYSIS

Paralysis caused by axillary crutches, though now rare, is so well known as to require little description. Prevention is best achieved by avoiding this type of crutch; the elbow crutch is safe. If for some reason it is unavailable the axillary crutch should be of such a length that when the patient presses firmly on the hand-bar the axillary pad exerts little or no pressure in the armpit. As with tourniquet paralysis, Wallerian degeneration can occur, as in the case illustrated in Figure **2**, 36 (p. 30).

NERVE DAMAGE DUE TO INJECTIONS

Solutions of drugs inappropriately injected may damage a nerve by virtue of their acidity or alkalinity, or—the sulphonamides, for example—their specific toxicity; but these distinctions have no practical significance.

The nerves chiefly affected by intramuscular injections are the sciatic and the radial, the buttock and the outer side of the arm being favourite sites for these injections. At the bend of the elbow the median nerve (Fig. **8**, 2) or the medial cutaneous nerve of the forearm may be damaged when there is leakage from an injection made into an antecubital vein.

A most curious injection injury, because of the route taken by the drug, is that of the sciatic nerve which occurs in the new-born. It has been described by (among others) Fahrni (1950), Hudson, McCandless and O'Malley (1950) and Kibel, Matheson and Stewart (1961). An analeptic drug is injected into the umbilical cord, but into an artery in mistake for the vein, the latter being perhaps collapsed. The fluid passes down the hypogastric artery to the internal

TABLE XIII—Twenty-four nerves damaged by injections

Sciatic (including 3 common peroneal)	10
Median at the elbow	6
Radial	5
Brachial plexus	1
Axillary	1
Medial cutaneous of the forearm	1

Agents

Intramuscular	
Sulphonamides (sulphapyridine 6)	7
Various analgesics	7
Heparin	1
Typhoid vaccine	1
Unknown	1
Intravenous	
Pentothal	3
Penicillin	1
Arsenical drug	1
Contrast medium for pyelography	1
Unknown	1

Paralysis

	Irritative symptoms	*Spontaneous recovery*	*Exploration*
Complete (15)	3	8	5*
Incomplete (9)	3	7	2

* Secondary suture in three of the five cases; imperfect though useful recovery in two.

iliac and so to the sciatic artery, the last being, before birth, a vessel of some consequence; and, of course, it is and remains the main nutrient vessel of the proximal part of the sciatic nerve. The paralysis can be accompanied by gangrene of the ipsilateral buttock. In Liverpool there was no further trouble after the use of cycliton was stopped; but nikethamide seems to be equally noxious. Even fatalities have been recorded; but in most cases the paralysis diminishes in time.

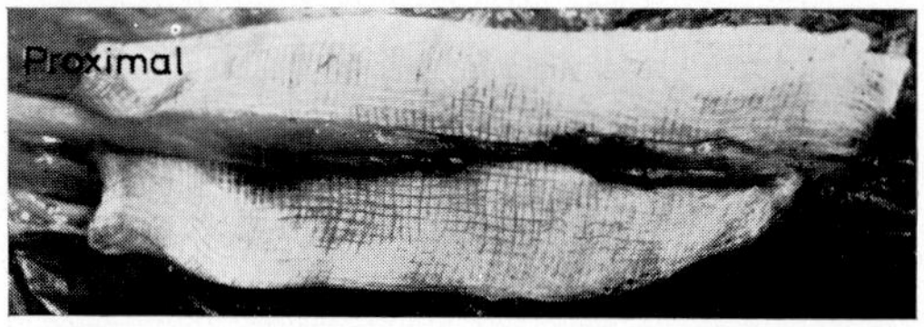

FIG. **8**, 2. Sodium pentothal was inadvertently injected into the median nerve. Twelve months later (there was sepsis in front of the elbow after the injection) resection and suture was performed. Gap after resection: 6·9 cm. Poor recovery, but better than permanent total paralysis. (Reproduced by kind permission from M.R.C. Special Report Series, No. 282, 1954.)

When intramuscular injection is indispensable, as is often the case, the injection must be made at a safe site. The outer side of the arm, particularly in a muscular person, is acceptable, provided the needle is well above the line of the radial nerve and below the axillary. Injections into the buttock are best avoided completely; it is far safer to give them into the middle of the outer side of the thigh, though even this requires caution in an infant and in an emaciated adult because there may be little muscle to protect the sciatic nerve.

The conscious patient usually complains immediately of very severe pain in the distribution of the affected nerve; and there is always burning pain within 24 hours which may continue for several weeks. It can be very persistent, especially if a sulphonamide drug has been injected. It is possible that the immediate type of pain is due to the injection having been made into the nerve, and that a delayed onset is due to the drug having diffused around and finally into it. It will be recalled (p. 4) that there is little obstruction to the intraneural diffusion of fluids; and a depressing feature of these lesions is their great longitudinal extent.

The paralysis may be partial, but more often complete. There is a good prospect of some spontaneous recovery if the paralysis is incomplete and some even if it is complete. When the paralysis is incomplete there is no indication for exploration, even if there are irritative symptoms. The two such operations listed in Table XIII—both fruitless—were done in our unenlightened days.

When there is complete paralysis it is desirable to consider the information contained in Table XIII before embarking on exploration of the nerve. Of the 15 totally paralysed nerves five were explored and in three the destruction was so obvious (Fig. **8**, 2) that it seemed that resection and suture were worth attempting. There was some recovery, enough to be useful, in two; in the third there was none and the persistent pain that plagued this patient became worse.

A nerve severely damaged by an injection shows intense intraneural fibrosis (Figs **8**, 3 to **8**, 5), and—a discouraging feature—this scarring extends far along the nerve with suppression of regeneration of its fibres in the proximal part (Fig. **8**, 5).

These 24 cases provide little evidence in favour of exploration; but it is just warranted if there is complete paralysis.

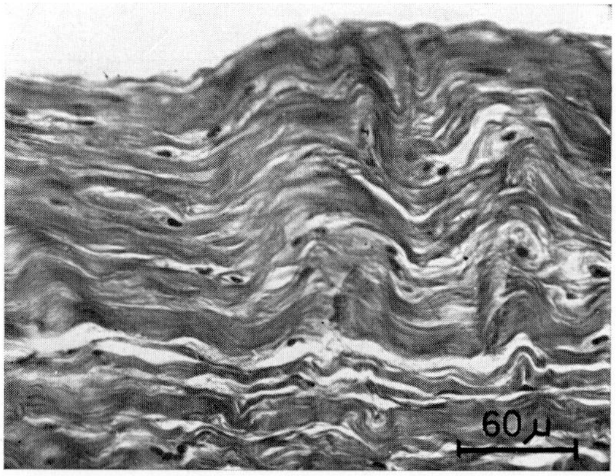

FIG. **8**, 3. The patient suffered immediate sharp pain and sciatic paralysis after an injection of sulphanilamide into the buttock. The nerve was explored 12 months later and the tibial division found to be fibrotic over a length of about 4 cm. Resection and suture were performed. This longitudinal section through the central part of the lesion shows complete collagenization. Fourteen years later there was no recovery.

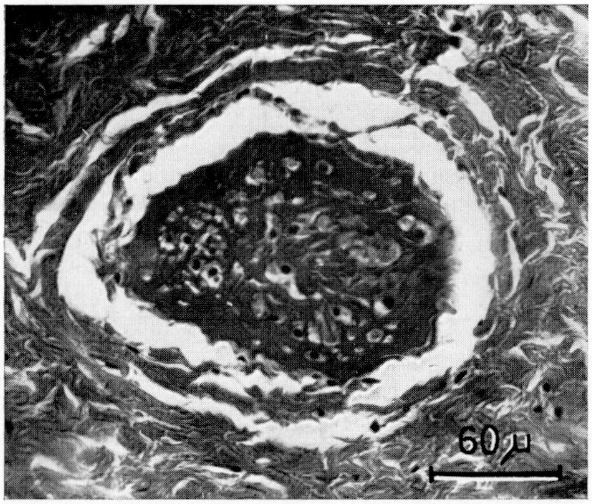

FIG. **8**, 4. Transverse section at the mid-point of the lesion: extensive extra- and intra-funicular collagenization.

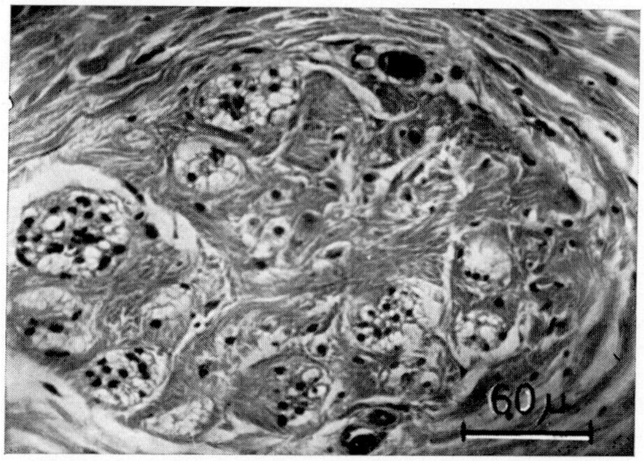

FIG. **8**, 5. Transverse section at the site of proximal resection which exposed apparently normal funiculi. There are very few myelinated fibres; this may be due to the severe damage to the intraneural vessels of which there was ample evidence in other sections.

NERVE INJURIES CAUSED BY PHYSICAL AGENTS

A *burn*, if deep enough, can damage a nerve. There is an unusual element of urgency in the treatment of these cases because the skin defect will require repair with a flap or tube-pedicle graft before the nerve can be explored. The damage to the nerve is likely to be rather more extensive than the skin loss and thus repair may be difficult. The surrounding muscles will certainly be fibrotic and the bed for a nerve graft, if one proves necessary, may be unsatisfactory.

Electrical burns. These have been well described by Dale (1954) and DiVincenti, Moncrief and Pruitt (1969). They are such deadly affairs that to dwell on the incidental nerve injuries is unbalanced. The damage caused by the current goes very deep and muscle in particular becomes necrotic. To make matters worse there may be a flame burn as well. DiVincenti *et al.* advised early fasciotomy over the damaged muscle to relieve swelling. Dale, with good reason, was strongly opposed to early excision because it is impossible accurately to determine the extent of the damage to muscle and other tissues. Moreover, when the time comes for the necrotic mass to be removed it is sometimes found that the nerves traversing it (most commonly the median and ulnar) are apparently intact. Good spontaneous recovery has been observed after the defect in the skin has been repaired with a tube-pedicle or flap graft.

Irradiation. This can cause a particularly vicious kind of nerve damage. The paralysis comes on gradually, months, sometimes many months, after treatment with X-rays. It is due to intraneural fibrosis which on account of its longitudinal extent does not lend itself to surgical repair. If, in addition, there has been damage to the surrounding soft tissues there is extraneural fibrosis as well. A curious feature noticed by Bateman (1962), which I confirm, is the absence of a neuroma. This is enough to discourage anyone from attempting to repair the nerve: a neuroma is an indication of regenerative potential. Plastic replacement of the scarred skin and subcutaneous tissues may be followed by some amelioration of the paralysis, as in the case illustrated in Figure **8**, 6.

These injuries have to be accepted as unavoidable evils when irradiation is required for malignant disease. The lamentable cases are those in which an innocent condition has been treated. I have seen a medical student who had warts on the back of both wrists. They were irradiated; he developed bilateral median nerve paralysis.

Cold. Although the experimental refrigeration of a human nerve by Waller (1862) was far removed from the accidents that damage nerves so commonly in warfare and occasionally, as in mountaineers, during times of peace, he was the first to show that cold can damage a peripheral nerve directly.

The conditions under which the extremities can be injured by cold are most varied, and it is remarkable that immersion foot and trench foot —which are much the same—can occur at temperatures as high as 12°C. We are not concerned with those extreme cases in which a part is frozen solid, with total destruction of all tissues,[1] but rather with the much more common disorders in which the hand or foot survives with at most some superficial sloughing.

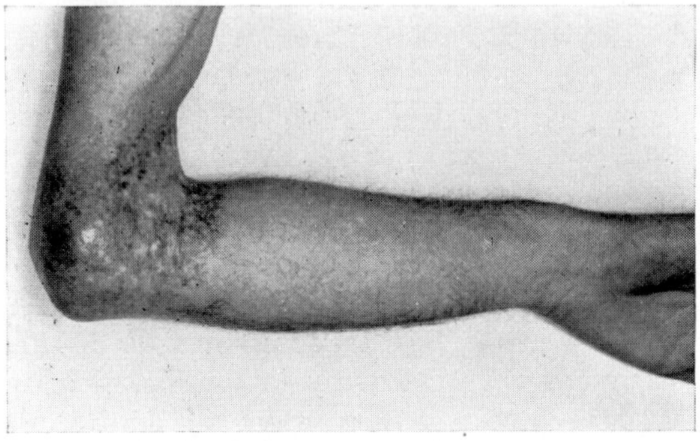

FIG. **8**, 6. This X-ray burn completely encircled the elbow and was followed by paresis of the median and ulnar nerves. Elaborate plastic operations were required to replace the scarred skin and subcutaneous tissues with a healthy covering. After this had been achieved there was some recovery in the nerves: so some of the paralysis was due to extraneural scarring.

Anyone who has experienced mild frostbite knows that the most conspicuous effect is loss of sensibility with annoying paraesthesiae during the period of recovery. Ungley and Blackwood (1942) have described the clinical manifestations of immersion foot, with particular reference to the neural changes. Immediately after exposure the skin is discoloured. At first it is usually red, then pale, a sickly yellow, mottled, or even blue or black. There is total loss of sensibility which has a sock (or glove) distribution; the muscles in the affected part are paralysed. The foot, or hand, is swollen. The succeeding hyperaemic stage lasts for 6 to 10 weeks. The patient complains of tingling, aching, throbbing, and shooting pains, often worse at night, which may be so severe as to require analgesics. A curious feature is that the disturbance of pain sensibility is more extensive than that of touch. There may be exaggerated responses to cutaneous stimuli (p. 145). Within the affected part there is motor paralysis and absence of sweating. Blisters appear where there had been swelling, and there may be superficial gangrene. The third stage, the post-hyperaemic, lasts for weeks or months. The characteristic feature is that the extremity is unduly sensitive to cold, as if it were affected by Raynaud's disorder. Sensibility and voluntary power gradually return to normal, but there may be excessive sweating for a long time.

Although the most striking morphological changes are vascular (Friedman, 1946), nerve is specifically affected (Denny-Brown, Adams, Brenner and Doherty, 1945), and according to Blackwood and Russell (1945) muscle too. The degree of damage to nerves depends on the intensity and duration of exposure to chilling or cold. In the milder cases there is no more than demyelination, affecting chiefly the larger nerve fibres, corresponding to neurapraxia in other conditions. Recovery is fairly rapid. However, there may be Wallerian degeneration; this is usually followed by regeneration, and with it there is more or less satisfactory re-innervation of the affected muscles.

[1] A freakish form of acute frostbite of the hands that occurred in high-altitude airmen was described in 1943 by Davis, Scarff, Rogers and Dickinson.

9. Nerve Injuries Causing Pain

BECAUSE THE PARALYTIC manifestations of nerve injury are so obtrusive the pain that accompanies them tends to be disregarded unless it is severe. Yet at some stage pain and other unpleasant disorders—paraesthesiae, excessive sensitivity and, rarely, phantom sensations—are experienced by almost every patient, though fortunately these disturbances usually subside sooner or later. We are concerned here with the kinds of pain that are disabling; but categorizing them is not easy because one type may merge with another.

In a series of some 1,250 cases observed during the war period 1940-43, fairly severe pain was experienced by about one patient in 10; injuries of the sciatic, digital and median nerves (in that order) leading the field. Many of the patients had suffered missile wounds, though most of the brachial plexus injuries, a number of which caused considerable pain, were due to traction. One cannot obtain figures more precise than these; much depends on the time after injury when a detailed history is first taken, and also on the patient's memory and probably on his sensitivity to pain. The incidence of comparable pain is much less in injuries encountered in civil life.

Immediately after an injury it is common for a patient to feel that the injured part is not there; he has to look at his finger, hand or leg to assure himself that it has not been severed. But very soon he begins to feel pain in it which is usually tolerable; sometimes it is distracting and very occasionally agonizing. A few days later, in the average case, the initial pain is subsiding but, as has been mentioned elsewhere (p. 39), the patient notices that stimuli falling on the margin of the area of sensory loss are most unpleasant; even the toughest subject may withdraw his hand or foot when the clinician is about to examine him. He also begins to experience spontaneous sensations, pricking, formication, pins and needles. These tend to persist for many weeks, whereas the over-reaction to cutaneous stimuli usually fades rapidly.

If a nerve injury has been extensive, total paralysis of the brachial plexus above all, phantom sensations may very occasionally be experienced, in no way different from those commonly felt after amputation of a limb.

During recovery, whether spontaneous or following repair of a nerve, there is sometimes a recrudescence of over-reaction as cutaneous sensibility returns, one of the features that led Head to formulate his hypothesis of protopathic and epicritic sensibility. This, too, is usually a passing phenomenon, though not in some cases in which regeneration is very imperfect.

We must now consider the significant departures from this pattern of subjective sensory disturbance and they are: (1) causalgia; and (2) what for want of a better term are called irritative nerve lesions, with painful digital nerve injuries, painful amputation stumps and painful phantoms as important sub-groups.

CAUSALGIA

Although causalgia is rare it occupies so prominent a place in our minds that the term is sometimes used to describe almost any persistent pain after nerve injury, occasionally with unfortunate consequences. Something of the sort had been recognized in the early years of the nineteenth century (Denmark, 1813) and by Paget in 1864, but causalgia—although the word was not used until 1867—was first clearly described by Weir Mitchell, Morehouse and Keen in their pioneer monograph on nerve injuries that appeared in 1864 and contained an account of their experiences in the American Civil War. This has justifiably been called the first modern war, and not the least significant of the many innovations was the employment of high-velocity missiles. Although causalgia means burning pain, it does not carry us very far because, as Richards (1967) points out, burning pain is also a feature of erythromelalgia, which has nothing to do with causalgia. And Mitchell and his colleagues used the latter term to describe burning pain that was sometimes almost trivial.

The best definitions have come from the two (British) Medical Research Council Reports (M.R.C.R., 1920, 1954), though in the latter Barnes regards the burning quality of the pain as less significant than its other features. His definition is as follows:

'In this survey the term causalgia has been reserved for pain, following an injury of a nerve trunk, which has the following characteristics:

1. It is severe, spontaneous and persistent.
2. It usually has a burning quality.
3. It may spread beyond the territory of the injured nerve or nerves.
4. It is invariably aggravated by both physical and emotional stimuli.'

He goes on to observe that 'this definition differs in one important detail from the description of Weir Mitchell. He regarded burning pain as an essential feature of causalgia. Although most of these patients did complain of burning pain it was not considered one of the essential criteria of diagnosis. There were some patients who described the pain as throbbing, bursting, clamping, stabbing, tearing or gnawing in quality. Aggravation of the pain by emotional stimuli was regarded as far more important in the diagnosis of causalgia, for this feature excluded a number of other painful post-traumatic lesions of the peripheral nerves, which are not relieved by sympathectomy.'

INCIDENCE

It is hardly surprising that in the reporting of the incidence of a predominantly subjective phenomenon there have been wide variations; in the list compiled by Richards (1967) it ranges from 1·8 to 13·8 per cent of all war-time nerve injuries. Much depends on when the records are made; causalgia can regress spontaneously. Yet there were striking differences as between the combatants in the Second World War. It was part of our business to review a number of German and rather fewer Russian reports. The Germans were careful to differentiate causalgia from what they called hyperpathia: yet one surgeon (Moser, 1943) could report 24 cases—the total number of nerve injuries was not given—whereas no surgeon in charge of any one of the five large nerve injuries centres in Britain encountered anything like that number. Chlenov (1944) considered that the Russian figure was between 0·5 and 2 per cent. In the British Army the rate given by Nathan (1947) was 13·8 per cent; he was in Palestine and saw his patients soon after injury. By contrast Slessor (1948), working under somewhat similar conditions in India, found an incidence of 4·2 per cent. Perhaps White, Heroy and Goodman's (1948) figure is as good as any: causalgia occurs in 5 per cent, or rather less, of all war wounds of *major* nerves.

The greater frequency of causalgia in the upper limb may be no more than could be accounted for by the preponderance of missile injuries of the upper as compared with the lower limb.

Clinical Features

Although my experience of causalgia is limited to 16 cases it is unforgettable. I have seen brave men reduced to a state of pathetic misery by this dreadful pain.

Pain. This dominates everything. It is felt chiefly in the hand or foot, though deep in the limb as well, and is not confined to the distribution of the affected nerve; the patient may even complain of pain in the contralateral or ipsilateral limb. The characteristic sensation is burning, but it may be described as throbbing, aching, clamping or 'pressure', stabbing or knife-like, twisting, crushing, tearing or gnawing (Kirklin, Chenoweth and Murphey, 1947; Barnes, M.R.C.R., 1954). The pain is spontaneous and persistent. Mercifully, it eases when the sufferer becomes sleepy and he may get a good night's rest. An essential feature is that the pain is aggravated affectively. Sudden noise, such as a door slamming; the passage of an aeroplane close overhead; excitement, as when watching the cinema; mental distress, as when a letter brings bad news: these are a few examples of the sort of stimuli that exacerbate the pain.

Dryness of the painful part is avoided because it aggravates the pain or the sensitivity of the affected part. The hand is wrapped in a towel usually soaked in cold water. But warm moisture may be comforting; Philippides (1942) described a patient who put his hand into his soup or coffee before he could use it at table. These oddities of behaviour may lead the uninitiated clinician to suspect some sort of mental derangement; but before the injury almost all of these patients were normal folk, and they become so again after the pain has been relieved.

Stiffness. Because use of the extremity is avoided stiffness develops with alarming rapidity, and no physiotherapist can attempt to mobilize the hand or foot.

The skin. There are no constant 'trophic' changes but the hand may be pink or cyanotic, the skin thin and shiny, the finger pads wasted so that the nails are unduly prominent. The growth of hair is excessive. Sweating may be pronounced, but sometimes the skin is dry.

Sensibility. Accurate examination is impossible because of the exaggerated response to any form of cutaneous stimulus; but when the pain has been relieved the patient presents the diminished sensibility of an incomplete nerve lesion. However, in the exceptional cases in which a nerve is completely severed (Nathan, 1947; Sunderland and Kelly, 1948) there is the usual loss of sensibility in its area of distribution.

Motor power. Here too accurate examination is difficult because of the patient's reluctance to move the part but it is usually possible to determine that the paralysis is partial; rarely, complete. The muscles waste rapidly.

Bones. A high degree of porosis has often been remarked but it has no specific features and is compatible with the inactivity of the limb.

Time of Onset: Duration

In over half of the cases reported by Barnes (M.R.C.R., 1954), though in only a third of those reported by Freeman (1947), the pain began within the first 24 hours which excludes sepsis and intraneural scarring as contributory factors. In the remainder, causalgia develops at any time up to about 45 days and in these the pathogenesis may be different.

Causalgia may regress without treatment. Hirschmann (1943) found that it ceased in half of his cases; and in the British Armed Forces the incidence of causalgia was higher in hospitals near the front than in the home-based nerve injuries centres to which almost all cases of any severity were ultimately referred. But the pain can drag on for years, as was found by Weir Mitchell's son, John (1895) and by others since. This has a bearing on treatment.

Severity

The picture that has been presented is that of severe causalgia; yet it can be only moderately disabling and not enough to demoralize the patient. The risk of labelling any painful sequela of a nerve injury as causalgic has already been mentioned; but it is equally reprehensible not to diagnose causalgia because the patient is not prostrated by the pain. This delicate topic will be considered more fully in the discussion of treatment.

Nerves Injured

Barnes alone (M.R.C.R., 1954) has drawn attention to the frequency of multiple injuries, such as of the median and ulnar nerves above the level of the elbow. This sometimes makes it difficult to connect causalgia with one nerve rather than another. Nevertheless, there is general agreement that the nerves most frequently affected are the median, the tibial division of the sciatic, and the lowest trunk of the brachial plexus. The level of injury is usually proximal. In Richards's (1967) collected figures, 88 per cent of nerve injuries with causalgia were caused by wounds at or proximal to the elbow or knee.

Pathogenesis

Until the Second World War it was denied that severance of a nerve was ever followed by causalgia. Now we must concede that this can happen, though rarely. A missile wound of a nerve, especially one caused by a high-velocity projectile, is the sort most likely to provoke causalgia. But traction injuries of the brachial plexus can do so; and cases have been reported after stab and incised wounds, though Richards (1967) says only one of each. He also refers to a few well-authenticated cases in which causalgia developed after a fracture of the pelvis that injured the sciatic nerve.

Only one of the theories propounded has survived, that of Doupe, Cullen and Chance (1944) and it is powerfully supported by Nathan (1947). In brief, it postulates the formation of what the proponents call an artificial synapse between the autonomic and sensory fibres in the damaged nerve. It is simpler and more exact, because it is probably not a true synapse, to call it a short circuit. That a confluence of axons can occur in a damaged nerve has been demonstrated by conduction studies (Granit, Leksell and Skoglund, 1944), and J. Z. Young once showed me some striking photomicrographs of axons that had fused laterally over a short distance. Let us consider the implications of this.

Causalgia is rare. In Chapter 2 evidence has been presented of the toughness of the basement membrane that invests a nerve fibre; it can withstand extremely heavy crushing. Quite apart from the Schwann cells it is the ultimate insulating structure. It can be damaged by severance, as in incised or lacerated wounds. But such injuries always cause more or less retrograde degeneration and the intact proximal axons remain within undisturbed sheaths, composed of basement membrane, Schwann cells and, in all except the smallest fibres, myelin. The stroma—fibroblastic and Schwann-cell—into which the regenerating fibres will grow, forms rapidly and well ahead of the outgrowing axons; thus the axons are insulated not only at the time of injury but throughout regeneration. The chances of fusion of contiguous axons are remote.

A high-velocity projectile that just misses a nerve injures it by violent displacement (p. 70) and thus, very occasionally, the stroma could be partially ruptured without all the contained axons being disrupted as well. A traction injury can certainly act in this way. In either case lateral axonal fusion could then occur, more particularly of fibres with a thin myelin sheath or none at all, that is to say, fibres mediating pain and autonomic fibres.

Thus there is a plausible explanation of the rarity of causalgia; of its association with high-velocity missile wounds and, to some extent, with traction injuries; and of its extreme rarity as a consequence of incised or lacerated wounds. The nerve injury is likely to be a partial one; this also accords with the facts. And if—as we believe—the part played by autonomic nerve fibres is crucial it is only to be expected that the median nerve, the tibial division of the sciatic, and the lowest trunk of the brachial plexus would be the nerves most commonly affected; they carry the greater part of the autonomic supply to the limbs. Moreover, if, as is the case, 9 out of 10 patients with causalgia suffer a wound in the proximal part of a limb the chances of autonomic fibres being involved are all the greater; they have not yet fanned out towards their ultimate distribution.

The mechanism whereby pain is produced is illustrated in Figure **9**, 1. It is assumed that the autonomic fibres are entirely efferent and there is ample evidence for this. Except during sleep an unceasing though variable stream of autonomic impulses passes down our limbs, in response to changes of temperature, painful stimuli, sudden noise and a wide range of emotions. If there is a short circuit with somatic nerve fibres mediating pain (and the hypothesis probably holds good even if the specificity of sensory nerve fibres is denied) then the efferent autonomic impulse provokes an afferent impulse in the conjoined sensory fibre. There is no reason why the short circuit should not form almost immediately and come into action rapidly. Causalgia can start within 24 hours of injury. Because the autonomic impulses are unremitting, so is the pain—during waking hours. And the sudden exacerbations are explained too. What matters more than any hypothesis is that sympathectomy almost invariably relieves the pain: the efferent pathway is interrupted.

However, there are difficulties.

1. Why should the extremity be so hypersensitive? It is possible that the stimulus coming across the short circuit travels centrifugally (antidromically) as well as centripetally. It has long been known (Lewis, 1942) that stimulation of the distal part of a severed nerve can cause pain. Lewis postulated that this was due to the release of a pain-producing substance. More recently Chapman, Ramos, Goodell and Wolff (1961) isolated what they call neurokinin, which when injected produces burning pain and vasodilatation.

2. This goes some way towards explaining the puzzling observation of Doupe *et al.*, that in some cases blocking the nerve with a local anaesthetic distal to the lesion relieves the pain temporarily; they called this *distal causalgia*. If as a result of the short circuits two kinds of impulse can be set up in somatic fibres—centri-

petal and centrifugal (antidromic)—both causing pain, the first directly and the second by the release of neurokinin peripherally, it is conceivable that one mechanism might sometimes predominate. If the antidromic impulses are particularly strong then distal anaesthetization of the nerve would interrupt them and so arrest the production of the pain-producing substance.

3. It has been alleged that resection of the damaged segment of nerve does not abolish

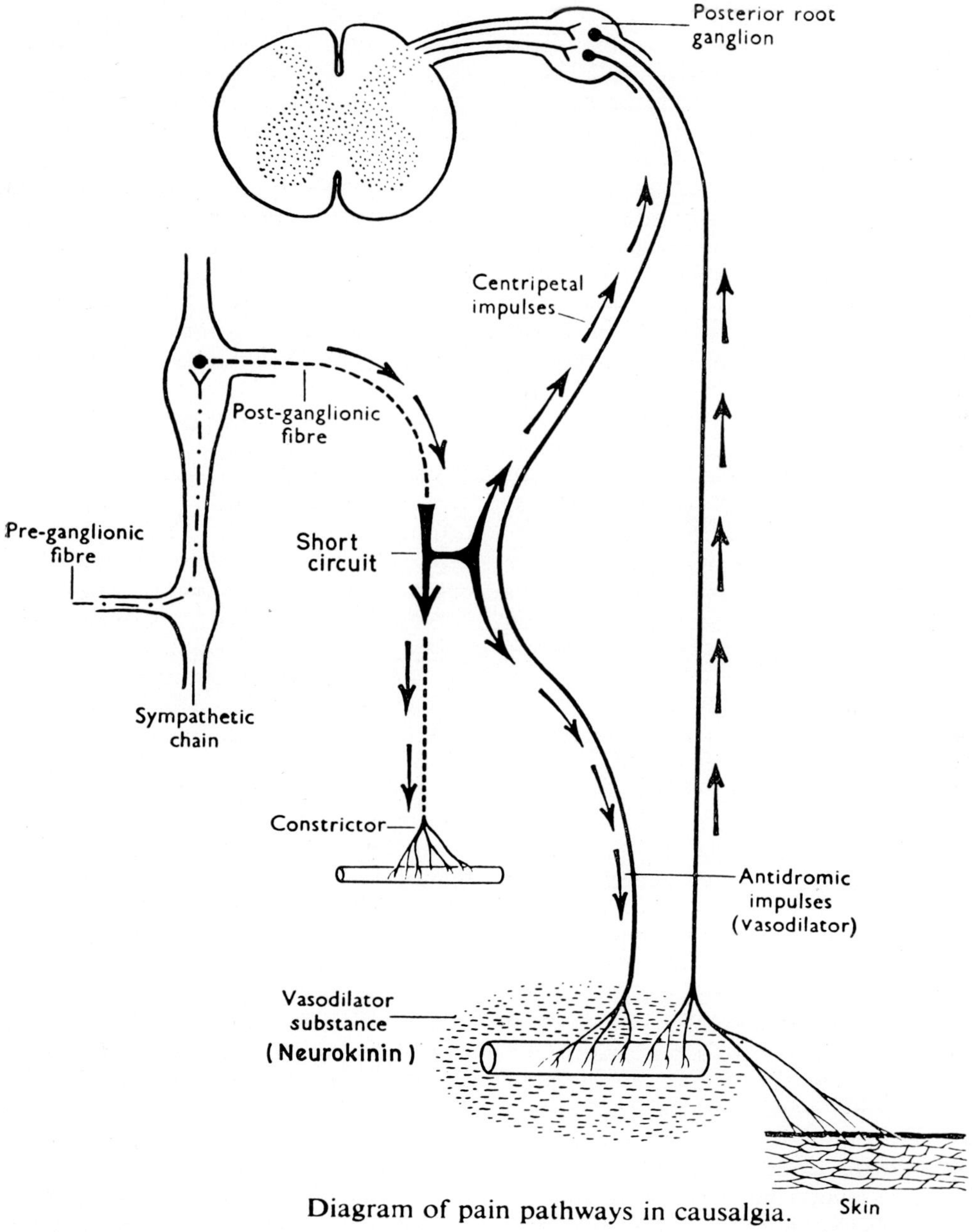

FIG. 9, 1. Diagram to illustrate Doupe's theory of the pathogenesis of causalgia. (Reproduced by kind permission from Barnes, R. (1954) in M.R.C. Special Report Series No. 282, p. 156.)

causalgia. The evidence for this is unconvincing. Moreover, it is pertinent to question the adequacy of the resection of the nerve in these cases. It has already been explained (p. 69) that a high-velocity missile wound causes widespread commotion of tissue, and the sort of damage—rupture of basement membranes without interruption of axons—that could permit the fusion of contiguous axons, the formation of the short circuit, is likely to be remote from the point of greatest damage. In dealing with an ordinary nerve injury caused by a high-velocity missile that requires repair it is sometimes necessary to resect the stumps generously before macroscopically normal funiculi are exposed; and occasionally, because of the difficulties of closing a large gap, one is obliged to be content with a resection that is inadequate. If this is the state of affairs when the aim is simply the exposure of funiculi that appear normal to the naked eye, how much greater a resection would be required to encompass the minute lesions—that a skilled microscopist would have the utmost difficulty is detecting—which are *ex hypothesi* responsible for causalgia? Barnes shrewdly observed that because injury of more than one nerve trunk is common in cases of causalgia it is possible that the wrong nerve may have been resected in some cases. Finally there are the records of successful resections (Platt and Bristow, 1924; Freeman, 1947).

4. It has been remarked that to define a certain type of pain by reference to its response to one form of treatment, namely sympathetic interruption, is artificial. This is unreasonable. If a theory of origin postulates the involvement of certain nervous pathways, then patients whose pain is relieved by interruption of one of them may properly be described as suffering from causalgia.

Before considering the second group of nerve injuries causing pain, it is necessary to contrast the views expressed in this chapter with those expounded in Chapters 34 to 37 of Sunderland's (1968) monumental work. He makes no distinction between causalgia and what are here described as irritative nerve lesions. It appears that although Sunderland concedes that sympathectomy relieves pain in some of the cases which he groups under the general heading of causalgia, he rejects the hypothesis set out above, largely because it fails to explain the facts in all cases. The generally accepted British view is that in the absence of a comprehensive explanation of why certain nerve lesions cause pain we do well to be content, for the time being, with a hypothesis that could account for the pain in some of them—those here described as causalgia. This attitude is at least helpful in the management of these distressing disorders.

IRRITATIVE NERVE LESIONS

We come now to an aspect of peripheral nerve injuries that is profoundly unsatisfactory: the painful syndromes that lack the distinctive features of causalgia. There is not even any accepted terminology; neither is there a working hypothesis as there is for causalgia. Yet, as will be seen from Table XIV, the number of patients presenting with these non-causalgic states far exceeds the number of patients with causalgia; they cannot be ignored.

The term *irritative nerve lesions* is unsatisfactory because it is too wide: it should include causalgia. On the other hand, the alternative, *hyperpathia*, is even more objectionable. It was employed by Foerster (1927) in connection with nerve injuries, and used by Büdinger and Kolmer (1943) to describe painful states that were not causalgic. An erudite description of hyperpathia was given by Walters (1959); it can occur in seven groups of disorders of the nervous system apart from peripheral nerve injuries. It is applied here to the exaggerated and very painful response to mechanical stimulation of the skin of the affected extremity. But this is a constant feature of causalgia. On the other hand, there are painful states following injury of a nerve in which the skin is not hypersensitive; there is no hyperpathia. So unless good reasons emerge for regarding the latter as a separate entity it seems expedient—no more than that—to apply one label to them all, and *faute de mieux* we may as well refer to these puzzling disorders as *irritative*.

CHARACTERISTICS

1. Whereas causalgia is almost exclusively a consequence of injury of the median nerve, of the tibial division of the sciatic or of the brachial

plexus, irritative nerve lesions may affect any nerve (Table XIV).

2. The interruption of the nerve in causalgia is almost always incomplete; in irritative lesions this is not invariably so, particularly when, as in complete brachial plexus paralysis, the pain is deep-seated, with no cutaneous hypersensitivity.

3. The pain is of two kinds, deep and superficial. A patient may complain of one or the other, or of both.

4. The deep pain, though usually present from the first, may not begin until months or years after the injury. This late pain may afflict a man who had become well adjusted to his paralytic disability and had been well content with his occupation. Whether coming on early or late the deep pain is more or less continuous, is affected by barometric changes and is less obtrusive if the patient's attention is held by work or by pleasant diversion. The pain is described as a deep aching, or as if the part were being crushed, or, rarely, there is a burning quality. The pain may be felt deep in an otherwise insensitive limb, as in some traction injuries of the brachial plexus. It can occur in limbs that have been severely damaged by ischaemia. Unlike the pain of causalgia it is but little influenced by sudden noise or emotional stress. It may be aggravated by cold.

5. The superficial pain is well described as hyperpathia. The gentlest stimulus applied to the affected part provokes a violently disagreeable response, though a sudden firm gripping of the hand or foot may fail to do so.

6. Both deep pain and hyperpathia are a feature (in one-third of the cases) of nerve injuries due to the injection of drugs.

7. Dryness or moisture of the hyperpathic part are without effect on its sensitivity. But a smooth moderately yielding surface is more comfortable than a hard one against which there is some friction. Many patients with hyperpathia of the foot required no treatment other than a well-fitting insole in the boot or shoe.

8. Unlike causalgia the pain of an irritative nerve lesion does not provoke pain in the contralateral or ipsilateral limb.

9. Hyperthermia of the affected part and

TABLE XIV—Comparative frequency of causalgia and of irritative nerve lesions

NERVE	NUMBER OF CASES STUDIED	CAUSALGIA		IRRITATIVE NERVE LESIONS	
		Number	%	Number	%
Brachial plexus: supraclavicular	180	2	1·1	25	13·9
Brachial plexus: infraclavicular	81	1	1·2	10	11·1
Median	489	5	1·0	29	5·9
Ulnar	586	—	—	39	6·65
Radial	236	1	0·4	5	2·1
Sciatic or its tibial division	242	7	2·9	29	12·1
Common peroneal	102	—	—	6	5·9
Posterior tibial	31	—	—	5	16·1
CUTANEOUS NERVES					
Digital	68	—	—	43	63·2*
Others	59	—	—	14	23·5*

If only major nerves are considered the frequency of causalgia is 0·82 per cent

* These proportions are misleadingly high; a number of patients with otherwise unimportant cutaneous nerve injuries were referred to us on account of pain

excessive sweating are uncommon. Usually the skin is as dry and cool as would be expected from the paralysis or paresis alone.

10. There are no striking dystrophic changes in the skin, nails or bones, and there is little tendency towards stiffness of the joints.

11. A patient with an irritative nerve lesion can be peevish, even miserable, like a man with a whitlow or a blistered foot. But he is never utterly demoralized and broken down by pain as is, more often than not, the case with causalgia. On the other hand, as will appear immediately, he may—like the victim of causalgia—come to be regarded as temperamentally abnormal.

Types of Injury

Causalgia is almost invariably due to a high-velocity missile wound; irritative nerve lesions can be caused by any type of injury.

Missile injuries are important; for example, 5 out of 10 irritative lesions of the infraclavicular brachial plexus (Table XIV) were caused by missiles. On the other hand the supraclavicular irritative lesions were mostly due to traction; but at this site traction injuries of the plexus, even in times of war, are far commoner than missile wounds. Ischaemic nerve lesions in the lower limb often cause persistent severe deep pain (p. 107); and one-quarter of all nerve lesions caused by the injection of drugs are irritative. Incisions for the evacuation of pus in a finger and clean incisions that happen to have involved a cutaneous nerve are not uncommonly followed by most unpleasant sensory disturbances.

The Co-existence of Causalgia and an Irritative Nerve Lesion

There are a few patients whose symptoms and signs cannot be clearly categorized as due to causalgia or to an irritative nerve lesion. If, as is suggested here, there are two (there may be more) kinds of derangement of sensibility following a nerve injury it is possible that they can co-exist. It may be found that interruption of the autonomic nerve supply, either by local anaesthesia or surgically, gives partial though welcome relief. The symptoms and signs that persist are then more distinctly those of an irritative nerve lesion; the causalgic component has been abolished.

Prognosis

Of the 205 patients listed in Table XV, 52 were not operated on: three out of four of them became free of pain within a matter of months. If to them we add the 55 patients whose nerves were explored—and it is doubtful whether this operation, if intended to be a neurolysis, had any beneficial influence on the pain—the proportion of patients who became free of pain is almost exactly the same. If to those patients whose pain was completely relieved (without operation or after exploration) we add those whose pain diminished to a degree that was easily bearable —they appear in Table XV as 'improved'—we find that 99 out of 113 (88 per cent) made a perfect or tolerable recovery. So quite apart from the difference in severity of the pain these irritative nerve lesions are much more benign than causalgia. But in the minority of about 1 in 10 patients the pain is most persistent, and there are a very few in whom it resists almost all, and sometimes all, that surgical therapeutics has to offer. Careful observers, such as Livingston (1947*b*), hesitate to label these patients as psychopathic. This is wise. Before sympathectomy became established as an almost sovereign remedy for causalgia (and provided a tenable explanation of its pathology) the same facile attitude was sometimes adopted towards the victims of this dreadful condition who persisted in their misery. If we confess, as we should, that we are even more ignorant of the cause of irritative nerve lesions it would be expedient to regard the basis of the disorder as organic, though not denying (as in the occasional case of causalgia: see Doupe *et al.*, 1944) that the pain can lead to mental disorder or bring to light some previously latent instability.

Irritative Lesions of Digital Nerves

It will have been noted (Table XIV) that lesions of the digital nerves of the hand are particularly liable to be followed by pain. However, the general incidence must be much lower than the figure of 63·2 per cent given in the Table, for

TABLE XV—Results of treatment

CAUSALGIA		Relieved	Improved	Unchanged	
No operation	4	2	2		
Exploration	4	1	1	2 (1 sympathectomy subsequently)	
Sympathectomy	9	6	2	1	
16 PATIENTS IN ALL	—	9	5	2	

IRRITATIVE NERVE LESIONS	Number of patients	Relieved	Improved	Unchanged	Worse	Late result unknown
1. MAIN NERVES						
No operation	40	30	7	3	—	—
Exploration	55	40	9	5	—	1
Repair	33	24	6	2	1	—
Resection	11	8	2	1	—	—
Others*	9	8	—	—	—	1
TOTALS	148	110	24	11	1	2
2. DIGITAL NERVES						
No operation	9	8	—	1	—	—
Exploration	4	2	1	1	—	—
Repair	16	11	3	2	—	—
Resection	13	6	4	3	—	—
Other†	1	—	1	—	—	—
TOTALS	43	27	9	7	—	—
3. OTHER CUTANEOUS NERVES						
No operation	3	1	1	—	1	—
Exploration	2	—	—	1	1	—
Repair	1	—	—	—	1	—
Resection	7	—	4	3	—	—
Other†	1	—	—	—	—	1
TOTALS	14	1	5	4	3	1

NUMBER OF PATIENTS WITH IRRITATIVE NERVE LESIONS 205

* Almost all anterior transpositions of the ulnar nerve. † Removal of foreign body

many patients were referred to us solely on account of the pain they suffered.

The nerve (or nerves, because multiple lesions are not uncommon) may have been severed but the injury is usually partial. The finger, or part of it, may have been amputated (Fig. **9,** 2) and the source of the pain is then an amputation neuroma. If to these cases we add those in which an exquisitely tender scar follows an incision for the drainage of a whitlow or for some other condition we are faced with a fair number of patients.

Sepsis may play some part in the genesis of the pain. It had been present in 25·6 per cent of the cases of irritative lesions of the digital nerves (only cases of overt nerve injury are included in Tables XIV and XV) but in only 8·0 per cent of those that were painless. Clearly, as with irritative nerve lesions in general, there are other more significant and, at present, unknown factors.

There is invariably tenderness, which may be pronounced, not only at the site of the scar in the finger or of the amputation but of the surrounding skin, skin which may be normally innervated. If the nerve has been partially divided there is the usual hyperpathia in its area of distribution distal to the scar. The lightest touch will provoke the pain but, as with irritative lesions elsewhere, firm pressure may be tolerated. If severe, the pain is described as being like an

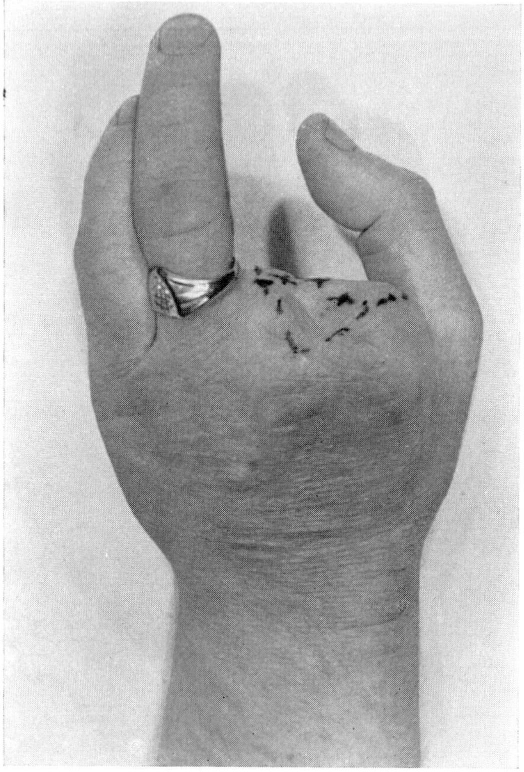

FIG. **9**, 2. The crosses indicate the tender neuromas; the broken line the area of hypersensitivity.

electric shock, milder pain usually as a sensation of pins and needles.

Some patients also complain of spontaneous pain, more particularly in the proximally situated lesions. It is an ache, very rarely a sensation of burning; it is always aggravated by cold but apart from that it can be spasmodic for no apparent reason.

The patients who suffer most severely generally show cyanosis of the tender area; the skin is a little cooler than normal, and there is no excessive sweating.

Painful Amputation Stumps

Amputation of a limb necessarily inflicts multiple nerve injuries. End-bulbs invariably form. They sometimes cause pain, which may be related to the far more frequent phantom sensations.

This awkward topic is not discussed here because it has to be considered as part of the whole subject of amputations and limb-fitting, which is outside the scope of this work.

Phantom Sensations and Painful Phantoms

Almost every patient who has suffered an amputation has phantom sensations, at least for a time. If we pause to think of it we are all aware of a body image; it is cortically represented (Head and Holmes, 1911; and see particularly Riddoch's (1941) superb essay), and the image persists after amputation. It usually shrinks, the image of the digits of the hand—which has a large cortical representation—continuing for longer than that of the rest of the upper limb, until the patient may feel that he has a short stump with some digits at the end of it. Amputation phantoms can be painful, though this is uncommon.

This topic concerns us here only in connection with complete lesions of the brachial plexus; the patient so afflicted sometimes has a phantom, and is startled to find that the position of it in no way corresponds with the actual position of his paralysed arm.

Of the patients with severe injuries of the plexus due to traction, 13 per cent noticed phantoms. In no case of missile injury were there phantom sensations, but the paralysis was invariably subtotal.

Provided that he is reassured by simple explanation of what is meant by the body image the phantom ceases to bother the patient whether the arm is retained or amputated. But painful phantom sensations, though uncommon, can be as great a nuisance to the patient who has suffered a brachial plexus injury as to one who has lost a limb. Only two patients had painful phantoms. In both the onset of the pain was long delayed; in one case it was tolerable, in the other a high cervical cordotomy was performed by M. A. Falconer (1953, 1966) with success.

TREATMENT

Causalgia

Whenever it is suspected that pain after a nerve injury is causalgic a diagnostic injection of a local anaesthetic should be made into the appropriate autonomic ganglia: alternatively the effect of a systemic sympathetic paralysant may be observed.

Upper limb. The injection is made into the region of the stellate ganglion by the anterior approach. The patient lies on his back with the head turned to the opposite side. If possible, the scalenus anterior muscle is palpated just lateral to the clavicular origin of the sterno-cleido-mastoid muscle. In this line a mark is made on the skin 2·5 cm proximal to the clavicle and here the needle is inserted. After the skin and deeper tissues have been infiltrated a number 22 gauge needle, 6·5 to 7·5 cm long, is inserted in such a way that it passes distally and medially at an angle of 45 degrees until at a depth of 3 to 5 cm it comes into contact with bone. About 10 ml of an appropriate local anaesthetic containing a trace of adrenalin are injected *slowly*.[1] The needle is then withdrawn a little and reinserted so that its point passes over the head of the first rib. When contact has again been made with bone, another 10 ml of the anaesthetic solution are injected. It is most important that the injections should be made at a rate not exceeding 5 ml a minute; serious and even fatal reactions have followed rapid injection. There is a slight but not alarming risk of pneumothorax.

Lower limb. The patient lies on his normal side and a 12-cm needle is inserted level with the upper edge of the third lumbar spinous process and at the outer border of the mass of the spinal muscles. The needle is advanced at an angle of 70 degrees with the coronal plane of the body until it touches a vertebral body. If it strikes the transverse process the needle is redirected to pass just distal to it. The point is advanced until it can be felt to glide tangentially past the antero-lateral surface of the vertebra; 20 ml of the anaesthetic solution are then injected slowly.

The paralysis being almost invariably partial, the clinician should not be satisfied unless signs of autonomic paralysis are apparent within 5 to 10 minutes: flushing of the skin, cessation of sweating and, in the upper limb, Horner's syndrome. True causalgic pain is abolished very quickly and the relief may persist for hours or several days. In mild cases the pain may be abolished permanently by repeated injection (Rasmussen and Freedman, 1946), and for this reason there should be no haste in resorting to sympathectomy; but this does not apply in severe causalgia because the response to repeated injections is disappointing.

The introduction of drugs causing paralysis of autonomic ganglia—such as tetraethyl ammonium compounds, then many others of which trimetaphan is a recent example—seemed to offer a way of avoiding the hazards of direct injection of the sympathetic chain. We have used these drugs diagnostically, often with success; but if their administration is not followed by rapid relief of pain thought to be causalgic it is wise to proceed to direct injection.

It would have been gratifying if in undoubted causalgia these ganglionic paralysants could have been employed therapeutically, especially as causalgia has a tendency to spontaneous regression. The patient's misery could have been mitigated, even abolished, while regression was occurring. Unfortunately, these drugs act on parasympathetic as well as on sympathetic ganglia and so give rise to various distressing symptoms. The boom in drugs used in the treatment of hypertension seems unlikely to benefit the victim of causalgia. They all (guanethidine, bethanidine and debrisoquine, for example) act peripherally by inhibiting the release of noradrenalin. If Doupe's theory of the pathogenesis of causalgia is correct, none of these drugs would relieve the pain. However, it would be of the greatest theoretical and possibly practical interest, in case the short-circuit theory is wrong, to investigate their action in proven cases of causalgia.

If in spite of an injection that has produced sympathetic paralysis there is no relief of pain, then—by definition—the patient is not suffering from causalgia and sympathectomy will be useless. There may, however, be substantial though not complete relief, in which case sympathectomy is likely to be worth while.

[1] A long-acting local anaesthetic, such as Marcain, is advantageous. Because it is about four times as potent as lignocaine it should not be used at a concentration exceeding 0·5 per cent.

Sympathectomy

In 1930 Spurling reported a case of causalgia following a missile wound of the brachial plexus that was cured by cervico-thoracic sympathectomy. Surgeons were slow to appreciate the significance of this experiment which not only rendered all other forms of surgical treatment obsolete but paved the way for a better understanding of the pathogenesis of causalgia. Resection and suture, even when successful, had been a heavy price to pay for the treatment of a paralysis that was almost always partial. Nevertheless it is necessary to define the conditions under which exploration of the damaged nerve is still called for.

The treatment of a patient with severe causalgia and a wound that is still open and possibly infected. Although the diagnosis has been confirmed by anaesthetization of the sympathetic chain the wound should be explored before sympathectomy is contemplated. The reason for this is that the local operation alone may relieve the pain, and more particularly if, as happens rarely, the nerve is found to be severed and should therefore be dealt with by resection and suture (Freeman, 1947). This is the one occasion when it is justifiable to explore and even to repair a nerve in the presence of infection, provided that the latter is not severe. The operation must include removal of all devitalized tissue, and the infection must be controlled by appropriate antibiotic therapy. The patient may be kept comfortable before and, if necessary, for a time after operation by anaesthetization of the sympathetic chain.

Exploration versus sympathectomy when the patient presents with a healed wound. This is a difficult question. As will be seen from Table XV, exploration alone was carried out in three of our patients; one was completely relieved, in another the pain was relieved to such an extent that it was not thought necessary to perform sympathectomy, and in one patient the pain remained unchanged. It is reasonable to explore the nerve before resorting to sympathectomy if the paralysis appears to be complete, or when a radiograph shows foreign bodies at the site of the nerve damage.

Technical aspects of sympathectomy. In the upper limb the preganglionic type of operation has usually been preferred, the technique being that devised by Smithwick (1940). The rami communicantes to the second and third thoracic ganglia are divided and the sympathetic trunk is severed distal to the third ganglion. For causalgia in the lower limb most surgeons have been content to remove the second, third and fourth lumbar ganglia; but some authors have occasionally found it necessary to remove the first ganglion as well, and even the lowest two thoracic ganglia.

Results of sympathectomy. The relief of pain may be immediate, but sometimes it can be delayed for as long as 10 days after the operation. The result is not jeopardized if there is long delay between injury and sympathectomy; it was almost seven years in the case of two prisoners-of-war described by Barnes (M.R.C.R., 1954). Nevertheless prolonged causalgia is demoralizing; it also leaves the affected limb in poor condition however gratifying the relief of the pain.

The final results have been well summarized by Richards (1967); sympathectomy is about equally effective in the upper and in the lower limb.

There are three reasons for some of the failures. The operation may have been inadequate, as can be revealed by a sweating test carried out subsequently. It is possible that in the lower limb the standard operation, though properly performed, has been insufficient, and it is in these cases that removal of the first lumbar ganglion and even the two lowest thoracic ganglia has proved necessary. It is possible that some failures have been due to the performance of sympathectomy for pain that was not causalgic, but this would hardly apply to any of the failures recorded in Table XVI; the surgeons concerned had been careful to establish the diagnosis by anaesthetization of the sympathetic ganglia.

Irritative Nerve Lesions

Digital Nerves

A few patients (Table XV) recovered spontaneously. Operative treatment should not, therefore, be undertaken unless disabling pain has been present for a considerable time.

Infiltration with a local anaesthetic is not

only useless, it is a most painful procedure. Open operation alone can give relief and only two types of intervention are valuable; resection and suture, or extensive resection.

Resection and suture. Most irritative lesions of the digital nerves are due to partial division, and it seems to be the lateral neuroma that is the source of pain. If resection and suture can be performed meticulously, normal channels are provided for the outgrowing fibres. This operation gives complete relief in almost three-quarters of the cases in which it can be performed, and substantial improvement in a further few cases.

Resection. Amputation or re-amputation of the painful part has long been practised; it rarely gives more than temporary benefit, and when the pain returns it is often worse than before. This operation should be avoided. Local resection of tender neuromas is also disappointing, except perhaps when there is an exposed and easily palpable neuroma to which the tenderness is confined. If resection is performed (this applies almost exclusively to cases in which a part or the whole of a digit has been amputated) it must be extensive. The nerve is traced into the palm and severed near its point of departure from the main trunk of the nerve, usually the median. This operation gives relief in about half the cases and acceptable improvement in over half of the remainder.

Chemical methods. It is convenient here to consider the chemical inhibition of neuroma formation. If it has been decided that resection is the appropriate treatment for an irritative lesion of a digital or other superficial nerve then it is logical to do whatever is possible to prevent the re-formation of a neuroma, which could be as troublesome as the one for which the resection had been performed. This subject was studied thoroughly by Guttmann and Medawar (1942). They found that fixatives alone inhibited neuroma formation and the development of adhesions to the tip of the severed nerve. Tannic acid is unsatisfactory because it does not spread within the nerve. Guttmann and Medawar recommend either formaldehyde, 20 per cent or stronger, or 1 per cent gentian violet. Because they are so potent—gentian violet is a most powerful protoplasmic poison—these agents must be handled with great care. Formaldehyde should be coloured with methylene blue so that the extent of its spread can be observed. The stump of the nerve to be injected is completely isolated from the surrounding tissues. A small sheet of impervious material such as jaconet is placed beneath the stump, which is then packed round with absorbent gauze or wool. A ligature is placed round the nerve not less than 2 cm from its cut end, but not closer than 1 cm to the parent nerve. It is tied moderately firmly, not tightly. The sclerosing solution is then injected beneath the epineurium, and into the substance of the nerve if it is larger than a digital or other cutaneous nerve. The danger is seepage of the fixative from the cut end of the nerve, but this can be avoided by the preliminary packing and by allowing seepage to occur into the absorbent material before it is removed. When the stump is replaced it should on no account be allowed to come into contact with a neighbouring nerve.

Experimentally, this chemical inhibition is effective for at least a year and adhesions do not form between the nerve and its bed. The question is whether this treatment is effective in dealing with painful neuromas. It seems logical to employ it if resection is indicated. We have used 40 per cent formalin, but because we had no adequate controls it could not be established that the chemical inhibition conferred any

TABLE XVI—Results of sympathectomy for causalgia

Collected from American and British sources.

		Excellent	Good	Poor
Upper limb	Cases	152	27	8
	Percentage	81·3	14·4	4·3
Lower limb	Cases	85	32	3
	Percentage	70·8	26·7	2·5

additional benefit. It appeared to inhibit the recurrence of tenderness; but some patients complained of aching in the hand and a few were troubled by hyperidrosis of the whole of the affected hand. Both these untoward sequelae regressed within a year or so.

Mechanical methods. These have been used to inhibit neuroma formation. We endeavoured to get the neuroma out of harm's way by drilling a neighbouring bone and drawing the end of the nerve into it so that any subsequent neuroma formation would be intraosseous. This operation was a failure, probably because the hole filled in with new bone and a new extraosseous neuroma formed. Caps of various inert materials have been used, but they also have proved ineffective (Poth, Fernandez and Drager, 1945).

Other Cutaneous Nerves

The incidence of these lesions is fairly high (Table XIV). The treatment is along the same lines as for irritative lesions of the digital nerves, but extensive resection has been employed almost to the exclusion of resection and suture. This, perhaps, may explain why the results have been indifferent; not one patient was completely relieved of his pain.

Major Nerves

These are the cases in which differentiation from causalgia is so important. The latter, as we define it, affects only major nerve trunks and not all of them. Unless accurate anaesthetization of the appropriate sympathetic ganglia abolishes the pain, or reduces it very substantially, sympathectomy will be ineffective. On the other hand the possibility that a patient's pain is causalgic should not be dismissed because it is not agonizing (Echlin, Owens and Wells, 1949).

There is no sovereign remedy for these irritative lesions of the major nerves. Fortunately, as has been explained on page 146, spontaneous improvement, even complete remission, is frequent.

Palliative measures. In the lower limb mechanical palliation can be useful. A patient with an irritative lesion of the sciatic or posterior tibial nerve may be sufficiently comforted by the fitting of an appropriate insole in his footwear.

Exploration. This operation, if dignified by the term neurolysis, has proved disappointing; but exploration of the nerve with a view to doing something more radical can be valuable.

Removal of foreign bodies. This is occasionally curative, especially if the foreign body is only just embedded in the nerve.

Burying the nerve. Formerly this applied only to ulnar nerve lesions at the elbow, where deep transposition gave good results (Table XV). There is now an attractive variant of this for the hand (Brown and Flynn, 1973) where painful neuromas may be protected by an overlying skin pedicle graft.

Resection and suture. Repair has given fairly satisfactory results; 24 out of 33 patients were completely relieved and a further six greatly improved. This is undoubtedly the treatment of choice, but it is sometimes inapplicable and then the last resort, so far as local operations are concerned, is resection.

Resection. If the resection is sufficiently extensive the result is likely to be satisfactory. However, there have been disappointments, notably in irritative traction lesions of the supraclavicular brachial plexus. A few patients suffering from total paralysis of the upper limb caused by damage mainly distal to the intervertebral foramina (infraganglionic), and who had been treated by amputation through the arm with arthrodesis of the shoulder, returned years later complaining of persistent pain in the stump. There were, of course, no amputation neuromas because the nerves were totally degenerate. It seemed possible that over a long period there had been progressive intraneural fibrosis and that longitudinal shrinkage of the plexus had irritated sensory axons proximal to the lesion. For all we knew what remained of the plexus was tethered distally. So in three patients the stump of the plexus was excised. It will be observed in Figure **11**, 19 (p. 188), which was typical of all three cases, that the resection was barely adequate proximally. Yet this hardly accounts for the return of the pain after a period of relief, because posterior rhizotomy, which is certainly adequate anatomically, has proved equally disappointing.

We come now to those few unhappy patients who are not relieved by any sort of peripheral surgery. The only heroic remedy of which we have had experience is high cervical cordotomy, to which reference has already been made (p. 148).

Antidepressant drugs. It is now necessary to consider the work on painful nerve lesions of Merle d'Aubigné and his colleagues (1961), and Maurer, Tomeno and Comiti, (1973). Their experience of these disorders is exceptionally great; the policy they are following in dealing with them is very different from that of most other centres; but their views must necessarily command respect. Although their classification of cases into five—more recently six—groups seems forbidding three at any rate are generally familiar: the local lesion (e.g. Fig. **9**, 2); the painful phantom limb, with which we have not concerned ourselves, except in relation to total brachial plexus injuries (p. 148); and causalgia. In neither of their two main studies, before 1961, and after that year, were they greatly perturbed by the first group; a local operation—suture if indicated, otherwise neurolysis or resection—usually gave relief. In the other groups of cases surgical intervention was all too frequently disappointing. Causalgia, for example, was relieved by sympathectomy in only 30 to 40 per cent of cases, an experience which led these surgeons to question the much greater proportion of successes reported by others.

The gravity of complaint in patients referred to them increased and this, together with the futility of much surgical endeavour, impelled them to seek the aid of psychiatrists. The success of the latter in the use of antidepressant drugs, such as imipramine plus promazine and amitriptyline (with adjuvants such as diazepam and chlorpromazine as required) led to a marked change in the plan of attack on all but the first tractable group of cases. It is first essential to categorize the pain in the difficult groups 2 to 6, and to ensure that the patient is not psychotic, sometimes no easy matter. The antidepressant drugs (thymoanaleptiques) are then given along with such surgical measures as may be indicated. The side-effects of these drugs can be disastrous; so this aspect of treatment needs to be embarked on 'advisedly, soberly, and in the fear of God'. The possible combined programmes of treatment may be studied in the 1973 paper. The results, though not spectacular, have been good enough to encourage these surgeons endowed with healthy scepticism. What is remarkable is that pain caused by a lesion so patently organic yields at all to such measures. We are further than ever from understanding the nature of these painful traumatic nerve disorders.

10. Nerve Tumours

THIS DISCUSSION OF nerve tumours is written from the clinical standpoint, although oncological terms must necessarily be used to describe the several varieties. The trouble about these tumours is that they are just common enough to come within the experience of almost all surgeons and rare enough to cause embarrassment in diagnosis and treatment. A patient presents with an isolated lump. Removal of it seems a simple affair; then there is consternation for patient and surgeon when it is subsequently discovered that there is paralysis of a major nerve. A child who came under the care of D. M. Brooks had had an innocent nerve tumour removed from the side of the neck: result, total paralysis of the arm. In one of my cases partial removal of a similar swelling had left an irreparable gap in the upper trunk of the brachial plexus. When it is found that the tumours are innocent and could have been shelled out with at worst a transient paresis the situation is deplorable. A surgeon, acting with the best of intentions, has been involved in litigation leading to heavy damages (Medical Protection Society, 1968).

But there are even more tragic cases. A lump that turns out to be malignant has been removed by circumscribed excision, such as is suited only to an innocent tumour. It recurs: a further excision is performed and before long the patient is dead, with metastases. Although not even amputation well wide of the tumour can guarantee survival, there is no doubt that malignant tumours of nerve have to be treated with almost the same ruthlessness that is needed in dealing with osteosarcoma; and with this disheartening difference, that whereas some primary malignant tumours of bone may be radiosensitive, malignant tumours of nerve are not.

Soft-tissue tumours in the limbs, including those of nerves, often present formidable diagnostic problems. In consequence there is a temptation to resort to diagnostic biopsy. As will be explained later this impairs the prospects of dealing satisfactorily with a neurilemmoma, the one tumour that can be enucleated.

Biopsy may be harmless, though we cannot be sure, in the investigation of what may prove to be a malignant nerve tumour; except in two respects: that it wastes valuable time, and that there is the possibility that malignancy developing in a previously innocent neurofibroma may not have spread as far as the piece removed. It is usually possible to make a provisional diagnosis on clinical evidence alone, and if the exploratory operation is properly planned a firm diagnosis can be made from what the exploration reveals: then an appropriate excision can be carried out forthwith. The surgeon should rely first on what he himself discovers. The role of the pathologist is to confirm or refute the provisional operative diagnosis; the histological evidence allows one to judge the propriety of the action already taken.

NOMENCLATURE

This, as perusal of Stout's (1949) classical monograph reveals, is singularly confusing; this is due mainly to the intractability of the material, though there also seems to be an element of semantic perversity, of which I may not be entirely guiltless. One example will suffice. One of the most important distinctions to be made is between neurofibroma and neurilemmoma, yet in their excellent account of the experience of innocent nerve tumours at the Mayo Clinic (Dodge and Craig, 1957) the authors say 'we have chosen to refer to these tumours as neurofibromas or neurilemmomas' and it is not until the reader is well into the paper that he realizes that they are in fact writing entirely about the latter. Fortunately in Britain there is a wide measure of agreement about terminology.[1]

[1] The two most important recent classifications are those of:

I. *The International Union Against Cancer* (*1965*):

Neurinoma, neurilemoma, Schwannoma: benign
The same three synonyms: malignant.
Neurofibroma: benign.
So general a classification does not call for comment.

Here are the terms commonly used and, in brackets, the number of cases that have come to our attention at the Royal National Orthopaedic Hospital.

Benign

Neurilemmoma (47)
Neurofibromatosis: multiple (154)
(but only nine of them referred to here)
Neurofibroma: solitary (9)
Fatty tumours (3)
Haemangioma (1)

Malignant

Neurosarcoma (12)
Primitive neurectodermal tumours (1)

This collection has been made over a period of 25 years by H. A. Sissons, D. M. Brooks and myself and I am greatly indebted to my two colleagues. Tumours not occurring in the limbs have for the most part been excluded. But the distribution of nerve tumours is pretty well ubiquitous and this is why whatever may be a surgeon's particular hunting ground he will surely encounter them sooner or later. Two of the common peripheral nerve tumours, neurofibroma and neurilemmoma, are familiar denizens of the spinal canal.

II. *The World Health Organisation (1969)*:

1. *Benign*
   (*a*) Traumatic neuroma (amputation neuroma)
   (*b*) Neurofibroma
   (*c*) Neurilemoma (Schwannoma)
   (*d*) Neurofibromatosis.
2. *Malignant*
   (*a*) Malignant Schwannoma (neurogenic sarcoma, neurofibrosarcoma)
   (*b*) Peripheral tumours of primitive neuroectoderm.

Comments on the second classification.

1 (*a*) Not a tumour; why include it?

1 (*c*) Both terms unexceptionable, but recent evidence from electron microscopy (Russell and Rubinstein, 1971) is heavily in favour of neurofibroma also originating in Schwann cells. Schwannoma suggests an exclusive origin; therefore although, as these authors point out, neurilemma is a vague anatomical term, it has the merit of not being too emphatic. So neurilemmoma will be used here, with two m's: Greek λέμμα.

2 (*a*) Russell and Rubinstein distinguish between sarcoma developing in neurofibromatosis and the malignant Schwannoma. Apart from the manifest element of danger in any patient with neurofibromatosis the distinction is unhelpful to the clinician. Neurosarcoma covers both adequately.

2 (*b*) This wide description is unavoidable, but there is doubt as to the need for it (p. 169).

BENIGN TUMOURS

NEURILEMMOMA

This is the commonest of all true peripheral nerve tumours, and its importance is enhanced by the fact that it can be removed with no impairment of function of the nerve in which it has originated.

AGE DISTRIBUTION. It is uncommon in children and in the very old. It is seen mostly between the ages of 20 and 70 with a peak in the 20 to 30 decade.

SEX DISTRIBUTION. It is rather commoner in females than in males.

ANATOMICAL DISTRIBUTION. A neurilemmoma may arise almost anywhere in the body, but references will be made only to tumours in the limbs and to those involving the brachial and lumbo-sacral plexuses. The distribution as between major and minor nerve trunks is 43:20 *tumours*, roughly 2:1. The distinction is important. In the first group, treatment by enucleation is obligatory; in the latter, excision of the lump together with its nerve of origin is often appropriate.

MULTIPLICITY. The frequency of multiplicity is sufficient to require notice, though it rarely approaches that seen in neurofibromatosis.

Apparently single tumours	40
Locally multiple	3
Tumours in more than one limb	1
Locally multiple and also in more than one limb	1
Multiple tumours in one limb and multiple spinal neurilemmomas	1
Tumour in one limb, one beneath the mandible and two in the spinal canal	1
Number of patients	47

Intriguing diagnostic problems can arise, as in the last patient listed, who was under the care of my colleague, E. L. Trickey. This man had a small lump beneath the mandible and another over one lateral femoral condyle. Both were excised and proved to be neurilemmomas. Then there were disturbing signs of spinal cord compression; neurilemmomas were discovered at two levels. Because several tumours, one of which may be large and the others small, can be found in one nerve trunk, and because a tumour may appear—perhaps after several years—at a slightly different level in a nerve trunk from which a neurilemmona has already been removed, there is reason to question reports of recurrence after complete enucleation. Once, at the conclusion of the enucleation of a sizable neurilemmoma, a vigilant assistant noticed a slight fullness of the nerve a few centimetres proximal to the site of operation. It was found to be due to another, very small tumour; if it had gone undetected its later appearance could easily have been attributed to recurrence.

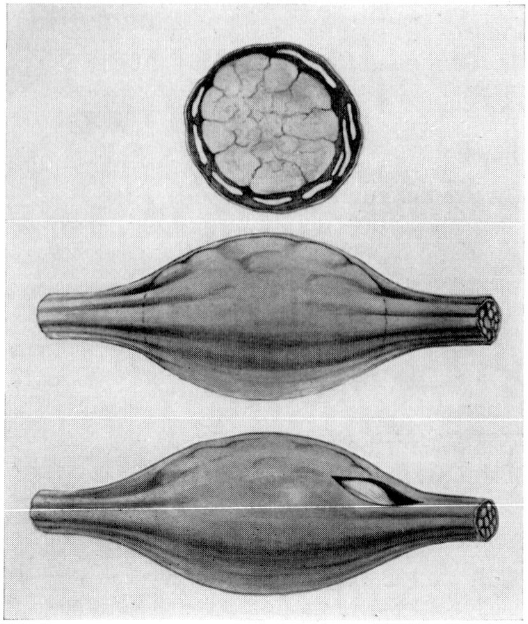

FIG. **10**, 1. Diagrammatic representation of a neurilemmoma. The tumour displaces and flattens out the nerve bundles. It is usually eccentric and the epineurium should be opened, as shown, where the tumour is most superficial and just where the ballooning of the nerve begins.

Pathology

GROSS STRUCTURE. The tumour, always encapsulated, grows slowly within a nerve trunk, displacing but not apparently invading the funiculi. Although it may be slightly lobulated this is not always apparent until the tumour has been enucleated. The mass is egg-shaped and its greatest dimension does not usually exceed 2·5 cm; however, we have removed one that was 9 cm long. Smith (1849) in his vivid description of nerve tumours, some of which were undoubtedly neurilemmomas, writes happily of lumps the size of a melon (variety not stated), a 'moderate-sized cocoa-nut' and a pineapple, the last being undoubtedly a neurilemmoma; but this was early in the nineteenth century, when patients were slow to complain.

The nerve bundles are, of course, greatly attenuated (Fig. **10**, 1), and those most severely stretched are like gossamer. The tumour is usually eccentric, and on the side where it protrudes most there may be no bundles at all (Fig. **10**, 2); it is covered only by its capsule and by the epineurium. One sometimes finds that the tumour has worked its way clear of all the funiculi, and removal is then very simple. It is unusual for the epineural vessels to be dilated, because they too are stretched. Nevertheless, they may be con-

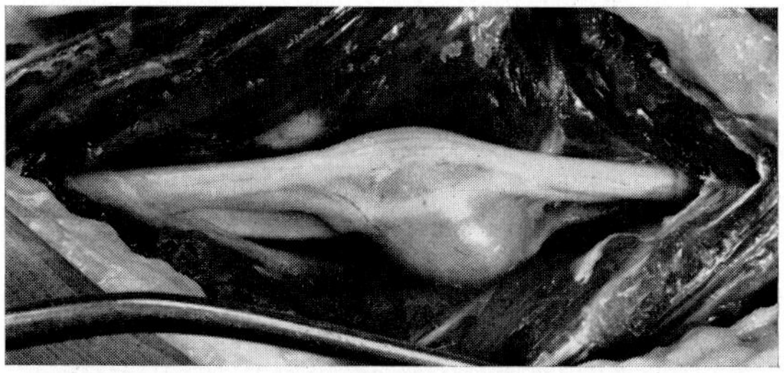

FIG. **10**, 2. The eccentricity of this neurilemmoma is well shown. (By courtesy of Mr D. M. Brooks.)

spicuous (Fig. **10**, 3), and the surgeon must not be misled into thinking that this is an indication of malignancy. If he finds that the tumour has not burst through the epineurium, if its extremities are rounded rather than tapering, if bundles can be seen coursing over it he should take courage and enucleate the mass.

These lumps are sometimes firm, sometimes oedematous (Fig. **10**, 4), sometimes more or less

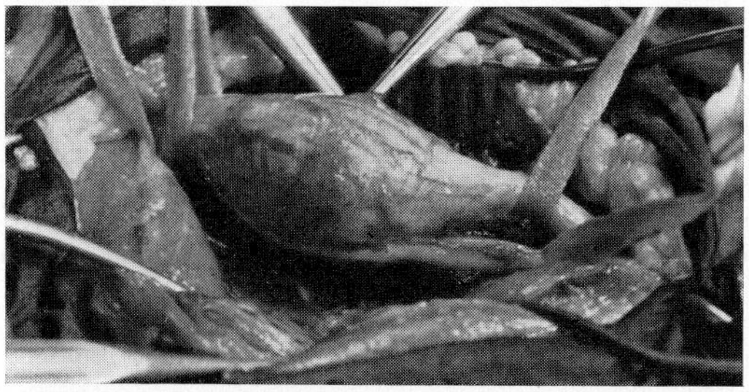

FIG. **10**, 3. A neurilemmoma more central than usual; epineural vessels very dilated.

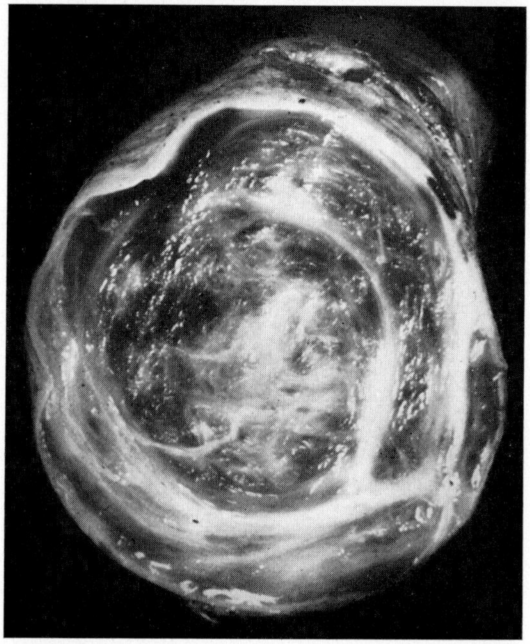

FIG. **10**, 4. A neurilemmoma shelled out from a nerve. The capsule is well shown; the tumour is oedematous and in places cystic.

cystic (Fig. **10**, 5) which explains why they may be transilluminable. Unless the lump is cystic—when it may look like any other cyst—its colour is greyish pink, yellow or brown.

HISTOLOGY. There seems no reason to question the arguments of Murray and Stout (1940) and others that these are Schwann-cell tumours; the evidence from tissue culture is impressive. Nevertheless, the term neurilemmoma has the advantage of being less specific than Schwannoma in that it means merely a tumour arising from the

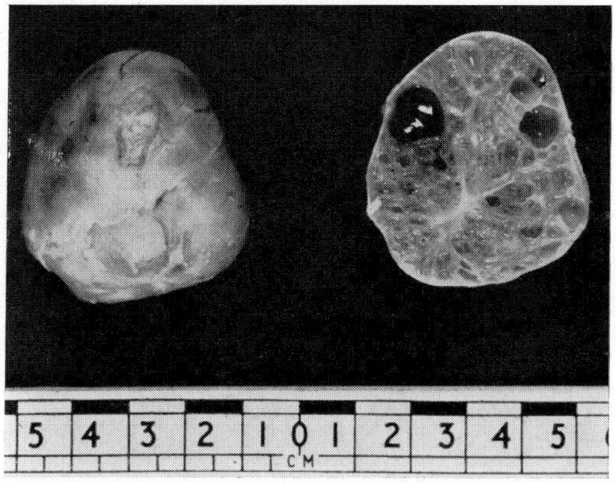

FIG. **10**, 5. Cystic neurilemmoma.

neural sheath without specifying which cellular component.

The histological features, which are distinctive, are as follows. The more solid parts of the tumour are composed of what look like Schwann cells arranged in clumps, mingled with fine connective tissue elements. The long nuclei may lie parallel with each other, an appearance described as palisading (Fig. **10**, 6). We come now to two names that persistently appear in pathological reports, Verocay (1910) and Antoni (1920). Verocay described agglomerations of Schwann cells bearing some resemblance to the more elaborate cutaneous sensory end-organs. What Antoni described as type A tissue are the compact masses of Schwann cells; and as type B tissue the much more loosely and irregularly arranged Schwann cells with spaces between them, perhaps actual cysts, and patches of what look like degeneration (Fig. **10**, 7). Other incidental features are the presence of mast cells and phagocytes containing lipoid material. The degeneration and cyst formation may be very pronounced so that the characteristic cells can be found only in the wall of the tumour.

Although Stout (1949) found occasional nerve fibres in the periphery of neurilemmomas, which he thought were due to mechanical damage inflicted by the tumour on the stretched funiculi, it has been generally believed that a neurilemmoma, unlike a neurofibroma, is normally devoid of nerve fibres. This view is supported by the comparative ease with which the lump can be enucleated from between the funiculi. Yet we

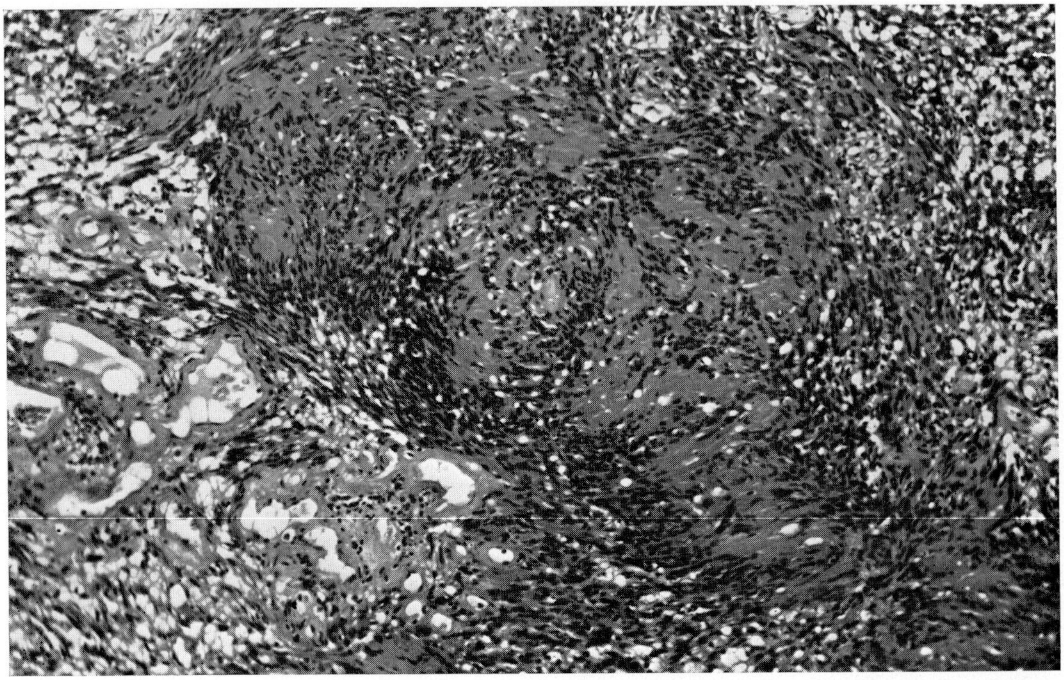

FIG. **10**, 6. Neurilemmoma. The densely staining cells (Antoni A) in the centre show palisading. On the left and at the top right are the irregularly disposed B cells.

have sometimes noticed that however painstaking the dissection has been one or two funiculi were found to be severed by the time the removal of the tumour was completed. Byers and Darby (personal communication, 1969) searched diligently for nerve fibres well within the substance of neurilemmomas, and they found them (Figs **10**, 8 and **10**, 9), though not invariably.

Clinical Features

Swelling. As might be expected the lump is often the presenting feature. Most neurilemmomas lie in the line of a nerve trunk and if there is room for them to move their mobility is only from side to side. But the tumour can easily be mistaken for other types of swelling such as a ganglion, a lipoma or, in the axilla, an enlarged lymph node. In countries where leprosy is endemic and, rarely, in those—such as Britain—with an immigrant population from the tropical zone, the disease may present as an isolated swelling of one nerve (Hoare, 1968). The local condition mimics a neurilemmoma; the lump has much the same shape and is tender. However, a disturbance of

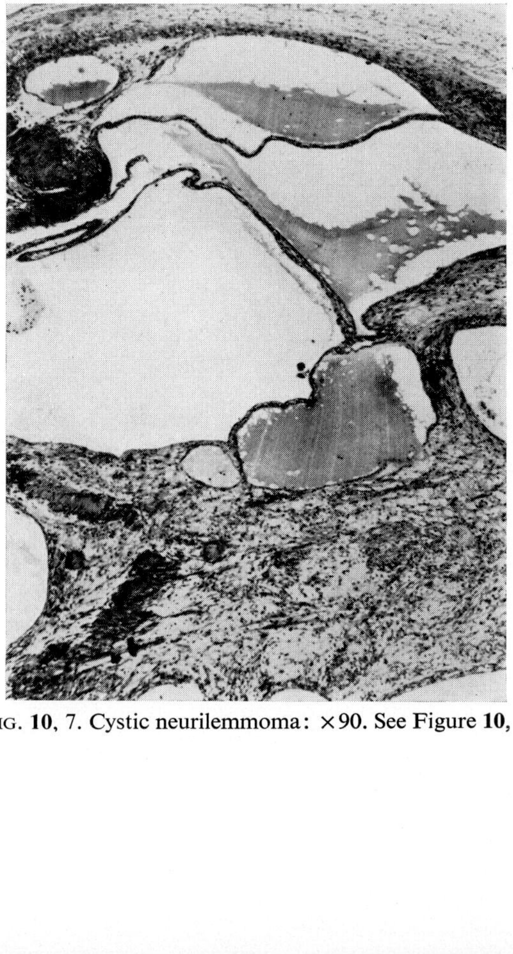

FIG. **10**, 7. Cystic neurilemmoma: ×90. See Figure **10**, 5.

sensibility within the distribution of the affected nerve should suggest the possibility of leprosy. Moreover, on exploration the fusiform swelling is found to involve the whole thickness of the nerve, with no displacement of unaffected funiculi; the swelling and the nerve are both hyperaemic and the latter is thicker than normal.

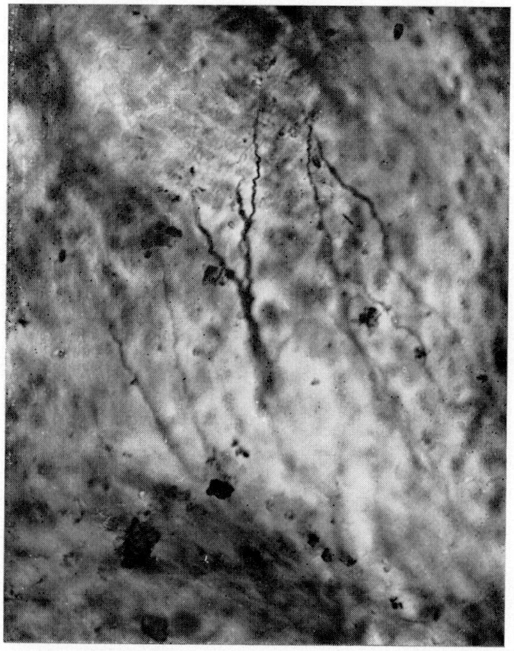

FIG. **10**, 8. Nerve fibres deep in a neurilemmoma. (Figs **10**, 8 and **10**, 9 by courtesy of Dr P. D. Byers and Dr A. J. Darby.)

When there is the slightest suspicion that a swelling may be a neurilemmoma—or any other nerve tumour—a long incision should be made, so that the relationship of the tumour to neighbouring nerves can be clearly established. It is a tragedy when, after excision of an obscure swelling, a patient is found to have, say, median paralysis.

Swelling was a notable feature in four-fifths of our cases and two-thirds of those reported by Dodge and Craig (1957).

Pain. Sensory symptoms are often prominent even when the tumour has ample room in which to expand. Pain was the presenting symptom in two out of five of our patients. There is vague local pain, and almost invariably a distinctive distal radiation of pain, or a sensation like an electric shock, when the lump is palpated. But if the swelling is more or less confined it may never be noticed by the patient, and can elude the most vigilant examiner. The only complaint is pain, which may be localized or diffuse. We have seen patients with neurilemmomas of the proximal part of the sciatic nerve who for long periods had been regarded as suffering from prolapse of an intervertebral disc. Vague pain in the forearm caused by a neurilemmoma has, after fruitless though perhaps inadequate examinations, led to a patient being referred to a psychiatrist. A neurilemmoma in the pulp of the heel, where there are tight fascial compartments, can cause excruciating pain exactly like that produced by a glomus tumour. A patient of ours had complained of it for 40 years.

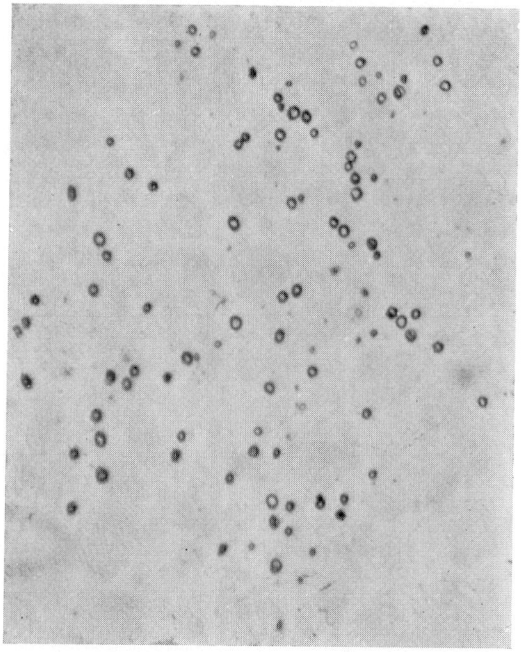

FIG. **10**, 9. Nerve fibres in a neurilemmoma: stained to show myelin.

As might be expected the mode of presentation is inconstant. Fifty tumours in 47 patients presented in the following way:

1.	Swelling alone	18
2.	Pain alone	10
3.	Swelling followed by pain	10
4.	Pain followed by swelling	12

Paralysis. Unlike those arising in the spinal canal, neurilemmomas in the limbs are rarely so confined as to cause paralysis of the affected or any other nerve. We have seen one example of common peroneal paresis due to a tumour situated just distal to the head of the fibula. It is very doubtful if ganglia causing paralysis (p. 125) are in fact cystic neurilemmomas; the two described by Jenkins (1952) certainly were not.

Dodge and Craig (1957) record a number of bizarre manifestations ranging from displacement of one eye to rectal bleeding; but these were in cases in which the tumour had arisen in the head or body cavities.

Very rarely a neurilemmoma presents as a *bone tumour* (Fig. **10**, 10) which may cause a fracture (Hart and Basom, 1958). In a recent paper, the most authoritative so far, Fawcett and Dahlin (1967) described seven cases in a series of nearly 4,000 primary bone tumours; in four the tumour was in the mandible.

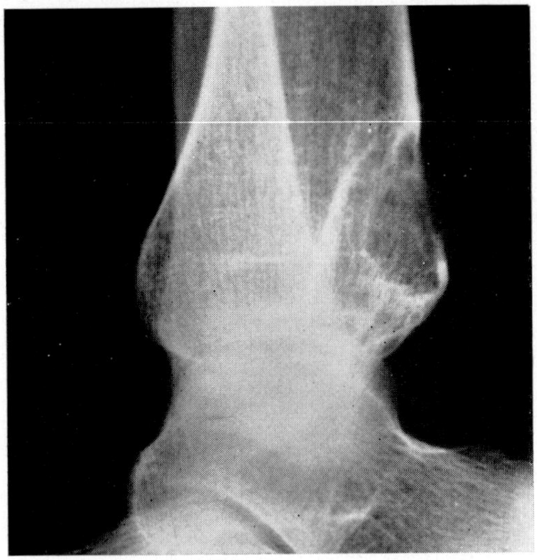

FIG. **10**, 10. Neurilemmoma in the lower end of the tibia. (Courtesy of Mr M. H. Carr.)

Treatment

The correct treatment for a tumour arising in a major nerve is enucleation, and for this an ample incision is required. It is best to expose a neurilemmoma in a bloodless field, but if this is not possible bleeding from the nerve may be controlled by the application of rubber-covered arterial clamps proximally and distally. If, as is usual, the swelling is asymmetrical, the epineurium should be breached in the concavity between the nerve trunk and the arc of greatest convexity (Figs **10**, 1 and **10**, 11); this is where the epineurium is likely to be lifted up leaving a small space between it and one pole of the tumour. It is then easy to find the plane of cleavage between the capsule and the funiculi; and when this has been done the enucleation may proceed. It has to be extremely delicate where the funiculi are thinnest and it is advisable to use the magnifying spectacles referred to on page 274. Nevertheless, one may find at the finish that one or two bundles have been cut; but this causes no appreciable impairment of function and need cause no alarm. If a biopsy has been performed the dissection will be difficult, and there may be some permanent impairment of function after the enucleation.

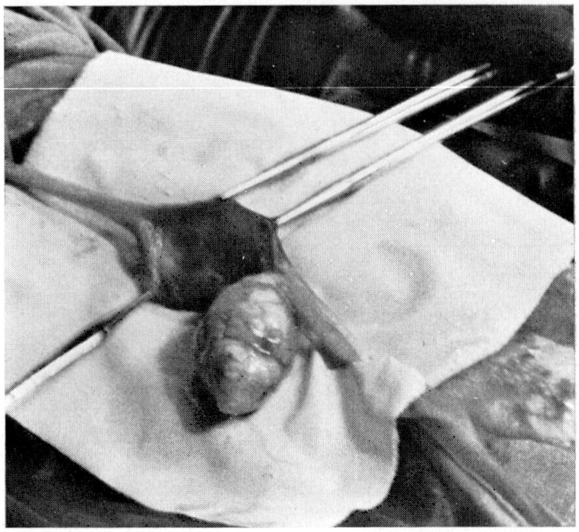

FIG. **10**, 11. Neurilemmoma. Enucleation from the ulnar nerve almost completed. No post-operative paralysis.

We have seen one recurrence, but have encountered several cases in which a second lump appeared which was not exactly at the site of the tumour that had been removed. It may have been there originally, too small to be detectable, or the incision may not have been adequate enough to reveal it (p. 156).

matosis, but the latter was known long before his day. Perhaps the clearest description of it is in Smith's celebrated monograph, published in 1849. It is like an atlas, measures 28 inches by 19 inches (71 cm by 48·3 cm) with 15 superb plates, some of the illustrations being life-size, and written in the most felicitous English.

TABLE XVII

RESULTS

	Number of operations	Period of post-operative observation (years)			
		1-3	4-10	11-15	16-20
Excision of tumour arising from an unimportant nerve	10	4	3	1	2
Resection (unwarranted) of a tumour arising from a major nerve	4	4			
Enucleation of a tumour from a major nerve	37	21	6	8	2

In the last group the incidence of post-operative paralysis or paresis was as follows:

Permanent paralysis	1
Permanent paresis	2
Paralysis followed by moderate recovery	1
Paralysis or paresis followed by complete recovery	5

In two cases the final result was marred by an initial biopsy; in both there was paresis before the tumour was removed.

Supervention of malignant change. We have never seen this and some of our patients have been followed for as long as 20 years. However, the development of sarcoma at the site of operation is mentioned as having occurred in two, possibly three, cases out of Dodge and Craig's 343, but they give no details. We do not regard this as an adequate reason—nor do they—for abandoning an operation that has the supreme advantage of avoiding loss of function. The question of malignancy *ab initio* is considered on page 169.

MULTIPLE NEUROFIBROMATOSIS

Von Recklinghausen, in 1882, was the first to associate molluscum fibrosum with neurofibro-

Tilesius (1793) described a patient with molluscum fibrosum but with no other manifestations of neurofibromatosis.

We should not, therefore, use the eponymous term. There are, however, objections to using neurofibromatosis, because it is inadequate. The *skin* may exhibit *café au lait* spots, a warty hypertrophy and naevi; the *subcutaneous tissues*, nodular and plexiform neurofibromas, various types of angioma, and diffuse hypertrophy; in *deep tissues* and the *body cavities*, localized and diffuse neurofibromatous changes; the *skeleton*, a great variety of disorders of which scoliosis and hypertrophy of the limb bones are commonest; and there are numerous manifestations of the disease in the *central nervous system*. But we

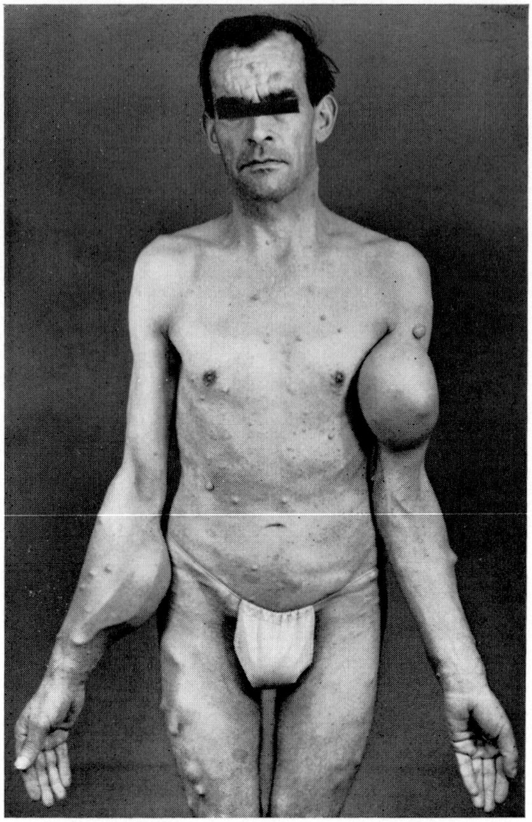

FIG. **10**, 12. Neurofibromatosis. *Café au lait* spots. Numerous subcutaneous nodules and two large swellings arising from deep structures, which were malignant. The sarcoma in the right forearm (Fig. **10**, 23) arose from the median nerve: that in the left arm from the medial cutaneous nerve of the forearm.

cannot change to *Smith's disease*; so *faute de mieux* we must be content with neurofibromatosis.

The disease, as Thomson (1900) recognized, is genetically determined. It is inherited as a Mendelian dominant, about half of the offspring of affected individuals showing signs of the disorder. Neurofibromatosis is said to afflict 1 in 3,000 of the population (Crowe, Schull and Neel, 1956). Gardner and Turner (1940) in their study of bilateral acoustic neurofibromas, found 38 cases of neurofibromatosis in five generations of a family of 217 members. In many the manifestations are minimal with no detectable swellings of nerves. And even in a hospital where

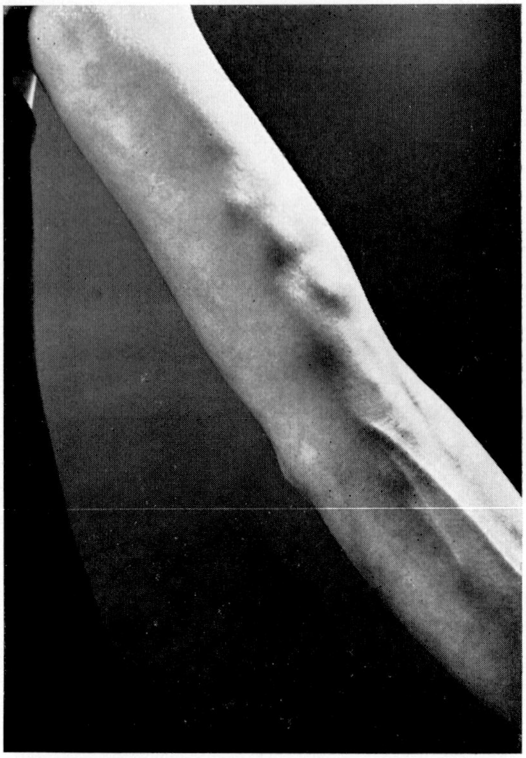

FIG. **10**, 13. The patient presented many swellings in the neck and both upper limbs. Most of them were tender. She had no *café au lait* spots.

a considerable number of cases are seen for one reason or another, few patients present themselves with disorders arising specifically in peripheral nerves. There were only nine such patients among 154 who attended the Royal National Orthopaedic Hospital on account of their suffering from neurofibromatosis.

Pathology

The lesions are sometimes called hamartomas rather than tumours, because they are tissue malformations, not neoplasms.

Neurofibromas can present in several ways:

1. Subcutaneous nodules (Fig. **10**, 12), which may be very numerous (molluscum fibrosum).
2. More or less uniform swelling of many nerves, to which the term plexiform neuroma may be applicable. This swelling may be localized, like a mass of worms.

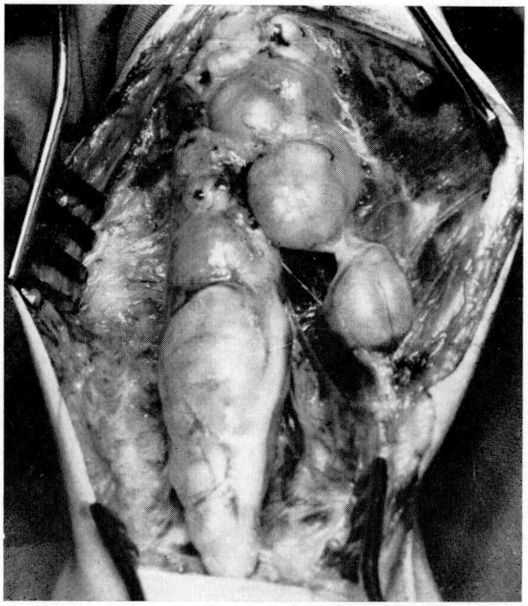

FIG. **10**, 14. Exploration of the arm of the patient shown in Figure **10**, 13. The nerve at the left is the median: upper right, the medial cutaneous nerve of the forearm.

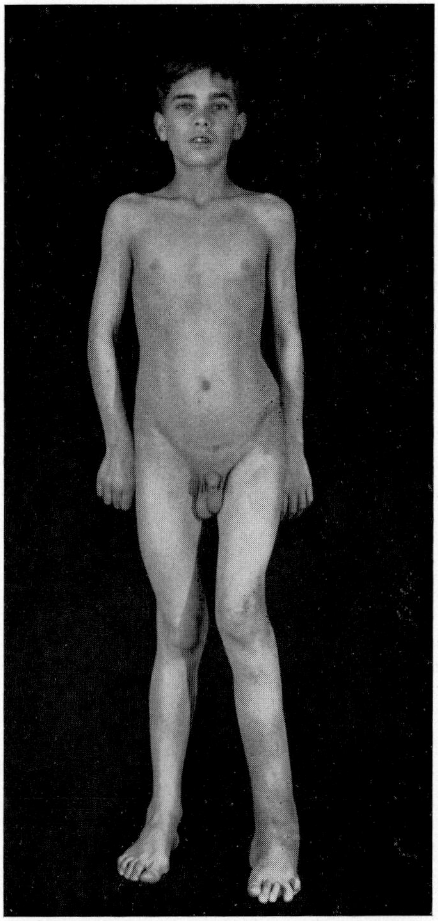

FIG. **10**, 15. This boy of 16 had 3·5 cm lengthening below the left knee, paresis of all the muscles and the deformity shown. On this account, and because it was certain that there were tumours of the nerves, the leg was amputated. The specimen was found to contain at least five sizable though not palpable innocent growths.

3. Many swellings of a nerve (Figs **10**, 13 and **10**, 14).

If the malformation has appeared early in life, any of the widespread lesions of main nerve trunks may be associated with gross changes in the whole limb (Figs **10**, 15 and **10**, 16). Some of these children are pathetic; the affected limb is not only enormously enlarged but it is or soon becomes completely paralysed. The bones, normal at first, fail to develop (Fig. **10**, 17). Amputation may be obligatory, though it may not avert malignant changes in the stump. Although some children are born with obvious neurofibromatosis of a limb the swellings and even the *café au lait* spots do not usually appear until adolescence or later. The swellings are almost always painless and grow very slowly: except in the young paralysis does not develop, unless the neurofibroma is within a confined space. They are soft to moderately firm lumps and never become cystic.

These neurofibromas in the limbs seem docile enough, no more than a blemish or a mechanical nuisance. But with the exception of the most superficial lumps, they are potentially dangerous, because at any age they may become malignant (p. 168). This means that even though a patient with neurofibromatosis may need no treatment he must be warned to watch for any rapid increase in size of a swelling, or the onset of pain. Paralysis is another, though later, indication of malignancy.

The superficial neurofibroma has no well-defined capsule and, microscopically, a uniformity of appearance that alone is almost sufficient to distinguish it from a neurilemmoma (Fig. **10**, 18). It is composed of spindle cells which occasionally show a palisade arrangement. On histological grounds alone it is occasionally difficult to distinguish a neurofibroma from a neurilemmoma. And some tumours in neurofibromatosis are undoubtedly neurilemmomas, especially those affecting the auditory nerves (Willis, 1962).

The origin of the cells composing a neurofibroma has been earnestly debated; but it is now generally agreed that they are derived from Schwann cells, which are therefore capable of producing two very different kinds of benign growth.

When the neurofibroma is in an identifiable nerve trunk it is, unlike the neurilemmoma, placed centrally; it can be fusiform or globular (Fig. **10**, 14), not ovoid. The nerve bundles, which themselves may be enlarged, merge into the swelling, and the lump cannot be shelled out. On histological examination the reason is clear enough; the nerve fibres ramify throughout the mass, the pathological process is interstitial. If a neurofibroma has to be removed the nerve from which it arises must be cut across. The resultant gap is so large that repair is likely to be impossible, though at any rate, in the young neurofibromatous nerve is capable of satisfactory regeneration. There is hardly ever any justification, apart from malignant transformation,

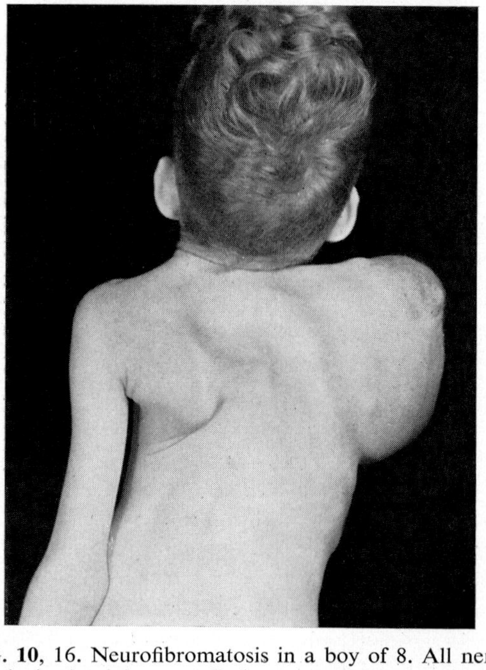

Fig. **10**, 16. Neurofibromatosis in a boy of 8. All nerve trunks in the right upper limb were enormously enlarged (plexiform neuroma). It was completely paralysed and so was amputated. But a sarcoma developed in the stump.

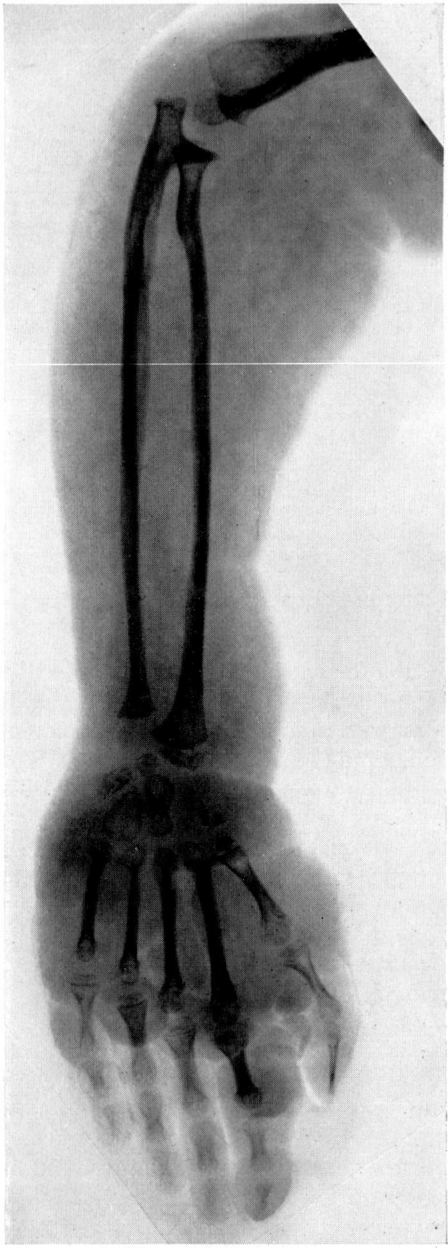

Fig. **10**, 17. Radiograph of the amputated arm. In infancy the bones had appeared to be normal. (Fig. **10**, 16 is a later photograph of the patient.)

for removal of a neurofibroma arising in a main nerve trunk. But others may be tackled with impunity provided that removal is complete. This may be difficult, as in a case of mine where a neurofibroma in the upper thorax was compressing the brachial plexus.

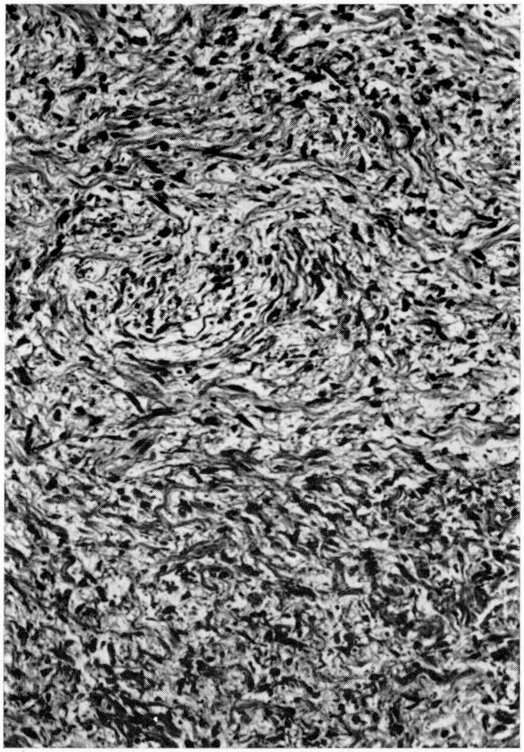

FIG. **10**, 18. Neurofibromatosis: plexiform neuroma of the face. Spindle cells predominate and show no sort of orientation (×145).

The generalized thickening of nerves is due to cellular proliferation and again the Schwann cells are regarded as responsible. There is collagenous overgrowth as well. The result is that the nerve fibres are widely separated (Figs **10**, 19 and **10**, 20).

SOLITARY NEUROFIBROMA

A neurofibroma may be found in the absence of stigmata of multiple neurofibromatosis. In the large collection of cases studied by Heard (1962) there were 46 such peripheral tumours, mostly superficial. They are sometimes painful. The age incidence is different from that of the neurilemmoma in that they are commonest in the first 10 years of life. These tumours are entirely benign. We have removed some superficial ones,

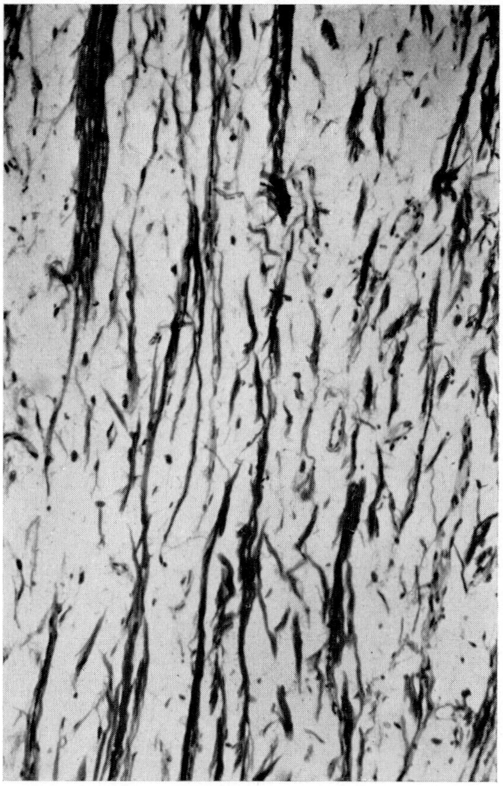

FIG. **10**, 19. Neurofibroma. The nerve fibres are widely separated. (Dr A. J. Darby.)

but those involving important nerve trunks (Fig. **10**, 21) have been left alone and it has been gratifying to find that they did not continue to grow. A curious feature is that six out of the nine tumours were in the hand, four involving the median nerve near the wrist.

FATTY TUMOURS

There are four kinds of fatty tumour involving nerves and although they are rare they deserve to be discussed in some detail, because they are puzzling.

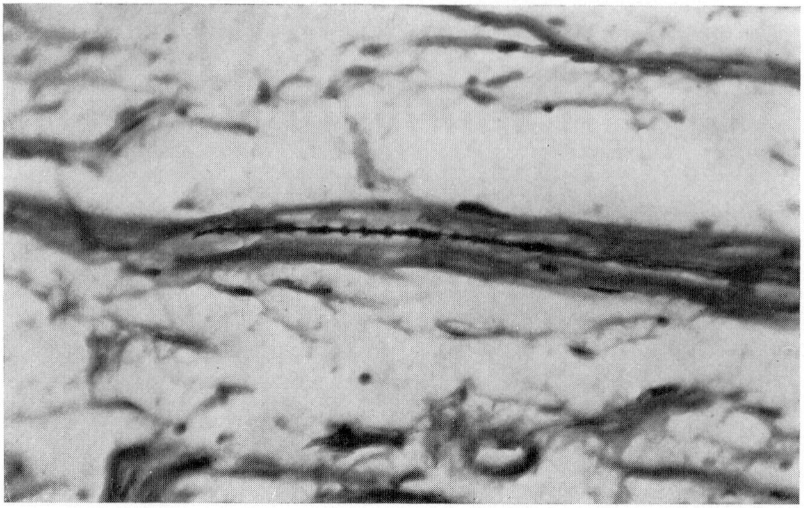

FIG. **10**, 20. Neurofibroma. A nerve fibre, the axon standing out unusually well. The fibrocytic proliferation involves the endoneurium. (Dr A. J. Darby.)

Compression of a nerve by a lipoma. This differs in no way from compression by any other innocent tumour. The lipoma is deeply situated, and if in a confined space such as the spiral groove of the humerus or the carpal tunnel is likely to cause mild symptoms. The main interest is diagnostic and the treatment is straightforward.

Macrodystrophia lipomatosa. This is the resounding name given by Werthemann (1952) to overgrowth of part of the hand, starting early in life, in which there is fatty infiltration of the subcutaneous tissues and of the median nerve and its branches, all of which may be enormously swollen. The only possible treatment is cosmetic. As will be shown presently this curious disorder may be related to another that has been regarded hitherto as distinct.

Until recently fatty tumours growing within and confined to peripheral nerves were unknown: then, in 1964, five short papers appeared in the British issue of the *Journal of Bone and Joint Surgery*, all concerned with fatty tumours of nerves; since then there have been a few further reports. An astonishing feature is that in every case the lesion involved the median nerve at the wrist or in the palm.

Encapsulated lipoma of nerve. These tumours (Morley, 1964; Watson-Jones, 1964) were found

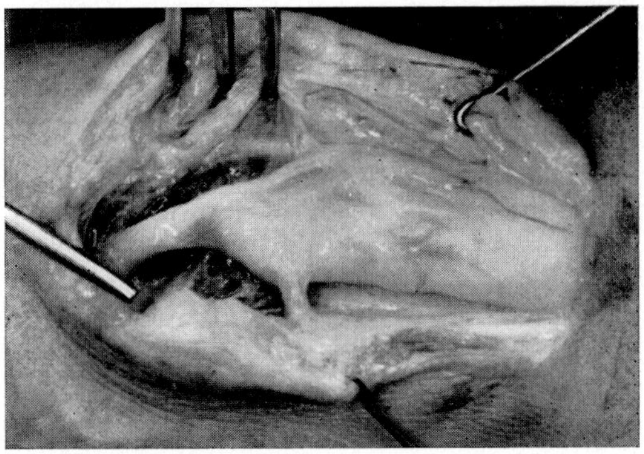

FIG. **10**, 21. Solitary neurofibroma in a child aged 5, just proximal to the wrist. Observed over a period of 14 years: no increase in size, no disturbance of function.

in adults, within the nerve; one was 7·5 cm long. They caused no more than trivial impairment of sensibility, and were shelled out without difficulty or ill-effect.

Lipofibromatous hamartoma of nerve. This term, introduced by Johnson and Bonfiglio (1969) in their excellent review, is used to describe a condition in which fat infiltrates a nerve interstitially and usually extends into its branches. The nerve fibres are as inextricably involved as in a neurofibroma and there is nothing that can be enucleated. The histological appearance is not uniform; there may be patches of fibrous tissue and areas (Pulvertaft, 1964) that look neurofibromatous.

In most cases the swelling appears early in life and may be present at birth. The patient suffers no more than some discomfort and the main anxiety is about the nature of the swelling. However, J. M. P. Clark (personal communication) has seen a man, 43 years old, who presented with what appeared to be the usual sort of compression of the median nerve in the carpal tunnel. On exploration he found 'gross hypertrophy of the median nerve extending from the mid-point of the forearm down to the palm and into the palmar branches. The thenar branch of the median nerve had increased to nearly the size of the main trunk in a normal man. The branches in the forearm appeared to be normal, and the ulnar nerve was normal.' A biopsy specimen showed collagen and fat, and two minute nerves that appeared normal. In all cases the median nerve and some of its branches (in one case—Yeoman, 1964—a digital branch alone) are ballooned out with fat. The surface of these swellings is usually smooth, but in one of my cases, reported by Yeoman (Fig. **10**, 22), it was lobulated.

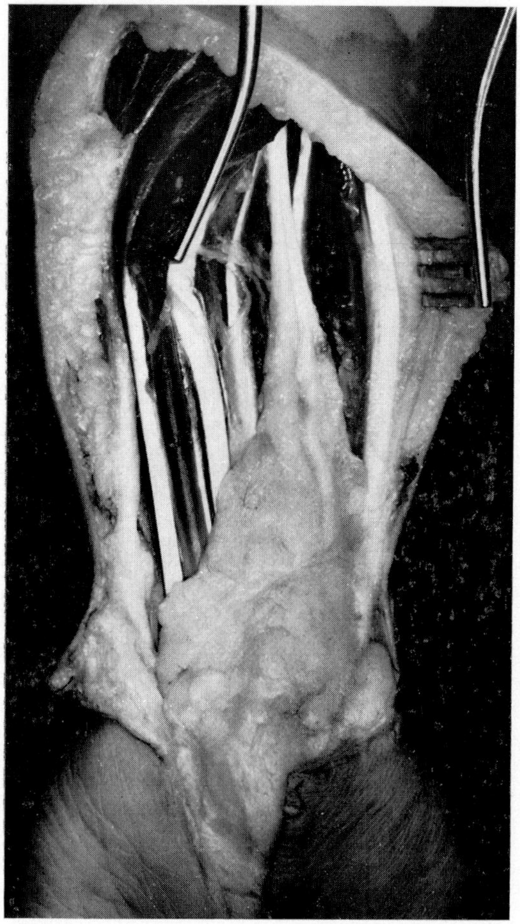

FIG. **10**, 22. Fibrolipomatosis of the median nerve. No paralysis. Macroscopic and histological examination showed that the fat lies between nerve fibres, a diffuse infiltration. (By kind permission of *J. Bone Jt Surg.*, **B**).

There are no other relevant abnormalities; in particular, no signs of neurofibromatosis. In all but one of the patients studied the fibrolipomatous mass was left undisturbed, apart from the essential exploration and the informative biopsy. This was wise. There would have been no possibility of repairing the gap after excision and, as it turned out, the fibrolipomatous tissue ceased to grow. Thus we may conclude that this disorder is a hamartoma.

The subsequent history of one of my patients (Case 1 in Yeoman's paper, 1964) is illuminating. Sixteen years after her first attendance, by which time she was a married woman of 27, two digits of the affected hand showed moderate hypertrophy, with soft swellings in the line of the digital nerves. There was no change in the original fibrolipomatous mass, no deterioration of function, and no abnormality of any other part of the body. During her adolescence the condition had developed into macrodystrophia lipomatosa, and it may eventually prove that the second and fourth disorders that have just been described are in fact related.

HAEMANGIOMA OF NERVE

A haemangioma near a nerve—in, say, a neighbouring muscle—may cause some minor disturbance of nerve function. A haemangioma in the substance of a nerve, which Purcell and Gurdjian (1935) and Stout (1949) rightly describe as very rare, may also cause mild symptoms. These two types of hamartoma may be indistinguishable clinically. They are likely to become manifest early in life; a vague, soft swelling, which it may be possible to obliterate by compression, and perhaps pain and paraesthesia.

I have come across only two cases in each group (four in all).

Only by exploration is it possible to determine the site of the angioma. Excision is the proper treatment if it is extraneural. If intraneural the most that is permissible is ligation of all the vessels connected with the affected part of the nerve.

MALIGNANT TUMOURS

There are three kinds: (1) sarcoma supervening in a patient with neurofibromatosis, (2) sarcoma of a nerve occurring in the absence of other abnormalities, and (3) the rare neurectodermal tumours. There is no justification for using the term malignant Schwannoma or malignant neurilemmoma and, as will be explained presently, there is some doubt about the third category, the neurectodermal tumours.

Sarcoma in Neurofibromatosis

In this disease this is perhaps the most serious threat to life. The incidence of malignant transformation has been estimated as 13 per cent by Hosoi (1931) and by Stout (1949), and as 17 per cent by Heard (1962). However, Heard points out that his figure is based on the incidence of sarcoma in hospital cases and he suspects that the true figure is considerably under 10 per cent in all patients with neurofibromatosis.

Sarcomatous change can occur any time between childhood and old age. The patient depicted in Figure **10**, 16 was 8 years old and the oldest patient reported by Hosoi was 70. The highest incidence is in the third, fourth and fifth decades.

Heard (1962) found that superficial nerves were affected in only four out of 37 reported cases that he had studied (see Fig. **10**, 12). The patient shown in this figure illustrates another though uncommon feature, that sarcomatous transformation can occur at more than one site.

It has been alleged that surgical interference with a neurofibroma can precipitate malignant change though the evidence is inconclusive. A case for this could be made out from reports such as the following.

A youth of 17 with obvious neurofibromatosis presented with two sizable swellings, one in the left occipital region (which need not concern us), the other in the left popliteal fossa. In the two months before he was seen the popliteal swelling had increased in size and the patient said that he had had pain below the knee for about two years.

A swelling 15 cm long by 6 cm in diameter was found on the tibial division of the sciatic nerve and an endeavour was made to remove it without severing the nerve. Sections of the material removed showed an innocent neurofibroma. Ten months later the swelling recurred, which suggested that something untoward was happening. A block resection was therefore performed, and the tumour removed was a sarcoma in which spindle cells predominated.

It can be argued either that the incomplete removal had precipitated the malignant change or that the partial resection had failed to include the part of the tumour that had become malignant.

Pathology

This description is applicable also to isolated neurosarcoma. A neurosarcoma may have a false capsule (Figs **10**, 23 and **10**, 24) or it may be diffusely infiltrative (Fig. **10**, 25). It is liable to spread inside the nerve well beyond the obvious swelling (Figs **10**, 25 and **10**, 26). There may be central necrosis (Fig. **10**, 23). The tumour tissue has the appearance either of a fibrosarcoma or of a spindle-cell sarcoma with no specific histological features suggesting its having arisen from nervous tissue. The regional lymph nodes are rarely affected—I have seen this in one patient with neurofibromatosis and in one other with an isolated neurosarcoma—but pulmonary metastasis is frequent.

Symptoms and Signs

Malignant transformation of a neurofibroma is heralded by a rapid increase in size and, to a considerably less extent, by pain, either local or referred. The swelling is firm, even hard, and it may be immovable. Muscle weakness and sensory disturbance are uncommon, but unless a nerve tumour is growing within a confined space they are a sure indication of malignancy.

Prognosis

Sarcoma occurring in neurofibromatosis is a lethal condition, and the mortality rate is about 90 per cent (Preston, Walsh and Clarke, 1952;

Heard, 1963). Three out of five of our patients have died; nearly 10 years have elapsed since operation in one survivor, the other was followed up for three and a half years. We shall shortly be considering whether the prognosis might be improved by more radical treatment.

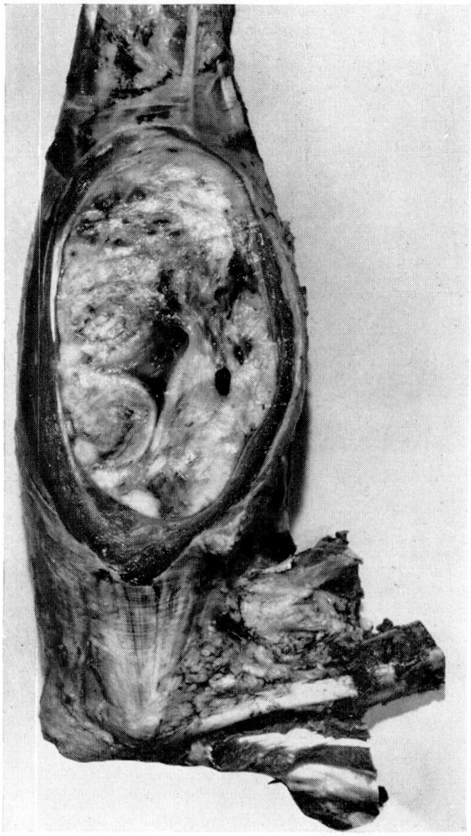

FIG. **10**, 23. Neurosarcoma in multiple neurofibromatosis. (See Fig. **10**, 12.)

ISOLATED NEUROSARCOMA

We have seen seven patients with apparently isolated sarcoma of a main nerve trunk; none had arisen in a superficial nerve. Not one of the patients presented any clinical evidence of neurofibromatosis; but a post-mortem examination was made of only one of the four patients who had died, and although this failed to disclose any evidence of neurofibromatosis it is perhaps unwise to affirm that the others were free of it.

Apart from the tumour appearing as an isolated phenomenon its characteristics are much the same as in neurosarcoma arising in neurofibromatosis. Pain is rather more pronounced as a presenting feature, and when the lump is deeply seated it may be the pain that leads to discovery of the tumour. The swelling is usually firm to hard, though in one case it was soft. Disturbance of nerve conduction is uncommon.

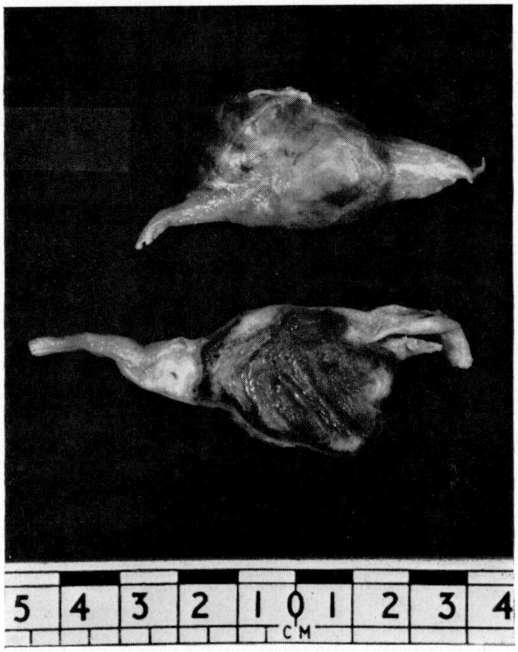

FIG. **10**, 24. Isolated neurosarcoma of the median nerve, treated by radical excision. Much of the tumour tissue is necrotic and haemorrhagic.

Prognosis

Four out of the seven patients have died.

RARE NEURECTODERMAL NERVE TUMOURS

Stout (1949) accepts that a very few primary tumours of nerve are neurectodermal in origin, like the tumours of this variety commonly seen in the central nervous system. Their existence is questioned by Willis (1960), who maintains that in the absence of conclusive post-mortem evidence, which he says has not yet been forthcoming, we should regard these rare tumours of nerve as possibly metastatic. For patients and clinicians this is important, and until this question has been answered we shall remain ignorant about prognosis and treatment. Only one case of this sort occurred in our series.

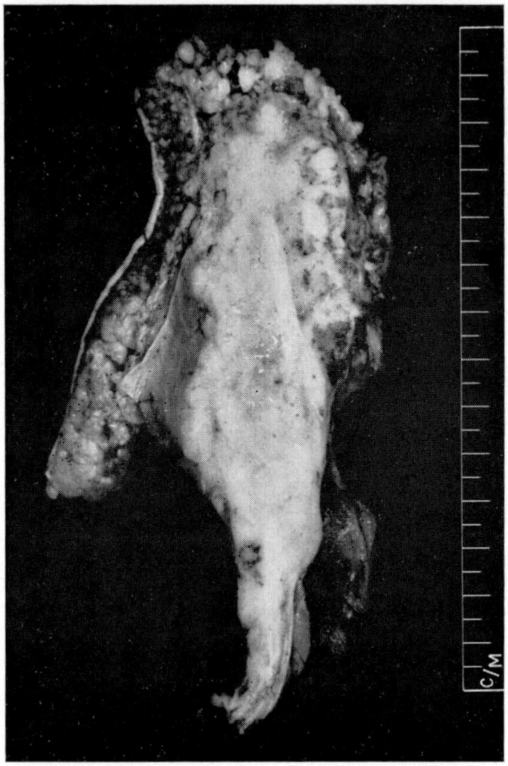

FIG. **10**, 25. Isolated neurosarcoma of the sciatic nerve. The tumour is infiltrating the adjacent muscle and fat.

A woman, 28 years of age, came under the care of my colleague, D. M. Brooks. For about a year she had had pain in the leg which was soon followed by drop-foot and then by the appearance of a swelling of the common peroneal nerve near the knee. On exploration he found a soft spreading tumour which was dealt with by block resection. Metastases appeared rapidly in the brain and in the bone marrow and she died six months after the operation. The section of the tumour shows what is called a neurepithelioma (Fig. **10**, 27).

Treatment of Neurosarcoma

We are in no position to consider the treatment of the last rare category, the so-called neurectodermal tumours. This discussion is confined to sarcomas arising in neurofibromatosis or as isolated tumours.

Biopsy. Heard (1963) favours biopsy on the grounds that 'in those cases in which the his-

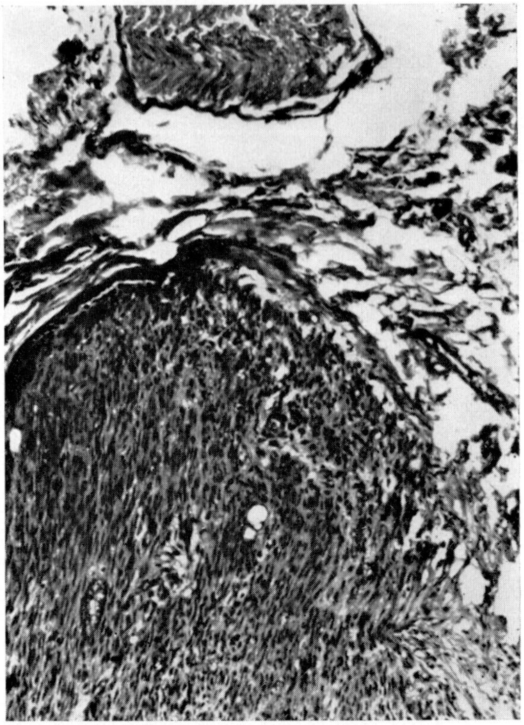

FIG. **10**, 26. Neurosarcoma of the sciatic nerve treated by what was thought to be adequate block resection. But at the proximal site of resection tumour cells were present in the upper left area of the large bundle, which is unusually cellular. These cells were not identifiable at the magnification shown (×80). Much higher magnification and a discerning eye were necessary. The nerve should have been transected even further away from the tumour. The patient died eight months later with abdominal metastases.

tology implies that malignancy may not be high (and this would be especially likely in the more superficial tumour), a fairly conservative procedure may be acceptable'. I question this on two grounds. Heard himself makes the point that in these usually very vascular tumours the blood spaces are often found to be partly lined by malignant cells and that metastasis by the bloodstream is common. Hence he favours a superficial biopsy which does not involve manipulation of the tumour; but this—particularly in cases of neurofibromatosis—could fail to disclose the true nature of the tumour. Because the proper treatment for a neurosarcoma should not be less than a radical excision the biopsy should be of the whole specimen and of a considerable length of the nerve trunk on either side of it—provided it is possible to make the diagnosis of malignancy on the clinical evidence and on the appearances disclosed at operation. A history of increasing pain, of a fairly rapidly developing swelling, the finding of a hard lump in the line of a nerve strongly suggest a neurosarcoma. When the swelling is exposed it can (quite apart from the history) be only one of three things; a neurilemmoma, an innocent neurofibroma or a neurosarcoma. The appearances of a neurilemmoma are unmistakable; a neurofibroma may be the same shape as a neurosarcoma but it is soft. The neurosarcoma is either firm or hard.

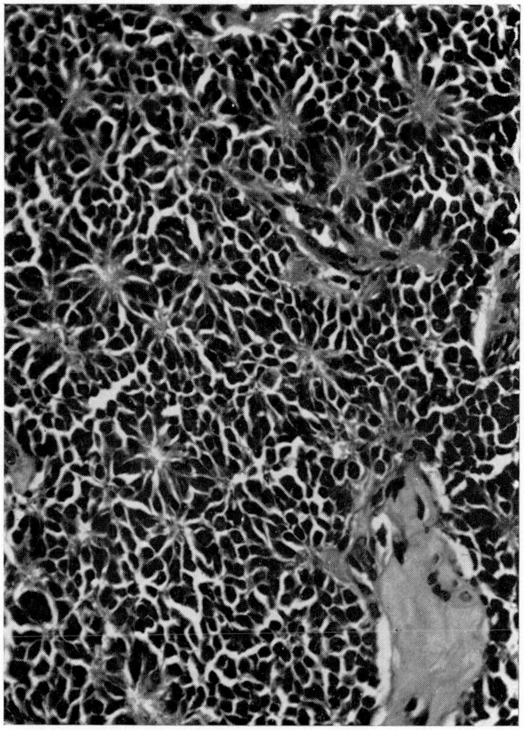

FIG. **10**, 27. Highly malignant neurepithelioma: the cells with their large deeply staining nuclei are arranged in the form of rosettes. This floral appearance is unmistakable (×300). (By courtesy of Mr D. M. Brooks.)

It may happen that a tumour is so extensive (Figs **10**, 12 and **10**, 23) that immediate amputation is appropriate, but in general it would appear that the primary treatment should be a block resection if this is anatomically practicable; by this is meant resection with a fair margin of the surrounding tissues. We may contrast two patients who presented with a neurosarcoma at the level of the knee. One affected the tibial division of the sciatic nerve, and it was possible to remove it with an enveloping layer of connective tissue and muscle. Happily, there was no encroachment on the popliteal vessels; but I was prepared to do an amputation if they had been involved. This boy has survived for nine years. Another patient (under the care of G. M. Lloyd Roberts) had a similar tumour behind the head of the fibula. A block resection would have been difficult and almost certainly mutilating, perhaps damaging the knee joint seriously. In this case an amputation was done and this patient has survived for seven years.

Until more information becomes available about the results of treatment all recommendations must be tentative; but with such a high mortality rate it is surely justifiable to approach these dreadful tumours with something approaching the ruthlessness that has been forced on us in the surgical treatment of bone sarcoma, the more so because neurosarcoma does not respond to radiotherapy. It has not been possible to find any report of a series of cases of neurosarcoma successfully treated by irradiation.

It is certainly reasonable to regard amputation as imperative if there is a local recurrence after a block resection.

11. Lesions of Individual Nerves: Upper Limb

INTRODUCTION TO CHAPTERS 11 AND 12

A FAIR KNOWLEDGE of the anatomy of the limbs is required for the accurate diagnosis of disorders of peripheral nerves. More detailed and rather different knowledge is necessary in operative treatment. The surgeon is required to expose the site of damage without undue disturbance of neighbouring structures; he may also have to deal with injured blood vessels, bones and tendons. Observations on operative exposure will be found in Chapter 15, pages 253 to 261.

In this chapter, and in Chapter 12, we are concerned with the regional application of the methods of examination that have been described in Chapter 3. There are excellent descriptions of muscle action,[1] so no attempt is made here to set out methods of examination of all muscles. But there are pitfalls, and these will be described together with the simple methods of examination required in dealing with a patient suffering from the immediate effects of injury, which may be grave.

Most clinicians use charts for recording motor and sensory paralysis. The latter presents no difficulty; suitable outline diagrams are available. Not so with muscle charts. After some 30 years' work on poliomyelitis and peripheral nerve injuries I have recently redesigned muscle charts; but I am beginning to suspect that ideal charts are unattainable. If a chart is anatomically comprehensive the recorder spends as much time in searching for a particular heading as in the elicitation of a particular movement. Moreover, certain muscles are either clinically unimportant or their actions such that they cannot be demonstrated satisfactorily. Sometimes it is difficult even to ascertain the power of an important muscle normally readily accessible to examination. A useful muscle chart must be selective; and when the inclusion or exclusion of muscles is under consideration there is ample scope for disagreement.

The charts set out below, and for the lower limb on page 215, represent an amalgam of three sets of charts, each with defects, that I have used over long periods. They are commended to the reader with great diffidence.

It has finally to be considered whether the columns for the recording of muscle power should be set out as in Figures **11**, 1 and **11**, 2, or with columns for right and left as in Figure **12**, 1 (p. 215). Patients with injury of the same nerve on each side are rare, and therefore the first type of chart, with about eight columns, should suffice. However, if the charts are also required for the documentation of cases of poliomyelitis, division into right and left sides is essential. But for this purpose the charts shown are inadequate because the muscles of the trunk are omitted; these muscles are few in number and can be added to the chart shown in Figure **12**, 1, the chart most frequently required in the examination of patients with poliomyelitis.

UPPER LIMB

In this chapter much attention has been paid to injuries of the brachial plexus. The reason is that this aspect of our subject has only recently emerged from obscurity. A rational approach to these injuries calls for more elaborate investigation than is required in the management of other disorders of the peripheral nerves.

ACCESSORY NERVE

After leaving the skull this nerve passes obliquely and distally, deep to the sterno-cleido-mastoid, which it supplies, to reach the upper part of the posterior triangle of the neck where it is superficial for a short distance before running beneath

[1] Kendall, H. O., Kendall, F. P. and Wadsworth, G. E. (1972). *Muscle: Testing and Function.* 2nd edition. Edinburgh and London: Churchill Livingstone. Medical Research Council Memorandum (1975). *Aids to the Examination of the Peripheral Nervous System.* London: Her Majesty's Stationery Office.

NECK, SHOULDER AND ARM

EXAMINER						
DATE						
SIDE						
TYPE OF OBSERVATION *						
DIAPHRAGM						
STERNOMASTOID						
TRAPEZIUS						
LEVATOR SCAPULAE						
RHOMBOIDS						
SUPRASPINATUS						
INFRASPINATUS						
SERRATUS ANT.						
PECTORALIS MAJOR { UPPER / MIDDLE / LOWER						
DELTOID						
TERES MAJOR						
LATISS. DORSI						
TRICEPS						
BICEPS						
BRACHIALIS						

0 No contraction.
1 Trace of contraction.
2 Active movement with gravity eliminated.
3 Active movement against gravity.
4 Active movement against gravity and resistance.
4+ Intermediate between 4 and 5
5 Normal power.

* V = Voluntary power. E = Electrical excitability.

FIG. **11**, 1. Upper limb. Neck, shoulder and arm.

the trapezius muscle which it supplies and in which it terminates. Rarely, the nerve runs superficial to the sterno-cleido-mastoid and is then most vulnerable. The branches of cervical 3 and 4 that are distributed with the accessory are entirely sensory.

This nerve suffers chiefly at the hands of surgeons. Fourteen patients have come under my observation, one of them with bilateral trapezius paralysis; in eight the nerve was injured in the course of an operation in the posterior triangle of the neck, though in one case the nerve was cut anterior to the sterno-cleido-mastoid with the result that this muscle also was paralysed. As if to add insult to injury the diagnosis of paralysis of the trapezius

FOREARM AND HAND

EXAMINER						
DATE						
SIDE						
TYPE OF OBSERVATION*						
BRACHIORADIALIS						
EXTENSOR CARPI RADIALIS LONG.						
EXTENSOR CARPI RADIALIS BREV.						
EXTENSOR DIGITORUM COMMUNIS						
EXTENSOR CARPI ULNARIS						
ABDUCTOR POLLICIS LONG.						
EXTENSOR POLLICIS LONG.						
EXTENSOR POLLICIS BREV.						
PRONATOR TERES						
FLEXOR CARPI RADIALIS						
PALMARIS LONGUS						
FLEXOR DIGITORUM SUPERFICIALIS						
FLEXOR DIGITORUM PROFUNDUS 1 2						
FLEXOR POLLICIS LONGUS						
THENAR MUSCLES: FLEXOR BREVIS						
THENAR MUSCLES: ABDUCTOR BREVIS						
THENAR MUSCLES: OPPONENS						
FLEXOR CARPI ULNARIS						
FLEXOR DIGITORUM PROFUNDUS 3 4						
HYPOTHENAR MUSCLES						
INTEROSSEI: MASS ACTION						
FIRST DORSAL INTEROSSEOUS						
ADDUCTOR POLLICIS						

FIG. **11**, 2. Upper limb. Forearm and hand.

(Figs **11**, 3 and **11**, 4) was rarely made within reasonable time; in only one case was it possible to carry out secondary suture, giving, as might be expected with a purely motor nerve, a good result. The other six injuries were due to more usual open wounds, and in one case the long

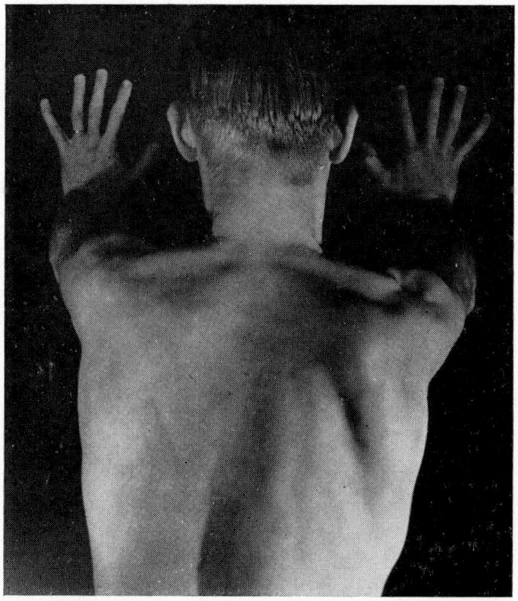

FIG. **11**, 3. This patient had weakness of the upper third of the right trapezius and paralysis of the lower two-thirds. The lower margin of the active left trapezius is just visible.

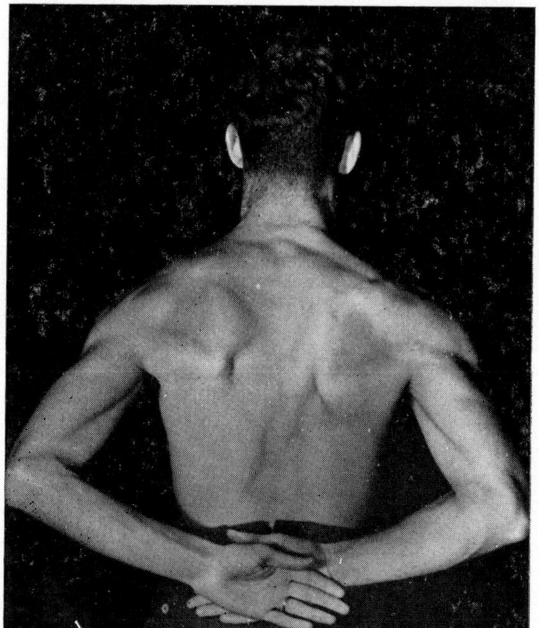

FIG. **11**, 4. If both hands are pressed against the lumbar spine the trapezius can always be felt and sometimes—as on the right in this patient—be seen to contract.

thoracic nerve was injured too. In five of these cases the nerve was explored and found to be in continuity; and in four satisfactory recovery occurred.

Fortunately the levator scapulae and the serratus anterior can sometimes compensate for paralysis of the trapezius. But some patients complain of a dragging ache in the shoulder and are unable to abduct it more than about 60 degrees; Henry's (1927) fascial sling operation usually gives relief.

BRACHIAL PLEXUS

The anatomy of the brachial plexus is illustrated in Figures **11**, 5 and **11**, 12 (p. 182); the motor branches with no clinical significance have been omitted.

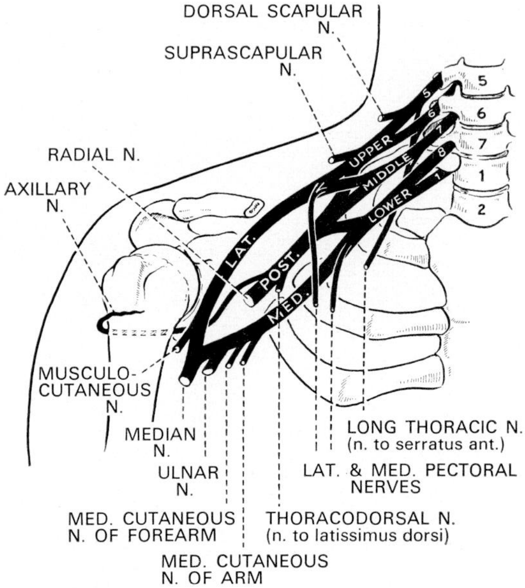

FIG. **11**, 5. The brachial plexus. Branches having no clinical significance (such as the nerve to the subclavius muscle) have been omitted. (Adapted from Haymaker, W. and Woodhall, B., (1953), *Peripheral Nerve Injuries*, p. 210. Philadelphia: Saunders. By kind permission of the publishers.)

The most important anomaly is in the origin of the roots. Sometimes the plexus arises one vertebra more proximal than usual, the upper trunk being formed by the confluence of C4 and C5; this is called pre-fixation. In the other abnormality, post-fixation, the plexus is shifted down one vertebra, the lower trunk arising from T1 and T2. In pre-fixation T1 takes no part in the formation of the plexus; in post-fixation C5 is excluded from it. These abnormalities are hard to detect. Myelograms showing traumatic meningoceles reveal only the level at which roots have been avulsed from the spinal cord, *but not which roots of the plexus;* an instructive example of this is shown in Figure **11**, 24 (p. 189).

Motor Branches

Phrenic nerve (C3, 4 and 5). Although this nerve arises from the cervical plexus, paralysis of the ipsilateral half of the diaphragm sometimes occurs in extensive traction injuries of the brachial plexus, the damage being near or proximal to the cervical transverse processes.

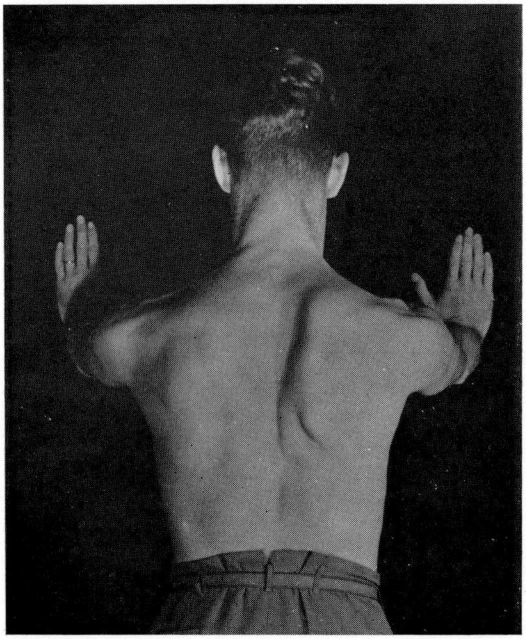

Fig, **11**, 6. Long thoracic nerve. This patient had paralysis of the right serratus anterior, and when he pressed his hands against a wall there was dorsal protrusion of the scapula.

Long thoracic nerve (C5, 6 and 7). This nerve arises from the three nerve roots, and courses distally behind the brachial plexus to end in the serratus anterior, which it supplies. Paralysis of this muscle causes winging of the scapula when the patient presses his extended arms against a wall (Fig. **11**, 6).

Isolated paralysis of this nerve is uncommon and is rarely due to injury; I have seen one case that followed a heavy blow on the shoulder and another due to a missile wound. The paralysis usually occurs spontaneously, is sometimes accompanied by pain, and so is usually ascribed to 'neuritis'. There is little to be done about it apart from avoidance of movements that stretch the serratus anterior. Three of our seven patients,

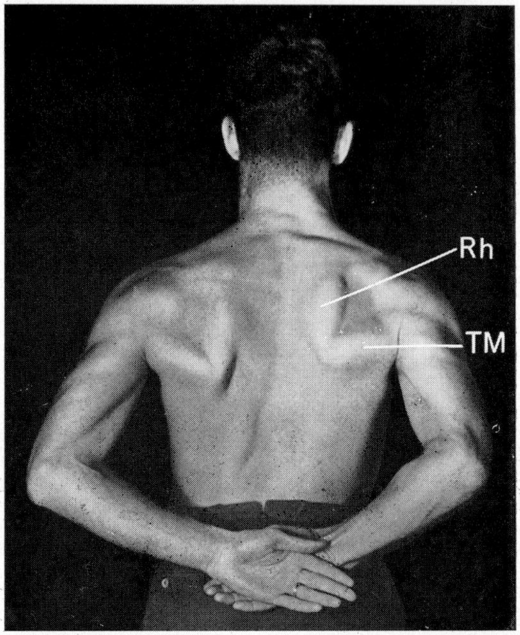

Fig. **11**, 7. In this test the hands are pressed away from the trunk. This is usually done against the hands of the examiner and the effect on the vertebro-scapular muscles is symmetrical. But this manœuvre would have interfered with taking the photograph, so this patient pressed the *right* hand back against the resistance of the left. This brought about the desired effect on the right side only, where the rhomboids and teres major stand out.

who were all adults, recovered almost full power in the muscle.

The long thoracic nerve is infrequently involved in injuries of the brachial plexus. If it is the prognosis is hopeless.

Dorsal scapular nerve (C5). Paralysis of the rhomboid muscles, which this nerve supplies, does not appear to occur in isolation. The diagnostic importance of the dorsal scapular nerve is in indicating the level at which the brachial plexus is damaged. A method for demonstrating the action of the rhomboids is shown in Figure **11**, 7.

Suprascapular nerve (C5 and sometimes a contribution from C6). This nerve supplies the supraspinatus and infraspinatus muscles. Direct examination of them is difficult because they are largely overlapped by other muscles. The main

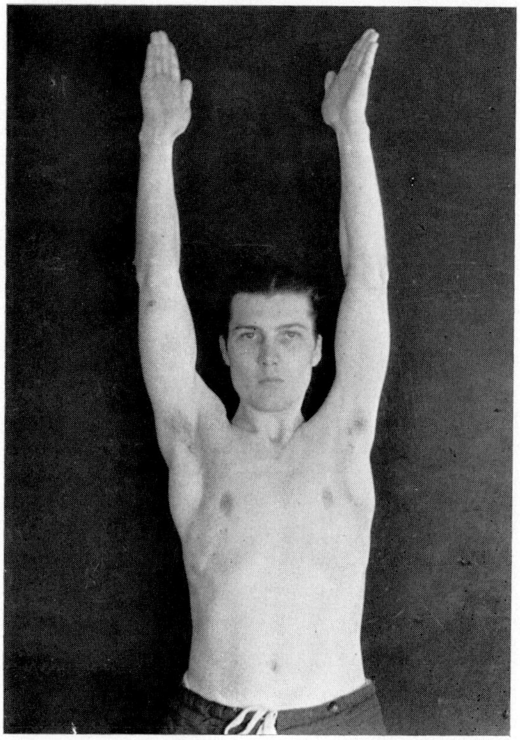

FIG. **11**, 8. This patient's left deltoid was completely paralysed, yet abduction of the shoulder was full. That this was due to the action of supraspinatus was proved by anaesthetizing the suprascapular nerve. This perfect abductor action of the supraspinatus is rare; it is more usual to find abduction to about 155 degrees, with the arm a little in front of the coronal plane of the body.

function of the supraspinatus is to anchor the head of the humerus during abduction of the shoulder by the deltoid. Thus, even when the deltoid is normal, abduction is defective if the supraspinatus is weak or paralysed. The supraspinatus alone is sometimes capable of abducting the shoulder (Highet, 1942; Fig. **11**, 8).

The simplest way of assessing the function of the suprascapular nerve, with no distinction between the two spinati, is to examine the power of lateral rotation of the shoulder.

Isolated paralysis of this nerve is rare, but it can be damaged by traction along with the axillary nerve. The suprascapular nerve can also be injured by a fracture through the blade of the scapula.

Lateral and medial pectoral nerves. These nerves contain fibres arising from every root of the brachial plexus: lateral, C5, 6 and 7; medial, C8 and T1.

Pectoralis minor is inaccessible clinically, but examination of pectoralis major can be most informative. The clavicular portion is supplied by C5 and 6, the sternal portion by C7 and 8, and by T1. No other muscle so faithfully reveals the state of the components of a damaged brachial plexus.

Thoraco-dorsal nerve (mainly C7). This nerve arises from the posterior cord of the plexus, runs distally with the subscapular artery, and supplies the latissimus dorsi.

Subscapular nerves. Only the lower (mainly C7) is significant clinically: it supplies the teres major (Fig. **11**, 7).

The importance of these two muscles is twofold: they reveal the state of the posterior cord of the brachial plexus; and if active they are used for the tendon transplantation that restores lateral rotation of the shoulder when the spinati are paralysed.

AXILLARY (CIRCUMFLEX) NERVE (C5 and 6)

This nerve, arising from the posterior cord of the brachial plexus, winds round the back of the neck of the humerus to supply the deltoid muscle and an area of overlying skin which may be only a few centimetres across but which may extend well above the acromion. The usual autonomous area is shown in Figures **11**, 9 and **11**, 10. The abductor action of the deltoid is dependent on the integrity of the supraspinatus. Sometimes, the supraspinatus alone is an efficient abductor of the shoulder; so in some suspected paralytic disorder the normal range of abduction must be demonstrably produced by the deltoid before it can be established that the latter is not paralysed (Fig. **11**, 8).

The causes of lesions of the axillary nerve are shown in Table XVIII. Skeletal injuries, to which

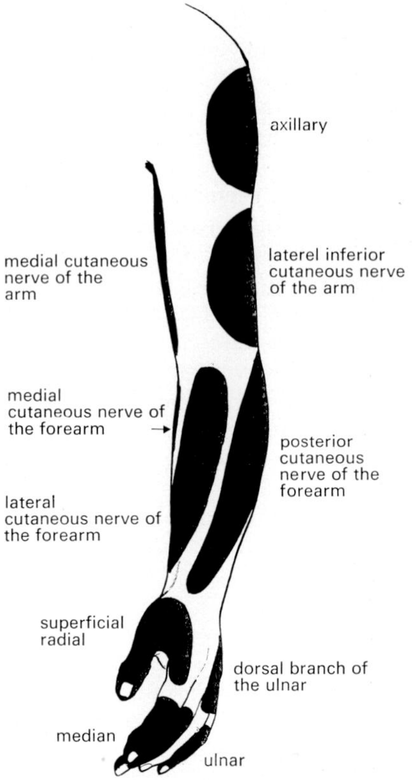

FIG. 11, 9. Autonomous areas of cutaneous sensibility in the upper limb. Lateral view.

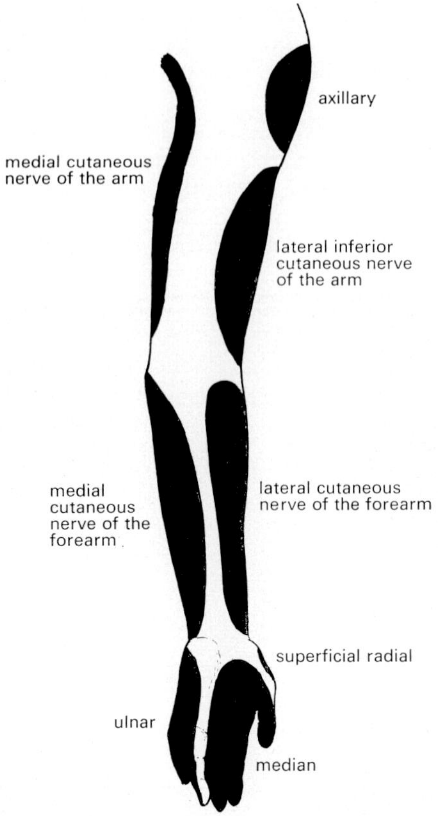

FIG. 11, 10. Anterior, or ventral view of Figure 11, 9.

TABLE XVIII—Lesions of the axillary nerve

TYPE OF DAMAGE		RECOVERY				
		Near normal	Impaired	Poor	Bad	Not known
Dislocation, fracture, fracture-dislocation: all closed injuries	15	6	4	1	2	2
Traction	6	4	—	2	—	—
'Neuritis'	2	2	—	—	—	—
Compression:						
acute	1	1	—	—	—	—
prolonged unconsciousness	1	1	—	—	—	—
Injection of drug	1	—	—	—	1	—
Missile	1	—	—	—	1	—
	27					

detailed reference has already been made (p. 81), are by far the commonest cause of damage.

The prognosis is uncertain because there is an element of traction in some of these injuries of the axillary nerve. Exploration in two cases revealed appearances exactly like those found in traction injuries—in continuity—of the common peroneal nerve.

Six injuries ascribed to traction occurred in the absence of demonstrable bony injury; but there may have been momentary dislocation of the shoulder (Codman, 1934).

Sensory Branches

Medial cutaneous nerve of the arm (N. cutaneus medialis brachii). This nerve supplies a strip of skin on the medial side of the arm (Figs **11**, 9 and **11**, 10). Because it arises from T2, which makes this one insignificant contribution to the brachial plexus, it is almost invariably spared in lesions of the brachial plexus. If it is involved, post-fixation of the plexus should be suspected.

Medial cutaneous nerve of the forearm (N. cutaneus medialis antebrachii). This terminal branch (C8.T1) of the medial cord of the plexus courses down the medial side of the arm beneath the deep fascia close to the brachial vessels and the median nerve. A little above the elbow it divides into anterior and posterior branches and pierces the deep fascia alongside the basilic vein. The two branches supply the area of skin shown in Figure **11**, 10.

The medial cutaneous nerve of the forearm is often injured by wounds damaging the median or ulnar nerve, or both, proximal to the elbow. But isolated injuries occur, and they commonly cause irritative symptoms (p. 147). On account of its accessibility, and because it has no significant branches proximal to the elbow, the medial cutaneous nerve of the forearm is an excellent source of material for autologous nerve grafting (p. 296). Moreover, the ultimate loss of sensibility is negligible because of the ingrowth of fibres from adjacent areas.

INJURIES OF THE BRACHIAL PLEXUS

If incised wounds of the sort that so often damage the median and ulnar nerves were at all common in the region of the brachial plexus it would be possible to localize the site of damage with unusual precision. But most of the injuries are of a blunderbuss kind, whether due to penetrating wounds or to traction; so even the most careful examination yields no more than an approximate assessment of the damage that the brachial plexus has suffered.

Neurapraxia. Short-lived paralysis may occur after missile injuries or traction. It can be confined to one part of the plexus, the remainder suffering more severely. Reference has already been made (p. 133) to neurapraxia resulting from injury to the plexus on the operation table. Of Yeoman's (1963) 10 cases of traction injury causing neurapraxia alone, eight were due to falls in the home (Table XXI, p. 185): the degree of violence was minimal.

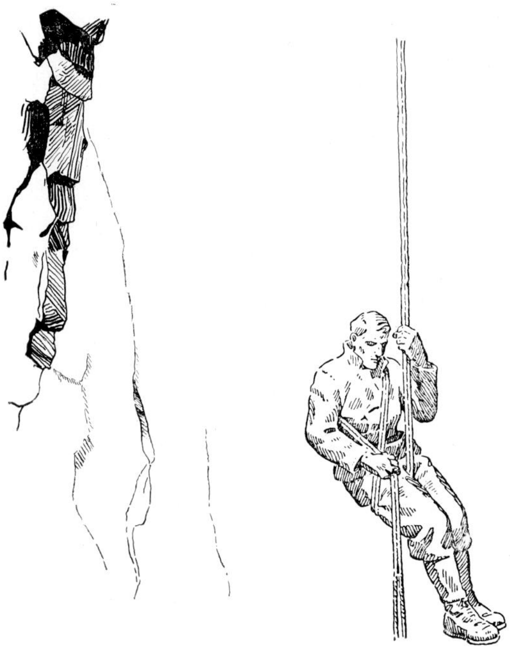

FIG. **11**, 11. The *abseil* or *rappel*. The climber prevents himself from tipping over by keeping his right thigh firm in the position shown and by gripping the rope above him with his left hand. He controls his descent with the right hand; the rope slides round the back of his body, over the left shoulder—the danger point—and behind the right thigh. (Reproduced by kind permission of the Association of British Members of the Swiss Alpine Club.)

Another variety can be serious. Gailland (1967) has described how pressure by a climbing rope over the posterior triangle of the neck may produce paralysis of the whole arm. Climbers sometimes descend the steep face of a mountain by means of a technique called *abseil* or *rappel*. If the angle of a rock face is less than vertical much of the climber's weight is borne by his feet; this is safe. But if there is an overhang he descends in mid-air like a spider (Fig. **11**, 11), with the rope tightly drawn across his chest, over one shoulder, and firmly held in the opposite hand. He hangs free, and unless he is adequately padded there is likely to be great pressure over the brachial plexus. There have been fatal falls for which no explanation has hitherto been offered. In some cases this pressure paralysis may have been the reason.

Traumatic asphyxia, the result of crushing accidents, can be accompanied by brachial plexus paralysis (Leach and Cuthbert, 1972). The latter may not in itself be serious, but it may be difficult to recognize in a semi-conscious patient; if he can be induced to stir a little the movement of his limbs should be carefully observed. The mechanism causing the injury is uncertain.

Degenerative lesions. We come now to the far more serious and more common degenerative lesions. Because the damage of one part of the plexus may be due to neurapraxia while another part has suffered damage causing a degenerative lesion, the initial paralysis, which may be total, is no certain guide to what may be its later, significant extent. The means of recognizing the element of neurapraxia have been described on page 33; here it is sufficient to recall that it is predominantly motor and that the paralysed muscles retain their normal electrical excitability.

It is necessary to distinguish supraclavicular from infraclavicular paralysis. This is simple when small wounds—and some large ones, as when the axilla has been sliced by broken glass—involve the plexus. But traction injuries are extensive longitudinally; the most one can say then is that the main site of damage is above or below the clavicle.

Useful localizing guides are as follows:

1. *The action of muscles deriving their nerve supply from the supraclavicular plexus:* the diaphragm, the serratus anterior, the rhomboids and the spinati, though the first two are paralysed only if the damage is close to the spinal cord. If there is a fracture in the region of the shoulder it may at first be difficult or impossible to ascertain the state of these muscles, except the diaphragm, which is observed by radiographic screening.

2. *Concomitant fractures.* If there is skeletal damage in the region of the shoulder there is a strong presumption that the injury of the plexus is infraclavicular (pp. 81-83). On the other hand, fracture of the cervical transverse processes is a sure indication of supraclavicular damage, and fracture of the clavicle points in the same direction.

3. *Horner's syndrome* indicates supraclavicular paralysis.

4. *Sensory paralysis* extending well above the clavicle indicates involvement of the cervical plexus and that the paralysis of the brachial plexus is supraclavicular.

5. *A swelling above the clavicle* is a sign of supraclavicular injury, but its absence has no significance.

Supraclavicular Paralysis

Clinical Features

There are four main types of paralysis. They involve (1) the fifth and sixth cervical nerve roots, or the upper trunk of the brachial plexus; (2) C5 and C6, plus the seventh cervical nerve, which continues as the middle trunk of the plexus; (3) the eighth cervical and first thoracic nerve roots, which form the lower trunk of the plexus, and (4) the whole plexus.

1. Cervical 5 and 6 (Upper Trunk)

Motor paralysis. The distribution of the paralysis is shown in Table XIX and Fig. **11**, 12. The chief movements lost are abduction and lateral rotation of the shoulder, and flexion of the elbow. Sometimes, especially in birth injuries of C5 and 6, (p. 130), the paralysis is wholly or predominantly motor, the largest nerve fibres having been damaged selectively.

Sensory paralysis. The area of cutaneous insensibility is shorter distally as well as narrower than the C5 and C6 dermatomes as usually described (cf. Figs **11**, 13 and **11**, 14).

2. Cervical 5, 6 and 7 (Upper and Middle Trunks)

Motor paralysis. In addition to the motor loss just described there is paralysis of about the upper half of the pectoralis major, of the teres major and latissimus dorsi, of the triceps, of all the muscles in the extensor compartment of the forearm, and sometimes of the flexor carpi

TABLE XIX—Distribution of motor paralysis in relation to the sites of damage of the supraclavicular plexus

<table>
<tr><th>C3</th><th>C4</th><th>C5</th><th>C6</th><th>C7</th><th>C8</th><th>T1</th></tr>
<tr><td colspan="3">Diaphragm</td><td></td><td></td><td></td><td></td></tr>
<tr><td></td><td></td><td>Rhomboids</td><td></td><td></td><td></td><td></td></tr>
<tr><td></td><td></td><td colspan="3">Serratus Anterior</td><td></td><td></td></tr>
<tr><td></td><td></td><td colspan="2">Spinati</td><td></td><td></td><td></td></tr>
<tr><td></td><td></td><td colspan="2">Pectoralis Major (clavicular)</td><td></td><td></td><td></td></tr>
<tr><td></td><td></td><td colspan="2">Deltoid</td><td></td><td></td><td></td></tr>
<tr><td></td><td></td><td colspan="2">Biceps</td><td></td><td></td><td></td></tr>
<tr><td></td><td></td><td colspan="2">Brachialis</td><td></td><td></td><td></td></tr>
<tr><td></td><td></td><td colspan="2">Brachioradialis</td><td></td><td></td><td></td></tr>
<tr><td></td><td></td><td colspan="2">Extensor Carpi Radialis Longus</td><td></td><td></td><td></td></tr>
<tr><td></td><td></td><td colspan="2">Pronator Teres</td><td></td><td></td><td></td></tr>
<tr><td></td><td></td><td colspan="2">Flexor Carpi Radialis</td><td></td><td></td><td></td></tr>
<tr><td></td><td></td><td></td><td></td><td>Triceps</td><td></td><td></td></tr>
<tr><td></td><td></td><td></td><td></td><td>Teres Major</td><td></td><td></td></tr>
<tr><td></td><td></td><td></td><td></td><td>Latissimus Dorsi</td><td></td><td></td></tr>
<tr><td></td><td></td><td></td><td></td><td>Pectoralis Major (middle fibres)</td><td colspan="2">Pectoralis Major (lowest fibres)</td></tr>
<tr><td></td><td></td><td></td><td></td><td>All muscles on dorsum of forearm except ext. c. rad. long.</td><td colspan="2">All muscles in flexor compartment of forearm except pron. teres and flex. carpi radialis</td></tr>
<tr><td></td><td></td><td></td><td></td><td>Flexor Carpi Ulnaris</td><td colspan="2">Intrinsic muscles of hand</td></tr>
</table>

Muscles that are sometimes paralysed are shown in *Italic type.*

This list should not be regarded as challenging the anatomists', though theirs show variations. What appears above are the observed consequences of damage to the three parts of the brachial plexus, only the clinically important and accessible muscles being listed. What is remarkable is the fair constancy of the patterns of paralysis, although the injuries—traction and missile—are by nature so variable.

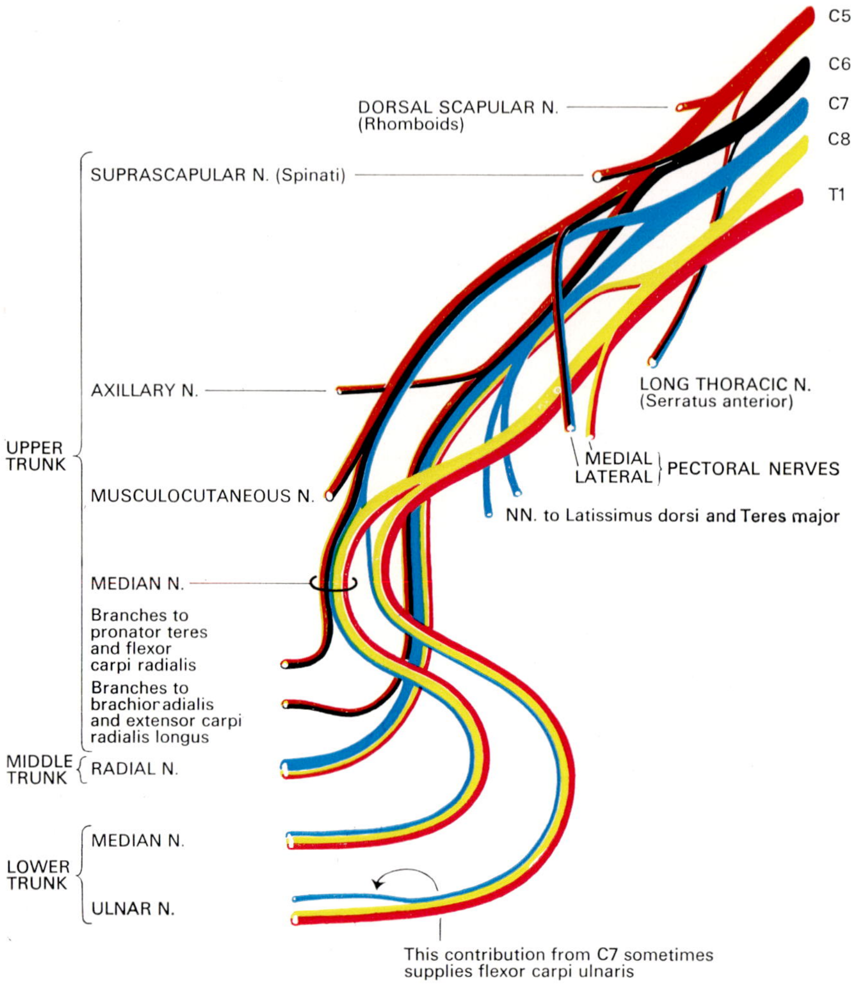

FIG. **11,** 12. The brachial plexus showing the distribution of nerve fibres in the five roots of origin. Anatomical textbooks are at variance about the root-origin of some nerves, and not one of them agrees in every detail with the information derived from clinical observation. This diagram is necessarily synthetic, but is in accord with what has been learned clinically.

ulnaris. There may be slight weakness of the flexor digitorum superficialis, of the lateral half of the flexor digitorum profundus and of the thenar muscles. In addition to the movements lost in paralysis of C5 and 6 there is loss of extension of the elbow, the wrist and the digits. The latissimus dorsi and teres major are unavailable for transplantation to restore lateral rotation, and sometimes the flexor carpi ulnaris is useless for transplantation into the extensors of the digits.

Sensory paralysis. The area of loss due to interruption of C5 and 6 now extends distally to include the palmar and dorsal surfaces of the thumb and index (Fig. **11**, 14).

Supraclavicular swelling. In injuries of C5-6 or C5-7 thickening or a fusiform swelling may be palpable in the line of the plexus.

3. Cervical 8 and Thoracic 1 (Lower Trunk)

Motor paralysis. This has much the same distribution as paralysis of the median and ulnar

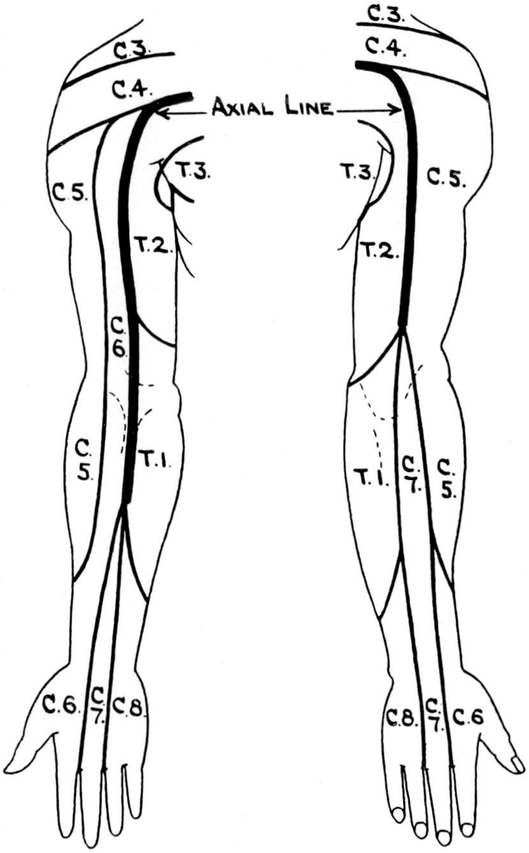

Fig. 11, 13. The dermatomes of the upper limb as usually described. Clinical evidence does not support the distribution of C6 to the thumb and index finger, or of C7 to the middle finger.

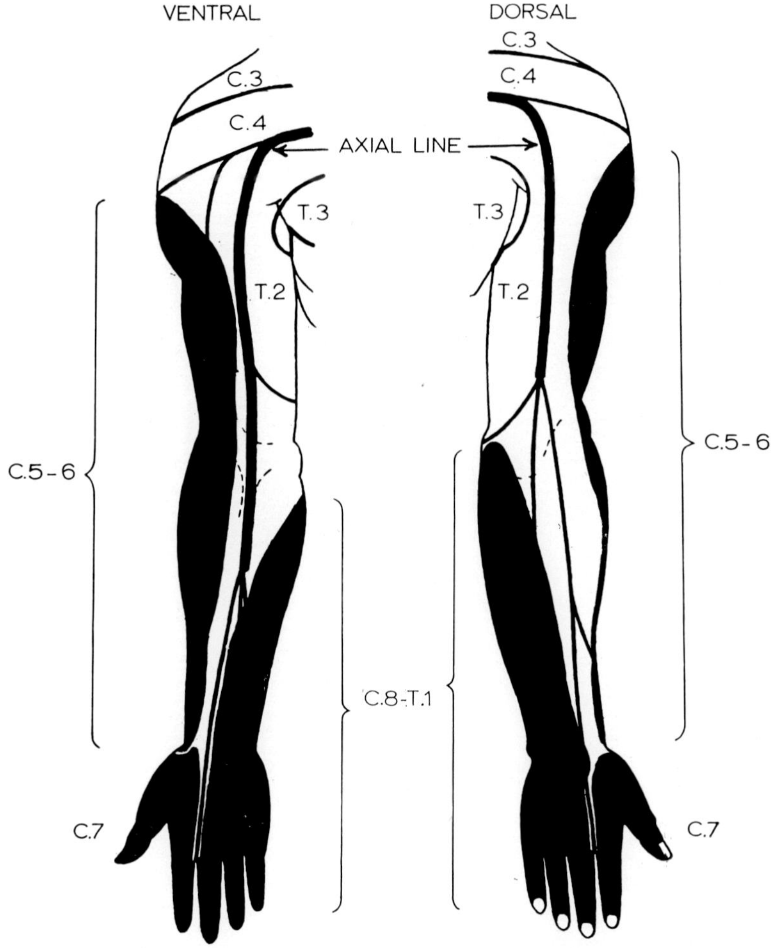

Fig. 11, 14. The area of sensory loss after lesions of C5 and 6 never extends distal to the wrist. On clinical evidence C7 supplies the palmar and dorsal surfaces of the thumb and index finger. In lesions of C8 and T1 the middle finger is insensitive.

nerves except that the pronator teres and flexor carpi radialis, being supplied by C5 and 6, are spared. The disability is grave.

Sensory paralysis. This is approximately as shown in Figure **11**, 14.

Horner's syndrome. This is often found with traction injuries involving C8 and T1 (p. 193). There are narrowing of the palpebral fissure, a small pupil, and unilateral loss of sweating of the head and neck (Fig. **11**, 15) extending as low as the second rib. There may be unilateral stuffiness of the nose due to flushing of the mucous membrane. This syndrome indicates severe proximal damage of C8 and T1 and is a most unfavourable sign.

4. Cervical 5 to Thoracic 1 (Total Paralysis)

Motor paralysis. All the muscles distal to the shoulder girdle are inactive; the limb is paralysed.

Sensory paralysis. Except for a narrow strip extending from the axilla to just above the inner side of the elbow, which is innervated by T2, the upper limb is insensitive distal to the acromion process (Fig. **11**, 16).

Horner's syndrome is frequent.

Oedema and stiffness. Oedema of the distal part

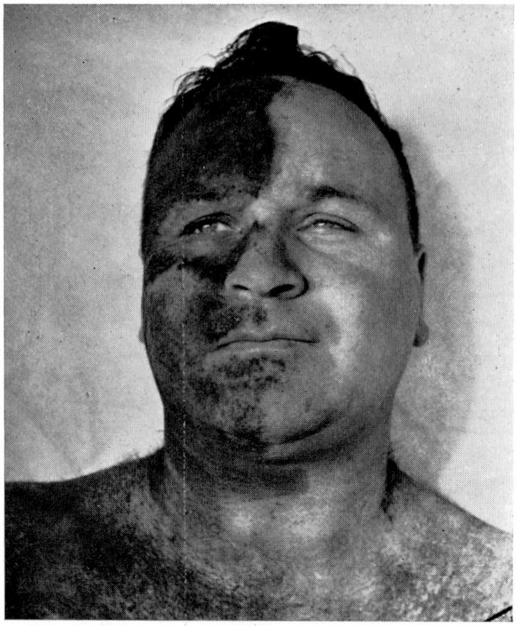

11, 15

FIG. **11,** 15. Horner's syndrome. Distribution of sweating demonstrated by quinizarin method.

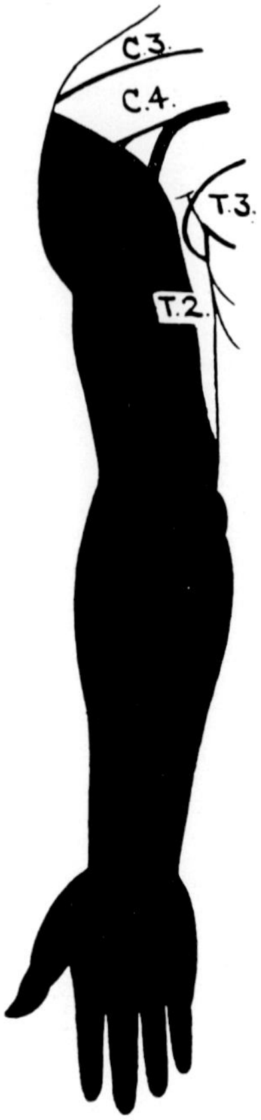

FIG. **11,** 16. The area of cutaneous sensory loss in total supraclavicular brachial plexus paralysis.

11, 16

of the limb is common, and this contributes to rapidly developing stiffness of the hand.

The paralysis sometimes involves the cervical plexus. The ipsilateral half of the diaphragm is paralysed, and the area of sensory loss extends well above the clavicle.

If the roots of the plexus have been damaged the most proximally innervated muscles, that is the serratus anterior and the rhomboids, are also affected; it may be found too that the area of analgesia is greater than that of anaesthesia.

In all four types of paralysis loss of sweating is co-extensive with loss of sensibility, though if Horner's syndrome is present it extends up on to the neck and face (Fig. **11**, 15) where sensibility is normal. Patients with brachial plexus injuries may suffer more or less severe pain (Table XIV, p. 145), but causalgia occurs only with lesions of C8 and T1. Associated injuries are common, and sometimes of such severity as to dictate the programme of treatment.

CAUSES OF SUPRACLAVICULAR BRACHIAL PLEXUS PARALYSIS

These are shown in Table XX. Birth paralysis has been omitted; on page 131 it is explained why our figures are worthless.

TABLE XX—Causes of supraclavicular injuries of the brachial plexus

Traction	123
Missile wounds	37
Miscellaneous	14
	174

Traction injuries predominate. This was so even during the Second World War. We dealt with 72 cases of traction injury, mostly in men in the armed forces and usually due to road accidents; in the same period there were 35 missile injuries, one being suffered by a civilian.

Traction Injuries

Traction injuries have certain peculiarities; on this account, and because they are common—particularly in countries where motor-cycles are popular—they require detailed consideration.[1]

Age groups and sex (Yeoman). Most of the patients are between 16 and 25 years old at the time of injury, and almost all male.

TABLE XXI—Types of accident causing traction injuries of the brachial plexus (Yeoman)

TYPE OF ACCIDENT	NEURAPRAXIA ALONE	DEGENERATIVE LESIONS: transient paralysis (neurapraxia) excluded				TOTALS
		C5 6	C5.6.7	C8.T1	C5.-T1	
Motor cycle	—	16	25	2	65	108
Pedal cycle	1	2	3	—	15	21
Fall at home	8	1	1	5	4	19
Automobile	1	3	3	—	6	13
Others	—	3	4	3	9	19
TOTALS	10	25	36	10	99	**180**

Type of accident (Table XXI). Motor-cycle accidents account for two-thirds of the degenerative lesions of the plexus, whether incomplete or complete, with the exception of injuries confined to C8 and T1. The cyclist shoots off his machine, striking the ground (or something else equally unyielding) obliquely. He is not killed by the all too frequent head injury because he is wearing a crash helmet; but the impact falls on and depresses his unprotected shoulder. The neural damage occurs first in C5 and 6, then in descending order in the other roots of the plexus until perhaps all are affected.

Damage falling primarily on C8 and T1 results from the opposite mechanism. The most dramatic example of this was in a patient who fell through the floor of a room, one arm being held up; in Yeoman's analysis half of the injuries of C8 and T1 were the result of accidents at home.

Bilateral plexus paralysis is rare.

On page 76 it was pointed out that before a nerve could suffer a traction injury some important structure, bony or ligamentous, must give way. The one exception to this is the brachial plexus; the great mobility of the neck and of the shoulder girdle permits longitudinal stretching of the plexus. Moreover, nerve roots lack the tough stroma of nerves in the limbs (p. 4) and so are more easily damaged. Nevertheless fractures occur in the more violent injuries. Fracture of the clavicle is by far the most important because this bone is the main safeguard against excessive depression of the shoulder. Yeoman found that avulsion of the cervical transverse processes occurs only in paralysis of the whole plexus. If these processes or the neck of the first rib are broken the corresponding nerve roots are severely damaged. The anchorage of the cervical spine which these bony bollards and their attached muscles provide is the last line of defence. When it has gone the cervical spine can open up laterally (Fig. **11**, 17) by rupture of an intervertebral disc. Roaf (1963)

[1] I owe a great debt to two friends, formerly my assistants, George Bonney and Philip Yeoman. Their contributions to our understanding of these injuries have dispelled the uncertainties that bedevilled this topic. Yeoman has not published his thesis (1963) for the Cambridge doctorate of medicine, for which, in the following year, he was also awarded the Robert Jones Prize of the British Orthopaedic Association. He has been kind enough to allow me to use some of the information it contains. There is some lack of correspondence between his statistics and mine. There are three reasons for this. Yeoman's thesis was concerned with traction injuries without distinction between supraclavicular and infraclavicular lesions; in this connection there are also differences of interpretation, though we were using much the same corpus of material; and, lastly, there was some difference in the timing of our analyses.

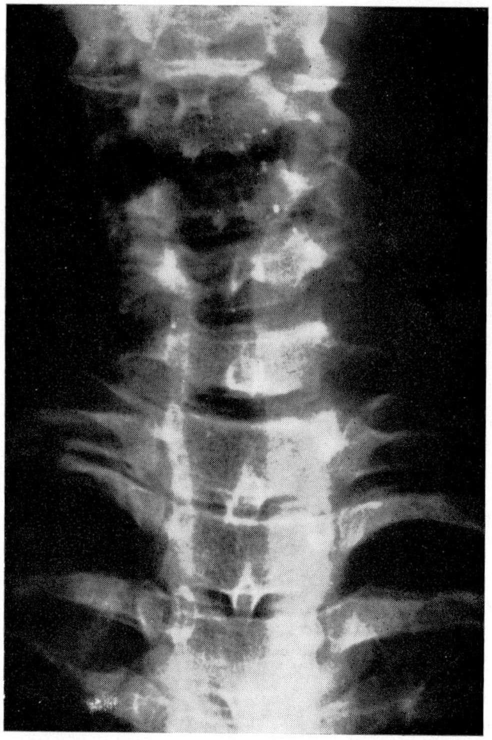

FIG. **11,** 17. Lateral tilt of the cervical spine: severe injury of the left brachial plexus (P. M. Yeoman).

described this tilting of the cervical spine in patients with the gravest injuries of the spinal cord accompanied by tearing of the brachial plexus on the side that opens up. Yeoman found this lateral tilt, which was easily visible, in 26 of the severest cases of traction injury of the plexus.

Skeletal injuries in the region of the shoulder joint are much more a feature of infraclavicular paralysis (pp. 81 to 83), and the nerve damage is relatively benign. Moreover, the mechanism is different. The shoulder is pushed in rather than depressed; the joint dislocates or a bone breaks. If the head of the humerus is dislocated the plexus may be stretched, but otherwise it is injured directly by the bony fragments, though only rarely to the point of severance of one of the cords.

The Varieties of Damage to the Plexus and to the Spinal Cord

The most important varieties of traction injuries are shown in Figure **11**, 18. The crucial point is whether the lesion is proximal or distal to the posterior root ganglia. The infraganglionic lesions (Figs **11**, 19, **11**, 18: 2 and 3), whether the nerve trunk remains in continuity or is ruptured, are like other traction injuries, which have already been described on pages 72 to 78. except in one respect, that owing to the relative fragility of the stroma of the nerve roots the damage nearest to the spinal cord is mainly intra-funicular (see Fig. **5**, 20, p. 75).

If the tear is between the spinal cord and a posterior root ganglion the peripheral axons of the ganglion cells usually survive (Fig. **11**, 18, 4 and 5; Figs **11**, 20 and **11**, 21); this gives rise to several phenomena by means of which these supraganglionic lesions can be recognized. But

1. Normal nerve root.
2. An injury in continuity distal to the posterior root ganglion. All axons degenerate; axon reflex tests are negative and there is no nerve conduction. Some recovery is possible if the regenerating axons can penetrate the intraneural scar.
3. The same, but there has been disruption of the nerve. Repair may be impossible on account of the extensive intraneural damage; (2) and (3) are distinguishable only by exploration in the posterior triangle of the neck.
4. A recent supraganglionic lesion. The nerve root has been torn out of the cord, and there is an intrathecal effusion which shows as a filling defect in the myelogram. The posterior root ganglion cell bodies are intact. Whereas their central connections degenerate (there is no way of demonstrating this) their peripheral axons are intact, as can be shown by axon reflex tests and by nerve conduction.
5. The same, but the rent in the dura mater has healed and the myelographic appearance is normal.
6. If the rent in the dura does not heal a saccular protrusion forms, a traumatic meningocele, easily visible in the myelogram. The nerve root here is shown as having suffered extensive interstitial damage, sufficient to destroy the posterior root ganglion cells. Axon reflex tests and nerve conduction would therefore be negative, suggesting an infraganglionic lesion—but for the myelographic demonstration of a meningocele.
7. A rare distortion of the spinal cord, a late consequence of a supraganglionic rupture of the nerve root.

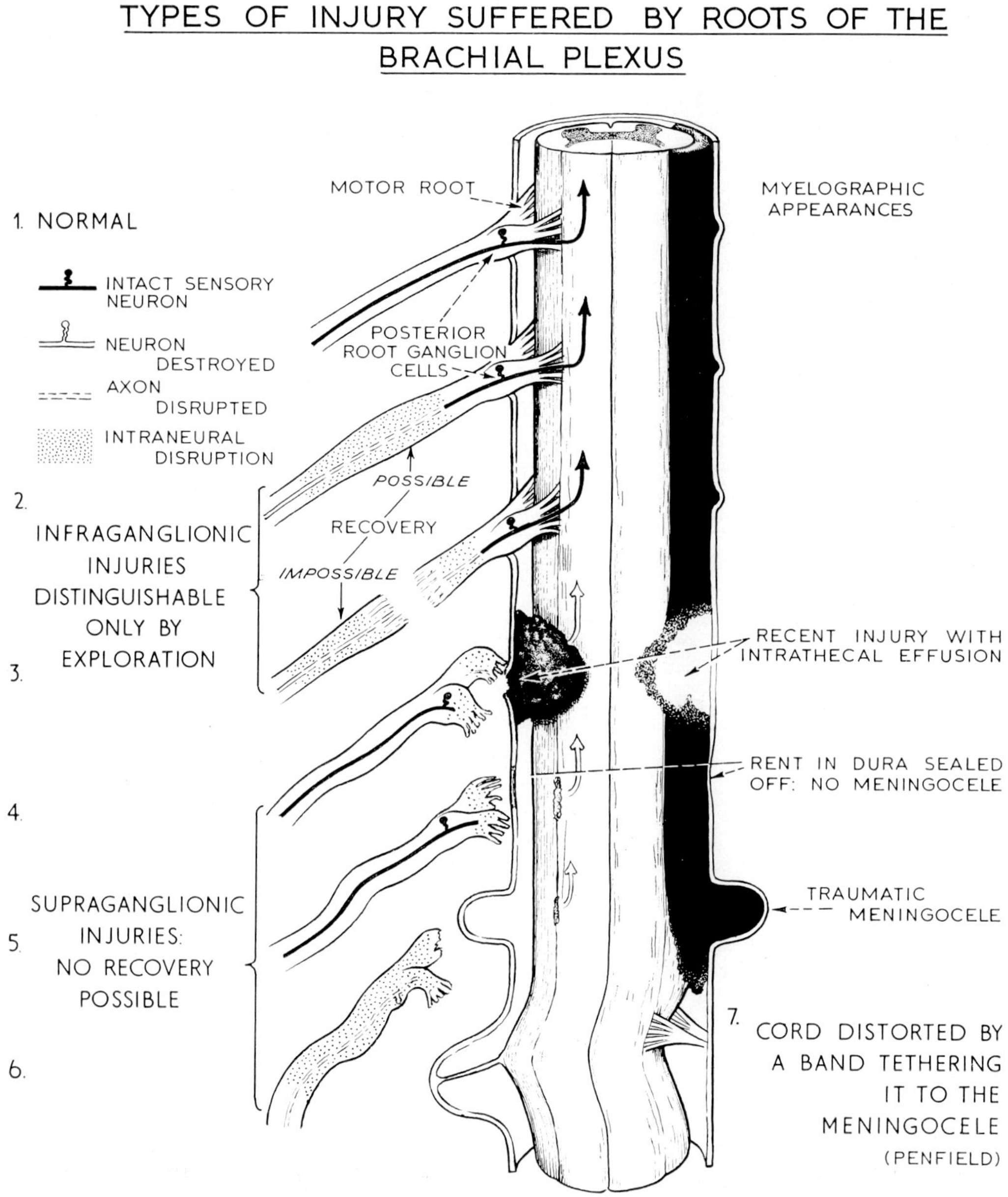

FIG. **11,** 18. Diagrammatic representation of the types of traction injury that can be suffered by a root of the brachial plexus. The spinal cord is viewed from behind.

(*See opposite page for key*)

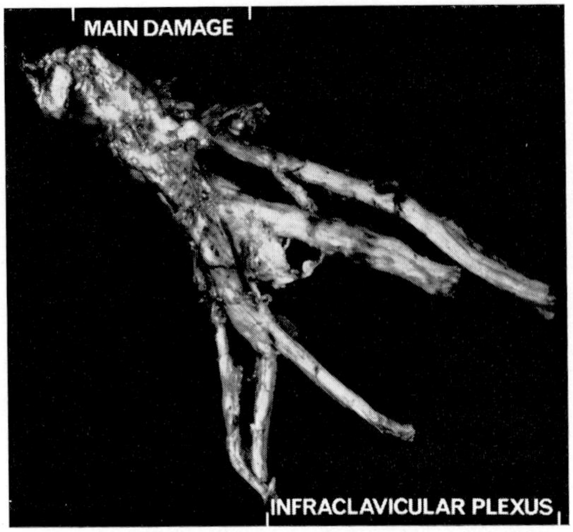

FIG. **11,** 19. Infraganglionic rupture of the brachial plexus. The provenance of the specimen is described on page 152.

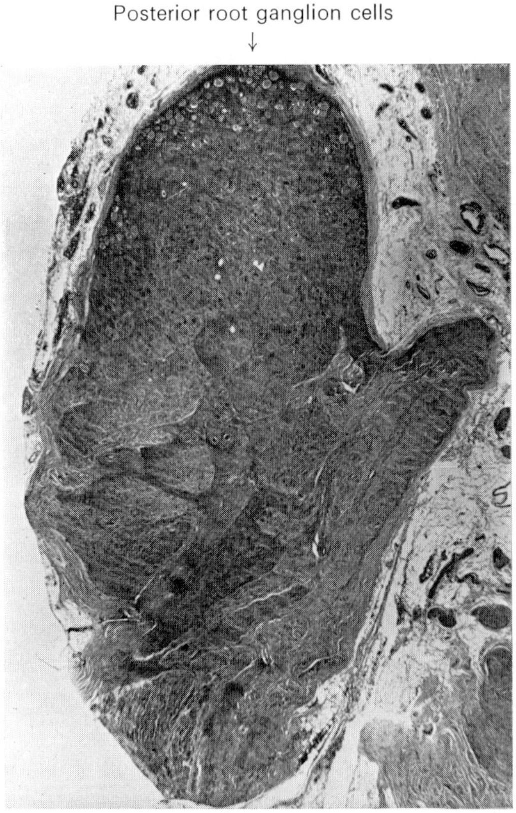

FIG. **11,** 20. Transverse section through part of an avulsed brachial plexus showing, at the top, a cluster of posterior root ganglion cells.

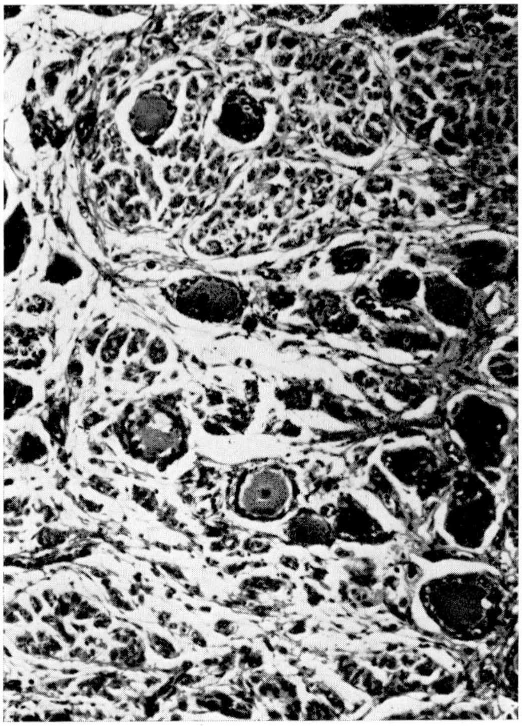

FIG. **11,** 21. Another section from the same specimen showing a mass of posterior root ganglion cells which were found just proximal to the clavicle. (× 50.)

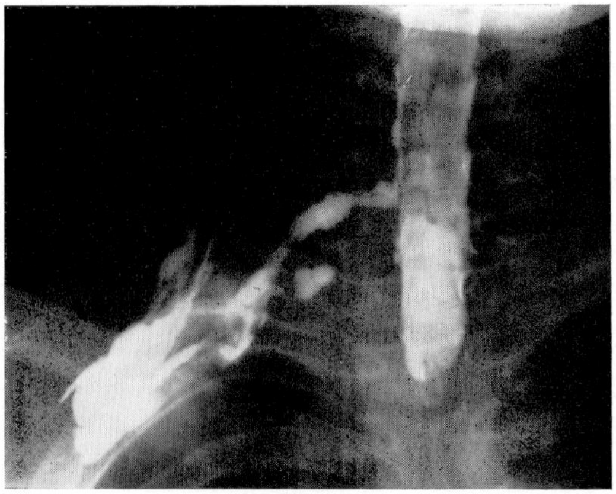

FIG. **11,** 22. A myelogram was carried out soon after the injury: the contrast medium leaked through a dural rent as far as the apex of the axilla. (Reproduced by kind permission of the author and Editor from Fulford, G. E., 1970, *Physiotherapy*, **56**, 285.)

the posterior root ganglion cells may be destroyed (Fig. **11**, 18, 6); there is then degeneration of their peripheral axons, as in the infraganglionic injuries, and myelography alone will reveal that the damage is in fact supraganglionic.

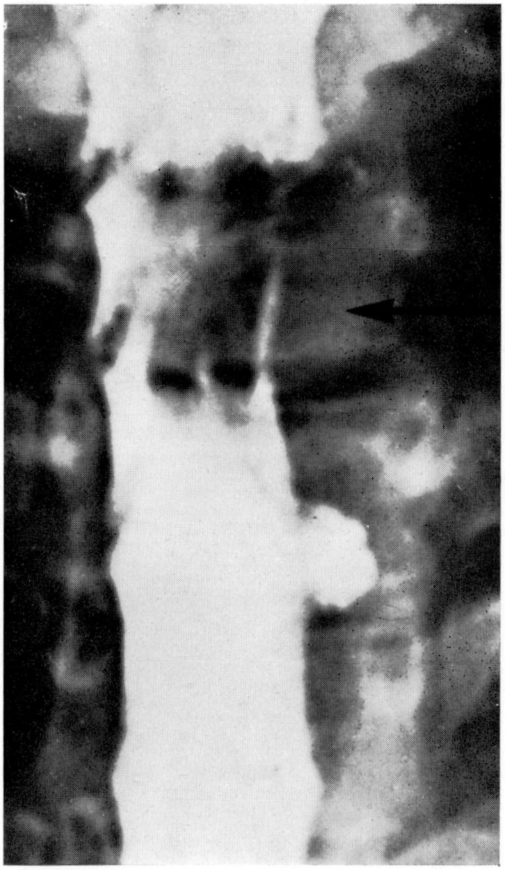

FIG. **11,** 23. The arrow indicates encroachment on the subarachnoid space by a traumatic exudate. A small meningocele is visible below. (P. M. Yeoman.)

Inevitably the meninges and cord are damaged. Leakage occurs through the rent in the dura mater (Fig. **11**, 22). There may also be intrathecal bleeding; but on account of the frequency of concomitant head injury, which itself can cause haemorrhage into the cerebrospinal fluid, it is rarely possible to demonstrate intrathecal bleeding due solely to injury of the brachial plexus (Yeoman). Before long a localized effusion—which may become organized—occurs at the site of the meningeal tear (Figs **11**, 18, 4 and **11**, 23). The rent in the dura mater may be sealed off leaving no myelographic abnormality. Haftek (1967b) has shown by laminectomy that a meningocele can be filled in by adhesions; the myelogram may then be normal. The commonest

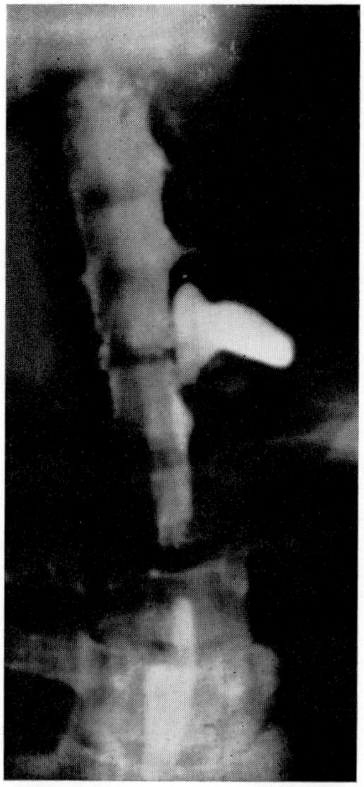

FIG. **11,** 24. The traumatic meningocele appears to be at C8, but this was not borne out by the subsequent history. A boy of 16 fell 12 feet and suffered total paralysis of the left brachial plexus, a fracture of the scapula and of the upper ribs. Horner's syndrome was present but disappeared within three months, although the complete motor and sensory paralysis had persisted. The boy then began to make a useful recovery *except in the distribution of C7*, so evidently his brachial plexus was post-fixed: a demonstration that localization of the damage should not be based on myelographic evidence alone (Mr D. M. Brooks's patient).

finding is, however, a traumatic meningocele such as is shown in Figures **11**, 18, 6; **11**, 24 and **11**, 25.

The various parts of the plexus may be injured in different ways, and Yeoman found that meningoceles are more frequent in the lower part of the plexus (Fig. **11**, 26).

In some patients who have suffered intractable pain total avulsion of the nerve roots has been

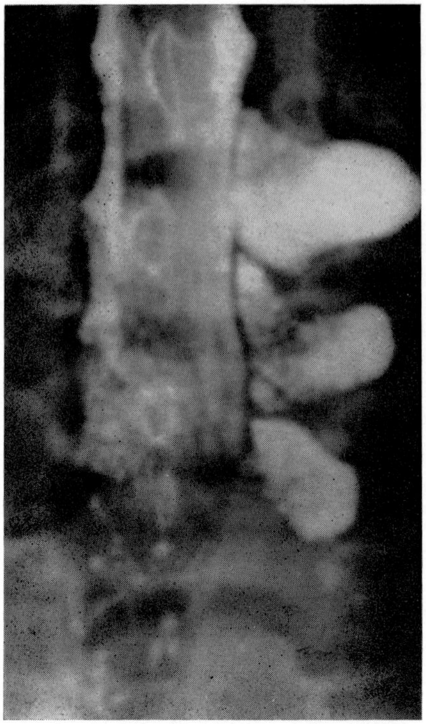

FIG. **11,** 25. Multiple meningoceles.

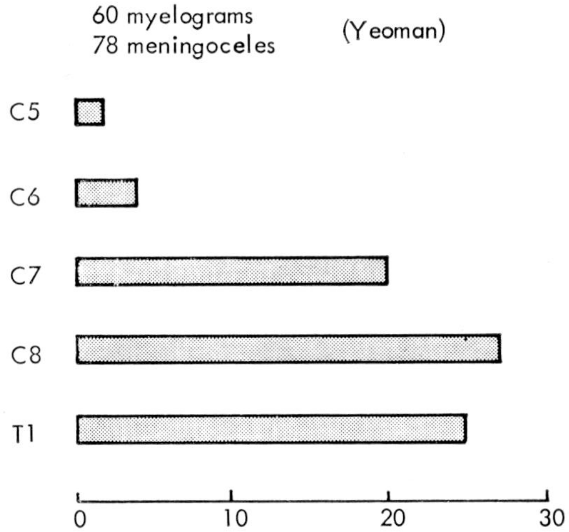

FIG. **11,** 26. The lower the traction injury the greater is the frequency of traumatic meningocele: and, therefore, the worse the prognosis.

demonstrated by laminectomy; there could be no doubt that the pain was due to intramedullary damage. Occasionally there is other evidence of injury to the cord: retention of urine and disordered sensibility in the lower limb. The spinal cord may be severely damaged by the same violence that injures the plexus (Roaf, 1963).

A remarkable late consequence of brachial plexus injury was described by Penfield (1949): the spinal cord becomes distorted and damaged (Fig. **11**, 18, 7) as a result of its being tethered to the fundus of a meningocele.

Associated injuries. These are very common and most varied. Head injuries occur in about half the patients and they range from slight concussion to damage causing prolonged unconsciousness. Tracheostomy may be required. Many of these injuries—to the head, chest, abdomen, pelvis and femur—must take precedence over the brachial plexus in the plan of treatment.

Clinical Features and their Prognostic Significance

It may be impossible to obtain a clear history of the accident, though even if the patient is brought in unconscious there is usually someone available who can say whether or not the victim was travelling at speed. This has an important bearing on the prognosis. A comparatively minor affair, such as a domestic accident short of falling downstairs, is a favourable factor.

In addition to the general features of supraclavicular brachial plexus paralysis that have already been described the following are particularly significant in traction injuries:

1. A swelling in the neck in the line of the plexus.

2. Sensory loss extending above the point of the shoulder.

3. Horner's syndrome (see p. 183). This is a most unfavourable sign, indicating that the lowest roots of the plexus have been avulsed from the cord (Barnes, 1949; Bonney, 1959). It was present in 78 of the patients studied by Yeoman, most of whom had been involved in high-velocity motor-cycle accidents, and who finished up with flail arms or forearms. Only one patient with Horner's syndrome recovered power in the muscles innervated by the lower trunk of the plexus; but there was permanent paralysis of those supplied by C7, at which level there was a traumatic meningocele. A possible explanation of this curiosity was that the patient had a haemothorax and fractures of the upper ribs; that is to say, the causation of the plexus

lesion and of the Horner's syndrome were separate and, up to a point, different (see also the case illustrated by Fig. **11**, 24).

4. Pain. When there has been a severe injury of the plexus most patients complain from the first of great pain in the whole of the upper limb. In some cases (p. 145) this pain persists—rarely as causalgia, more often as what we have called an irritative nerve lesion. Yeoman found that pain was severe in 32 of the 46 patients who suffered permanent paralysis of the whole plexus. Pain was also pronounced in 22 of the 40 patients who had total paralysis initially but who later showed some recovery proximal to the elbow.

Investigations and their Prognostic Significance

Radiography. In addition to obvious fractures, such as those of the clavicle, radiography may reveal avulsion of the cervical transverse processes, fracture of the neck of the first rib or, rarely, slight separation of a pair of vertebral bodies on the affected side. All are bad prognostic signs.

In severe damage, involving the cervical plexus, paralysis of the diaphragm may be revealed.

Myelography. The first radiographic demonstration of meningoceles resulting from traction injuries of the brachial plexus was reported in 1947 by Murphey, Hartung and Kirklin, and since then a number of other papers have appeared. Yeoman (1968) described the findings in 60 patients investigated at the Royal National Orthopaedic Hospital.

Technique. White and Hanelin (1954) used up to 9 ml of contrast medium injected by the lumbar route; it was removed subsequently, but even so a few of their patients suffered minor disturbances of function of the spinal cord. In our patients 5 ml of Myodil have proved satisfactory; the contrast medium was not removed and there have been no ill effects. The pressure of the cerebrospinal fluid is measured and a specimen is examined microscopically. After the injection of the contrast medium the patient is placed on a tilting viewing couch. Filling of the pouches is facilitated if the patient lies on the affected side, but some do not fill until he coughs.

The distribution of the meningoceles is shown in Figure **11**, 26. In eight cases the myelograms were normal and in all of them recovery of the paralysis occurred. In 24 cases there were single meningoceles, in 30 there were two and in 24 three. Filling defects (Fig. **11**, 23) were found in six cases; it was proved by laminectomy that this abnormality was due to subarachnoid fibrosis. In two patients Yeoman found a curious loculus in the subarachnoid space that communicated with a neighbouring meningocele; the contrast medium could be decanted from one to the other. If myelography is carried out within 10 days of the accident no well-defined pouches are found; the contrast medium leaks out through the meningeal tear, travelling some distance into the root of the neck (Fig. **11**, 22).

The prognostic significance of meningoceles will be considered below in conjunction with the results of other investigations.

Axon reflexes. Myelography provides anatomical evidence of avulsion of a nerve root from the spinal cord—that is to say, of damage proximal to the posterior root ganglion. Bonney (1954, 1959) provided what might be called physiological evidence of supraganglionic damage. The basis of the tests to be described is that the distal axons arising from the posterior root ganglion cells are intact. During the Second World War we found histological evidence of this from biopsies carried out on nerve trunks distal to the clavicle, our endeavour being to avoid time-consuming exploratory operations on the plexus. In some cases the nerve trunks contained a fairly large population of myelinated fibres, and in consequence the outlook was thought to be favourable. However, these patients failed to recover; we lacked the wit to grasp the significance of what was, in fact, a bad prognostic sign.

Bonney applied Lewis's well-known work on axon reflexes to brachial plexus injuries.

HISTAMINE RESPONSE. If 1 per cent histamine acid phosphate is pricked into normal skin it produces a triple response: local vasodilatation, then the formation of a weal (an oedematous patch) and a further widespread vasodilatation described as a flare. The sign is negative in denervated skin: there may be local vasodilatation, even a weal, but no flare. In 1948 Bonney observed a positive response in a patient with complete and permanent brachial plexus paralysis. This suggested that there must be some intact axons and that the damage was therefore proximal to the posterior root ganglia.

An attraction of this test is its simplicity and the ease with which it may be applied to the various dermatomes; but it cannot be used in the hand.

COLD VASODILATATION RESPONSE. This method of demonstrating axon reflexes is more elaborate and time-consuming, and the reader wishing to use it should consult Bonney's (1954) paper. It can be applied only to the finger-tips; but the prognosis for function of the hand is more important than anything else in the upper limb.

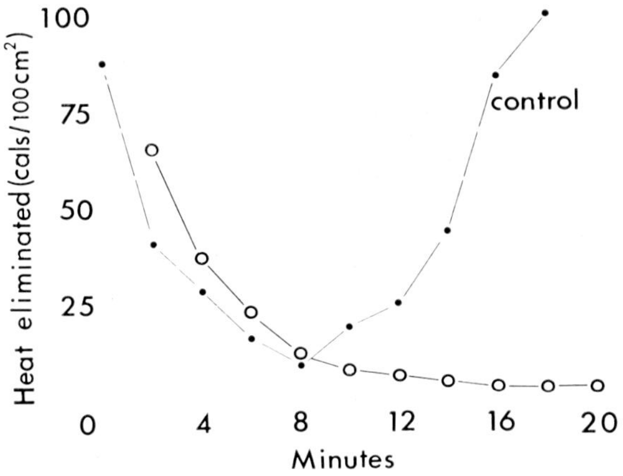

FIG. **11**, 27. In the ordinary degenerative nerve lesion—and in the infraganglionic brachial plexus lesion—there is no reactive vasodilatation.

The principle of the response is illustrated in Figures **11**, 27 and **11**, 28. The method is based on the work of Greenfield, Shepherd and Whelan (1951), and modified for investigation of brachial plexus injuries. If normal fingers are immersed in water at 5°C they cool rapidly; 5 to 10 minutes later there is vasodilatation and a considerable rise in the local skin temperature. This does not happen in a denervated digit, provided that there has been time for axonal degeneration to occur (Fig. **11**, 27). In supraganglionic lesions of the brachial plexus the response is like that in a normal digit. It has nothing to do with the autonomic nervous system. The reflex depends on the integrity of sensory axons; it is present in the normal hand if the appropriate nerve is anaesthetized proximally.

Sensory nerve conduction. It follows that in a supraganglionic lesion it should be possible to find evidence of conductivity in the intact sensory axons. This has been done by Bonney and Gilliatt (1958).

Posterior cervical electromyography. This test has an anatomical basis. The deep muscles at the back of the neck are supplied segmentally by nerves arising from the main roots just lateral to the intervertebral foramina. Their state can be determined electromyographically (Bufalini and Pescatori, 1969). If motor-unit action-potentials are absent, or if fibrillation action-potentials are picked up by the concentric needle electrode,

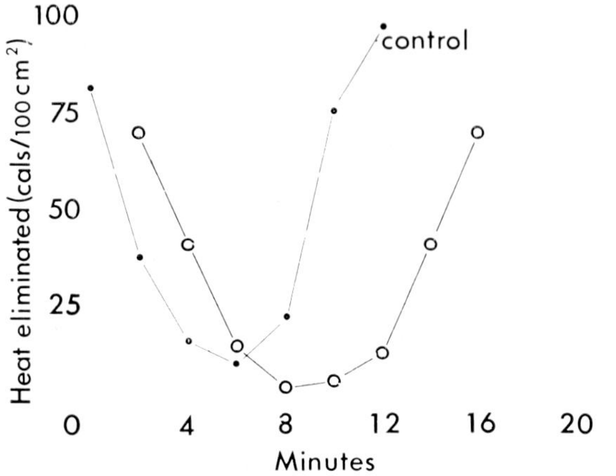

FIG. **11**, 28. In the supraganglionic lesion the reaction is much the same as in the normal limb.

then the damage to the nerve root in question is close to the spinal cord. The prognosis is bad. A normal electromyogram indicates that the lesion is distal to the intervertebral foramina, that is, infraganglionic.

Significance of the Tests Used to Determine the Level of Damage in Relation to the Posterior Root Ganglia

The reliability of the tests that have just been described is important because prognosis and treatment depend upon them.

Traumatic meningocele demonstrated. The demonstration of a meningocele indicates that a nerve root has been avulsed from the spinal cord and that no recovery in it is possible. But which root? We cannot be certain because a brachial plexus may be pre-fixed or post-fixed, as in the case illustrated in Figure **11**, 24. This question is, however, unimportant when two or more meningoceles are found; the prognosis for the whole plexus is then hopeless, and no time should be wasted on conservative treatment. Cervical myelography demonstrates the state of the nerve roots; the histamine and cold vasodilatation tests are applied peripherally and they have, therefore, a localizing value that myelography sometimes lacks. We have to consider the correlation between these two tests and myelography. In 16 of our cases with meningoceles Yeoman found that the histamine and cold-vasodilatation tests were negative. This could mean that there was a lack of correspondence between the dermatomes and the nerve roots that had suffered avulsion. A more likely explanation—though complete proof is lacking—is that the violence was so great that in addition to nerve roots being avulsed the posterior root ganglia were destroyed, so leading to total axonal degeneration peripherally (Fig. **11**, 18, 6). That the outcome was bad in every case of this sort suggests that this is the correct explanation. Yet a lack of correspondence between the level of *one* meningocele and the results of the axon reflex tests should make one hesitate before embarking on either of the two very radical operations that are described later (pp. 195 to 196).

No meningocele demonstrated. Yeoman analysed 14 cases with positive axon reflex tests, indicating supraganglionic damage, but with no corresponding meningoceles. It has been already pointed out that a meningocele may be obliterated by fibrosis, and it is significant that in eight of Yeoman's cases there was a traumatic meningocele of the root above the one under consideration; in two other cases a traumatic meningocele was found one nerve root below, and in the remaining four there were doubtful though possibly abnormal radiographic findings.

It will now be evident that in these cases of extremely disabling paralysis the clinician is obliged to take every piece of evidence into account before formulating a prognosis. The following considerations are relevant.

1. *Neurapraxia.* This benign paralysis was not found in one case of motor-cycle accident. The electrical reactions of the muscles at 21 days show whether the plexus has escaped damage sufficient to cause a degenerative lesion of all the nerve roots or of some.

2. *The more extensive the paralysis the worse the prognosis.* If the cervical as well as the brachial plexus is affected the outlook is extremely bad.

3. *Horner's syndrome.* This is a most unfavourable sign as far as the roots of C8 and T1 are concerned. Table XXII, column 7, shows Horner's syndrome was present in 91 per cent of cases of total brachial plexus paralysis that failed to recover and (column 6) in 80 per cent of cases of total paralysis in which there was no recovery in C8 and T1. However, very exceptionally, Horner's syndrome may be due to a separate lesion, caused by skeletal damage in the upper thorax. It may regress spontaneously and then has no sinister significance.

4. *Severe and persistent pain.* Table XXII, columns 6 and 7, shows that severe and persistent pain occurs in total and permanent brachial plexus paralysis and in a slightly smaller proportion of cases of total paralysis in which some recovery ultimately occurs proximal to the elbow. Quite apart from the distress this pain causes the patient, it is an unfavourable prognostic feature.

5. *Radiography.* Plain radiography may reveal one or more of the following unfavourable features: (*a*) if there is a lateral tilt of the cervical spine (Fig. **11**, 17, p. 186) the prognosis is hopeless; (*b*) avulsion of transverse processes is a most unfavourable sign and (*c*) fracture of the clavicle moderately unfavourable.

When all this evidence has been collected, together with the results of myelography and axon reflex tests (we have no experience of electromyography of the posterior cervical muscles—see p. 192—but it appears to be a valuable test), the clinician has to consider whether anything will be gained by exploration of the plexus. Before myelography and the axon reflex tests were introduced we carried out a fair number of exploratory operations, sometimes exposing the whole plexus. The need for this has gone, and exploration is now confined to cases in which there is an infraganglionic lesion of C5.6—and 7, provided that myelography shows no more than one meningocele at a lower level. If a complete rupture is found there is then no hope of spontaneous recovery. Yeoman noted that if the upper trunk of the brachial plexus was in continuity but attenuated it was equivalent to a complete tear. The surgeon must then decide what to do: attempt to repair C5 and 6 by autologous grafting, secondary suture being impossible; or deal with the paralysis by reconstructive surgery.

If he finds C5.6 (and 7) unmistakably in continuity, with little or no irregularity of form or consistence, then a hopeful attitude is proper. The nerve trunks are, of course, stimulated electrically; a positive response in any muscle is a matter for rejoicing.

TABLE XXII—Spontaneous recovery after traction injuries of the brachial plexus (Yeoman)

					TOTAL PARALYSIS INITIALLY (99 patients)		
	1 Neurapraxia	2 C5.6	3 C5.6.7	4 C8.T1	5 C5.T1 Axonotmesis	6 C5.T1 Recovery in C5.6 (and C7)	7 C5.T1 No recovery
Number of cases	10	25	36	10	13	40	46
Motor-cycle accidents	0	64%	70%	20%	23%	62·5%	80%
Pain	—	—	—	—	—	55%	70%
Horner's syndrome	—	—	—	40%	—	80%	91%
Recovery	Complete	—	—	Motor recovery in three	Good motor recovery in seven, imperfect in six	—	—
Deltoid	—	64%	39%	—	—	7.5%	—
Flexors of elbow	—	67%	44%	—	—	67%	—
Triceps	—	—	68%	—	—	42·5%	—
Forearm extensor group	—	—	83%	—	—	—	—
Sensibility		Unimportant	Good or fair recovery in all	Recovery in three	Return of protective sensibility	Recovery proximal to elbow	None

Prognosis

The fate of the 180 cases studied by Yeoman is shown in Table XXII together with the incidence of three of the more important prognostic features. There were 99 patients who had total degenerative paralysis of the plexus, and we may therefore say that some 13 per cent of them made a good or imperfect recovery. But 40 per cent showed recovery only in muscles proximal to the elbow, being left with the forearm and hand totally paralysed and insensitive (Fig. **11**, 29); in 46 per cent there was no recovery at all.

Treatment

In Britain, more particularly since the nature of traction lesions of the brachial plexus became well understood, there has been little enthusiasm for reparative operations. We do not share Bateman's (1962) attachment to neurolysis. In all traction injuries the main damage is intraneural, and in injuries of the brachial plexus, on account of the mechanical weakness of the stroma of the nerve roots, the brunt of the damage is borne by the funiculi (Fig. **5**, 20, p. 75).

In our early days we repaired five infraganglionic lesions of the upper trunk by autologous grafting. Useful recovery occurred in two patients. However, Clark's (1946) transplantation of the pectoralis major into the biceps which, in combination with arthrodesis of the shoulder, usually restores satisfactory function, seemed preferable. Infraganglionic lesions of C5,

6 and 7 were treated conservatively at first if exploration revealed a favourable lesion in continuity.

But the new enthusiasm for a more radical approach to brachial plexus injuries demands appraisal and it will be considered later in this chapter after discussion of open wounds of the supraclavicular plexus and injuries of the infraclavicular plexus.

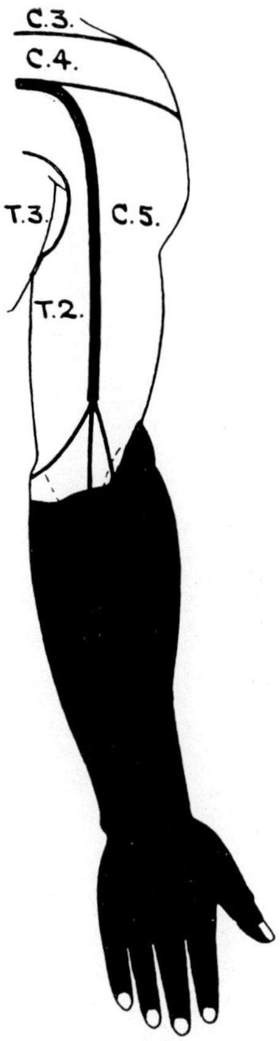

FIG. **11**, 29. If there has been a complete lesion of the plexus, but some recovery in C5 and 6 the patient is left with total paralysis below the elbow.

To return to patients with traction injuries of C5 and 6—and 7—and what has been the standard management. During the time when signs of recovery are awaited—if they do not appear within 12 months hope must be abandoned—a patient can be fitted with apparatus that will control the elbow. This may be a simple ratchet type of splint, permitting the elbow to be locked in whatever degree of flexion is required, or power-driven apparatus which will give the patient active control of the joint (Fig. **11**, 30).

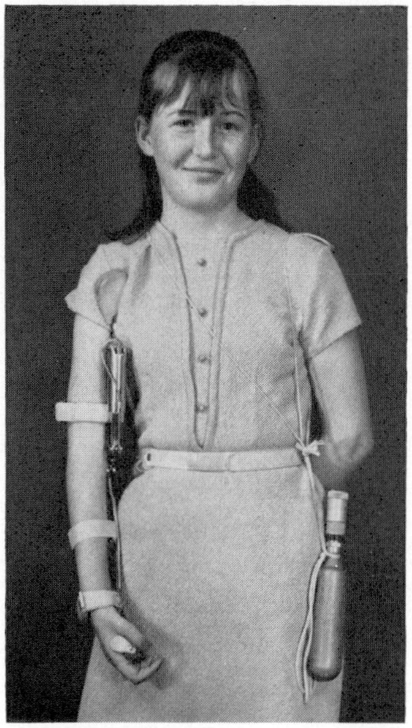

FIG. **11**, 30. This girl's paralysis was due to poliomyelitis, but we have used identical apparatus for patients with paralysis of the flexors of the elbow due to injury of the brachial plexus. A cylinder like that of a steam-engine is incorporated in the splint. Power is supplied by compressed air (the storage cylinder is shown), with separate controls for flexion and extension of the elbow. (Reproduced by kind permission of the Editor from *Br. J. Surg.*, 1966, **53**, 836.)

The loss of control of the shoulder is awkward, but it can be overcome to some extent by a proximal extension of the splint as in Figure **11**, 31. If no recovery occurs then reconstructive surgery is necessary.

Total paralysis of the plexus. The prospects of recovery have already been set out in Table XXII (p. 194). So far as recovery in the forearm and hand is concerned—and this matters most—the outlook is very gloomy. There is a danger

(Yeoman and Seddon, 1961) that under a prolonged conservative regime a patient may resign himself to being functionally one-armed. If, finally, amputation is performed—either above or below the elbow, depending on whether any recovery has occurred in C5 and 6—he will have no interest in making use of a prosthesis, however satisfactory it may appear mechanically. paralysed limb is painful. It is very difficult for the patient to use a prosthesis, and it appears that if, when the pain is severe, he can grip the paralysed limb he feels some relief.

The drift into the one-armed attitude can be checked to some extent by encasing the flail arm in an appliance that enables the patient to make some use of it (Fig. **11**, 31B).

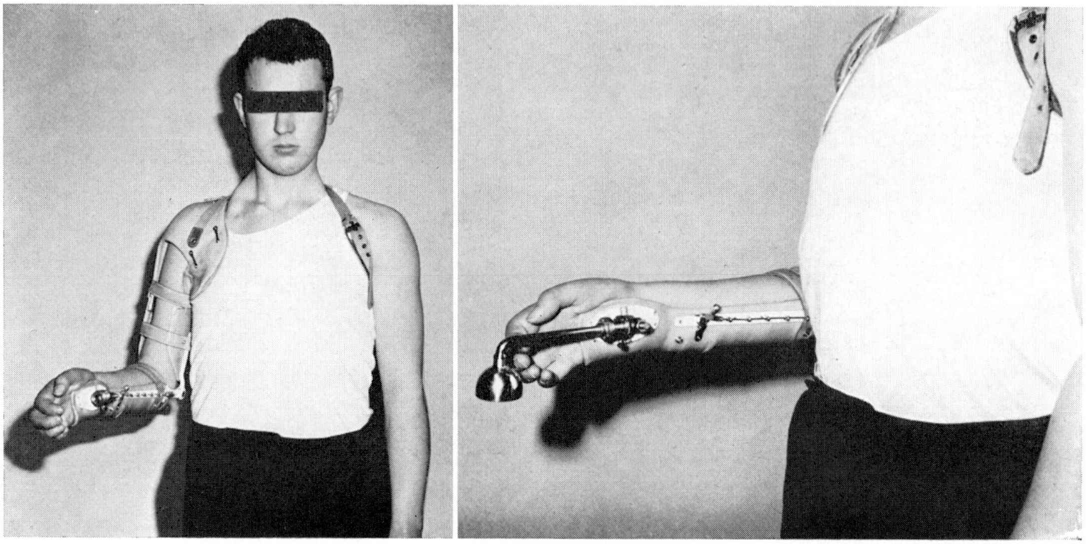

A B

FIG. **11**, 31. Splint for a patient with a flail arm. The shoulder is steadied by a polythene cap. Below it there is a device that allows the limb to be rotated; the position of the elbow can also be varied. A socket attached to the palmar part of the splint takes various fitments. The attachment shown in B allows the patient to shift the gear control of an automobile. (Reproduced by kind permission of the author and Editor from Fletcher, I., 1967. *Physiotherapy*, **53**, 362.)

This is why Yeoman and I somewhat hesitantly reached the conclusion that early amputation, with arthrodesis of the shoulder, should be considered if every piece of evidence pointed to a hopeless prognosis. Yet even then—as in cases in which this radical operation was performed much later, when there was manifestly no recovery—we limited amputation-arthrodesis to patients with some mechanical ability, patients who could be relied on to make good use of an artificial limb.

Arthrodesis of the shoulder is, of course, valueless unless the scapula is strongly controlled by the serratus anterior and by the trapezius. Fletcher (1969) is opposed to amputation if the

If there is no shadow of doubt that the plexus is completely destroyed it is possible to restore flexion at the elbow by an ingenious though formidable operation suggested by Yeoman, which he and I have performed together on four occasions. The technique is outlined in the legend to Figure **11**, 32; and see also p. 199.

Patients with total paralysis initially but useful proximal recovery. In these cases the forearm and hand are useless, and, subject to the proviso just mentioned, there are benefits in performing amputation through the forearm. The flexors of the elbow are useful: the trouble in these cases is that the extensors remain paralysed, as does the deltoid. Arthrodesis of the shoulder is desirable, and despite the loss of active extension of the elbow it is then possible to fit a prosthesis that some patients will use (Fletcher, 1969).

Open Wounds

Open wounds of the supraclavicular brachial plexus are caused by missiles, by stabbing and by operation. Apart from a very few cases in which removal of a neurilemmoma damaged the plexus (p. 154) our experience has been limited to 37 cases, in all of which the plexus was injured by a missile. Strict comparison with the experience of others—for example Brooks (M.R.C.R., 1954), and Nulsen and Slade (in Woodhall and Beebe, 1956)—is not possible because their reports dealt with infraclavicular as well as supraclavicular injuries.

A few clinical features call for comment. Most of the injuries are confined to the upper trunk or, less commonly, to the lower trunk; a complete lesion of the brachial plexus above the clavicle would inevitably be accompanied by severance of the subclavian vessels which would be rapidly fatal. Concomitant vascular injuries were present in only nine of our cases, the patients presenting with aneurysms. As they enlarge, these aneurysms can produce Horner's syndrome, which has nothing to do with the injury to the plexus.

Open wounds of the upper trunk of the plexus, especially those due to stabbing, should lend themselves to repair by suture. Yet only four repairs were reported by Brooks in the 170 open injuries of the plexus (above and below the clavicle) dealt with at the five Nerve Injury Centres established in Britain during the Second World War. A satisfactory result was obtained

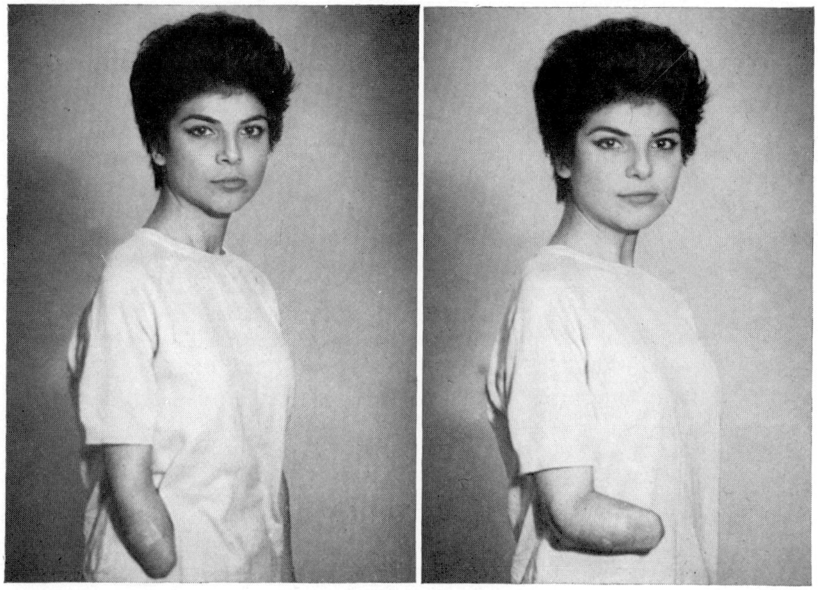

FIG. **11**, 32. The first patient with total traumatic brachial plexus paralysis to be treated by amputation through the forearm, arthrodesis of the shoulder and a nerve graft, a length of the degenerate and otherwise valueless ulnar nerve being used to unite the third and fourth intercostal nerves with the musculocutaneous. The photograph shows active flexion of the elbow, which was strong when the girl took a deep breath. If there is to be any hope of success the operation must be done within three to four months after the injury. Regeneration through the very long graft should be complete before irreversible collagenization has occurred in the degenerate graft or in the denervated flexors of the elbow. Thus the operation is justifiable only if one can be sure, at an early date, that there is no prospect whatever of recovery. (Reproduced by kind permission of the Editor from *J. Bone Jt Surg.*, 1963, **45B**, 460.)

in only one case. Bateman (1962) reported 12 repairs with useful recovery in all. Nulsen and Slade collected the records of 19 cases of suture and the results were moderately encouraging. Merle d'Aubigné and Deburge (1967) described 17 cases of open wounds (above and below the clavicle) of which five were due to surgical operations. What impressed us, as it did them (it is the same with infraclavicular injuries—see Table XXIII), is the frequency with which exploration reveals a lesion in continuity; it is difficult to correlate the operative findings with the subsequent recovery, and exploration does little to clarify the prognosis.

TABLE XXIII—Lesions of the infraclavicular brachial plexus

TYPE OF INJURY	TOTAL	RECOVERY			
		Near normal	Impaired	Poor	Bad
Shoulder: skeletal damage, all closed	45	33	10	1	1
Wounds					
1. Missile *a.* 30 in continuity, 24 proved by exploration		8	15	5	2
b. 2 severed and repaired	32	—	1	1	—
2. Other wounds: one glass cut, one at operation	2	Treated by reconstructive surgery			
Traction					
1. Due to fracture of shaft of humerus	3	—	1	1	1
2. No known bony injury	7	1	4	1	1
Irradiation	3				
TOTAL	92				

INFRACLAVICULAR PARALYSIS

Although some authors make little distinction between supraclavicular and infraclavicular plexus lesions (which in the case of open wounds is justified), examination of Table XXIII shows how different are the injuries suffered by the infraclavicular plexus. Firstly, traction injuries are rare; they can occur as a result of a fracture of the humerus and even of the forearm bones, with distraction of the limb (p. 76). Injury of the plexus due to a fracture or dislocation in the region of the shoulder is, by contrast, fairly common and, as the Table shows, the prognosis is excellent. This type of injury has already been fully discussed in Chapter 5, pp. 81 to 83. The open wounds have two characteristics: the first is the frequency with which the nerves are damaged in continuity; secondly fair spontaneous recovery usually occurs, in general far better than could be expected after nerve repair at this level.

Reference has already been made to the means of distinguishing between supraclavicular and infraclavicular paralysis. Sometimes there is no difficulty: wounds of entry and exit which indicate that the plexus could be damaged only below the clavicle; not infrequently, too, the paralysis is partial and explicable only in terms of infraclavicular damage. But when there is no wound and the arm is almost completely paralysed the distinction between damage above and below the clavicle requires care. It may be necessary to wait until the immediate effects of the injury have passed off. Much depends on it: in general, supraclavicular injuries, particularly traction injuries, have a poor or bad prognosis; on the other hand the prospects of recovery after infraclavicular damage are good.

Vascular Injuries

Concomitant damage to the axillary artery and vein are not uncommon. They are usually caused by penetrating wounds, but can occur after closed injuries, and a careful watch must be kept for some time after a patient has suffered a severe injury of the shoulder (p. 83). Indeed, the paralysis may come on late as a result of a large haematoma or aneurysm forming. Vascular injuries were present in 13 of the 92 cases listed in Table XXIII: most were caused by missiles.

Indications for Exploration

It will be noted that in six of the cases of missile injury no exploration was performed; it is sometimes unnecessary.

A woman was injured by a sports gun at close range; a large number of pellets lodged in the axillary region, her arm was totally paralysed, but there was no vascular damage. She was very thin, and after the reaction to the injury had subsided it was possible to palpate along the course of the plexus high into the axilla. At no point was there any tenderness or thickening of a nerve trunk. It was therefore concluded that the plexus was in continuity and no exploration was performed. She made an excellent recovery except in the thenar muscles.

There were two fractures near the shoulder that damaged the plexus in which exploration should have been performed. Signs of recovery in the most proximal of the paralysed muscles did not appear at the expected time; the opportunity of carrying out what might perhaps have been a useful repair was missed.

A Further Review of the Repair of Brachial Plexus Injuries

The reader will by now have gathered that attempts to repair the brachial plexus are by no means new; that the only method which at present offers any hope of success is autologous grafting, but that interest in its employment has fluctuated. With increasing age and experience surgeons have tended to lose their enthusiasm. Indeed, in Britain between the world wars they discouraged all forms of nerve grafting. This must not happen in the specific case now before us.

Two patients in whom exploration should have been performed with a view to repair have been mentioned above. This omission was deplorable. By contrast Yeoman successfully seized the opportunity presented by what was virtually a complete infraclavicular brachial plexus lesion (pp. 287-289). Even a devastating traction injury (Fig. **16**, 12, p. 295) could be salvaged. If this is possible at the lower border of the axilla then one can hardly withhold repair of more proximal infraclavicular lesions and indeed some supraclavicular ones distal to the cervical transverse processes.

It is therefore encouraging that a determined start has been made by Narakas (1972). All one asks is that in the light of many past failures technical skill should be restrained by what is now certainly known of the limitations to which the process of nerve regeneration in Man is subject. There is room here for the same kind of dispassionate observation of results as is mentioned on page 314 under the subject of controlled clinical trials.

MUSCULOCUTANEOUS NERVE

One could almost wish that this nerve rather than some others were injured more commonly because the results of repair (p. 306) are better than those of any other nerve in the body; our experience of it, although small, may not be atypical.

The musculocutaneous nerve arises from the outer cord of the brachial plexus, usually deep to the pectoralis minor. Its divergence from the lateral head of the median nerve is the site of several variations, but they are unlikely to embarrass an alert surgeon. After supplying and traversing the coracobrachialis it runs between the biceps and the brachialis, both of which it supplies.

The sensory continuation emerges lateral to the tendon of the biceps and, as the lateral cutaneous nerve of the forearm, supplies the area of skin shown in Figures **11**, 9 and **11**, 10 (p. 178).

Examination of the Recently Injured Patient

This is simple: the biceps and the brachialis are paralysed, and there is loss of sensibility in the area referred to above. The only caveat concerns the brachioradialis, which is supplied by the radial nerve; it is a flexor of the elbow, sometimes powerful. So the clinician must palpate the biceps and brachialis; otherwise he may fail to recognize that they are paralysed.

Lesions of the Musculocutaneous Nerve

TABLE XXIV—Lesions of the musculocutaneous nerve

Incised wounds	3	Results of repair all satisfactory
Missile wounds	7	
Fracture-dislocation of the shoulder	1	Almost full spontaneous recovery
Traction injury	1	
Other lesions	2	

Not surprisingly the musculocutaneous nerve is usually injured along with others, the median nerve especially.

Treatment and Results

There should be no hesitation about attempting repair of the nerve either by suture or autologous grafting (see Fig. **6**, 3C, p. 94) when the nerve has been injured by an open wound, unless flexion of the elbow by the brachioradialis is very powerful. It was so in one of the two cases listed in Table XXIV as *other lesions*, the cause being regarded as a neuritis. The results of repair are excellent.

RADIAL NERVE

Motor distribution. The radial nerve supplies the extensor muscles of the upper limb in the following order:

Main Trunk	*Posterior Interosseous Nerve*
Triceps { long head, inner head, outer head	Extensor Carpi Radialis Brevis
(Anconeus)	Supinator
Brachioradialis	Extensor Digitorum Communis
Extensor Carpi Radius Longus	Extensor Digiti Minimi
	Extensor Carpi Ulnaris
	Abductor Pollicis Longus
	Extensor Pollicis Longus
	Extensor Pollicis Brevis
	Extensor Indicis

1. In proximal lesions the heads of the triceps may need to be examined separately, because only part of the muscle may be paralysed.

2. Brachioradialis has only one action. It is a supplementary flexor of the elbow and always contracts when the joint is flexed strongly. This action is sometimes so powerful that the muscle is an adequate substitute when the biceps and brachialis are completely paralysed. It is a difficult muscle in which to detect feeble contraction; the brachialis and the tendon of the biceps lie medial to the upper part of the belly of the brachioradialis, and when the prime flexors of the elbow contract they produce a movement of the overlying fascia which is hard to distinguish from feeble contraction of the brachioradialis.

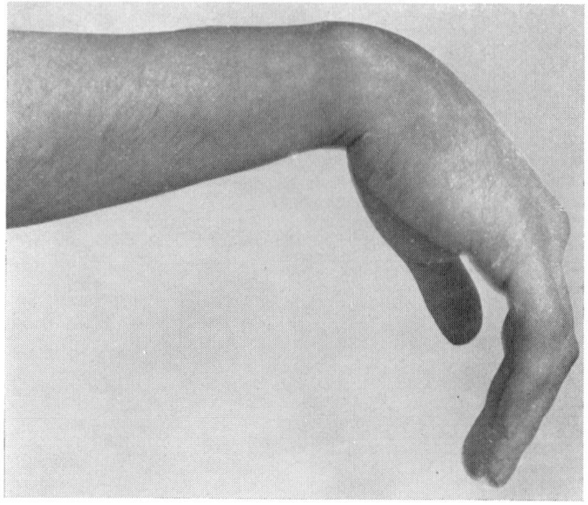

FIG. **11,** 33. Radial paralysis with some contracture of the extensor digitorum communis.

3. Supinator. Activity of this muscle is said to be revealed by the ability of the patient to supinate the forearm with the elbow fully extended.

4. Extensor digitorum communis. Although this muscle is primarily an extensor of the fingers at the metacarpo-phalangeal joints it extends the proximal and, to a lesser extent, the distal interphalangeal joints when the metacarpo-phalangeal joints are held in flexion. If there is a contracture of this (paralysed) muscle, flexion of the wrist produces extension of the fingers (Fig. **3**, 4, p. 37), and flexion of the fingers causes the wrist to extend (Figs **11**, 33 and **11**, 34).

5. Extensor carpi ulnaris. Feeble activity of this muscle is difficult to detect, and the most careful palpation of the tendon is required at a point just distal and lateral to the ulnar styloid. E.C.U. contracts synergically on radial abduction of the thumb.

6. Abductor pollicis longus can flex the wrist (Fig. **11**, 35).

7. Extensor pollicis longus. In complete radial paralysis it is not uncommon to find that extension of the interphalangeal joint of the thumb can be brought about by a slip from abductor pollicis brevis that is inserted into the terminal phalanx. One cannot be sure that this movement is produced by E.P.L. unless movement of its tendon can be seen and felt.

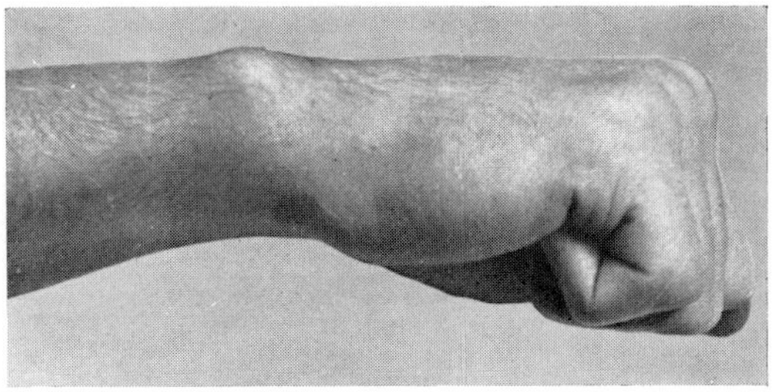

FIG. **11**, 34. When the digits are flexed the tightening of E.D.C. causes the wrist to extend.

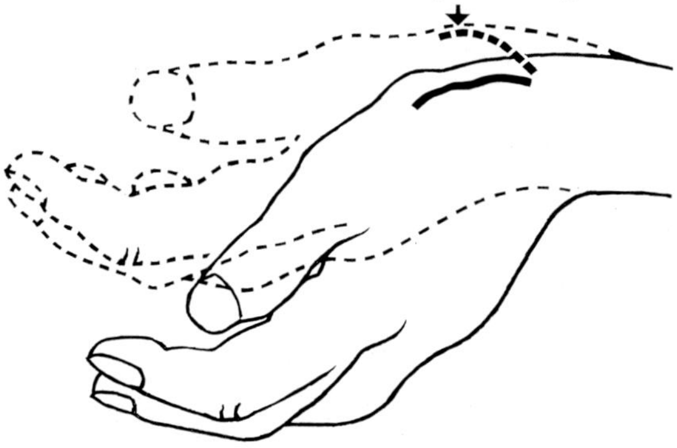

FIG. **11**, 35. Flexion of the wrist from full extension to the neutral position by abductor pollicis longus: in this case all three of the wrist flexors were paralysed.

8. Extensor pollicis brevis. This muscle runs with abductor pollicis longus and diverges from it to be inserted into the base of the proximal phalanx. The muscle and its tendon are sometimes so poorly developed that it may be impossible to assess its activity.

CONTRACTURES. Contractures are due almost entirely to faulty splinting, and it is the extensor digitorum communis that suffers most. The contracture shown in Figure **13**, 2 (p. 233) was so severe as to be only partially remediable by capsulectomy of the metacarpo-phalangeal joints.

Sensory distribution. The radial nerve has four sensory branches: the posterior cutaneous nerve of the arm, which supplies an insignificant area of skin; the lateral inferior cutaneous nerve of the arm; the posterior cutaneous nerve of the forearm; and the terminal superficial radial nerve. The areas supplied by these branches are

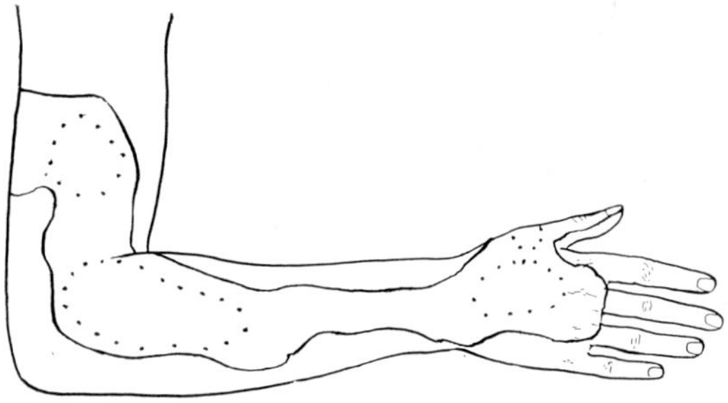

FIG. **11**, 36. Confluent areas supplied by the lateral inferior cutaneous nerve of the arm, the posterior cutaneous nerve of the forearm and the superficial radial nerve.

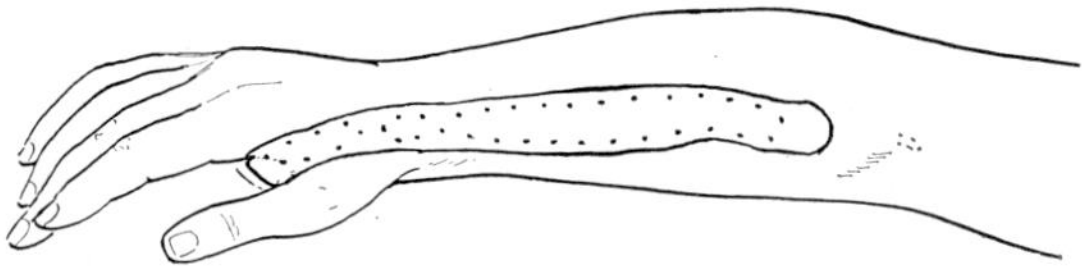

FIG. **11**, 37. Small but confluent areas supplied by the posterior cutaneous nerve of the forearm and by the superficial radial nerve.

most variable (Stopford, 1918). They may merge as in Figures **11**, 36 and **11**, 37, or be separate as in Figure **11**, 38 (see also Figs **11**, 9 and **11**, 10, p. 178). The area supplied by the superficial radial nerve may be large, as in Figures **11**, 36, **11**, 38 and **11**, 39; the area shown in Figure **11**, 40 is about average; it can be very small, as in Figure **3**, 5 (p. 39) or even non-existent. Preservation of sensibility in the superficial radial area is valueless diagnostically.

Examination of the Recently Injured Patient

This should be only motor. The patient is asked to extend the wrist, then the digits. If neither movement is possible there is a lesion of the radial nerve; if the wrist but not the digits can be extended the posterior interosseous nerve is damaged.

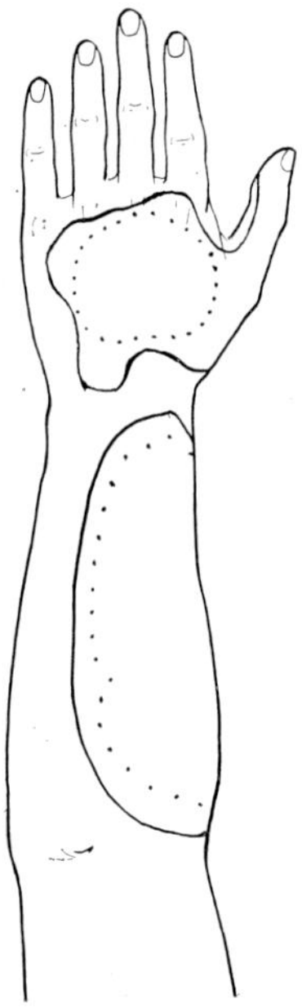

FIG. **11,** 38. Larger, but separated areas supplied by the same nerves as in Figure **11,** 37.

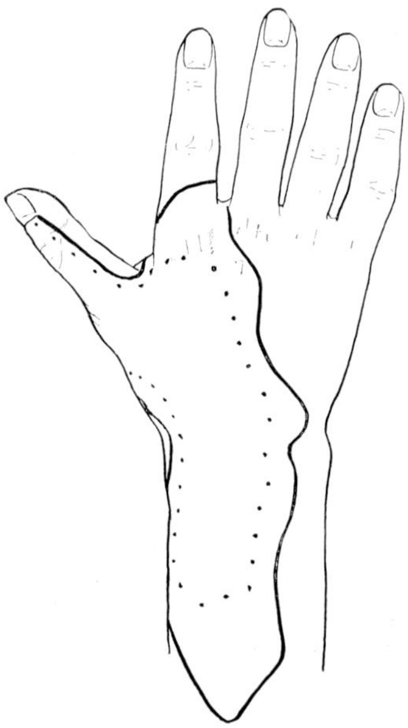

FIG. **11,** 39. A large area supplied entirely by the superficial radial nerve.

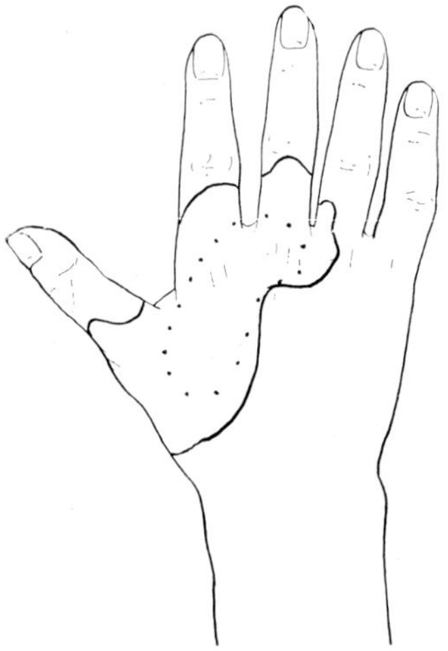

FIG. **11,** 40. The usual distribution of the superficial radial nerve.

Lesions of the Radial Nerve

Axillary injuries are uncommon; they are usually caused either by missiles or by the pressure of faulty axillary crutches. The pressure paralysis need cause no alarm because spontaneous recovery will occur, though slowly (Fig. **2**, 36; p. 30). If the nerve is severed near the axilla, repair can be so difficult that tendon transplantation may be preferable if the necessary muscles are available.

TABLE XXV—Lesions of the radial nerve

Incised wounds and lacerations	13
Missile wounds	68
Injury in the course of surgical operations	16
Skeletal injuries, mostly fractures of the humerus	74
Traction injuries	2
Other lesions (ischaemia, injections, innocent tumours, etc.)	37
	210

Fracture of the shaft of the humerus. This is the commonest cause of radial paralysis. The appropriate treatment is conservative, whether the fracture is closed or open (see pp. 79 and 83). But the nerve may have been severed, and if signs of recovery fail to appear at the expected time (see Figs **14,** 1 and **14,** 2, pp. 246-7) the nerve should be explored. There may be a case for early intervention—open reduction of the fracture and exploration of the nerve—if there is an oblique fracture of the lower half of the humerus, producing a trough in which the nerve can be trapped (Fig. **5**, 30, p. 84).

Injury in the course of surgical operations. The radial nerve is at risk in the spiral groove; if open reduction of a fracture of the humerus is necessary it is best to begin by formal exposure of the nerve. The danger is not only that the nerve may be cut if the exposure of the humerus traverses tissues distorted by swelling or scarring; it can be injured simply by the subperiosteal insertion of retractors, which stretch it.

Treatment and Results

Because the radial nerve is predominantly motor, and, unlike the ulnar, does not innervate muscles that perform delicate movements the results of repair are gratifying (Table XLVI, p. 306) and fortunately there is a most satisfactory tendon transplantation in reserve if suture is impossible or should fail.

Posterior Interosseous Nerve

Paralysis of the posterior interosseous nerve differs from that of the radial in two respects. There is no disturbance of sensibility; and because the long radial extensor of the wrist is supplied by the radial nerve just above its terminal bifurcation the joint can be extended, though usually with some radial deviation because the other two wrist extensors are paralysed. The digits cannot, of course, be extended; they, as well as the wrist, must be examined if paralysis of the posterior interosseous nerve is not to escape recognition.

Lesions of the Posterior Interosseous Nerve

Table XXVI—Lesions of the posterior interosseous nerve

Incised wounds and lacerations	9
Missile wounds	33
Injury in the course of surgical operations	16
Skeletal injuries	8
Other lesions	3
	69

Treatment and Results

Cuts, lacerations and missile wounds. Because posterior interosseous paralysis can be treated satisfactorily by tendon transplantation there is a tendency to ignore the possibility of repair by suture. Admittedly, on account of the shortness of the main trunk of the nerve before it fans out and disappears into the slit in the supinator muscle, the occasions when repair is possible are infrequent. Yet, because the posterior interosseous nerve is purely motor, the results of suture are gratifying. There is no point in exploring the nerve when there has been a deep and destructive wound, but in favourable circumstances it should be inspected if only to establish the propriety of carrying out tendon transplantation forthwith; it is embarrassing if, after the performance of a tendon transplantation, spontaneous recovery of the nerve occurs, as is otherwise possible. One may, of course, wait 6 months to be sure that spontaneous recovery is excluded; but this is a waste of time when the state of the nerve can, without much difficulty, be determined by direct observation.

The proper procedure, therefore, is to explore the nerve whenever there has been an open wound of less than devastating proportions. If conditions are favourable the nerve is repaired; if it is in continuity and no intraneural scar is palpable it should be left alone because there is a possibility of spontaneous regeneration; if there is total destruction, then tendon transplantation may be performed forthwith. The nerve was explored in 15 of the 58 cases referred to in this and in the following paragraph; on six occasions secondary suture was carried out with satisfactory results in five cases and a fair result in one.

Injury in the course of operations on the head of the radius. This is the second commonest cause of injury of the posterior interosseous nerve; the reason for it is an inadequate incision for exposure of the head of the radius. The incision recommended is the same as that used for exposure of the nerve, and the risk of damaging it is then minimal whatever the distortion of the radius.

Skeletal injuries damaging the nerve. These injuries should be treated conservatively. Of the eight examples that we have seen six were followed by normal recovery: in one recovery was somewhat impaired; in one (the nerve was explored) it was bad.

Reference has already been made (p. 117) to compression lesions of the posterior interosseous nerve.

Superficial Radial Nerve

Isolated injuries of this nerve occasionally attract attention on account of irritative symptoms. It may be necessary to perform secondary suture. The nerve is particularly at risk in operations for stenosing tenosynovitis (de Quervain's disease).

MEDIAN NERVE

In the leg the flexor muscles are supplied by a single nerve trunk. In the forearm there are two nerves for the flexors, the median and the ulnar. If we imagine that they parted company reluctantly—in pre-mammalian phylogeny there is a common ventral nerve trunk—it may make us more conscious of the frequency of variations in the distribution of the median and ulnar nerves and of the anastomoses between them (Mannerfelt, 1964). Certainly, the clinician who clings to traditional anatomical descriptions will soon be led astray, with unhappy consequences. Alike in the examination of patients and in the exposure of nerves we must expect anomalies (see Fig. **15**, 1, p. 254).

Motor distribution. The commonly accepted distribution is as follows:

Forearm	*Hand*
Pronator teres	Abductor pollicis brevis
Flexor carpi radialis	Opponens pollicis
Palmaris longus	Flexor pollicis brevis
Flexor digitorum superficialis	Lumbricals: index and middle fingers
Flexor pollicis longus	
Flexor digitorum profundus (lateral half)	
Pronator quadratus	

1. Flexor digitorum superficialis. Some persons are able to flex the proximal interphalangeal joints of the fingers without flexing the terminal joints; that is to say, they can produce an isolated contraction of the superficial

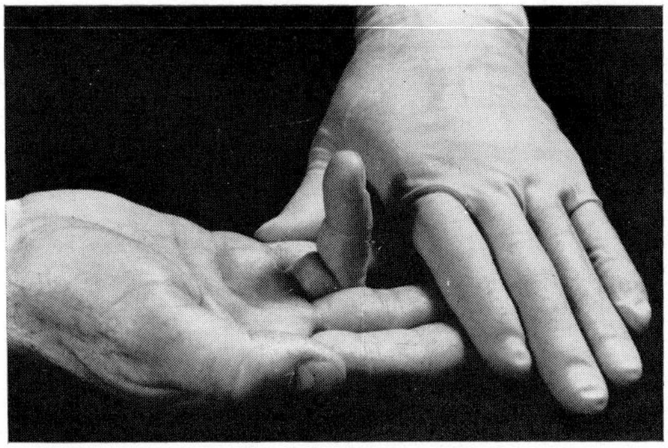

FIG. **11,** 41. The only satisfactory method of examining the flexor digitorum superficialis.

muscle, even of its component parts. There is then no difficulty in recognizing whether the flexor digitorum superficialis is active. However, when it is found that the superficial and deep flexors act together the action of F.D.S. must be isolated by means of the manoeuvre shown in Figure **11**, 41.

2. Flexor digitorum profundus. The part of this muscle supplied by the median nerve usually controls the index and middle fingers, but it is not uncommon to find it flexing only the index, the remaining three parts being supplied by the ulnar nerve. This anomaly is often associated with ulnar innervation of the whole of the flexor pollicis brevis and sometimes with a small—two-and-a-half digits—cutaneous distribution of the median nerve in the palm. Each finger should always be examined separately, the interphalangeal joints of the others being held in extension. If the distal I.P. joints of the ring and little fingers are allowed to flex, there will usually be moderate flexion of the terminal joint of the middle finger as well, even though the part of F.D.P. controlling it is paralysed. The ulnar half of the muscle pulls the adjacent paralysed part with it, and so moves the corresponding tendon. F.D.P. is inaccessible to electrical stimulation.

3. Pronator quadratus. There is no reliable test for activity of this muscle apart from electrical stimulation. Bipolar electrodes are used and are applied to the lowest quarter of the forearm dorsally and ventrally. The current then passes straight through the muscle, the activity of which is revealed by obvious pronation.

4. Abductor pollicis brevis. This is an important muscle diagnostically because it is the thenar muscle most likely to escape innervation by the ulnar nerve. Its action is palmar abduction (distinct from radial abduction, the function of abductor pollicis longus), that is abduction of the thumb in a plane perpendicular to the surface of the palm (Fig. **11**, 42). It can extend the terminal joint of the thumb (see radial paralysis, p. 201).

5. Opponens pollicis. Careful observation of the action of this muscle is necessary: it rotates the thumb through 90 degrees, towards the little finger, without flexing the metacarpo-phalangeal joint. The other muscles of the thumb, long and short, acting in concert, can produce a similar movement; but when the palmar surface of the hand is viewed, the whole of the thumb nail never becomes visible, as it does in true opposition; or, as in Figure **3**, 3 (p. 36) the whole of the nail is seen only because the metacarpo-phalangeal joint is flexed.

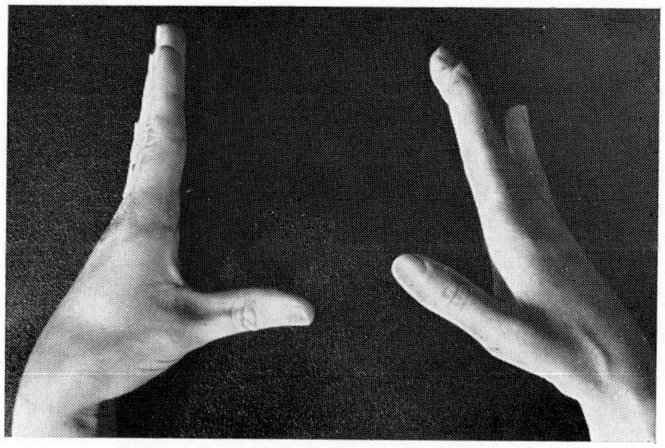

FIG. **11**, 42. Palmar abduction of the thumb. Action of abductor pollicis brevis on left: wasting of the paralysed muscle on right.

ANOMALOUS INNERVATION. This intriguing topic may be considered under two headings: anastomotic bridges between the median and ulnar nerves; and variations in the innervation of the intrinsic muscles of the hand. They are interconnected.

The best known anastomosis is that described by Martin (1763), which according to Mannerfelt (1964) is present in at least 15 per cent of persons. A branch runs from the median to the ulnar nerve in the forearm (Fig. **15**, 1, p. 254); it seems to be purely motor and to be distributed with the deep branch of the ulnar nerve. In a case in which stimulation of the anastomosis was possible the first and second dorsal interossei and the adductor pollicis contracted.

Variations in the innervation of the thenar muscles were studied in our patients by Rowntree (1949), and they are illustrated in Figures **11**, 43 to **11**, 48. It is immediately apparent that the flexor pollicis brevis is supplied most commonly by the ulnar nerve, and also that there is a wide range of variation in the innervation of the thenar and neighbouring intrinsic muscles.[1] Ignorance of this has sometimes led to a lesion, usually of the median nerve, being regarded as incomplete when it was not; and on this account exploration and repair have been delayed.

Blocking a nerve with a local anaesthetic (p. 55) finds its best application in the investigation of cases that appear to present some anomaly of innervation of the intrinsic muscles of the hand.

DEFORMITY AND CONTRACTURES. In total thenar paralysis the thumb is in the plane of the palm, which makes the hand look flat. Neglect of passive movements and splinting leads to the development of an adduction contracture of the thumb, and the web between it and the index may become so narrow that freeing of the shortened muscles and a fairly elaborate plastic operation on the skin are needed to correct the deformity.

Thenar paralysis due to poliomyelitis occurring early in life can cause subluxation of the carpometacarpal joint. It is rare after median nerve injury, because repair is usually performed.

Sensory distribution. There are variations in the cutaneous distribution of the median nerve (Stopford, 1918; Figs **11**, 49 and **11**, 50). In one case of proven total ulnar paralysis there was no loss of sensibility in the palm or digits: the median nerve supplied all of them. Loss of deep sensibility is generally confined to the distal halves of the index and middle fingers.

Trophic changes. In most median nerve lesions of more than a few weeks' standing there is atrophy of the soft tissues of the index finger and sometimes of the ring finger. Atrophy of the thumb is uncommon. The digital skin becomes thin and shiny, and cyanosis is frequent. In older patients slight limitation of movement of the interphalangeal joints may develop in spite of almost uninterrupted activity. This stiffness has been seen in a middle-aged physiotherapist who took great pains to maintain mobility of his joints from within one week of the time of division of the nerve at the wrist.

Examination of the Recently Injured Patient

Sensory examination—a pin will suffice—is essential; it should include the thumb, index

[1] That this catalogue of anomalies is incomplete is demonstrated by a vivid episode. An able and careful surgeon telephoned me in distress to say that he had just performed a difficult operation on an elbow and had severed the ulnar nerve. Conditions were unfavourable for primary suture. When the patient had sufficiently recovered we found that all the intrinsic muscles of the hand were active except the hypothenars; the little finger was insensitive. We were uncertain about the state of the flexor carpi ulnaris and the ulnar half of the flexor digitorum profundus. When I suggested that there was, at most, division of a few funiculi of the ulnar nerve the surgeon replied: 'I am not in the habit of cutting the ulnar nerve, but I know when I have done it'. I was present when, some weeks later, the nerve was explored. It was completely severed; there must have been an exceptionally large median-to-ulnar anastomosis in the upper forearm.

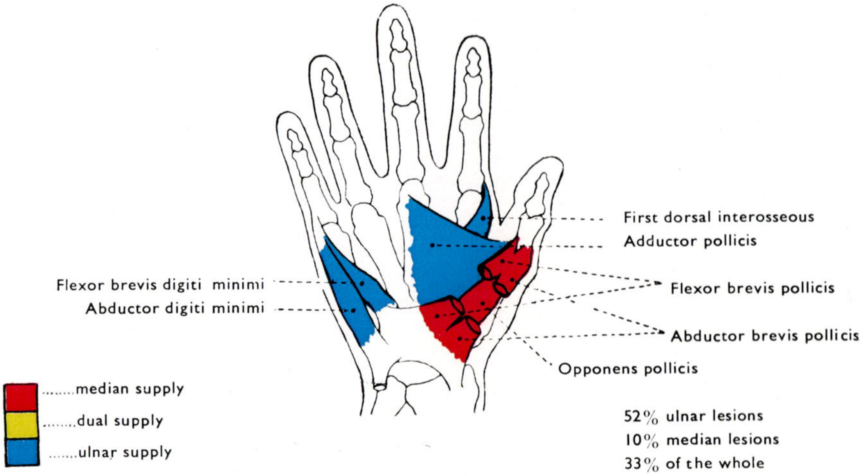

FIG. **11,** 43. All the muscles of the thenar eminence—but not the adductor—are supplied by the median nerve. Anatomical textbooks describe this as the usual arrangement, but it was present in only one-third of our patients. (Figs **11,** 43 to **11,** 48 reproduced by kind permission of the author and Editor from Rowntree, T., 1949, *J. Bone Jt Surg.*, **31B,** 505.)

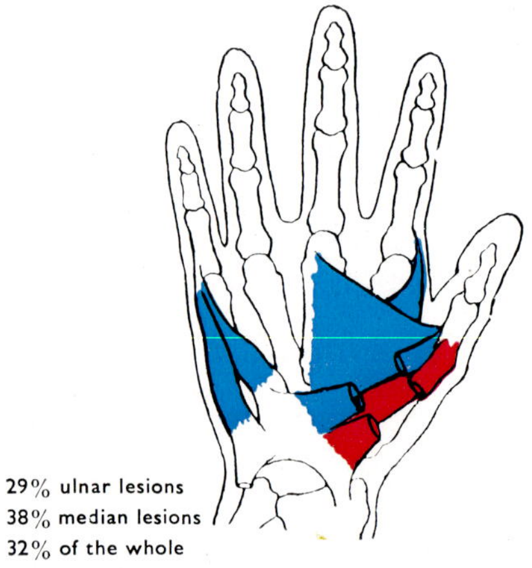

FIG. **11,** 44. An equally common arrangement is innervation of the flexor pollicis brevis by the ulnar nerve.

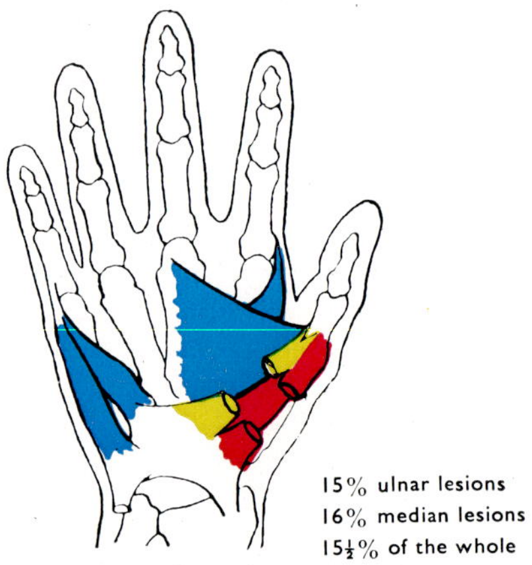

FIG. **11,** 45. The flexor pollicis brevis not uncommonly has dual innervation.

and middle fingers, as otherwise a partial division (Fig. **15**, 32, p. 277) may be overlooked. In the motor examination the thenar muscles should be examined first, the patient being asked to approximate the thumb and little finger. If this movement cannot be performed the thenar muscles are paralysed. But in view of the frequent anomalies of innervation, ability to perform this movement does not exclude a complete median nerve lesion. Then, if relevant, the proximal muscles are examined.

One must be on the look-out for damage confined to the anterior interosseous nerve. A man's forearm was penetrated by a splinter of glass. There were none of the usual signs of median paralysis. Later, he was found to have paralysis of the flexor pollicis longus, of the radial half of the flexor digitorum profundus and, on electrical

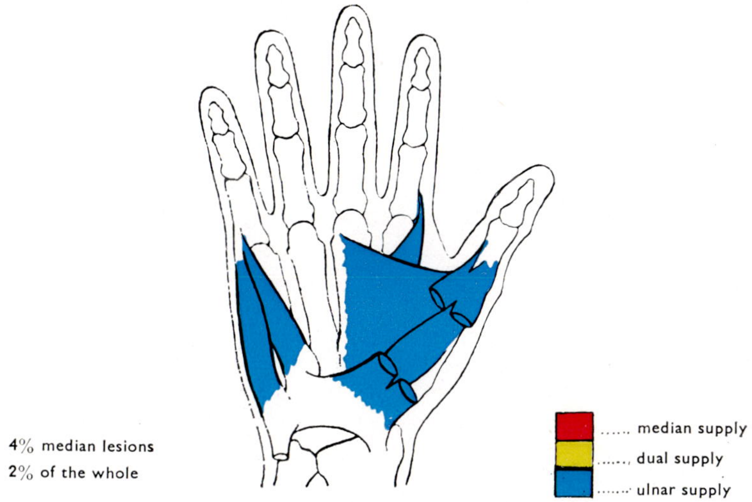

FIG. **11,** 46. All the short muscles of the thumb are supplied by the ulnar nerve: rare.

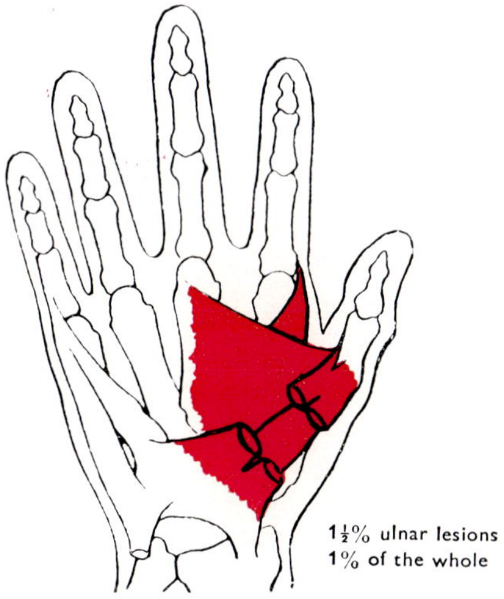

FIG. **11,** 47. The median nerve supplies all the short muscles of the thumb and the first dorsal interosseous muscle: rare.

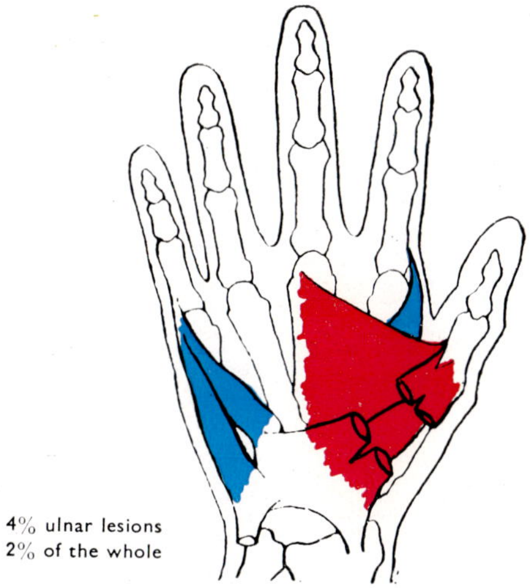

FIG. **11,** 48. All the thenar muscles and the adductor pollicis are supplied by the median nerve: rare.

examination, of the pronator quadratus (p. 204), indicating complete paralysis of the anterior interosseous nerve.

Lesions of the Median Nerve

A glance at Table XXVII shows that the median nerve is usually damaged by an *open wound*; in war by missiles, at any level in the upper limb; in peace by something sharp, broken glass above all (80 per cent of the 172 cases), and usually at the wrist. Most of the *skeletal injuries* are near the elbow, and spontaneous recovery is the rule; but there are exceptions, as has been mentioned in Chapter 5. The group of *ischaemic injuries* merely reflects a personal interest in Volkmann's

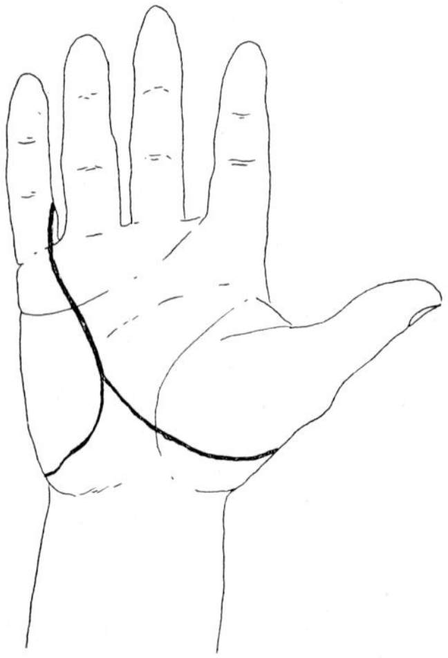

FIG. **11,** 49. The palmar distribution of the median nerve is larger than normal, and the ulnar area is correspondingly smaller.

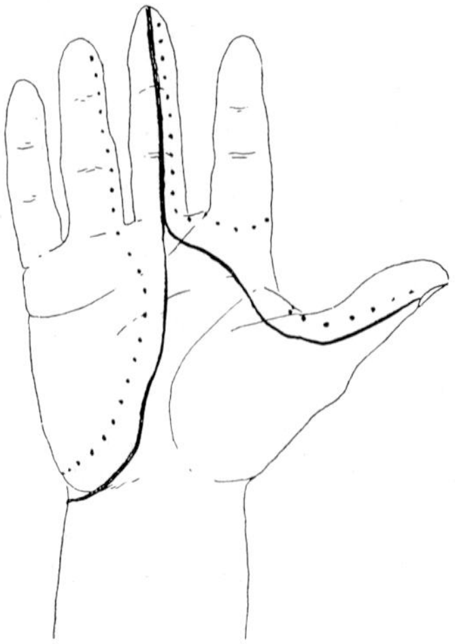

FIG. **11,** 50. The opposite state of affairs: large ulnar area, small median.

ischaemia. Table XXVII is also unrepresentative in that there is no great number of cases of *compression of the nerve in the carpal tunnel:* they are included under the last heading.

Injuries of nerves in the digits (see p. 213) are grouped separately, along with the digital branches of the ulnar nerve. Among the palmar injuries are a few in which a small penetrating wound severs the motor division of the nerve alone; exploration is usually fruitless because the distal end of the thenar division is cut off short, and repair is impossible. It is best to remedy the

TABLE XXVII—Lesions of the median nerve

	LEVEL OF LESION					TOTALS
	Axilla	Mid-arm and elbow	Forearm	Wrist	Palm	
Incised wounds	1	13	26	119	13	172
Lacerations	—	3	10	12	—	25
Missile wounds	28	93	68	21	8	218
Injuries in the course of surgical operations						1
Skeletal injuries	2	17	3	3	—	25
Traction injuries						6
Ischaemia						22
Other lesions mentioned elsewhere						35
						504

paralysis by tendon transplantation if no spontaneous recovery occurs. Injury of the sensory branches in the palm sometimes presents a formidable problem (Fig. **11**, 51) and multiple autologous nerve grafting is often necessary.

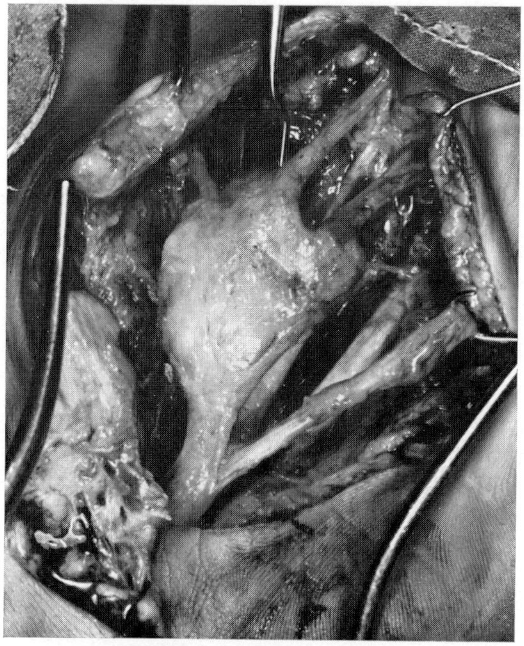

FIG. **11**, 51. A large neuroma involving all but one of the digital branches of the median nerve in the palm.

Treatment and Results

Exploration of the injuries caused by open wounds is usually necessary; the results of repair are given on page 307. The question of primary repair is important and this is discussed on pages 275 to 278.

The compression lesions at the wrist (pp. 119 to 122) present an entirely different problem, and diagnosis is sometimes difficult.

Injuries of the median nerve caused by fractures usually recover spontaneously, but there is a case for early exploration if the fracture is at the lower end of the humerus (p. 84).

ULNAR NERVE

As has been explained in the preceding section (p. 204) the median and ulnar nerves are closely associated; thus in considering variation in the distribution of the ulnar nerve some repetition is unavoidable.

Motor distribution. The commonly accepted motor distribution of the ulnar nerve is as follows:

Forearm	*Hand*
Flexor carpi ulnaris	Palmaris brevis
Flexor digitorum profundus (medial half)	Hypothenar muscles
	The two medial lumbricals
	All the interossei
	Adductor pollicis

1. Flexor carpi ulnaris. Feeble action of this muscle is difficult to detect, particularly in a well-covered forearm. It is best to ask the patient to flex the wrist in ulnar deviation. The tendon must be felt to tighten.

2. Flexor digitorum profundus. The part of this muscle innervated by the ulnar nerve often controls the middle as well as the ring and little fingers; in frequent association with this the flexor pollicis brevis is innervated by the ulnar nerve, and two digits instead of the usual one-and-a-half are supplied by the sensory part of the ulnar nerve. In examination of the flexor digitorum profundus, each digit is tested separately, the interphalangeal joints of the others being held in full extension.

3. Palmaris brevis. This tiny muscle is sometimes useful in localization of the site of damage because it is the only muscle to be supplied by the superficial division of the ulnar nerve. Palmaris brevis helps to cup the palm, as when holding water or sand; it pulls the superficial part of the hypothenar eminence towards the centre of the palm, so elevating it.

4. The hypothenar muscles are difficult to examine. When the ulnar nerve is damaged distal to the branch to flexor carpi ulnaris a curious trick movement may be found. When the patient endeavours to abduct or oppose the little finger a feeble movement may be seen in the hypothenar mass, although there is complete paralysis of the hypothenar muscles. Movements of the little finger produced by the hypothenar muscles, especially abduction, are always accompanied by contraction of F.C.U. the purpose of which is to stabilize the pisiform bone. If the hypothenar muscles are paralysed, the proximal pull on the pisiform is unopposed, and this drag

on the hypothenar muscles may give an appearance simulating contraction of them. The trick is eliminated by testing for activity of the hypothenar muscles with the wrist in full flexion.

5. Interossei. These muscles should be examined as a group and then individually. They act together when the metacarpo-phalangeal joints are flexed and the interphalangeal joints extended. Isolated lateral movements may be observed when the hand is laid palm downwards on a table and the patient asked to adduct and abduct each digit in turn. This is a delicate test: the activity of each interosseous muscle, as well as of the abductor digiti minimi can be observed. In a well-developed hand it is sometimes possible to detect individual movement of the dorsal interossei, and this is always possible in the case of the first dorsal interosseous. But activity of the first dorsal interosseous muscle does not exclude ulnar nerve damage. It may be supplied by the median nerve (Sunderland, 1946: and Fig. **11**, 47, p. 207). Other variations, some remarkable, have already been mentioned.

6. Adductor pollicis. Examination of this muscle depends on its ability to adduct the thumb without producing flexion of the interphalangeal joint (Froment's sign).

7. Flexor pollicis brevis. Although, as has already been shown, this muscle usually receives its nerve supply from the ulnar nerve it is unusual, in ulnar paralysis, to find any wasting of the thenar eminence or to detect any weakness of flexion. This is because both may be obscured by the good development of the opponens and the abductor pollicis brevis. If F.P.B. is supplied by both nerves, weakness of the muscle cannot be detected in ulnar paralysis whereas in median paralysis isolated activity of part of F.P.B. is easily recognized.

DEFORMITY AND CONTRACTURES. The claw-hand is not typical of ulnar paralysis so much as of neglected paralysis. When mobility of the hand has been maintained the postural abnormality is moderate, and full passive correction is possible (Fig. **11**, 52). The patient complains chiefly about the persistent abduction of the little finger, produced by the unopposed pull of the extensor tendons, and an aggravating factor is its insensitivity. If the ulnar nerve is injured proximal to the flexor digitorum profundus the clawing is less pronounced because active flexion of the distal joints of the ring and little fingers is lost.

There is no situation in which correct splinting is more valuable. The sort of apparatus shown in Figures **13**, 6 and **13**, 7 (pp. 235-236) holds the metacarpo-phalangeal joints flexed and thus permits extension of the interphalangeal joints by the extensor digitorum communis. In some patients failure to prevent a claw-hand allows the dorsal hoods of the proximal interphalangeal joints to become stretched and then, however satisfactory the return of power in the interossei, ability to extend the digits has been permanently lost. The only remedy for this—and an indifferent one—is arthrodesis of the proximal interphalangeal joints in moderate flexion.

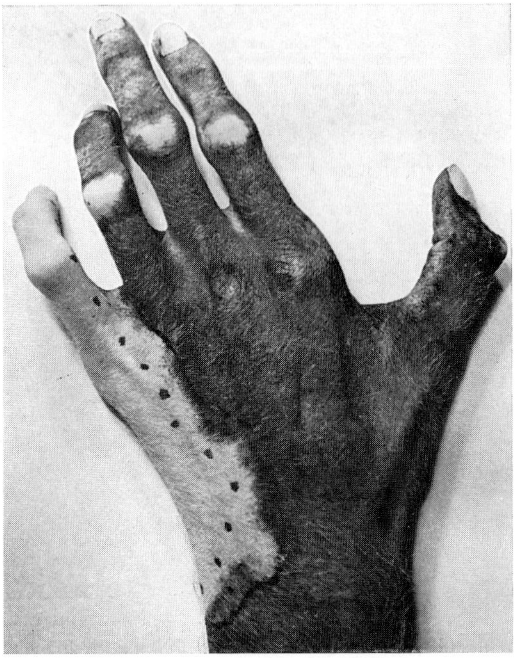

FIG. **11**, 52. Ulnar paralysis. The characteristic features are: wasting of the interossei; flexion of the terminal joint of the thumb, due to loss of the stabilizing action of the adductor pollicis; clawing of the ring and little fingers, the intact lumbricals preventing this almost completely in the middle and index fingers.

Sensory distribution. The sensory distribution of the ulnar nerve is in two parts. The dorsal cutaneous branch, which usually leaves the parent trunk about two-thirds of the way down the forearm, but may separate from it more proximally, supplies the medial border of the hand, the dorsum, the dorsal surface of the little finger and the dorso-medial surface of the ring finger, except for the terminal part supplied by the palmar cutaneous branches. The area supplied by the dorsal cutaneous branch can be extensive, and the nerve is then correspondingly large; or it may be small (Fig. **11**, 53).

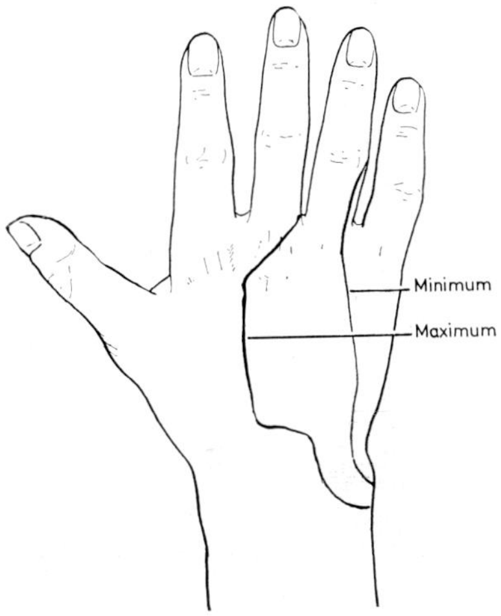

FIG. **11**, 53. Limits of the distribution of the dorsal cutaneous branch of the ulnar nerve.

The palmar cutaneous branches supply one-and-a-half digits; sometimes only the little finger.

Patients often complain of coldness of the little finger; if it is insensitive it is easily damaged, particularly by burning.

Examination of the Recently Injured Patient

If the palmar surface of the little finger is insensitive—the dorsum may be insensitive too—the ulnar nerve is injured. But normal sensitivity does not wholly exclude an ulnar nerve lesion, and it is wise to test the function of the interossei by inviting the patient to spread and approximate his *fully extended* fingers.

Lesions of the Ulnar Nerve

The ulnar nerve is injured or otherwise deranged more frequently than any other nerve in the body.

As with the median nerve, *open wounds* are commonest; similarly missiles can injure the nerve at any level. Incised wounds are usually at the wrist, broken glass being the chief offender. *Injuries inflicted by the surgeon* are more frequent than in the case of the median nerve. *Skeletal injuries* affect the nerve most commonly at the elbow. Spontaneous recovery is usual, but if a fractured medial epicondyle has been trapped in the joint operative replacement is necessary for satisfactory recovery both of the elbow and of the ulnar nerve. *Traction injuries* are rare, but can be devastating (p. 301). *Ischaemic damage* runs parallel with the similar median nerve lesions, but the prognosis is better because the ulnar nerve lies near the periphery of the ellipsoidal infarct, whereas the median nerve runs through its centre (Fig. **6**, 4, p. 95 and Fig. **6**, 6, p. 96). *Traumatic ulnar neuritis* is common: it has already been described (pp. 114 to 117). Pressure on the ulnar nerve by a *ganglion*, though rare, is particularly significant in the hand; it is the chief cause of paralysis of the deep palmar branch of the ulnar nerve (pp. 122 to 123).

Treatment and Results

Exploration of the ulnar nerve is frequently necessary, and so is repair. The results of suture, however well-executed, are rarely very good; not so much because the ulnar is a mixed nerve as on account of the confused re-innervation of the interossei which, except sometimes in children, prevents restoration of the independent action of these important little muscles.

COMBINED LESIONS OF THE MEDIAN AND ULNAR NERVES

Because of their close anatomical association, combined injuries of these nerves are very frequent—mostly between the axilla and the lower quarter of the arm, then at the wrist. There were combined lesions in about two-fifths of all our cases of median and ulnar nerve injury.

Clinical Features

If the nerves are completely interrupted proximal to the elbow all the muscles in the anterior compartment of the forearm are paralysed;

TABLE XXVIII—Lesions of the ulnar nerve

	LEVEL OF LESION					TOTALS
	Axilla	Mid-arm and elbow	Forearm	Wrist	Palm	
Incised wounds	1	31	40	143	10	225
Lacerations	1	9	11	19	2	42
Missile wounds	19	132	81	36	4	272
Injury in the course of surgical operations						17
Skeletal injuries	3	33	9	6	—	51
Traction injuries						5
Ischaemia						19
Traumatic ulnar neuritis		97				97
Pressure by ganglion	—	2	—	3	4	9
Other lesions mentioned elsewhere						45
						782

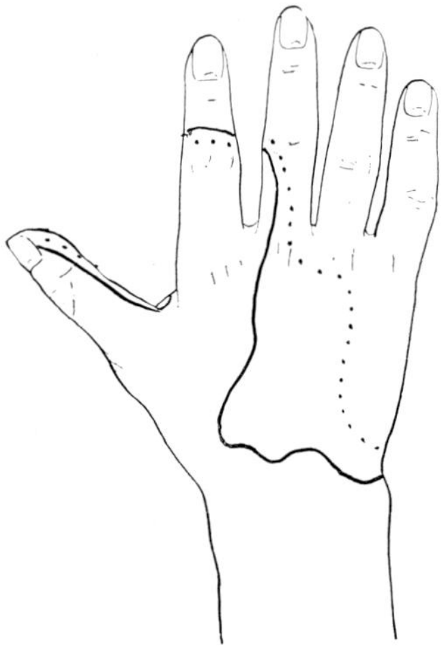

FIG. **11**, 54. The dorsal cutaneous sensory loss when the damage to the median and ulnar nerves is proximal to the dorsal cutaneous branch of the latter.

there is no clawing of the fingers and the hand has a flat simian appearance. Yet, it is still possible for the patient to flex the wrist; he uses the abductor pollicis longus (Fig. **11**, 35, p. 201). The dorsal area of sensory loss is shown in Figure **11**, 54. If the combined injury is distal to the level of innervation of the long flexors of the fingers severe clawing develops which must be controlled by appropriate splinting. If the combined injury is distal to the point at which its dorsal cutaneous branch leaves the ulnar nerve, the area of insensibility is as shown in Figure **11**, 55.

Vascular Injuries

A grave feature of these combined injuries, particularly those in the proximal part of the limb, is the frequency of damage to the main blood vessels; although this may not lead to frank ischaemia of the forearm muscles, the circulation in the limb is sufficiently depressed to impede nerve regeneration. If blood vessels as well as nerves are damaged, the primary treatment of these injuries is therefore of the utmost importance. Arterial repair should be carried out whenever possible.

At the wrist there is the familiar hazard of severance of most or all of the *flexor tendons* which adds considerably to the complexity of treatment.

DIGITAL NERVES

Digital nerve injuries in the palm are caused by deep cuts or lacerations, sometimes by missiles. The consequent scarring can be formidable. Primary repair should be attempted whenever possible because it is often extremely difficult to find the nerve ends later. If secondary repair is obligatory it may have to be by autologous grafting.

Injury of these nerves in the digits themselves has two distinctive features. No less than two-thirds of our patients had irritative symptoms (p. 146); this can hardly be the true incidence because many of them were referred on account of the disabling sensitivity of their digits. Nevertheless, digital nerves are singularly prone to this sort of misbehaviour. Secondly, severance of the neighbouring digital vessels can cause profound ischaemic changes in the distal part of the severed nerve (see p. 277 and Fig. **15**, 33). The best way of avoiding these troubles is primary suture; the nerve fibres are directed into their proper channels and revascularization of the nerve can occur across the suture line.

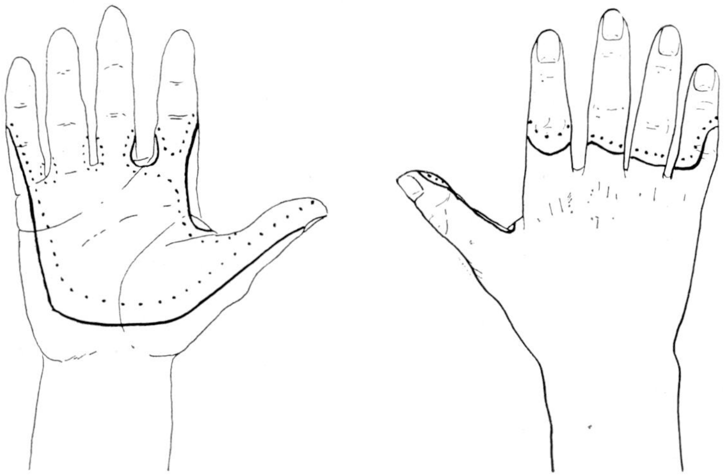

FIG. **11**, 55. Sensory loss in combined median and ulnar paralysis, the injury being distal to the emergence of the dorsal cutaneous branch of the ulnar nerve.

12. Lesions of Individual Nerves: Lower Limb

THE PRECEDING CHAPTER opened (p. 172) with some general observations that apply equally to peripheral nerve lesions whether in the lower or the upper limb. All we need add here is a specimen muscle chart (Fig. **12**, 1), which is so arranged that bilateral paralysis can be recorded; it may be desired to use the chart for the documentation of paralysis affecting both lower limbs—for example, that caused by peripheral neuritis or by poliomyelitis.

LUMBO-SACRAL PLEXUS

Unlike the brachial plexus the lumbo-sacral plexus is rarely damaged. *Traction injuries* at birth can occur (pp. 131 to 132). *Missile injuries* are sometimes encountered (Fig. **12**, 3). In all three of the patients who came to us the paralysis was incomplete; one patient recovered almost completely; in the other two there was imperfect but useful recovery. *Maternal obstetrical paralysis*, supposedly caused by foetal pressure on the lumbo-sacral trunk, has been discussed on pages 132 to 133; there is reason to believe that the cause is protrusion of an intervertebral disc.

LATERAL FEMORAL CUTANEOUS NERVE

The lateral femoral cutaneous nerve, arising from L2 and 3 (Fig. **12**, 2), has an extensive distribution (Fig. **12**, 4). At one time it was favoured as a source of material for autologous grafting, but it is unsuitable for this purpose because it begins to send off branches almost immediately after it emerges from beneath or through the outer attachment of the inguinal ligament. The most important affliction of this nerve is *meralgia paraesthetica* (p. 123).

It can be injured by the antero-lateral (Smith-Petersen) incision for exposure of the hip, and irritative symptoms may follow. One missile injury was seen.

SUPERIOR GLUTEAL NERVE

The superior gluteal nerve (L4-5, S1), arising from the roots of the common peroneal component of the sciatic nerve (Fig. **12**, 2), seems never to be affected alone. But the muscles it supplies are so important in locomotion that this nerve must be mentioned. After leaving the pelvis above the piriformis muscle the superior gluteal nerve passes laterally between the gluteus medius and gluteus minimus muscles, both of which it supplies. These muscles are the abductors of the hip, and at every step they balance the rest of the body as it pivots on the femoral head of the weight-bearing limb. The nerve terminates in and supplies the tensor fasciae latae, a muscle which is sometimes a passable substitute for the quadriceps femoris (Fig. **12**, 9).

If the sciatic nerve is injured high in the buttock, particular care is needed to avoid injury of the superior gluteal nerve during exposure of the lesion.

INFERIOR GLUTEAL NERVE

The inferior gluteal nerve (L5, S1-2) arises similarly from the common peroneal division of the sciatic nerve, emerges distal to the piriformis, and supplies the gluteus maximus. It may be injured, even totally destroyed, by an extensive wound of the buttock. It also has to be respected when the gluteus maximus is transected laterally, and reflected medially, for exposure of a proximal lesion of the sciatic nerve. Enucleation of a neurilemmoma at this level, which may prove to be large, can be an exacting operation because the inferior gluteal nerve, perhaps grossly distorted, must be preserved.

FEMORAL NERVE

The femoral nerve is formed from the dorsal divisions of L2, 3 and 4. Its main surgical interest is that it supplies the quadriceps femoris, a large area of skin in the thigh (Fig. **12**, 3) and, through its terminal saphenous branch, in the leg (Figs **12**, 3, **12**, 5 and **12**, 7).

Clinical examination, even in the recently injured patient, presents no difficulties.

HIP AND THIGH

EXAMINER												
DATE												
SIDE												
TYPE OF OBSERVATION *												
HIP FLEXORS												
GLUTEUS MAXIMUS												
ADDUCTORS OF HIP												
ABDUCTORS OF HIP												
TENSOR FASCIAE LATAE												
QUADRICEPS												
INNER HAMSTRINGS												
BICEPS												

LEG

TIBIALIS ANTERIOR												
EXT. DIG. LONG.												
EXT. HALL. LONG.												
EXT. DIG. BREV.												
PERONEUS LONGUS												
PERONEUS BREVIS												
CALF												
TIBIALIS POSTERIOR												
FLEX. DIG. LONG.												
FLEX. HALL LONG.												
ABDUCTOR HALLUCIS												
FLEX. DIG. BREV.												
INTRINSICS OF TOES												

0 No contraction.
1 Trace of contraction.
2 Active movement with gravity eliminated.
3 Active movement against gravity.
4 Active movement against gravity and resistance.
4+ Intermediate between 4 and 5
5 Normal power.

* V = Voluntary power. E = Electrical excitability.

FIG. **12**, 1. Lower limb. Hip and thigh: Leg.

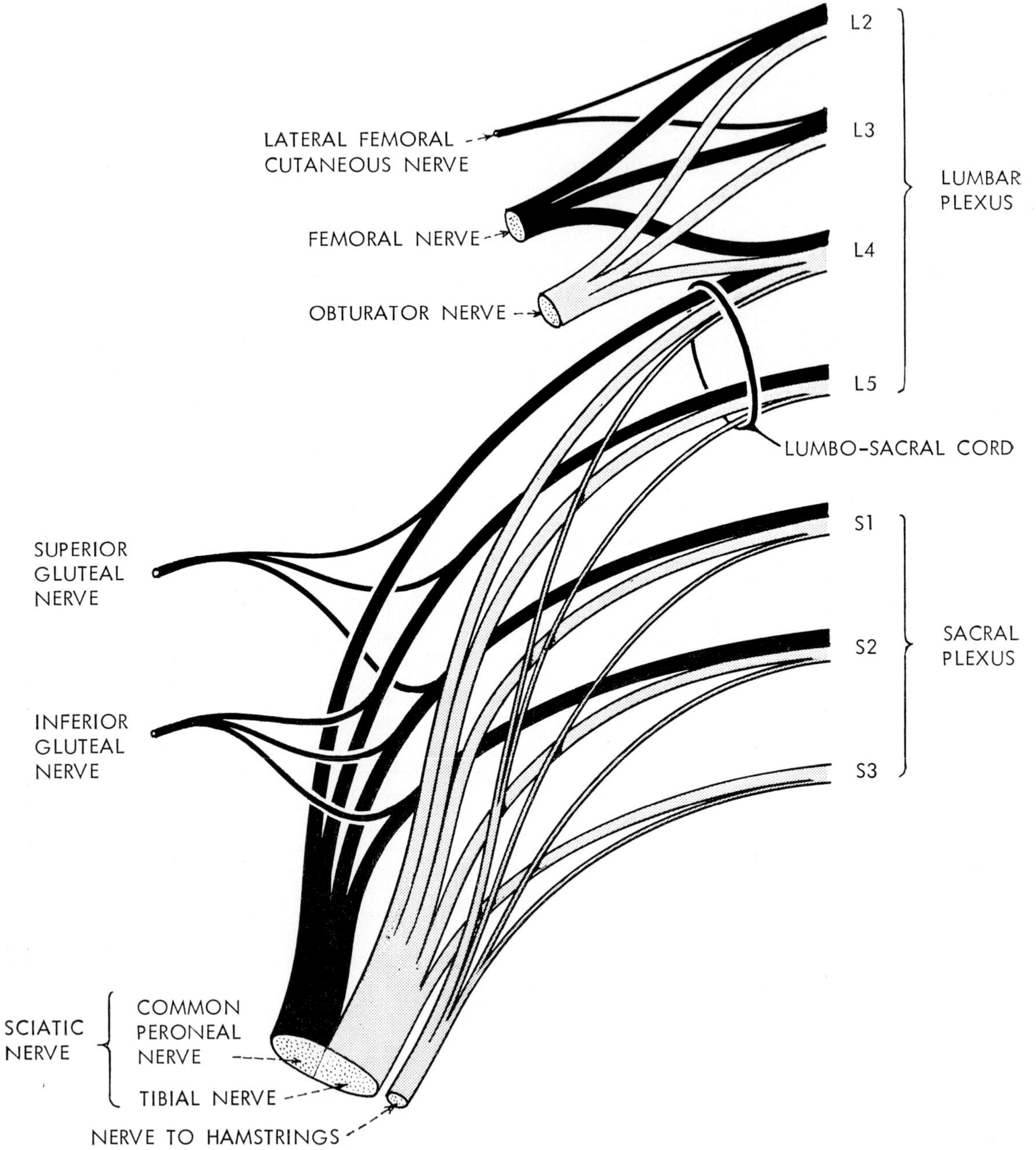

FIG. **12,** 2. Simplified diagram of the lumbo-sacral plexus.

Lesions of the Femoral Nerve

Seven injuries were caused by missiles. In one case secondary suture was performed with a poor result. Of the six other patients four made an excellent, and two a fair spontaneous recovery.

The femoral nerve was cut during the arrest of bleeding after an operation for femoral hernia.

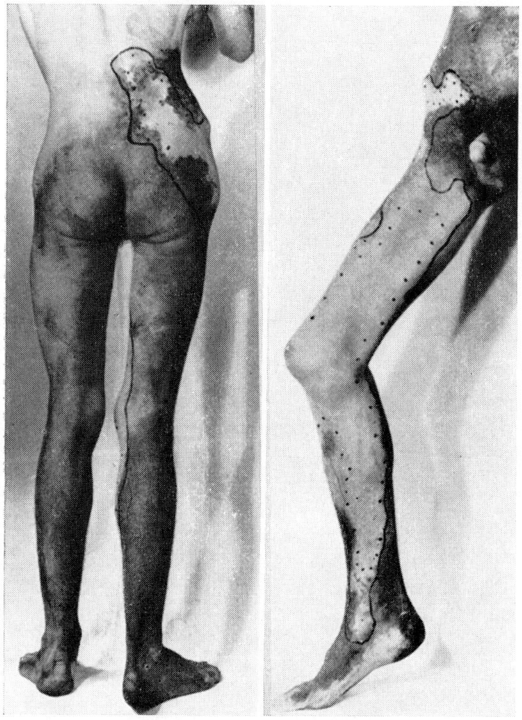

FIG. **12**, 3. Missile wound of the lumber plexus. *Motor*: weakness of the quadratus lumborum, ilio-psoas, quadriceps and the adductors of the hip. *Sensory*: loss of sensibility in the distribution of the dorsal primary divisions of the lumbar nerves; the ilio-inguinal, ilio-hypogastric and femoral nerves. The confluence of the two main areas of distribution of the femoral nerve, in the thigh and (saphenous) in the leg is well shown.

Secondary repair was impossible, but the functional result was good because the tensor fascia latae became a useful extensor of the knee (Fig. **12**, 9).

Saphenous Nerve. This nerve, which has a large area of distribution (Figs **12**, 3, **12**, 5 and **12**, 7), is rarely injured, though it is at risk in operations for varicose veins. The two cases that came to us did so because of irritative symptoms.

OBTURATOR NERVE

The obturator nerve, which arises from the ventral divisions of L2, 3 and 4, supplies mainly the adductor muscles of the hip, the adductor longus, adductor brevis, the part of adductor magnus arising from the inferior ramus of the pubis, and the gracilis.

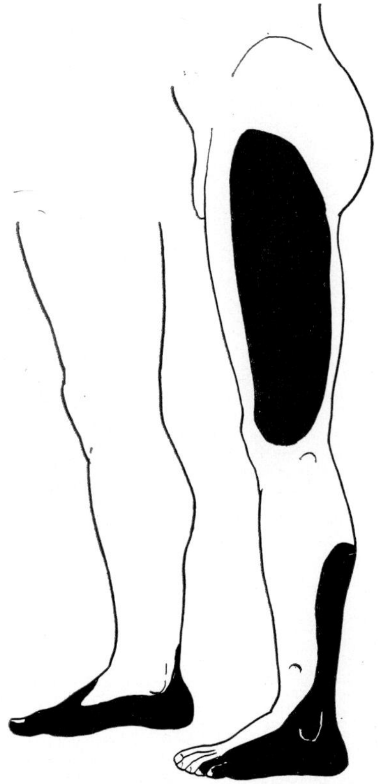

FIG. **12**, 4. *Upper right*: distribution of the lateral femoral cutaneous nerve; *Lower right*: maximal distribution of the sural nerve; the heel and the outer margin of the sole of the foot may not be included. *Lower left:* maximal distribution of the sciatic (tibial) nerve in the foot, medial aspect.

We have not seen one case of isolated injury of this nerve. Worster Drought (1921) found two among 544 nerve lesions in the lower limb; Sunderland (1968) one case in his series of 365 war injuries of nerves.

SCIATIC NERVE

The sciatic nerve is remarkable not only on account of its great size but because it is

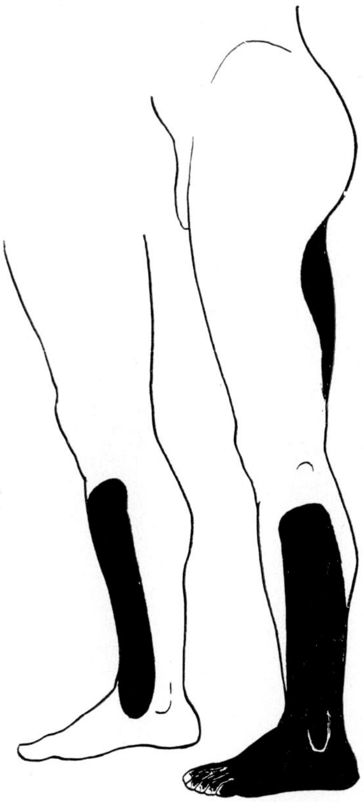

FIG. **12,** 5. *Upper right:* distribution of the posterior femoral cutaneous nerve. *Lower right:* usual area of loss of cutaneous sensibility after interruption of the sciatic nerve. *Lower left:* distribution of the saphenous nerve, medial aspect.

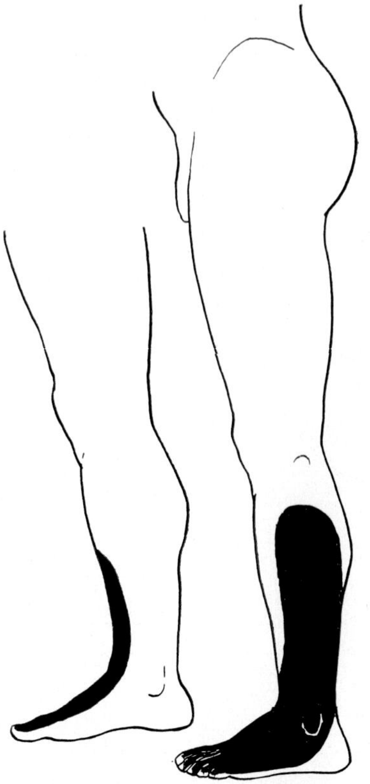

FIG. **12,** 6. Maximal cutaneous distribution of the common peroneal nerve.

composed of two entirely separate divisions. It emerges from the pelvis distal to the piriformis muscle, but sometimes the two divisions—the common peroneal and the tibial—remain separate throughout their entire course (Fig. **12**, 10), in which case the common peroneal division pierces the belly of the piriformis.

NERVE TO THE HAMSTRINGS

The nerve to the hamstrings (Fig. **12**, 2) is closely bound to the tibial division until, in the upper part of the thigh, it approaches its distribution to the long head of the biceps femoris, the semitendinosus, and semimembranosus and the ischial portion of the adductor magnus. The nerve to the hamstrings may be injured along with the sciatic by a deep wound of the buttock.

It is as necessary to consider the two main parts of the sciatic nerve separately, as in considering their homologues in the upper limb; the common peroneal nerve is the equivalent of the radial, and the tibial the equivalent of the median-ulnar nerve trunks.

COMMON PERONEAL NERVE

Motor distribution. The common peroneal nerve supplies the following muscles:

In the thigh: the short head of the biceps femoris.

DEEP PERONEAL (ANTERIOR TIBIAL) DIVISION:

Tibialis anterior
Extensor hallucis longus
Extensor digitorum longus
Peroneus tertius, and
Extensor digitorum brevis.

SUPERFICIAL PERONEAL (MUSCULO-CUTANEOUS) DIVISION

Peroneus longus and brevis.

Examination of all these muscles is straightforward, though it should be noted that except in persons with minimal subcutaneous tissue it is difficult to distinguish between peroneus longus and brevis. These two muscles can act as (plantar) flexors of the ankle, which may be valuable when the tibial nerve is paralysed.

Sensory distribution. The areas of skin supplied by the common peroneal nerve are the following:

1. Through its *fibular communicating branch*, which leaves the main nerve in the popliteal fossa, the area supplied by the sural nerve (see p. 220 and Figs **12**, 4, **12**, 7 and **12**, 8).

2. Through the *superficial peroneal nerve*, an area on the antero-lateral surface of the leg, which is occasionally large (Fig. **12**, 6).

3. Through the termination of the *deep peroneal nerve* the web between the first and second toes.

TIBIAL NERVE

Motor distribution. After supplying the two heads of the gastrocnemius and the soleus (triceps surae) the nerve descends deep to them (and—for convenience in a surgical context—being then described as the posterior tibial nerve), and supplies the tibialis posterior, the flexor digitorum longus and the flexor hallucis longus.

In dealing with disorders of the peripheral nerves there is no difficulty in the examination of these muscles, though in poliomyelitis it is essential to distinguish the action of the long flexors of the toes from that of the plantar intrinsic muscles. The long flexors must be seen and felt to flex the terminal joints of the toes. These same muscles are supplementary (plantar) flexors of the ankle, which accounts for inaction of the triceps surae—due either to rupture of the tendo calcaneus or, rarely, to paralysis of the triceps surae—being sometimes overlooked.

Beneath the flexor retinaculum the (posterior) tibial nerve ends by dividing into the medial and lateral plantar nerves; their exact distribution need not detain us because in relation to surgical disorders of the peripheral nerves it is significant only in plantar digital neuroma (pp. 126 to 129) and in the tarsal tunnel syndrome (p. 126).

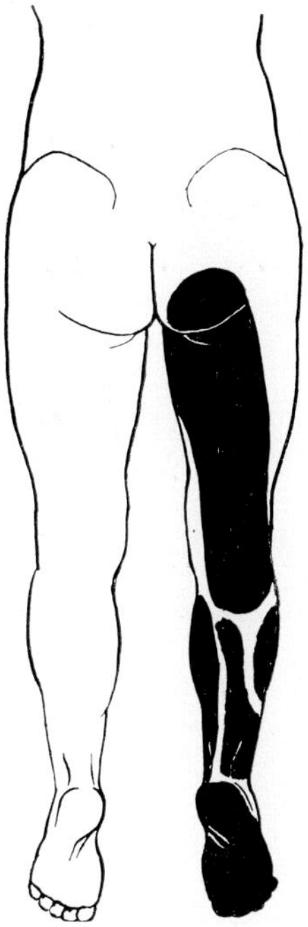

12, 7

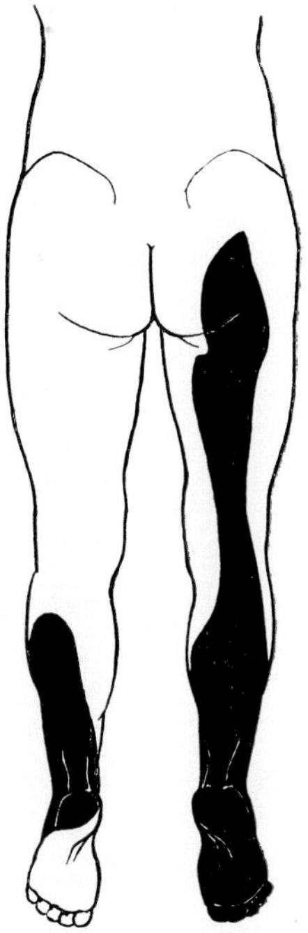

12, 8

FIG. **12**, 7. *Calf*: L to R; saphenous, sural and common peroneal areas. *Sole*; tibial area.

FIG. **12**, 8. *Right:* drawn from a clinical record: complete interruption of the sciatic nerve and of the posterior femoral cutaneous nerve. Missile injury in the buttock. *Left:* a large area, including the heel, supplied by the sural nerve.

DEFORMITY. The various deformities that can occur in paralysis of the sciatic nerve or of its terminal divisions are the same in every respect as those occurring in other kinds of peripheral paralysis affecting the leg; they are caused by an upset of muscle power. Thus in complete sciatic paralysis there is usually no deformity, though as a consequence of neglect the tendo calcaneus may shorten.

The commonest deformity is clawing of the toes, and it is almost always a consequence of paralysis or paresis of the tibial nerve. It is comparable with the claw hand of combined median and ulnar paralysis. Because (in our experience) the intrinsic muscles of the foot never recover after nerve suture it was seen in a fair proportion (31 per cent) of patients whose nerves had been repaired.

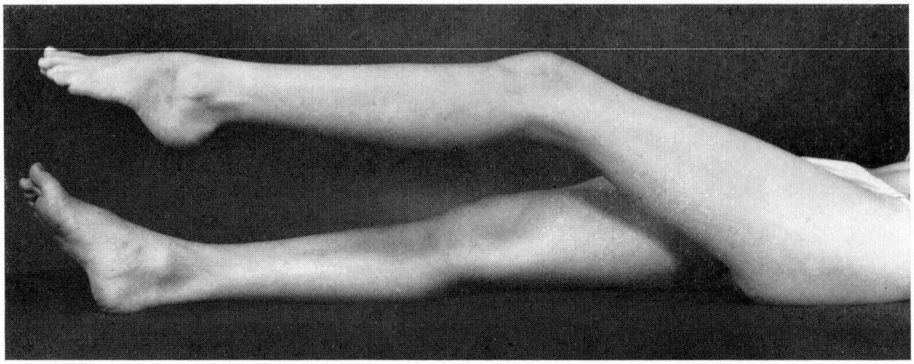

FIG. **12**, 9. The quadriceps was paralysed as a result of irreparable damage to the femoral nerve. Eighteen months after the injury the patient was able to extend the knee, though not fully against gravity, by means of the tensor fasciae latae.

It should be dealt with as in poliomyelitis; preferably by soft-tissue operation, but by interphalangeal arthrodesis—confined to the proximal joints—if the clawing is fixed.

Sensory distribution. The *sural nerve* arises from the tibial in the popliteal fossa and, after being joined by a communicating branch from the common peroneal nerve, supplies the area of skin shown in Figures **12**, 4, **12**, 7 and **12**, 8.

All of the five recorded cases of isolated injury of this nerve were due to missiles. In only one were irritative symptoms present. Its area of distribution (Figs **12**, 4 and **12**, 8) may extend over the heel, sometimes considerably; nevertheless it has become a popular source of material for autologous grafting (p. 299).

The terminal sensory distribution of the *tibial nerve* is extremely important. The typical area of sensory loss is shown in Figures **12**, 4, **12**, 7 and **12**, 8. Difficulty may be encountered in testing for pain; the skin of the sole is sometimes so thick that the examiner may find it necessary to refer constantly to the normal side so as to know the strength of stimulus (depth of needle-prick) required to elicit a painful response.

If the sole of the foot is insensitive it becomes vulnerable to injury. In nerve injuries of the posterior tibial nerve the triceps surae is active and the potentially dangerous loss of sensibility in the sole is sometimes overlooked.

Other Disturbances of Sensation After Lesions of the Sciatic Nerve

In addition to loss of sensibility there are certain more obtrusive sensory phenomena which have no parallel in the upper limb except after severe lesions of the brachial plexus and injuries of the digital nerves (p. 145).

Pain. About half the patients complain of pain, and its incidence is not greatly influenced by the level of the nerve injury or which division is affected, though a common peroneal lesion is slightly less likely to be troublesome.

Paraesthesia. About one patient in five complains of sensations described as tingling, pins and needles or burning.

Over-reaction. It will be recalled that the incidence of irritative nerve lesions is comparatively high after injury of the sciatic nerve (Table XIV, p. 145). The symptoms, which are far commoner in the distribution of the tibial nerve than in that of the common peroneal nerve, range from a very uncomfortable sensation when walking to complete inability to bear weight on the foot unless particular care is taken to protect it. There may be severe pain when walking in an ordinary shoe on irregular ground, and climbing a ladder may be impossible. The irritability of the sole does not diminish with the passage of time. The patient may resign himself to minor degrees of it. But some require a shoe (or boot) with a stout

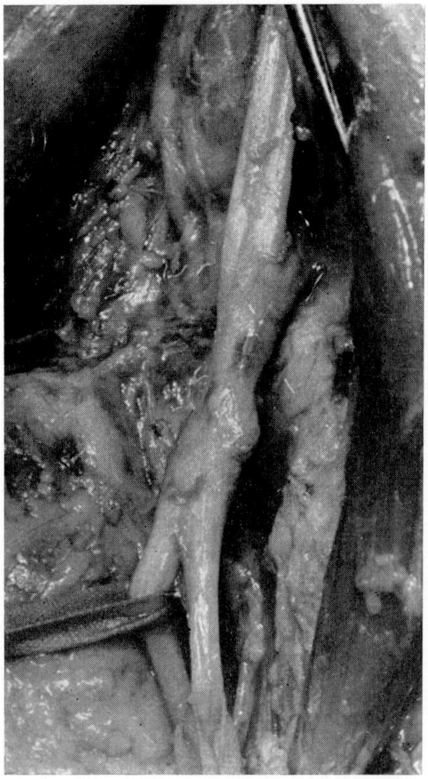

FIG. **12**, 10. The common peroneal and tibial divisions of the sciatic nerve are separate, though adherent at the point where they have been damaged by a missile.

sole, containing an insole made of Plastazote, which has the great advantage that it can be easily and accurately moulded to the sole of the foot. It should be 6 to 12 mm thick: any tendency to its compacting can be minimized by bonding a thin layer of sponge rubber to the upper surface of the insole.

When over-reaction is present the limb is sharply withdrawn when the affected area is stroked, or pricked with a pin. Thirty-five per cent of all patients—54 per cent of those with tibial nerve lesions but only 3·5 per cent of those with common peroneal lesions—present this sign. A few patients with total tibial nerve paralysis are troubled by excessive sensitivity at the junction of the area of sensory loss with the saphenous area at the inner side of the ankle.

Because over-reaction is disabling its absence or disappearance is one of the conditions for good sensory recovery. Over-reaction may be a troublesome feature after nerve repair at any level in the lower limb. After suture at the level of the hip or in the thigh the benefit from return of power in the muscles below the knee may outweigh the risk of over-reaction developing. But this consideration does not apply with nerve lesions below the knee; activity of the calf muscle is preserved and, moreover, as is apparent from Table XXIX, the incidence of over-reaction is highest of all with nerve lesions near the ankle, whether repaired or not. An anaesthetic sole may be of little consequence if the saphenous and sural nerves are intact. Furthermore, motor recovery in the plantar muscles after repair of the posterior tibial nerve—if it occurs at all—is so poor as to be useless. Patients who did not complain of over-reaction after repair of the posterior tibial nerve were the few treated by early secondary suture after a clean wound, or were children under the age of 12.

It will be noted that the incidence of over-reaction is far higher than the incidence of irritative nerve lesions given in Table XIV (p. 145). The difficulty is in deciding what constitutes an irritative lesion, over-reaction being usually (though, especially in brachial plexus lesions, not invariably) one of its most prominent features. There is every grade of disturbance. We decided —arbitrarily—to use the term irritative nerve

TABLE XXIX—Incidence of over-reaction in patients with lesions of the sciatic nerve in relation to the level of the injury

Level of injury	Percentage of all patients in each group with over-reaction
Hip	37
Thigh	55
Knee	40
Calf	47
Ankle	67

lesion when the irritative symptoms, as opposed to paralytic manifestations, were predominant, and the chief reason for the patient's seeking treatment.

Vasomotor and Trophic Disorders

In some patients with sciatic nerve injury the initial vasomotor and trophic changes disappear, whereas in others they become progressively more prominent.

We have to consider the degree to which these complaints may be disabling, and their relationship to other phenomena. One-third of all patients show some of the following changes. Most complain of coldness of the limb; others exhibit erythema, pigmentation, thin shiny skin, nail changes and oedema.

Although the skin temperature is raised at first, owing to the autonomic paralysis, after an interval of up to 3 months it becomes and remains subnormal. No patient shows increased warmth of the extremity except those with partial lesions who have been subjected to sympathectomy. Coldness of the affected limb is present in 95 per cent of patients with vasomotor or trophic complaints. It is often associated with an ache and, while never disabling, is an annoyance. Two-thirds of the patients with involvement of both divisions of the sciatic nerve exhibit vasomotor and trophic disorders. Seventy-one per cent of patients with tibial nerve lesions and 35 per cent of those with peroneal nerve lesions are affected. Patients with lesions in continuity have fewer complaints than those with complete division, regardless of the eventual degree of recovery. There is no relationship between motor recovery and the persistence of vasomotor and trophic disorders. There is some connection between sensory recovery and vasomotor and trophic disorders: when the latter are present good sensory recovery occurs in 46 per cent of the patients, whereas 85 per cent of patients without such complaints show good sensory recovery.

Vasomotor and nutritional changes are more severe in proximal than in distal lesions (Table XXX).

TABLE XXX—Vasomotor and trophic disorders

Level	Percentage incidence at each level
Hip	65
Thigh	58
Knee	34
Calf	42
Ankle	25

Pressure Sores

A pressure sore is a serious consequence of sciatic nerve injury, but the incidence is not high. Fourteen per cent of patients suffer from pressure sores at some time or other, mostly those in whom the main nerve is damaged. The sore usually appears within two years of the nerve injury. It may be caused by faulty encasement in plaster-of-Paris or by a splint. In such cases healing takes place rapidly, without recurrence, when the cause is dealt with. Fixed deformity of the foot is more grave and is present in all of the patients who continue to have troublesome sores; but if the deformity is corrected healing takes place. Although patients with no sensibility in the sole are twice as prone to ulceration as those with good sensory recovery, impairment or loss of sensibility is far less important than fixed deformity.

Examination of the Recently Injured Patient

Common peroneal nerve. It is sufficient to ask the patient if he can dorsiflex the foot, and if he can evert it.

Tibial nerve. If the wound is above the level of the knee it is sufficient to determine whether the calf muscle is working and whether there is sensibility of the sole. With wounds at or below the knee the surgeon should examine the flexors of the toes and the sensitivity of the sole.

Features Peculiar to Injuries of the Sciatic Nerve

1. The Relative Vulnerability of the Common Peroneal and Tibial Divisions of the Sciatic Nerve

It is universally agreed that an injury that might be expected to affect all parts of the sciatic nerve complex equally, tends to damage the common peroneal division more frequently and more severely than the tibial division. It has been generally supposed that the reason for this is anatomical. The common peroneal division is nearer to the surface of the body than the tibial division, and the nerve to the hamstrings is deeper than the tibial division. This might seem to explain the greater vulnerability of the common peroneal division and the relative immunity of the nerve to the hamstrings. Moreover, because the tibial division is about twice as thick as the common peroneal division it is less likely to be totally destroyed by a missile that had just failed to transect the nerve—a near miss; but this would not hold in respect of the nerve to the hamstrings. An excellent discussion of this phenomenon is given by Sunderland (1968; pp. 1076 to 1079). He reaches the conclusion that the vulnerability of the common peroneal division is due to a number of factors. They are summarized here, but the interested reader should consult Sunderland's work.

(*a*) He accepts the anatomical facts that have just been mentioned, but points out that the superficial position of the common peroneal division is confined to the buttock and the upper part of the thigh.

(*b*) Because the muscles supplied by the common peroneal nerve can so easily be overstretched by careless nursing or failure to supply toe-raising apparatus, it has been suggested that the apparent vulnerability of the peroneal division lies in the musculature, not in the nerve itself. Overstretching of paralysed muscle hinders recovery. However, this does not explain how it is that the initial paralysis is often greater in the common peroneal division than in the tibial.

(*c*) There is some evidence that the common peroneal division has a poorer blood supply than the tibial, but Sunderland remarks that this does not apply in the proximal part of the sciatic nerve; and there is no doubt that in the buttock and upper thigh, selective damage of the common peroneal division is frequently seen.

(*d*) The size, number and arrangement of the funiculi. This topic is very near to Sunderland's heart, and he suggests that the reaches of nerves in which the funiculi are large and tightly packed are particularly vulnerable. The displacement of a nerve caused by a high-velocity missile is considerable (p. 70), and in Sunderland's view small funiculi, surrounded by abundant connective tissue, yield readily to displacement. If the funiculi are large they, rather than the connective tissue, tend to give way. He has demonstrated that the peroneal division of the sciatic nerve is composed of fewer and larger bundles, with less connective tissue between them, than the tibial division.

(*e*) The last and possibly most significant difference between the two divisions is that whereas both are equally firmly tethered proximally the peroneal division is firmly anchored distally at the neck of the fibula, but the tibial division is comparatively free. This means that any stretching force—a near miss by a high-velocity missile or more overt traction—would tend to cause greater damage to the nerve anchored at both ends.

Distribution of Nerve Injuries

As is evident from Table XXXI (p. 226), missile injuries—that is, predominantly, war injuries—are those most likely to damage the sciatic nerve and its terminal divisions. The incidence of these injuries is far greater above the knee than it is below. This cannot be simply because the thigh presents a bigger target. Girth is irrelevant, since all that matters is more or less deeply placed nerve trunks. The greater length of thigh is insufficient to account for a 7 : 1 predominance of nerve injuries above the knee. It may be that the severe missile injuries of the leg shatter the bones and damage the blood vessels to such an extent that many of the patients end up with an amputation and are not therefore classified with patients who have nerve injuries. There is no proof of this but it is a reasonable supposition.

The Discrepancy between Neurological Recovery and Function

It has already been remarked (p. 9) that the results of repair of nerves injured proximally are, in general, inferior to distal nerve repairs and this is evident from Tables XLVII and XLIX (pp. 307 and 308). Thus, as in proximal injuries in the upper limb, recovery after even the best possible suture of the sciatic, common peroneal and tibial nerves is usually poor at the periphery. Fortunately, this does not mean that repair of these nerves is less worth while than repair in the upper limb. In 1959 D. K. Clawson devoted much time to studying the results of injury of the sciatic nerve (Clawson and Seddon, 1960*a*, *b*). It soon became apparent that restriction of attention to the results of repair gives an incomplete picture so far as function of the lower limb is concerned, which is why two papers were published.

A patient with total paralysis of one lower limb caused by poliomyelitis can always walk somehow. In severe neural leprosy, with sensory as well as motor paralysis below the knee, the patient can always walk provided that contractures have been prevented and sores dealt with. Complete sciatic paralysis usually causes no more than paralysis below the level of the knee; even if the nerve to the hamstrings has been destroyed the additional disability is not great; the knee can still be flexed by the gracilis muscle, which is supplied by the obturator nerve. Contractures and sores are menacing, as in leprosy, but both are avoidable. Chronic pain and over-reaction are a nuisance, but are usually tolerable. Thus if nothing is done, or if no recovery occurs after repair, a patient can still get about, and function may be very good (Figs **12**, 11 to **12**, 13). We have remarked elsewhere on some lack of correspondence between neurological and functional recovery; it is more pronounced in the case of the sciatic nerve than in any other. One

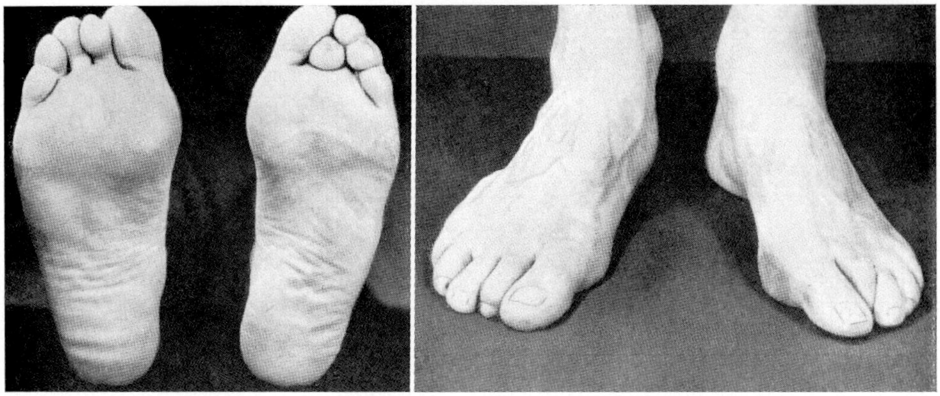

FIG. **12,** 11. Total left sciatic paralysis of 16 years' duration. Suture but no recovery. Function: grade II. Normal footwear: very active: work, panel wiring. (Figs **12,** 11 to **12,** 13 reproduced by kind permission from Clawson, D. K. and Seddon, H. J., 1960, *J. Bone Jt Surg.*, **42B,** 213.)

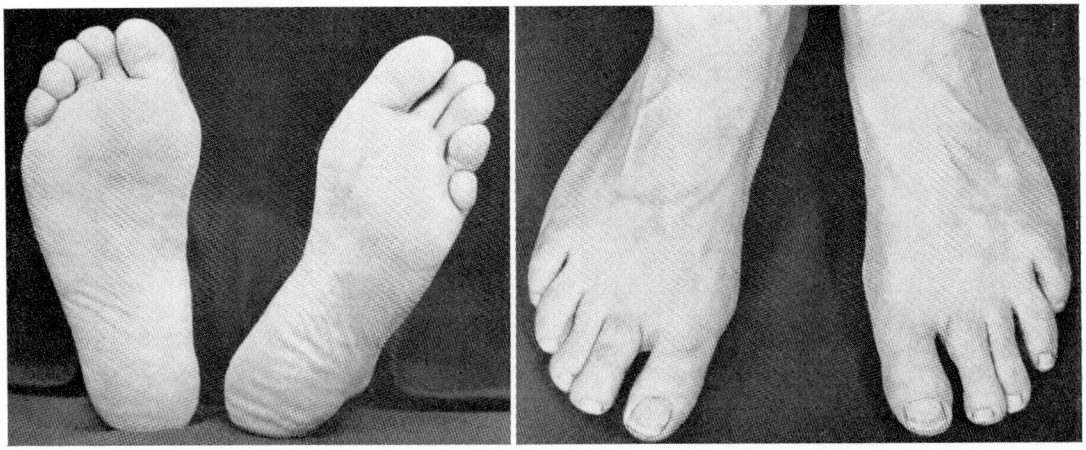

FIG. **12,** 12. Common peroneal paralysis of 13 years' duration: large, irreparable gap. Function: grade III. Wears toe-raising apparatus.

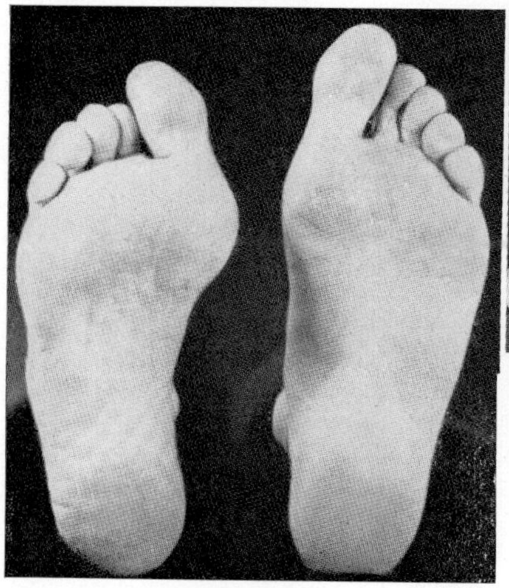

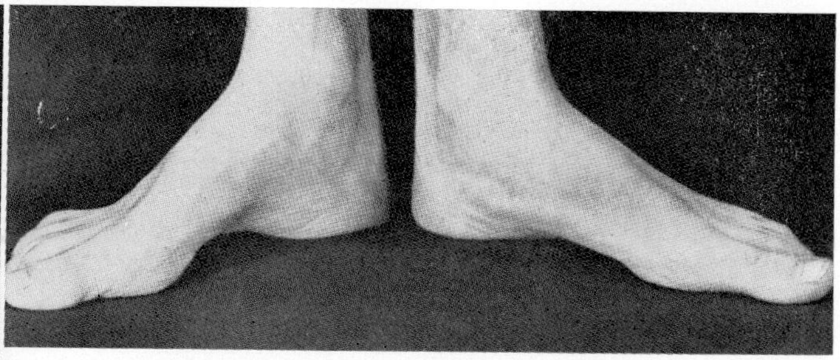

FIG. **12**, 13. Right tibial paralysis. No repair; no recovery. Function: grade II. Good push-off in walking from powerful peronei. Fully active, no complaints.

of our patients with total sciatic paralysis continued rock climbing and was able to tackle difficult routes. Another, with common peroneal paralysis, pilots a jet aircraft and enjoys playing eighteen holes of golf. These patients are not wildly exceptional. By contrast there were a few with only a slight neurological deficit who were very sorry for themselves.

This means that injuries of the sciatic nerve can be approached with restrained optimism. The indications for repair are no different from those for other nerves. Although regeneration entails the risk of the sole of the foot becoming hypersensitive, functional results are—as would be expected—better in patients who exhibit moderate or good neurological recovery (Clawson and Seddon, 1960*b*).

Lesions of the Sciatic Nerve and of its Terminal Divisions

Clean Wounds

There were only 13 clean wounds of the sciatic and common peroneal nerves, eight of them incised; there were none involving the tibial nerve alone proximal to the gastrocnemius. Although the quality of recovery after repair was well above average, two-thirds of these patients exhibited over-reaction.

Missile Injuries

In Table XXXI missile injuries are more common than all other lesions put together. Most of them occurred during the Second World War; sciatic nerve injury is chiefly a hazard of warfare.

Injuries in the Course of Surgical Operations

Operations on the hip can endanger the sciatic nerve. In upper femoral osteotomy, usually for osteoarthritis, the spike retractor inserted round the posterior (dorsal) surface of the femur may inadvertently be placed superficial to the sciatic nerve, with the result that the latter is severely compressed against the bone. The bone graft inserted in ischio-femoral arthrodesis may injure the sciatic nerve. The cement used to secure a metallic prosthesis in the operation of total replacement of the hip joint generates much heat as it sets; and if some of it leaks into the region of the sciatic nerve thermal damage can occur.

The common peroneal nerve is liable to be damaged by traction after operations for correction of flexion-contracture of the knee, and the sciatic nerve itself may suffer after an operation for lengthening of the leg.

Compression, Acute and Chronic

In seven cases of common peroneal paralysis due to external pressure, with complete RD in the affected muscles, there was good sensory recovery in all and satisfactory motor recovery in four (see Chap. 7, p. 124).

Injection of Drugs

This subject has been dealt with in detail in Chapter 8, (pp. 135-136). Ten cases of sciatic nerve paralysis were caused by injection into the buttock and in seven both divisions of the

TABLE XXXI—Lesions of the sciatic nerve and of its main components

	COMMON PERONEAL NERVE ALONE	SCIATIC NERVE BOTH DIVISIONS		TIBIAL NERVE ALONE
TOTALS	**136**	**209**		**20**
Incised wounds	6	2	2	—
Lacerations	4	1	1	—
Missile injuries, mostly war wounds	70	147	147	19
Injuries in the course of surgical operations	3	3	3	—
Compression, acute or chronic	7	3	3	—
Injection of drugs	3	7	7	—
Dislocation of hip, with or without fracture	3	18	18	—
Central fracture of acetabulum	—	5	5	—
Fracture of femur	11	11	11	—
Injuries of the knee causing traction lesions of nerves	26	11	11	—
Ganglia and tumours	3	1	1	1
	COMMON PERONEAL NERVE INJURIES **345**		TIBIAL NERVE INJURIES **229**	

nerve were involved. All patients showed some recovery but in none was it complete. The initial degree of paralysis bore no relation to the grade of final recovery.

Injection of analeptic drugs into the umbilical cord of the new-born child was once a serious though rare cause of lesions of the sciatic nerve (pp. 135-136), but we have seen no case of it.

Nerve Lesions Caused by Skeletal Injury

Dislocation of the hip, with or without fracture of the acetabular rim, injured the sciatic nerve in 18 cases and the common peroneal component alone in three. The results were as follows:

Dislocation alone: 5. Good or fair recovery in all.

Fracture-dislocation: 16. Good or fair recovery in 11, and poor recovery or none in five.

Quite apart from the nerve injury it is necessary to operate, and operate early, if a sizable fragment requires reposition; and it is in this sort of case that the nerve may be caught between the bony fragments. But otherwise the appropriate treatment is conservative.

In *central dislocation of the hip*, with fracture of the acetabulum, there is, by contrast, no element of traction, as there is in ordinary dislocation. If the sciatic nerve is injured—five cases are listed in Table XXXI—it is by pressure on it by a displaced fragment of bone: it may be that early operation would be beneficial. The results of late operation have been disappointing.

When a *fracture of the femur* has injured the sciatic nerve or the common peroneal division alone it is wise to explore the nerve without waiting for signs of spontaneous recovery to appear, even though the prognosis is, in general, favourable. The reasons for this have been given on page 88. Of the 22 patients listed in Table XXXI, 18 made a good or fair spontaneous recovery; in two the result was unsatisfactory;

and in the two cases in which the sciatic nerve was found to be transected, repair gave a most satisfactory result in one.

Traction Injuries

Traction injuries of the common peroneal nerve due to adduction of the extended knee were first described by Platt (1928): in 1943 a detailed description of the changes in the nerve was given by Highet and Holmes (see Chap. 5, p. 73). The tendon of the biceps is avulsed or the styloid process of the fibula breaks and is pulled upwards by the muscle. The fibular collateral ligament is always damaged, often ruptured, and violent injury tears the cruciate ligaments as well. If the knee is dislocated, with or without concomitant fracture—and this may result from any kind of violence, not adduction alone—the tibial nerve and the popliteal vessels may also be injured. This can cause most complex injuries (pp. 107 to 108): both main nerves are damaged by traction; the muscles of the leg are more or less ischaemic, and the distal reaches of the tibial and peroneal nerves are involved in the ischaemia. Thus there are double nerve lesions, due, at the level of the knee, to traction, and in the leg to ischaemia.

The commonest and most clearly defined injuries are those produced by adduction without dislocation of the knee. The common peroneal nerve can suffer every degree of traction injury up to complete rupture. One end of the nerve may be trapped in the lateral compartment of the joint (Platt, 1940). If the nerve is ruptured or if there is a severe lesion in continuity the longitudinal extent of the interstitial damage is so great that repair is impracticable.

If there is total paralysis the nerve should be explored. It may be that the damage is comparatively benign, as indicated by a little swelling and induration of the nerve extending over no more than a few centimetres. The nerve may then be left alone, though it may be expedient to repair the lateral ligament of the knee and the biceps. The best means of restoring the action of the biceps—unless an avulsed styloid process can be replaced—is to transfer the insertion of the semitendinosus to the fibula, and to stitch together the tendons of the biceps and semitendinosus.

In our 26 cases the results were: good or moderately impaired spontaneous recovery, 18; one impaired and two good recoveries after suture; in the remaining cases there was little or no recovery. An example of over-ambitious suture is illustrated in Figure **5**, 18 (p. 75) and Figure **5**, 21 (p. 77).

In the 11 cases in which both divisions of the nerve were damaged there was no recovery in the common peroneal component.

A traction injury of the common peroneal nerve remote from the site of skeletal damage may be caused by a fracture of the tibia and fibula, or by violent inversion of the ankle (Nobel, 1966).

Lesions of the Superficial Peroneal Nerve

This nerve is rarely injured. We have seen only two cases; in one there was an irritative lesion, in the other an incised wound had transected the nerve, which was sutured with a moderately satisfactory result.

Lesions of the Deep Peroneal Nerve

Involvement of this nerve is invariable in the anterior tibial syndrome and has been seen in 11 cases of Volkmann's ischaemia of the leg. The injuries encountered apart from these were as follows:

Incised wound	1
Missile injuries	5
Operation on an aneurysm	1
Fractures	3
Haematoma	1

We have already commented on the small number of missile injuries (p. 223). Considering how common are fractures of the tibia and fibula it is surprising that this nerve is not injured more frequently; but perhaps such injuries escape notice because they are often below the upper third of the leg and the tibialis anterior at least escapes paralysis. We have carried out only one exploration, we know nothing of suture of this nerve and there seems little need to worry about it because no less than eight of the patients listed above made a good recovery.

Lesions of the Posterior Tibial Nerve

Incised and lacerated wounds. Provided that mobilization is adequate, repair of these lesions is not difficult. But the results are disappointing because of the frequency of over-reaction when regeneration has occurred (see p. 221).

Missile injuries. In this series these were all due to war wounds, and the extent of the damage was most variable.

Skeletal injuries. It is remarkable how rarely the posterior tibial nerve is injured. Recovery occurs spontaneously and is usually good.

Ischaemia. The figure given in Table XXXII is artificially inflated, on account of a personal interest in Volkmann's ischaemia. Ischaemic nerve lesions in the lower limb have been considered in detail on pages 107 to 108.

TABLE XXXII—Lesions of the posterior tibial nerve

Incised wounds and Lacerations: clean	8
Missile injuries	28
Skeletal injuries	6
Ischaemia	11

Results of Sciatic Nerve Injury

From what has been written above (p. 223) it follows that even if a lesion of the sciatic nerve cannot be repaired the outlook is by no means bleak, provided that steps have been taken to avoid deformity and pressure sores.

Five grades of function have been devised which take no account of the neurological state of the limb (Clawson and Seddon, 1960*b*); the first three are regarded as satisfactory.

Grade I. Foot as good as the normal one.

Grade II. Able to walk any reasonable distance without pain; wears normal footwear and is fully active.

Grade III. Able to walk any reasonable distance with special shoes, pads or apparatus, with little or no pain; no disabling over-reaction to cutaneous stimuli; able to follow his occupation.

Grade IV. Able to walk no more than one mile; pain; troublesome over-reaction; forced to accept worse paid work because of the injury; pressure sores.

Grade V. Unable to work because of persistent pressure sores, or incapacitating pain; in a few cases, amputation.

In the 329 cases studied, which included 132 in which some form of surgical repair had been performed, the results were as shown in Tables XXXIII, XXXIV, and XXXV.

TABLE XXXIII—Results: total sciatic paralysis

GRADE OF FUNCTIONAL RECOVERY		PERCENTAGE OF CASES	
Satisfactory	I	0	64
	II	12	
	III	52	
	IV	27	
	V	9	

TABLE XXXIV—Results: common peroneal nerve

GRADE OF FUNCTIONAL RECOVERY		PERCENTAGE OF CASES	
Satisfactory	I	6	89
	II	38	
	III	45	
	IV	10	
	V	1	

TABLE XXXV—Results: tibial nerve

GRADE OF FUNCTIONAL RECOVERY		PERCENTAGE OF CASES	
Satisfactory	I	4	87
	II	30	
	III	53	
	IV	13	
	V	0	

If neurological and functional recovery are compared, startling results emerge (Table XXXVI, and Figs **12**, 11 to **12**, 13). The reader may well ask whether there is much point in embarking on surgical repair. The answer is in

TABLE XXXVI

Nerve	Neurological State		Percentage of patients with satisfactory function: Grades I-III
Sciatic	Motor recovery	good	65
		poor or none	50
	Sensory recovery	good	76
		poor or none	38
Common peroneal	Motor recovery	good	96
		poor or none	83
	Sensory recovery	good	92
		poor or none	80
Tibial	Motor and sensory recovery; good, poor or none		85

differences between the three grades described as satisfactory. Consider these grades as they concern the common peroneal nerve. Foot-drop can always be controlled by apparatus, and the patient is able to engage in most of his usual activities; this is Grade III. But a young man who, after an unusually satisfactory repair of the nerve, is able to ski, and ski well, is in a much higher category. Patients whose nerves are successfully repaired are, on the whole, much better off than those left with an appreciable neurological deficit.

Amputation. The amputation rate over a period of 18 years or more is 2·5 per cent. The reasons for amputation are stiffness of the foot with fixed deformity; pressure sores associated with the fixed deformity; and pain of some sort. The dissatisfied patients are those on whom amputation has been carried out on account of pain. This is not remarkable because there is little doubt that the cause of the pain is usually the nerve lesion, which is proximal to the level of amputation. However, amputation relieves the intractable pain that is sometimes a feature of ischaemic nerve lesions below the knee; this is discussed on page 108, and the patients in this category are excluded from the rate of 2·5 per cent just mentioned.

13. Forms of Treatment Required Apart from Repair of the Nerve

WHETHER OR NOT repair of a nerve is required, some of the forms of treatment described in this chapter are necessary in the management of all but the mildest nerve injuries (neurapraxia). Neglect of them may impair recovery that could have been good or even perfect. These methods of treatment pertain either to associated local injuries, or to the paralysed part, which is often remote from the site of damage.

TREATMENT OF ASSOCIATED LOCAL INJURIES

Wounds

Incised wounds. If a wound is recent and apparently clean, with no significant damage to other structures such as tendons, there is a case for primary repair of the nerve, and this topic will be considered later (p. 275).

Lacerated wounds that can be closed by immediate or by delayed suture. Primary repair of nerves in wounds of this kind is unlikely to succeed, and the treatment of the wound is therefore the same as if there were no nerve injury, apart from one manoeuvre. If a nerve or nerves are seen to be divided (no attempt should be made to hunt for them), they should be brought together in correct axial orientation with two sutures of, say, black silk which is easily identifiable later; if this is done, loss of length from retraction is prevented, secondary suture is facilitated and axial distortion is minimized. If the injury has been so violent that part of a nerve has been torn away it may be impossible to tack the ends together; but they should be anchored to some convenient neighbouring structure so as to prevent retraction. If it is feared that in spite of thorough treatment of the wound—opening it up adequately, and removal of contaminated and devascularized tissue—there is some risk of infection, it is better to use plain catgut for anchoring the nerve ends.

Lacerated wounds that cannot be closed. The treatment of the nerve or nerves, if visible, is the same as in the previous type of wound. The urgent matter here is repair of the skin defect because nerve suture, or grafting, cannot be undertaken until 3 to 6 weeks have elapsed after complete healing of the wound. If the wound is recent and is likely to heal without infection supervening then the raw surface may be covered immediately with a split-skin graft, or if suitably situated with a flap raised from the abdominal wall. Even apart from cosmetic considerations the latter is preferable if there is a nerve injury, because the subsequent approach to the nerve through an area that has been covered with split-skin grafts, and therefore lacks subcutaneous fat, is likely to be unsatisfactory. If the skin loss requires coverage by a tube-pedicle graft the delay before repair of the nerve can be undertaken will be greater. For this reason the first stage in the preparation of the tube-pedicle should be completed at the same time as the treatment of the wound, if the condition of the patient and other factors permit.

If there is doubt about the wound healing without infection a split-skin graft alone is permissible, to be replaced as soon as possible by a flap or tube-pedicle graft.

Missile wounds. In dealing with these wounds it is much less likely that the nerve will be encountered, and no attempt should be made to search for it. The wound is treated as if no nerve injury were present, though everything possible must be done to expedite healing not only of the soft parts (Fig. **13**, 1) but of any fracture that may be present. It has to be faced that when a bone such as the humerus or femur has been shattered the delay before the nerve can be explored is bound to be considerable.

Skeletal Injuries

Closed fractures (see pp. 78-88). When a nerve injury has been caused by a closed fracture the treatment of the fracture requires some modification. As has already been mentioned (p. 78) the nerve lesion is usually an axonotmesis or neurapraxia; in both, good recovery will occur spontaneously, in the latter very rapidly. It is important, therefore, to avoid aggravating the damage to the nerve; rough handling could convert a neurapraxia into an axonotmesis, and possibly an axonotmesis into a more serious lesion that might call for exploration and even repair of the nerve. Reduction is carried out gently; if it is found that manipulation is unsuccessful open reduction of the fracture should be considered with less than usual reserve; the nerve may be found trapped between the fragments. Open reduction can be combined with exploration of the nerve which, if found to be severed, may be tacked together.

Open fractures. Because open fractures are usually accompanied by more damage to the soft parts than are closed fractures, the prospects of spontaneous recovery in a damaged nerve are not so good, although they are still considerable: 65 per cent with open fractures compared with 83·5 per cent with closed fractures (p. 80). However, this difference is hardly such as to warrant a more radical approach than is required in the treatment of a closed fracture causing a nerve injury. Yet because there is a greater possibility of delayed or non-union of the fracture, that would delay exploration of the nerve—should this prove necessary—every effort is made to secure early union.

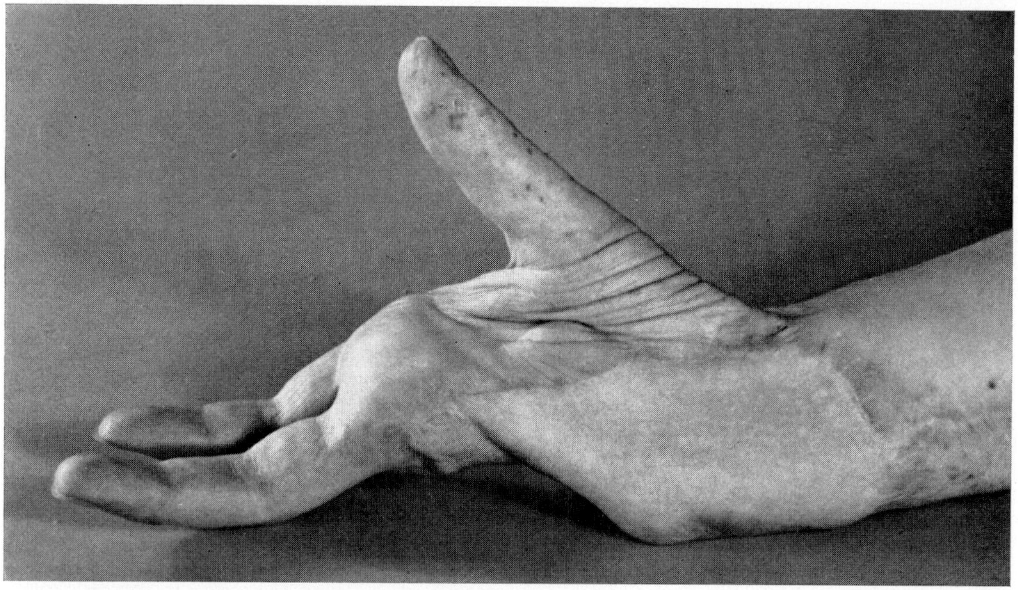

FIG. **13,** 1. The ulnar half of the hand was destroyed by a missile, and there was a large gap in the median nerve. After plastic repair of the skin defect a free graft taken from the ulnar nerve above the elbow was used to bridge the gap in the median.

Good sensory recovery, but the thenar muscles remained paralysed. Function was restored by tendon transplantation, which, as is shown here, was satisfactory.

In the light of knowledge acquired subsequently it would probably have been better to repair the median nerve by nerve-pedicle grafting.

Joint injuries. When a joint, especially the knee or the elbow, is injured along with a neighbouring nerve (or nerves) the treatment of the nerve will be greatly influenced by the nature of the wound. (1) If a clean, incised wound has opened a joint and severed a nerve, both injuries can sometimes be dealt with primarily, the nerve being sutured. (2) On the other hand there is the joint that is irreparably shattered by a missile; ankylosis in a functionally satisfactory position is the best that can be hoped for. If it is the knee or the elbow that has been destroyed the usual type of secondary repair of the nerve will be impossible, and therefore the objective is to secure sound healing of the wound as quickly as possible so that repair of the nerve by autologous grafting may at least be considered. If the wrist is ankylosed there is some hope of end-to-end suture because the nerve can be mobilized as far proximally as the lower third of the arm, the elbow then being flexed to 90 degrees—but not more (p. 270)—to permit apposition. (3) Between these extremes is a group of injuries in which some range of joint movement is regained. Whether this proves sufficient to permit secondary suture of the nerve depends not only on the range of movement but on the size of the gap revealed when the nerve is explored and also on which joint was injured. Whatever may be the range of movement at the knee full extension is necessary and the range of flexion may not allow the nerve ends to be brought together. At the elbow a limited range of movement is most useful if the mid-position of the joint is about 60 degrees of flexion; nerve suture is within the range of possibility.

Injuries to Blood Vessels (see pp. 89-94)

The only point to mention here is that if the damaged nerves are visible at the time when a blood vessel is ligated or repaired, their state should be noted with some care. If the nerves are in continuity there is a fair prospect of spontaneous recovery.

Tendon Injuries

The only situation that calls for comment is the deep incised wound over the front of the wrist that severs tendons and nerves. There is no uniformity of practice. If it is what they so aptly call a 'tidy' wound, Rank, Wakefield and Hueston (1973) repair tendons and nerves primarily. Bunnell (1964) repairs the nerves first, the tendons later. We have usually repaired the tendons first and the nerves secondarily. Much depends on the surgeon's attitude towards primary nerve suture, a topic that is fully discussed on pages 275 to 278.

TREATMENT OF THE PARALYSED PART

Prevention of swelling. Any severe injury of a limb may be followed by oedema. It is likely to be greater if there is a nerve injury, and greater still if there is a vascular injury. One important means of combating this oedema is to encourage the return lymph flow by active movement. But active movements are impaired or even impossible if there is considerable paralysis. This oedema leads so rapidly to disabling stiffness that it has to be tackled most vigorously. The two measures that help are elevation of the part, which in the upper limb usually calls for the use of an abduction splint; but equally important is frequent passive movement. I recall several patients with extensive wounds who had been treated expeditiously elsewhere, but whom I was obliged to admit urgently to hospital solely on account of oedema of the hand that could quickly have led to serious stiffness.

Maintenance of mobility. But stiffness can occur in the absence of oedema. We are now so accustomed to insist on the paramount importance of active movement of a hand or foot during recovery from injury to a limb—usually a fracture—that passive movement, which is admittedly less effective, is condemned. Yet a nerve injury may prevent the patient from carrying out active movements; passive exercise is then obligatory for maintenance of those movements that he himself cannot perform. The value of frequent mobilization of the joints of the hand cannot be over-emphasized. Indeed, when there is injury of more than one nerve in the upper limb the prognosis is often largely influenced by the treatment of the hand—or lack of it—in the period immediately following the injury. Neglect of passive movement is harmful enough but if, in addition, the paralysed part has been immobilized in a splint the consequent stiffness may be such that no later treatment will remedy it (Fig. **13**, 2). The most disappointing cases are those in which good spontaneous recovery has occurred in the damaged nerve but the hand remains more or less rigid.

Passive movement, along with elevation of the limb, is particularly necessary after injuries of the brachial plexus. Admittedly, in some cases the prognosis is so bad that the hand will be

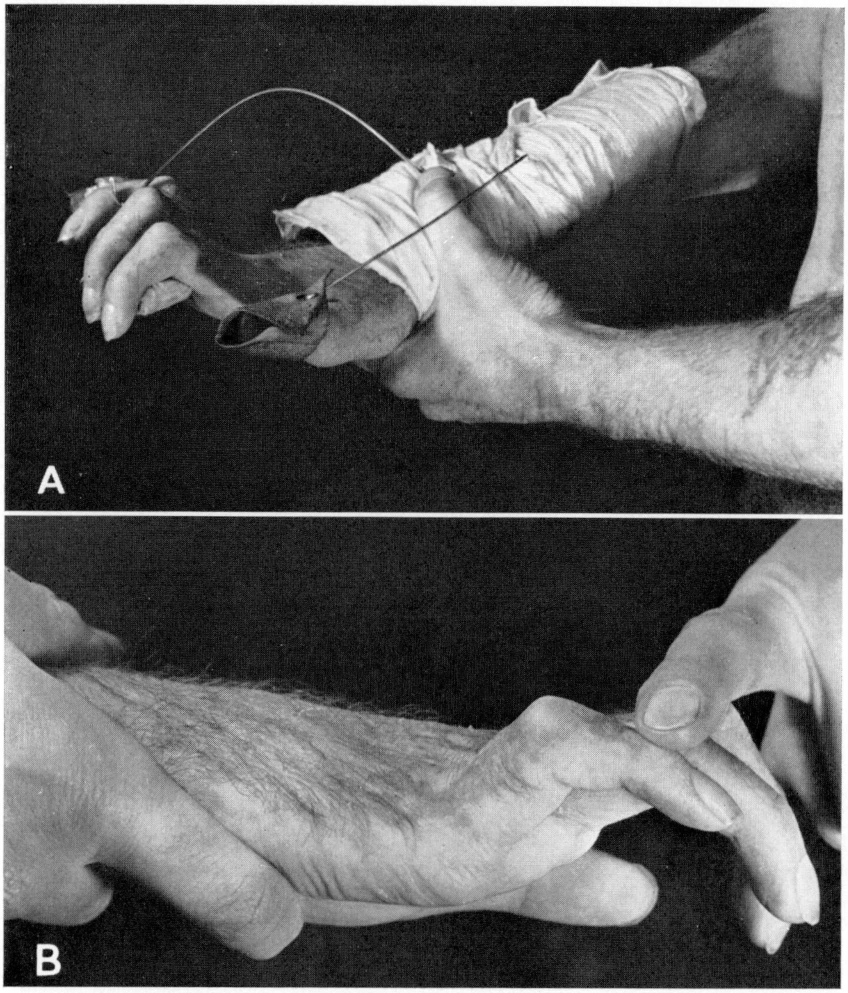

FIG. **13**, 2. A, This patient had radial paralysis and wore a crude ill-constructed splint. B, No precautions were taken to keep his joints mobile, and consequently he developed a contracture of the paralysed extensors of the fingers with shortening of the lateral ligaments of the metacarpo-phalangeal joints.

useless anyway. But this is not known at first—good recovery can occur—and it is in the early days when the mobility of the hand can so quickly be lost. The first patients we saw with severe brachial plexus injuries had received their primary treatment elsewhere; their hands were stiff, and even the most vigorous treatment resulted in only partial mobilization of the joints. It seemed that this stiffness was inevitable. When it became possible for us to treat patients with brachial plexus injuries from the first we found that the stiffness, which in the earlier cases had developed with such disconcerting rapidity, could be prevented; but it was necessary to mobilize all parts of the limb very frequently, up to five times a day. This intensive regime need not be followed for more than 3 weeks, this being the period during which stiffness can become so pronounced. Thereafter the frequency of mobilization can be progressively reduced, but not to less than two sessions a day.

Mobilization of a limb is hindered if movement causes pain. This is most strikingly seen in patients with causalgia, who may find any contact unbearable. As has already been explained (p. 141), this is probably why stiffness of the hand or foot is a feature of causalgia; it is not a direct result of the unusual nerve injury but occurs because the patient tends keep the part completely immobile. This is one reason why the treatment of causalgia is a matter of some urgency. In some other painful states, notably in patients with traction injuries of the brachial plexus, gentle handling of the part does not aggravate the pain but the physiotherapist must be skilful in order to achieve her ends.

Splints. It used to be thought that denervated muscle was in a peculiarly delicate state, a notion eloquently expressed by Keith (1919), who though not a clinician faithfully interpreted opinions that were widely held: 'Massage applied to the delicate and broken organization of a crippled muscle seems to me calculated to help in the work of destruction. If in any crisis of surgical treatment rest is necessary, it is in the early stages of degeneration of a paralysed muscle. . . .'

This wholly imaginary view underlay a system of splinting paralysed limbs that persisted into the Second World War. It had two elements: the maintenance of a paralysed muscle in a relaxed position; and immobilization of the muscle, which necessarily precluded all movement, active or passive. The latter may be quickly dismissed. Denervated muscle does not degenerate. It atrophies; and collagen is deposited between the fibres, a process which in the absence of passive movement can lead to permanent and disabling contractures. All the evidence shows that the more a paralysed muscle is exercised the less it atrophies. The problem is how to exercise it.

The other aspect, keeping a paralysed muscle relaxed, demands more serious attention. Let us compare recovery in muscles kept relaxed with those left in the normal neutral position. The deltoid muscle is a convenient example because it cannot be overstretched; the trunk prevents this. It can only be in the neutral position, the arm by the side, or relaxed on an abduction splint.

In 1956, Sharrard and Knowelden reported an investigation based on a study of 359 upper limbs in which there was abductor paralysis at the shoulder after poliomyelitis. Some patients were treated on abduction splints, others were not. Recovery in the patients who were splinted was slightly inferior to that in those who were left with the arm free, though the shoulder was mobilized regularly to prevent the development of an adductor contracture. Laxity of the capsule of the shoulder joint was related to the severity of the paralysis but was aggravated by splinting in abduction. The differences between poliomyelitis and peripheral nerve injury are not relevant here. Thus it appears that nothing is gained by keeping a muscle relaxed.

The recommendation that in birth paralysis of the upper part of the brachial plexus (Erb's paralysis) the shoulder should be splinted in abduction and lateral rotation (p. 130) is exceptional: this type of paralysis is unique in that from the first there is a vicious tendency for a contracture in medial rotation and adduction to develop, the nature of which has not yet been satisfactorily explained.

We need pay little attention to the harmfulness of keeping a paralysed muscle in a stretched position because there are two reasons, apart from the effect on the muscle itself, why it is undesirable. (1) Prevention of overstretching is usually a convenience to the patient. In paralysis of the common peroneal nerve toe-raising apparatus enables him to walk without catching his toe or walking with a high stepping gait. (2) Even more important is the prevention of a contracture in the normally innervated muscles. Admittedly, a contracture of the normal calf muscle (triceps surae) in a case of common peroneal paralysis can be prevented by regular passive dorsiflexion of the foot, but prevention is greatly simplified if toe-raising apparatus is used to counteract the tendency to shortening of the calf muscle. There are some situations in which important ligamentous structures may be irreparably damaged if overstretching of muscles is not prevented, notably in the proximal interphalangeal joints of the fingers in ulnar paralysis. If a claw hand is allowed to develop the dorsal envelopes of these joints become overstretched and the normal extensor action will never be regained even though good power returns to the interossei. If the metacarpo-phalangeal joints are held flexed the interphalangeal joints can still be extended by the extensor digitorum communis, and the extensor hoods are preserved.

Happily, the concept of the type of splint needed in the treatment of peripheral paralysis has undergone a profound change. Apparatus has been devised to permit useful movement of the affected part, while preventing the paralysed

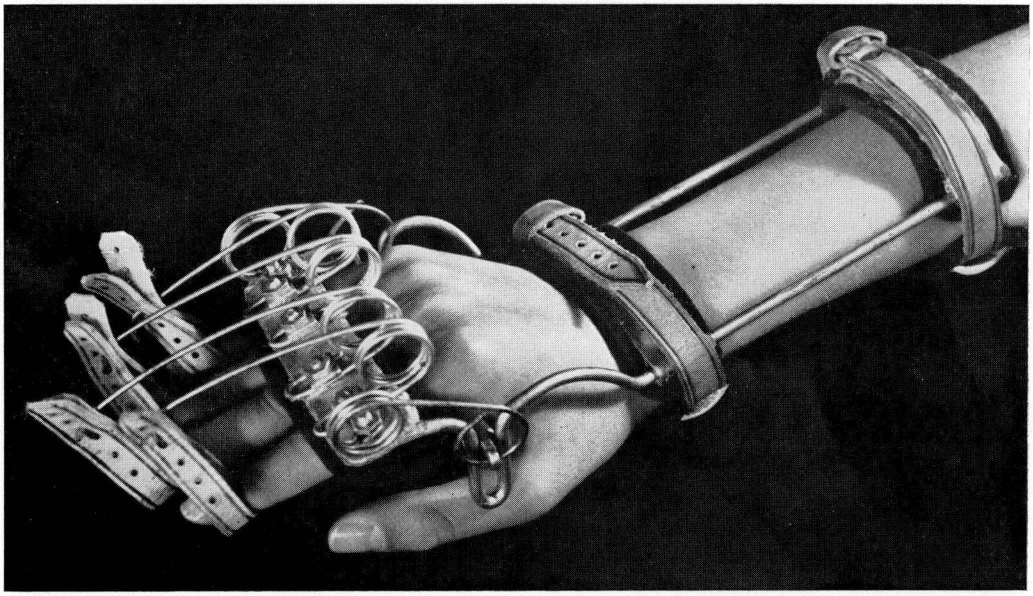

FIG. 13, 3. This splint for combined radial and ulnar paralysis is technically unexceptionable. It enables the patient to use the muscles supplied by the median nerve. Yet it is too bulky and elaborate to be completely acceptable.

muscles from being overstretched. Capener (1956), who among many others devised some excellent types of apparatus, coined the term 'lively splints' to describe them. The more elaborate the splint (Fig. **13**, 3) the less likely it is to be useful, that is, lively. Four types are selected for consideration; these are illustrated in Figures **13**, 4 to **13**, 9. A compromise in the interests of elegance has proved satisfactory (Tuck, 1966).

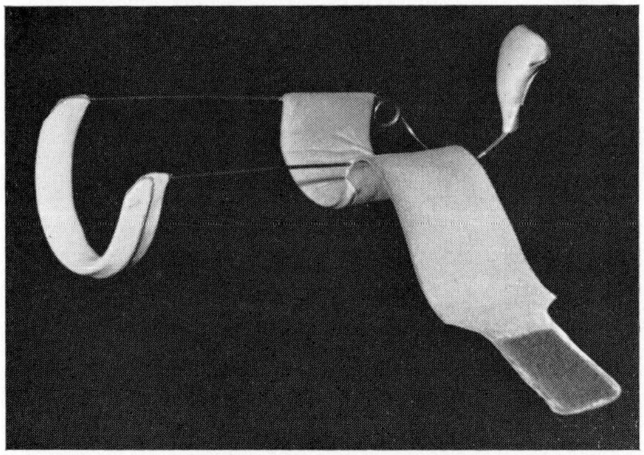

FIG. **13**, 4. A simple splint for radial paralysis. No attempt has been made to provide support at the metacarpo-phalangeal joints; this hardly matters because the extension of the wrist prevents the extensor digitorum communis from being overstretched. (Figs **13**, 4 to **13**, 7 are reproduced by kind permission from C. B. Wynn Parry and his colleagues, 1970, *The Hand*, **2**, 31.)

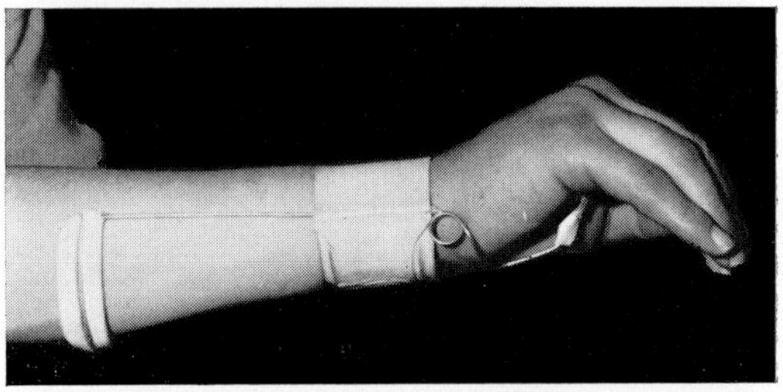

FIG. **13**, 5. The splint in position.

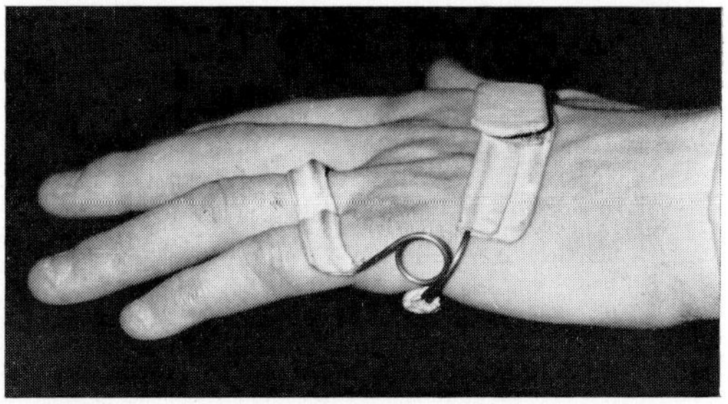

FIG. **13**, 6. A simple splint for ulnar paralysis. The lumbrical muscles controlling the index and middle fingers prevent clawing of these digits.

A splint made of a very tough plastic called Ortholen (Fig. **13**, 10) gives excellent and slightly springy support to the foot; it may be worn in an ordinary shoe and is inconspicuous.

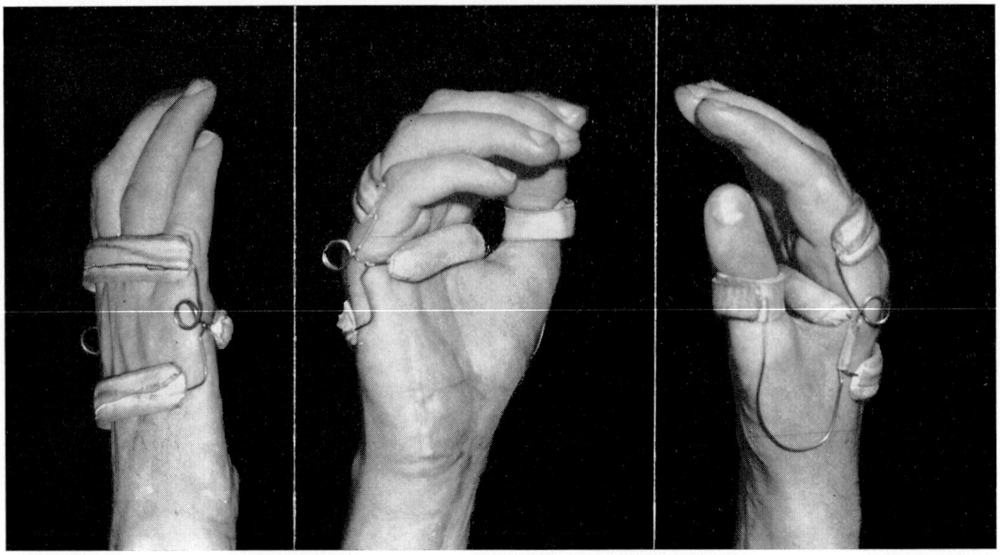

FIG. **13,** 7. A splint for combined ulnar and median paralysis.

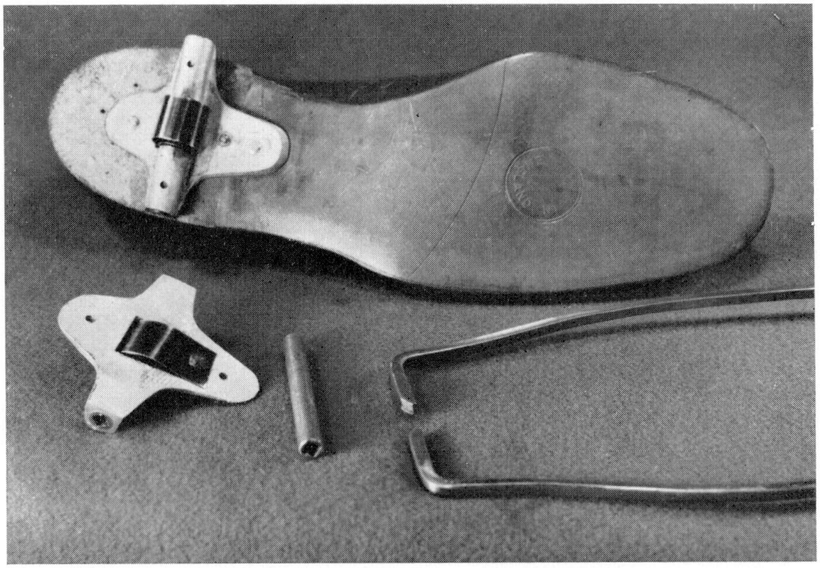

FIG. **13,** 8. Concealed clock spring toe-raising apparatus. (Figs **13,** 8 and **13,** 9 by kind permission from W. H. Tuck, *J. Bone Jt Surg.*, 1957, **39B,** 335.)

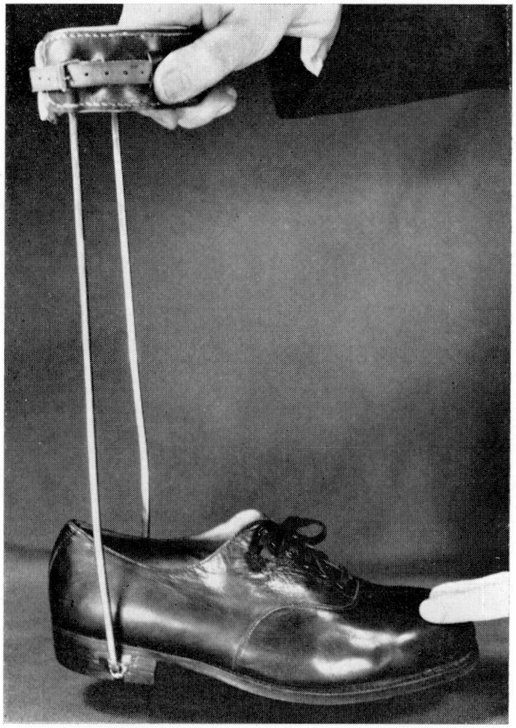

FIG. **13,** 9. The assembled concealed spring apparatus. Tuck (1962) devised something even better; in place of the metal spring there is a rubber torsion socket. Nothing can break or corrode.

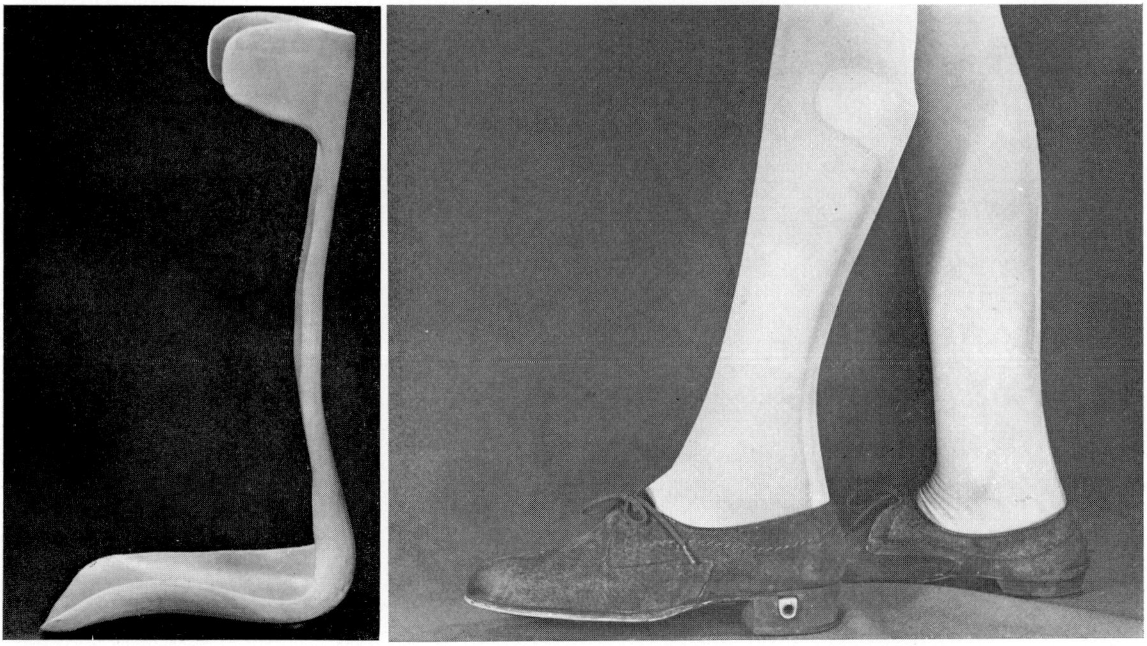

FIG. **13,** 10. Ortholen splint. (Reproduced by kind permission of the author and Editor from W. H. Tuck, *Physiotherapy*, 1966, **52**, 442).

Electrotherapy

There can hardly be any form of therapy in which the gulf between the results of animal experiment and their clinical application is so great.

It was necessary to investigate experimentally the value, if any, of stimulation of denervated muscle, and many physiologists applied themselves to this question. A convenient starting point is a paper by Fischer (1939), which contains an excellent review of earlier work. In small animals, stimulation of denervated muscle with an appropriate current prevents wasting.

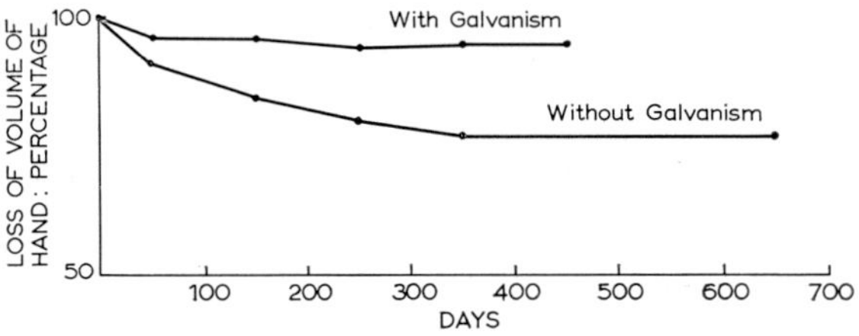

FIG. **13**, 11. The decline in the volume of the hand when the paralysed intrinsic muscles are not stimulated electrically. The muscles account for about a quarter of the total volume; so by the 350th day the atrophy is extreme.

The weight and volume of the muscle are maintained, and the interstitial fibrosis that always occurs otherwise in wasting denervated muscle is prevented (Gutmann and Guttmann, 1944). This is important because this fibrosis can be a serious hindrance to re-innervation (Gutmann and Young, 1944). It was shown by Langley and Itagaki (1917) that denervated muscle used more oxygen, which led them to conclude that the increased metabolism, which they associated with the ceaseless fibrillation, was burning up the muscle and so causing it to waste. However, Fischer (1939) found that electrotherapy increased the oxygen consumption still further, although preventing wasting; and that the electrical excitability of the muscle also increased. The strength of the electrically induced contraction is augmented (Hines, Thompson and Lazere, 1943). It has not been shown that galvanically induced exercise accelerates motor recovery, though Gutmann and Guttmann found that the quality of recovery was enhanced. A few workers have failed to demonstrate any beneficial influence from electrotherapy, but they are in a minority.

It would seem that there is a case for the clinical employment of electrical stimulation of denervated muscle, but there is little well-documented supporting evidence. Doupe, Barnes and Kerr (1943) studied a number of patients whose radial nerves had been repaired; six of them were treated with galvanism for nine months or longer at the rate of 15 to 30 'moderate contractions' of each muscle, five to six times a week, the electrodes being applied longitudinally to each muscle. This, which may be regarded as conventional treatment, proved valueless. Even when much more intensive stimulation was employed, more than is normally possible, there was only a slight increase in blood flow, which they chose as an index of the amount of exercise to which the muscles were subjected. Jackson (1945) reported a much larger series of cases in which the volume of the hand was measured in 92 patients with ulnar or combined median and ulnar paralysis. Half of the patients were treated daily with galvanism at the rate of 30 stimuli a minute to each muscle or muscle group—90 stimuli in all to each. She found that for a short period after denervation the volume of the hand decreased whether or not the muscles were stimulated, but the shrinkage was controlled thereafter in the patients receiving electrical treatment (Fig. **13**, 11).

However, even in the large group of cases observed by Jackson there were so many variables that it was not possible to show that the quality of recovery was superior in the patients whose muscles had been prevented from wasting.

One great hindrance to the clinical application of galvanotherapy is that it is not possible to stimulate muscles with the intensity and frequency employed by many laboratory workers. A powerful current is intolerably painful. Hines *et al.* treated their animals under anaesthesia, in the belief that the benefit was related to the amount of work done by the muscles. Doupe and his colleagues showed that in their conventionally treated patients the work done by the denervated muscles was small. Moreover, a unidirectional current causes ionization in the tissues beneath the electrodes, though this can be avoided by what Wickham (1948) calls balanced-pulse galvanism. A square-wave stimulus of relatively high amplitude is followed by one of opposite polarity, subliminal in amplitude but of prolonged duration so that the ionizing effect of the first stimulus is counteracted. Yet even so, with an ideal stimulus, the daily ceremonial (anything less frequent is ineffective) is time-consuming and burdensome. However, I have found it possible to supply conscientious and intelligent patients with portable machines that they can use themselves. An ingenious one was devised by Bateman (1947).

The bulk of the muscle to be stimulated is relevant. The experimental work was done on small animals; it is much simpler to stimulate the gastrocnemius in a rabbit than in man. It is likely, however, that with one electrode in the palm of the hand and the other applied to the dorsum so as to stimulate each group of intrinsic muscles in turn a strong current is effective in stimulating interossei and lumbricals, if one may judge by the briskness of the contractions produced. But it is a very different matter with bulky muscles and with long ones. The muscle is denervated, there is no motor point, and only the part of the muscle traversed by the current contracts. Even if the electrodes are applied at each end of a fairly long muscle mass, such as the radial extensors of the wrist, there is no certainty that the full thickness of the muscle is stimulated from end to end.

Good recovery can occur in the absence of galvanotherapy and many specialists in physical medicine are content with this. It is not possible to make any dogmatic recommendation, but it would seem desirable that the intrinsic muscles of the hand, at any rate, are worth treating, more particularly if on account of the proximal situation of the nerve lesion the time that must elapse before re-innervation can take place is long.

For those interested it may be useful to summarize some practical notes compiled by R. H. S. Holbourn and L. Guttmann but never published.

1. The strongest possible current should be used, the limiting factors being pain and the excitation of neighbouring normal muscles.

2. The electrode pads must always be kept moist. Hard water is best avoided because it is possible to deposit insoluble calcium in the tissues beneath the cathode. Common salt may be used or, better, a phosphate buffer solution: 25 g of Na_2HPO_4 and 12 g of NaH_2PO_4 in 1 litre of water, this being diluted with 5 to 10 times its volume before use. It has the effect of slightly reducing the risk of skin burns, though in this connection a balanced-pulse generator is far superior.

3. Pain is less if large electrode pads are used; the physiotherapist should, therefore, use the largest pads compatible with the anatomical situation.

4. Except in stimulation of the short muscles of the hand it is best to place the electrodes at each end of a muscle. The choice of anode or cathode at any particular site depends entirely on the strength of the response to stimulation, which must be judged not only by the amount of bellying of the muscle but also by the tightness of its tendon, if palpable, during the contraction.

5. The muscle should be treated in the stretched position; this increases the amount of exercise it will do on contraction.

6. The duration of the stimulus should be as short as possible, but not to the extent that the intensity has to be increased; between 0·07 and 0·01 second is about right. Metronomes dipping in pots of mercury are, for this reason, unsatisfactory.

7. A stimulation rate of 40 impulses a minute is probably satisfactory.

8. There is no risk of fatiguing a muscle by frequently repeated contractions (Hines *et al.*, 1943); 100 to 200 contractions is desirable.

9. A progressive current, taking about 4 seconds to reach its maximum and then dying away, produces a contraction only in denervated muscle; but it is useless therapeutically.

10. Treatment should be continued until re-innervation is well established as judged by the return of voluntary movement. Electrical treatment should then cease and voluntary movement be strongly encouraged.

Active Exercise

As soon as active movement is detectable it should be encouraged by appropriate exercises. These exercises present no difficulty to patients whose nerve damage has been an axonotmesis—as for example radial paralysis caused by a fracture of the humerus—because the pattern of re-innervation is undisturbed. But after nerve suture the inevitable confusion that has occurred at the suture line results in more or less cross re-innervation of muscles. This is seen most strikingly in the interossei after repair of the ulnar nerve; these muscles will contract well together but it is rarely possible for them to act separately except, for reasons that are still obscure, in the very young. Normal independent movement does not return after nerve suture. This is often disheartening for the patient, particularly if he has been accustomed to use his hand for fine work. In the lower limb it can be embarrassing too if, as sometimes happens with the common peroneal nerve, the peronei and the muscles in the anterior compartment of the leg contract simultaneously. Yet something can be achieved by deliberate training, and I have been greatly impressed by the functional improvement in the hands of intelligent women—to whom we had explained the nature of what had happened—after they had applied themselves assiduously to knitting and even to playing the piano.

TABLE XXXVII—Summary of physical treatment

TREATMENT	BEFORE AND AFTER NERVE REPAIR	AXONOTMESIS	NEURAPRAXIA
Prevention of oedema if paralysis is extensive	Imperative	Imperative	Rarely needed
Prevention of stiffness	Imperative	Imperative	Only if paralysis is extensive
Splinting	Desirable in some situations		No
Electrotherapy	Useful in the hand		No
Motor and, in some situations, sensory re-education	Yes	No	No

The treatment of the paralysis may be summarized as shown in Table XXXVII.

Rehabilitation and Resettlement

In this connection patients with nerve injuries present two significant features. Recovery is slow; and injury even of a single nerve may oblige the victim to change his occupation. Hence the patient's way of life deserves attention from the start. If, for example, he has radial paralysis due to a closed fracture of the humerus there is a strong probability of full recovery, and there is an excellent tendon transplantation available should the nerve not recover spontaneously or defy repair. The outlook is favourable. The other aspect of the problem may be illustrated by an extreme example.

A young soldier cut his right forearm near the wrist. The median nerve was damaged and it was sutured five weeks later. Six months after the accident he was discharged from the Army (presumably because his trigger finger was still insensitive) and he started work as a builder. Then he struck the wrist with a hammer; after that it felt weak, so he retired from this work to keep his father company in a hairdressing establishment for women. He found this boring. About a year after leaving the Army he was convicted, along with others, of breaking into a school and stealing a heavy safe. He was sent to prison.

Although this young man's turning thief cannot be condoned it cannot be excluded that but for the mismanagement of his nerve injury he might have continued to run straight.

His contacts with medical folk had been casual throughout. No one had explained to him what would be the consequences of the injury: no one took the trouble to advise him about the sort of work he would be fit to do immediately or ultimately: no one followed the progress of his recovery. He lacked a counsellor. There was no need for him to go to an elaborate rehabilitation centre; any well-organized hospital could have supplied what was required.

This is not the place to describe methods of rehabilitation: there are many excellent books on the subject. It may be added, however, that the functional as distinct from the neurological quality of recovery is enhanced in patients who have been encouraged to use the paralysed part from the earliest possible moment (Davis, 1949).

14. Factors Influencing Indications for Operation

THIS CHAPTER IS concerned chiefly with acute injuries. Chronic lesions of mechanical origin have been dealt with in Chapter 7, and nerve tumours in Chapter 10.

As will be evident in Chapters 15 and 16, there is much interest in the refinement of methods of nerve repair. Yet if the latter remained unchanged the lot of patients with damaged nerves could be immensely improved by more accurate appreciation of what is amiss, and of the consequent choice and timing of treatment. If, as is happily usual in traumatic cases, there is little or no delay in the detection of a nerve injury there are still two possible sources of error. The first is unnecessary intervention, though except in the case of inapposite primary suture this is rarely harmful. It is much more grievous to operate at a time when the prospects of obtaining a satisfactory result from repair of the nerve, should it prove necessary, have long since passed. The reasons why delay is harmful have been described in Chapter 2.

DELAY

Valuable information about the influence of delay on the prospects of recovery after nerve suture is given by Zachary (M.R.C.R., 1954, pp. 369 to 374 and Tables 91 to 99. Table 99 is reproduced here as Table XXXVIII) and by Woodhall and Beebe (1956, pp. 139 to 157, Fig. 12 and corresponding tables).

My own results appear in Table XXXIX. There are many gaps, which is not surprising. In the cases referred to there had been an interval of more than 12 months between injury and final repair. There are only 65 *nerves*: fewer patients, because some of the injuries were multiple. Where surgical practice is good, clinicians strive to avoid delay; thus undue delay is a consequence of exceptional circumstances such as, for example, a soldier having been a prisoner-of-war; the dehiscence of a sutured nerve (see Fig. **2**, 16, p. 19 and Fig. **15**, 28, p. 272), or a late secondary suture performed with a view to relieving the pain caused by an irritative nerve lesion, the result in terms of motor and sensory function being of secondary importance. In the 65 cases recorded, there were far more failures than successes; the periods listed under *delay* indicate only that exploration with a view to repair has some prospect of being successful.

Although we are not at liberty to generalize from these two tables, based as they are on exceptional happenings, other information enables us to take account of certain factors that bear on the question of delay.

Age

The prognosis is better in the young than in adults (Fig. **16**, 15, p. 276 and Fig. **17**, 2, p. 305); in children the capacity for regeneration is greater, and their limbs are shorter.

Level of the Lesion

The more proximal the site of damage the worse the prognosis and the shorter the *critical delay*. Retrograde changes, in motor structures particularly, will be advanced before regenerating axons reach the periphery (pp. 23 to 27); and there is what we have called axonal exhaustion (p. 9). Thus the element of urgency in nerve repair is particularly pressing if the lesion is at the root of a limb. Indeed in one situation, the middle and lower trunks of the brachial plexus, the prospects of success after suture are gloomy from the start, at any rate in adults. Early repair of the upper trunk of the plexus, which is distributed in the proximal part of the upper limb, is much more promising.

The prognosis varies from nerve to nerve, and even within the distribution of a nerve. For example, after repair of the sciatic nerve or of its tibial division recovery after suture is good in the triceps surae whether the delay before operation is short or as long as 23 months; far better than in any of the other muscles of like innervation, and better than could be accounted for by the fact that the triceps surae is proximal to them.

The periods of delay that we have been considering are to be avoided if possible. They indicate only that recovery *may* occur after suture is performed after so many months: it may not. Zachary showed that the prospects of recovery after suture performed within six months of injury are better than after six months. Woodhall and Beebe went further, and demonstrated that the decline is, as might be expected, progressive.

THE SITE OF THE LESION

This is not always self-evident. A fall on the shoulder can produce a traction injury of the

TABLE XXXVIII—Critical delay compatible with recovery to specific grade (Zachary)

NERVE AND SITE	GRADE OF RECOVERY	DELAY (months)
Ulnar (motor)		
proximal	M2	9
intermediate	M2 +	16
distal	M2 +	18
Ulnar (sensory)		
proximal	S3	9
intermediate	S3	24
distal	S3	31
Median (motor)		
proximal	M1 +	9
intermediate	M3	13
distal	M3	32
Median (sensory)		
proximal	S3	12
intermediate	S3	36 child; 17 adult
distal	S3	26 child; 9 adult
Radial (motor)		
proximal	M3	13
intermediate	M3	16
distal	M3	9
Common peroneal (motor)		
proximal	M1 (3)	12
intermediate	M1 (3)	13
distal	M1 (3)	12
Tibial (motor)		
proximal	M1 (4)	13
intermediate	M1 (4)	15
distal	M1 (4)	12
Tibial (sensory)		
proximal	S2	15
intermediate	S2	14
distal	S2	12

For grading of recovery see page 303.

brachial plexus and the prognosis is uncertain or bad. It can also cause dislocation of the shoulder, fracture of the upper end of the humerus or of the adjoining part of the scapula, or fracture-dislocation, any one of which can cause more or less extensive paralysis of the arm. Yet these latter nerve lesions are comparatively benign (p. 82); their management is conservative. In distinguishing between these two types of nerve damage—with such different prognoses—some help may be obtained from enquiry into the nature of the fall. A young man tossed off a motor cycle and landing on his shoulder suffers a traction injury of the brachial plexus; an elderly person falling in the street is likely to suffer an injury of the shoulder and a favourable type of nerve damage. But if someone falls down a flight of stairs either type of injury can occur. Although in the recently injured patient accurate examination of the muscles round the shoulder may not be possible, the clinical evidence may help. If the clavicle has been broken or if there is a telltale swelling above it then almost certainly there has been a traction injury of the brachial plexus. By contrast, if the paralysis of the arm does not correspond to one or other of the patterns of supraclavicular brachial plexus injury that have been described (pp. 180-184), then the probability is that the patient has a benign infraclavicular paralysis, and this diagnosis is certain if there is an injury in the shoulder region.

A patient may suffer two injuries, one of which is overlooked for a time. An unhappy example of this is shown in Figure **3**, 18 (p. 50).

TABLE XXXIX—Delay compatible with useful recovery after repair (author's series)

NERVE AND LEVEL	CHILDREN 16 years of age or younger			ADULTS		
	Number of patients	Best results recorded after repair	Delay (months)	Number of patients	Best results recorded after repair	Delay (months)
Ulnar						
axillary	—	—	—	—	—	—
mid-arm and elbow	—	—	—	7	M4 : S3	13
forearm	—	—	—	5	M3 : S4	13
wrist	1	M3 : S4	13	5	M2 : S3	15
palmar	—	—	—	—	—	—
Median						
axillary	—	—	—	—	—	—
mid-arm and elbow	—	—	—	5	M3 : S3	24
forearm	1	M3 : S2	22	5	M3 : S3	24
wrist	5	M3 : S3	48	13	M3 : S3	48
palmar	1	M4 : S4	28	—	—	—
Radial	—	—	—	2	M3 : S3	13
Common peroneal						
upper thigh	—	—	—	3	M3+no toe-raising }	16
lower thigh	—	—	—	4	M4+apparatus }	11
Tibial						
upper thigh	—	—	—	3	calf M4 : S3	16
lower thigh	—	—	—	4	calf M4 : S2	14

Sometimes there are multiple wounds, common enough in warfare, but by no means rare in civil practice. The distribution of the paralysis may enable the site of damage to be localized accurately. A tender swelling in the course of a nerve provides welcome evidence of the site of injury. Yet I have sometimes been obliged so to plan an exploration that the nerve was exposed at more than one possible site of injury, and I have found the lesion at an unexpected level. It is also worth remembering that a nerve can be injured in two or more places (Fig. **2**, 3, p. 11; and Fig. **15**, 10, p. 262).

THE TYPE OF PARALYSIS

Neurapraxia

It is important that this, the most benign form of nerve injury, should be recognized. It does not occur when the wound has been caused by a sharp object, and it is rare with lacerations; but in most other kinds of injury it is common. The features of neurapraxia have already been fully described (pp. 32-36). The paralysis is almost invariably partial, motor paralysis predominating; nerve conduction below the lesion persists and so does normal electrical excitability of the paralysed muscles. Thus, examination of nerve conduction after the third day and of the strength-duration curves after the second week can be crucial. Once neurapraxia has been eliminated we are concerned with those lesions in which there is partial or complete degeneration of the nerve.

Complete Paralysis

When the signs of this are unequivocal there is no difficulty, but it is possible to label paralysis as incomplete when it is in fact total. There are four sources of error:

1. *Trick movements.* The various kinds of trick movement have already been described (p. 37), but it is worth recalling one as an example; the supplementary flexor action of the abductor pollicis longus at the wrist, which may give the impression that combined lesions of the median and ulnar nerves above the elbow are incomplete (Fig. **11**, 35, p. 201).

2. *Anomalous innervation of muscle.* The most familiar example is in complete lesions of the median nerve where the persistence of power in the flexor pollicis brevis is due to its being innervated by the ulnar nerve. It may be possible to demonstrate this by stimulation of the ulnar nerve at the elbow, but unless this produces a contraction in the flexor pollicis brevis it will be necessary to resort to injection of a local anaesthetic into the ulnar nerve, using the technique described on page 55.

3. *A small area of sensory loss.* Sometimes the cutaneous distribution of a nerve is unusually small; indeed, the area supplied exclusively by the superficial radial nerve may be non-existent. If some time has elapsed since the injury, shrinkage of the area of sensory loss will always have occurred as a result of ingrowth of nerve fibres from the surrounding, normally innervated, parts. In neither of these cases will anaesthetization of the affected nerve produce any change in the size of the area of sensory disturbance; it may then be concluded that so far as sensibility is concerned the nerve is totally interrupted. If, however, the small size of the area is due to recovery—which can occur only if sufficient time has elapsed—blocking the affected nerve will produce a larger area of sensory loss. Moreover, the clinical features of returning sensibility are usually distinctive. Recovery manifests itself by recession of the *proximal* boundary of sensory loss. Furthermore, when recovery is occurring, pain sensibility returns well in advance of tactile sensibility, and the response to painful stimuli has that peculiarly unpleasant quality described as over-reaction (p. 43). Blocking the affected nerve is conclusive; if recovery is in progress the area of sensory loss after anaesthetization will be much larger, perhaps of almost normal dimensions.

4. *A positive Tinel's sign.* Even when a nerve has been completely severed a certain number of sensory fibres make their way across the gap, and sensory fibres can also grow into a completely decentralized distal stump of a nerve from adjoining blood vessels. Both can give a positive Tinel's sign and its presence should not be accepted as a contraindication to exploration.

Only when all these sources of error have been eliminated can it be decided that a paralysis is in fact incomplete.

Partial Paralysis

The theoretically possible combinations of neurotmesis, axonotmesis, neurapraxia and normally conducting nerve are bewildering. Fortunately, in practice, the significant combinations are few.

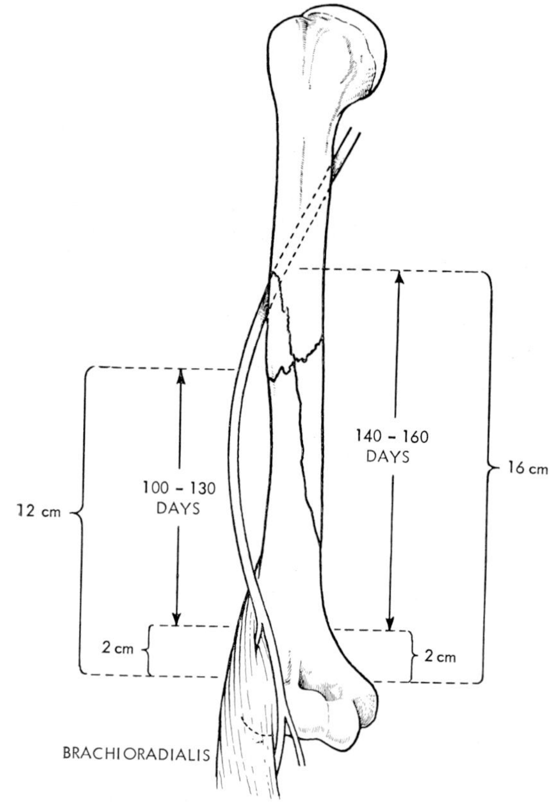

FIG. **14,** 1. *Left:* calculation of the time that must elapse before signs of recovery can be expected after a transverse fracture of the shaft of the humerus causing a degenerative lesion of the radial nerve. *Right:* the same for an oblique fracture. The nerve to brachioradialis enters the muscle about 2 cm above the lateral epicondyle.

Missile wounds and traction injuries can cause bizarre mixtures of nerve injury, and one component may be neurapraxia. It simplifies the elucidation of these injuries very considerably if time is allowed, usually six to eight weeks, for recovery to occur in that part of the nerve that has not undergone Wallerian degeneration. If this is done—and local conditions compel it if there is an open wound to be treated—we may confine our attention to the partial paralyses in which there is no element of neurapraxia. Clinically, and that is all we are concerned with here, a partial paralysis can take one of three forms:

1. *Funicular.* If there is a partial lesion of a nerve a short way proximal to a point at which an important branch or branches arise, the paralysis may be confined to the distribution of the branches, or the branches may be spared and the paralysis is limited to the more distal distribution of the nerve. It is much the same where a nerve is about to bifurcate. A small wound at the wrist, for example, may injure the terminal sensory or motor division of the ulnar nerve alone, and the same can happen with the median nerve. The paralysis is complete within an anatomically definable part of the distribution of the nerve.

2. *Generalized.* It will be recalled (p. 5) that in the proximal part of a nerve trunk, nerve fibres are very much mixed up in relation to their ultimate distribution. Thus a partial lesion of, say, the ulnar nerve in the upper arm will produce an effect throughout the whole distribution of the nerve; Sherren (1908) found that up to one-third of the thickness of a nerve had to be severed before any motor or sensory deficit could be detected clinically. Thus, if a proximally situated wound has caused diffuse paresis of a nerve the damage done must be considerable and in the cases I have seen it amounted to at least one-half.

3. *Modal or dissociated.* This unusual type of nerve involvement is produced by blunt injuries, by traction and by slow compression or friction as in entrapment lesions of the median or ulnar nerves. In general the motor fibres are the most vulnerable. Nevertheless loss of sensibility without motor paralysis has been seen in ulnar lesions though it has not yet been satisfactorily explained.

THE CAUSE OF THE NERVE INJURY

Even after the extent of the paralysis has been defined and neurapraxia has been excluded, the

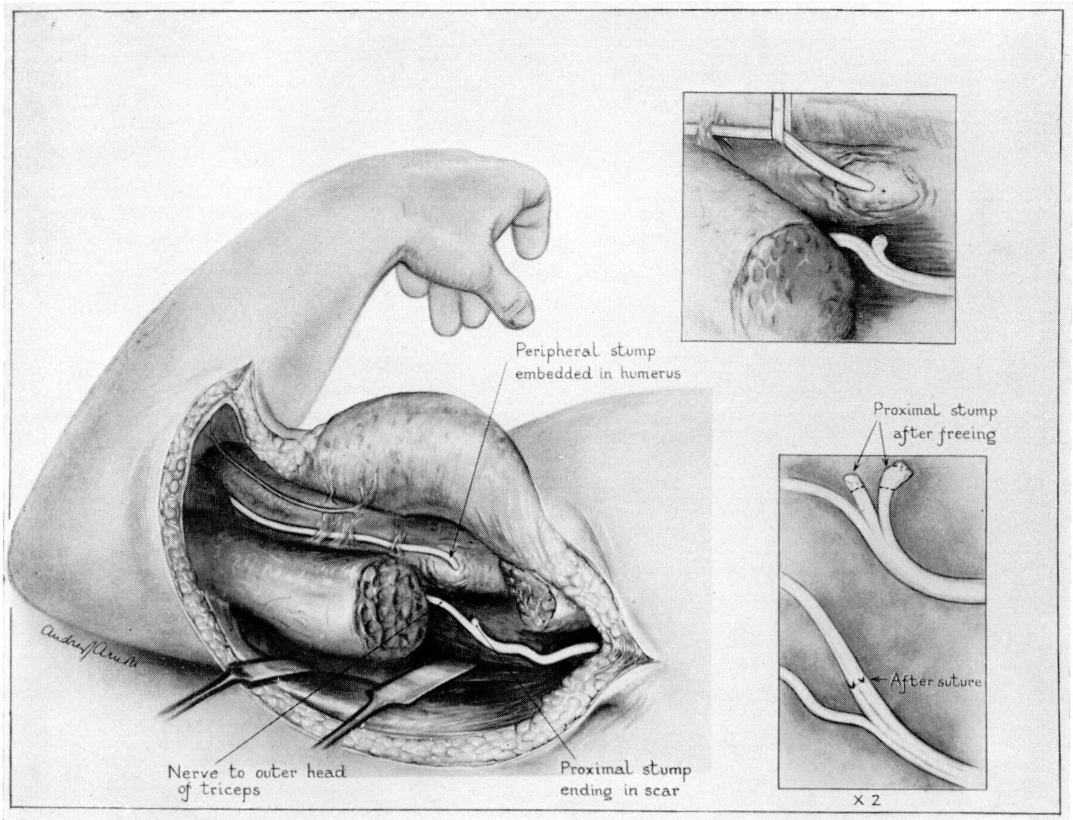

FIG. **14,** 2. This radial nerve had been caught between and severed by the fragments of the shaft of the humerus. Repair by suture. (Reproduced by kind permission from *J. Am. med. Ass.*, 1947, **135,** 691.)

surgeon is influenced as much by the nature of the injury as by the distribution of the paralysis in deciding whether the nerve should be explored. In Chapters 5 to 9 the indications for intervention have been discussed, but in view of the importance of nerve injuries caused by open wounds, traction, and fractures, a recapitulation is given overleaf, in tabular form, of what is generally and exceptionally advisable.

Table XL overleaf.

TABLE XL—Indications for operation: open wounds, traction injuries, skeletal injuries

TYPE OF INJURY	AFFECTED NERVES	APPROPRIATE TREATMENT	REASON	EXCEPTIONS	REFERENCES Chapter	REFERENCES Pages
INCISED, LACERATED AND MISSILE WOUNDS	All except lumbo-sacral plexus; and posterior tibial and plantar nerves	Exploration	9 : 1 probability of complete or partial division	1. Perhaps if there is *clinical* evidence of partial division	5 15	68 262
				2. If the interval since the injury is such that spontaneous recovery might become apparent within six weeks		
				3. If there is already evidence of spontaneous recovery		
				4. Injury of middle and lower trunks of brachial plexus—possibly	11	197
				5. Injuries of lumbo-sacral plexus		
				6. Posterior tibial nerve except in children, and	12	220
				7. Plantar nerves	12	221
TRACTION INJURIES	Brachial plexus: supraclavicular	In infraganglionic lesions, exploration to discover whether the nerve trunks are in continuity	To establish the prognosis: if the damage is supraganglionic it is hopeless anyway	Birth injuries: no exploration	8	131
	Radial, ulnar and median nerves	Exploration	To establish the prognosis, and in the case of the median nerve to attempt repair		16	295
	Sciatic nerve at the hip	No exploration	Useless	If there is a large bony fragment, i.e. a fracture-dislocation: explore	12	226

	Common peroneal at the knee	Exploration	To discover whether the nerve has been ruptured, and thus establish the prognosis: repair occasionally successful		12	227
NERVE INJURIES DUE TO FRACTURES	Brachial plexus: infraclavicular	No exploration	Spontaneous recovery almost invariably good	If signs of recovery are overdue	5	86
	Radial	No exploration	4 : 1 probability of spontaneous recovery	1. Explore if recovery is overdue	See Figs 14, 1 and 14, 2	
				2. Oblique fracture of lowest third of the humerus	5	84
	Median	No exploration	As above	1. Any fracture near the elbow	5	84
				2. At the wrist if recovery is overdue	5	80
	Ulnar	No exploration	As above	Any fracture involving the medial side of the elbow	5	84
	Posterior interosseous	No exploration	As above			
	Sciatic at the hip	Exploration probably worth while	The nerve may be trapped or otherwise embarrassed by bony fragments		5 12	86, 88 226
	Sciatic damaged by a fracture of the femoral shaft	Exploration	The time that must elapse before signs of spontaneous recovery could appear is dangerously long, if it turns out that repair is necessary		5	88
	Anterior and posterior tibial nerves	No exploration unless there are irritative symptoms	Spontaneous recovery probable		12	227

15. Operative Treatment: Exploration, Suture, Neurolysis

J'assurai le Roi que c'étoit l'opération qui faisoit le plus de peine au Chirurgien, et que s'il témoignoit de l'empressement de faire voir son adresse, c'étoit sur les opérations qui demandent de la délicatesse, et non pas sur celle-là qui . . . devroit être faite par un Boucher que par un Chirurgien.

Pierre Dionis
Cours d'opérations de Chirurgie
6me Edition Paris 1765

EXPLORATION

The wound. Unless primary suture is the proper treatment, a subject we shall presently be considering in detail, exploration of a nerve is not undertaken until the primary wound is soundly healed, and the tissues at the site of injury are supple.[1] The only possible exception to this, a very rare one, is in a case of causalgia with clinical evidence of complete interruption of the nerve as explained on page 150.

Position on the operation table. This requires forethought, so that the limb is not only conveniently sited for exposure of the nerve, but so that the position that may be necessary for suture—with, say, the elbow or knee flexed—is at least equally comfortable. This final position will need to be studied with particular care if the intention is to use an operation microscope.

The field of operation and towelling. The preparation of the field of operation should be generous. If there is the remotest possibility that autologous nerve grafting may be required the part from which the nerve graft might be taken is also prepared. In the upper limb this means a field of operation that includes the shoulder, because the favourite donor nerve is the medial cutaneous nerve of the forearm; the dissection needed to expose a sufficient length of it may have to extend almost into the axilla. The nature of the injury will suggest whether the question of grafting is likely to arise.

[1] That nerve repair can be carried out while a wound is still granulating was shown by Lebedenko (1943); but this is hardly justified even by the direst exigencies of war. He was more concerned about the wait-and-see policy of some of his colleagues.

Anaesthesia

1. General anaesthesia. This is usually preferred. If the anaesthetist uses a muscle relaxant he should be asked not to inject it until after the pneumatic tourniquet has been inflated: otherwise there is a risk that electrical stimulation of the nerve may fail to give the proper response.

2. Regional anaesthesia. I have no experience of this: the only possible objection to anaesthetization of the brachial plexus or to spinal anaesthesia is if the surgeon is anxious to use electrical stimulation of the nerve as a means of assessing sensory conductivity (p. 252).

3. Local anaesthesia. This form of anaesthesia was thrust on us during the Second World War by the volume of work and the shortage of anaesthetists. We used it in preference to regional anaesthesia because we were anxious to employ sensory stimulation when there was a possibility that the damaged nerve was in continuity.

Provided that the local anaesthetic solution is dilute—for example, 0·5 per cent lignocaine—and that adrenalin, one in 200,000 parts, is added so that the rate of absorption of the local anaesthetic is slow, and so that oozing from minor blood vessels is checked, extensive exposures are possible. On many occasions we used up to 200 ml of this solution, and there were no ill effects; but the recommended maximum for a patient weighing 70 kg is 100 ml. Local insensibility persists for at least three hours. The only contraindications are dense scarring, and a patient whose apprehension is such that it defies the usual pre-operative sedation.

If the injections are planned appropriately, conduction in main nerve trunks is unaffected (it is notoriously difficult to inject a local anaesthetic into the substance of a deeply situated nerve; and the superficial ones are easily avoided), and even in their branches for a time. However, the nerve to be explored should be exposed as quickly as possible proximal to the lesion, so that electrical stimulation can be carried out before the local anaesthetic has seeped into the small motor branches of the nerve. At this stage the lesion itself is not exposed because this can be time-consuming and may itself suppress conduction.

Exsanguination of the Limb Under General or Regional Anaesthesia

Whenever possible the exposure of the nerve should be made in a bloodless field; even then it can be difficult. A sterile rubber pressure bandage is applied first, and removed the moment the pneumatic tourniquet has been inflated. The proper pressure for the latter is about 180 mg of mercury in the upper limb, and 220 in the thigh; but much depends on the adiposity of the part. These pressures may safely be maintained for an hour and 40 minutes in the upper limb and two hours in the lower limb. If the complexity of the operation is such that the dissection has not been completed within these time-limits the pneumatic tourniquet should be released at the appointed time: re-establishment of the circulation is permitted for five minutes, during which time bleeding from small vessels can be arrested by diathermy; then the exsanguination of the limb can be repeated.

If the initial exsanguination proves faulty there is only one thing to be done: start again.

There are circumstances in which a pneumatic tourniquet cannot be used but a rubber bandage can because it can be sterilized;[1] for example, in the exploration of a nerve in the middle of the arm. There is no way of judging the pressure exerted by a rubber bandage used as a tourniquet, and cases of pressure paralysis have occurred (p. 133). The time-limits should be reduced to one hour and an hour and 20 minutes for the upper and lower limbs respectively.

Lastly, there are situations in which no exsanguination by pressure is possible, as in exposure of the brachial plexus, or of the sciatic nerve in the buttock. Here it is helpful to infiltrate the tissues with 1/200,000 adrenalin in normal saline solution. It is dangerous to use adrenalin if the patient is inhaling halothane; there is a risk of ventricular fibrillation. Whenever adrenalin is used even the smallest vessels require coagulation. Later, when the vasoconstriction has worn off, they can bleed vigorously.

[1] A sterile disposable pneumatic cuff has recently become available, but it is perhaps a little too early to judge its worth.

Instruments

The ordinary soft-tissue instruments suffice until the surgeon is nearing the nerve; after that he will need more delicate ones. Here we will consider the few required during exposure of the nerve; later (p. 273), those needed for nerve suture. Dura mater forceps are the best for picking up tissues other than the nerve and blood vessels. Watchmaker's forceps (Fig. **15**, 19, p. 267) are ideal for picking up the nerve when a blunt hook cannot be used; they seize no more than the epineurium. The most delicate pressure forceps are needed when dealing with blood vessels near a nerve, and the finest ligature material—not diathermy. But apart from this diathermy is indispensable. The gentleness and the thorough haemostasis that characterize neurosurgical technique are as necessary in dealing with the peripheral as with the central nervous system.

Nerve stimulator. It is astonishing that in this age of technological idolatry, exploration of nerves is still being performed without the aid of this instrument. Our surgical grandparents used a faradic coil; it is cheap, reliable, safe and can be calibrated sufficiently for a domain in which great precision is unnecessary. Any instrument will do that delivers a stimulus of a duration not exceeding a thousandth of a second, of controllable intensity, and preferably with an interval of half a second between the pulses. Bipolar stimulation should always be employed. The special forceps shown in Figure **15**, 19, p. 267, is convenient in many situations, but for very delicate work separate electrodes with fine points are necessary; diathermy needles are ideal, provided they are easily distinguishable from the electrode being used for diathermy. Electrical stimulation has four applications.

1. *Proximal stimulation of the nerve trunk, which is carried out before the lesion is exposed.* If the operation is being performed under local anaesthesia the nerve must first be anaesthetized by the injection of one per cent lignocaine, a few centimetres proximal to the point of application

of the electrodes. This, however, makes it impossible to study distal, sensory stimulation, and if the latter is contemplated (the reasons why it is rarely used are given later) it should be carried out first. The value of proximal stimulation is illustrated by the following case history.

A child of 3 cut her hypothenar eminence with broken glass: the wound was closed with three stitches. Seven weeks later it was discovered that there was ulnar paralysis. After a period of Micawberism (which, by chance, turned out to be justified) she came under our care, five months after the injury. The hypothenar muscles were normal, all other ulnar-innervated muscles distal to them paralysed, and there was diminution of sensibility in the palmar distribution of the nerve. The nerve was exposed proximal to the lesion and stimulated electrically. A weak current produced powerful contraction of the hypothenar muscles and moderate contraction of all the apparently paralysed muscles.

Clearly, spontaneous regeneration across an 'unaided union' (see p. 20) was well advanced. The wound was closed and good recovery followed. In an older patient this information could have been obtained by electromyography, though the needle would have had to be inserted into each group of paralysed muscles.

In this and in similar cases the motor fibres had made their way through the lesion and reached their destinations, and voluntary power would soon have become apparent clinically. But there was no certainty of this and exploration was necessary because there had been an incised wound. A positive response of this sort can be expected only if sufficient time has elapsed between injury and exploration to permit spontaneously regenerating motor fibres to reach the more proximal of the paralysed muscles. If there is, say, a proximal lesion of the sciatic nerve a negative response at any time up to 300 days would have no significance, because a period of this order must elapse before outgrowing motor fibres could make effective connection with the most proximal muscle, that is, the gastrocnemius. Such lengthy delay is harmful if the lesion turns out to be one that requires repair. Hence, it would be advantageous if some means could be found of detecting regenerating fibres distal to the lesion at a much earlier stage; sensory fibres could provide the necessary information.

2. *Distal stimulation of the nerve trunk*. If the nerve is exposed under local anaesthesia, distal to the site of damage, care being taken to avoid injection into the nerve itself, it is a simple matter to stimulate the unanaesthetized nerve and for the patient to record his sensations, if any. However, even in complete neurotmesis a certain number of regenerating fibres are usually present distal to the lesion within weeks of the injury. These fibres have either jumped the gap at the site of damage or grown in from surrounding blood vessels. Thus, if a sufficiently strong stimulus is used, some sort of response is likely to be obtained. The only significant result is absence of response on application of a strong stimulus, as in the following case.

Immediately after an injection of sulphanilamide into the buttock, a woman suffered great pain and paralysis of sciatic distribution. She was referred to us 320 days later because there was persistent paralysis in the tibial distribution of the nerve. There had barely been time for regenerating fibres to reach the gastrocnemius, and electromyographic examination was negative. The nerve was exposed under local anaesthesia in the proximal part of the popliteal fossa. There was no response whatever on strong electrical stimulation. Exposure of the lesion revealed total destruction of the tibial division of the sciatic nerve.

However, the field of application of this test is limited. It is unfortunate that the very high threshold of regenerating fibres has so far frustrated attempts to detect them by percutaneous conduction methods (but see p. 66).

3. *Identification of tissues*. During exposure of the lesion the surgeon may find himself in an anatomical jungle. Strands of tissue may be branches of the nerve; they may be only fibrous adhesions. They sometimes appear indistinguishable and here electrical stimulation is useful, though this usually applies only to motor branches proximal to the lesion.

4. Lastly, there is *electrical identification of funiculi preparatory to suture* (Hakstian, 1968), which will be considered later.

Exposure of the Damaged Nerve

Because it is usually wise to expose the lesion by working towards it from anatomically normal regions the incision must be generous. It is best to start with a long incision; extensions of a short one can so easily be untidy and inadequate. The recommended lines of incision are shown in Figures **15**, 2; **15**, 4; **15**, 5; **15**, 7 and **15**, 9, the surgeon choosing whatever segment of a line is appropriate in a particular case.

If there is a scar at the site of nerve injury, if there is possibly little tissue between it and the nerve, and especially if the scar is adherent to underlying structures there should be two incisions at first, one proximal, the other distal to the scar. An incision at the level of the scar could damage the underlying nerve if it is near the surface. It is safer to expose the nerve proximally and distally before completing the incision. If an area has been covered with a split-skin graft it is usually best to skirt it, provided that the preliminary proximal and distal exposures indicate that there will be a sufficient thickness of tissue beneath the graft when the exposure of the nerve is completed. If an extensive wound has been covered by a flap or pedicle skin-graft it does not matter whether the incision follows one of the previous scars or goes straight across the graft. The first is better cosmetically; the second involves less dissection.

No surgeon should embark on the exposure of a peripheral nerve unless he is sure that in any situation where anatomical relations have not been disturbed he can find the nerve or nerves requiring attention by the unhesitating use of a sharp knife, without recourse to the fumbling blunt dissection that betrays the indifferent anatomist. Furthermore, he must be capable of recognizing the nerve when he sees it.

The gross appearance of a normal nerve is so familiar as not usually to be confused with that of any other structure. Yet astonishing mistakes have been made. I have known the median nerve in the forearm used as a graft for repair of the severed flexor tendon of a finger; on several occasions I have exposed nerves that have been sutured to tendons. We cannot be too circumspect in identifying the structures we display. The ivory colour of a normal nerve, its funiculi and its blood vessels should distinguish it from all other elongated objects. A degenerate nerve looks different, slightly more translucent, purplish grey, sometimes smaller than normal, and the funiculi may not be easily distinguishable beneath the epineurium.

The nerve stimulator is constantly required, sometimes to identify a normal nerve and so exclude it from the search. Electrical stimulation of the damaged nerve should invariably precede exposure of the lesion because, however gentle the dissection, it may impair conductivity, and thus valuable information would be lost.

Having defined the nerve proximally and distally the operator carries the dissection towards the site of damage. If the injury is a simple one this will be easy, but if scar tissue is abundant he will need much patience and perseverance. In dissecting along the surface of the nerve it is better to pick up the surrounding tissues rather than the nerve itself. Tapes moistened with saline solution may be passed beneath the nerve on either side of the lesion and used as retractors. If the lesion is at a level where branches arise, the scalpel should cut proximally to distally, so that if a branch is encountered the knife will be carried away along its surface. Cutting in the opposite direction may easily sever a branch. There is a hazard peculiar to the upper forearm: there may be anastomoses between the median and ulnar nerves (Fig. **15**, 1). As the centre of interest is approached it may be found that the damaged part of the nerve is adherent to an important blood vessel, and the surgeon may find himself working along a narrowing cleft between the two. If the risk of damaging one or the other has to be taken the vessel should be spared; the severity of the nerve injury will certainly prove to be such that repair will be necessary.

Exposure of Individual Nerves

Upper Limb

Supraclavicular brachial plexus. If the aim is to expose the plexus thoroughly the L-shaped incision (Fig. **15**, 2) is the best. However, as has been pointed out earlier (p. 193), exploration is usually confined to the upper trunk, and an incision in the line of it suffices. If there is a possibility of the exposure's being continued below the clavicle—as in neurovascular injuries at this level—the straight incision is easily extended distally. If no more than limited exposure of the upper trunk is required a suitably sited collar incision is advantageous cosmetically.

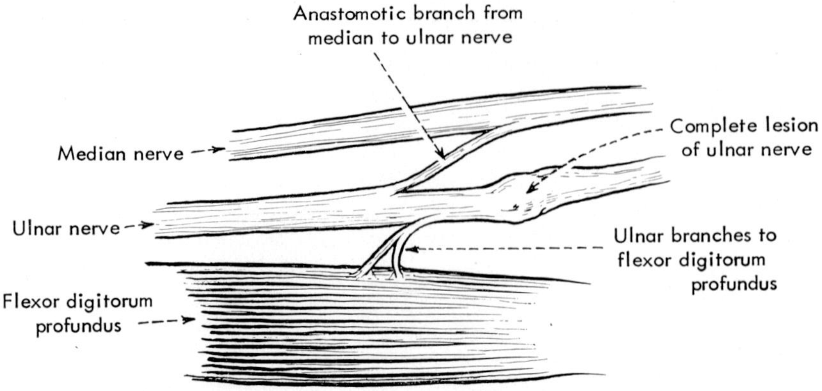

FIG. **15,** 1. This patient presented with an ulnar paralysis that was complete except for some action in the first and second interossei. These two muscles contracted on stimulation of the ulnar nerve at the wrist. The wound was near the elbow, and on exploration a complete lesion of the ulnar nerve was found: but at a point 2 cm distal to the lesion the ulnar nerve was joined by a branch from the median. Stimulation at and distal to this level evoked contraction of the first and second dorsal interossei and of the adductor pollicis.

When the L-shaped incision is preferred, its horizontal limb should lie about 2 cm below the subcutaneous surface of the clavicle. It is deepened to the surfaces of the sterno-cleido-mastoid and pectoralis major and the triangular flap is dissected off the muscles, so that all lymphatic tissue and fat are included in it. The external jugular vein comes into view and is ligated just above the clavicle. The next landmark is the posterior belly of the omohyoid, which is removed. The transverse cervical vessels are identified and ligated as far medially and laterally as possible, the intervening segments being excised. If the sterno-cleido-mastoid is well developed its clavicular head is cut transversely a few centimetres above the clavicle. At this stage the scalenus anterior appears, and pulsation of the internal jugular vein is visible in the deep cleft between this muscle and the sterno-cleido-mastoid. The next step is to identify the plexus. If the lesion lies low in the posterior triangle, so that the nerve trunks distal to it cannot be seen satisfactorily even when the shoulder is strongly depressed, the incision has to be extended distally in the direction of the coracoid process, as for exposure of the infraclavicular plexus. (This is when the straight incision is preferable.) The clavicle is then dealt with by one of the methods described below.

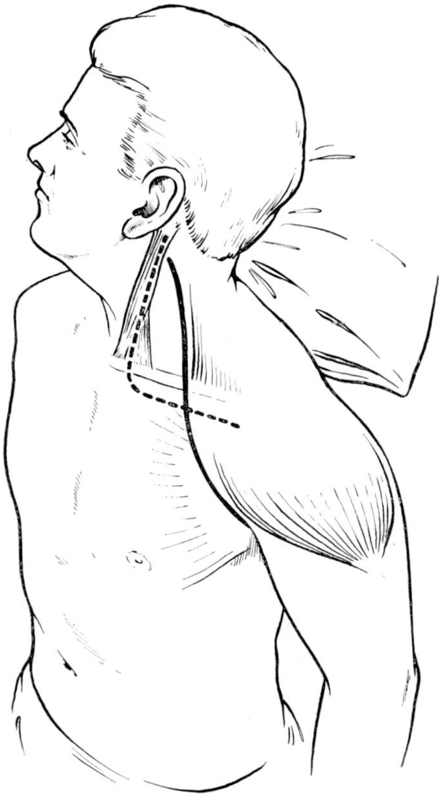

FIG. **15,** 2. The heavy line shows the incision for complete exposure of the brachial plexus. The L incision—broken line—gives a good exposure of the supraclavicular plexus. If exploration only of C5, 6 and 7 is contemplated a collar incision suffices.

If thorough exposure of the lower trunk of the plexus is required, the tendon of scalenus anterior is severed just above the first rib, care being taken first to identify the phrenic nerve and, on the left side, the thoracic duct.

In closing the supraclavicular wound the tissues are brought together layer by layer, care being taken to approximate the platysma; otherwise a thick ugly scar may develop.

Infraclavicular brachial plexus. Exposure of the infraclavicular part of the plexus is straightforward, but separation of the nerve trunks from the vessels may prove exacting. The exposure is shown in Figure **15**, 3, but there is no need to cut through the whole of the pectoralis major if the lesion is situated distally. Should it be necessary to sever pectoralis minor the tendon of the muscle is first isolated, and then cut through about 1 cm medial to the coracoid process. When these two muscles are retracted medially their nerve supplies, unless irreparably damaged by the injury, must be respected. The medial pectoral nerve is rarely in danger; the lateral runs some risk of being stretched because it arises from the outer cord of the plexus. If the lesion is high in the axilla it may not be possible to identify the proximal components of the plexus without extending the exposure above the clavicle. The incision is continued proximally. There are two ways of dealing with the clavicle, and it will quickly become apparent which is preferable in a particular case. Double ligatures are tied round the cephalic vein near its termination, and the vessel is cut between them. All the

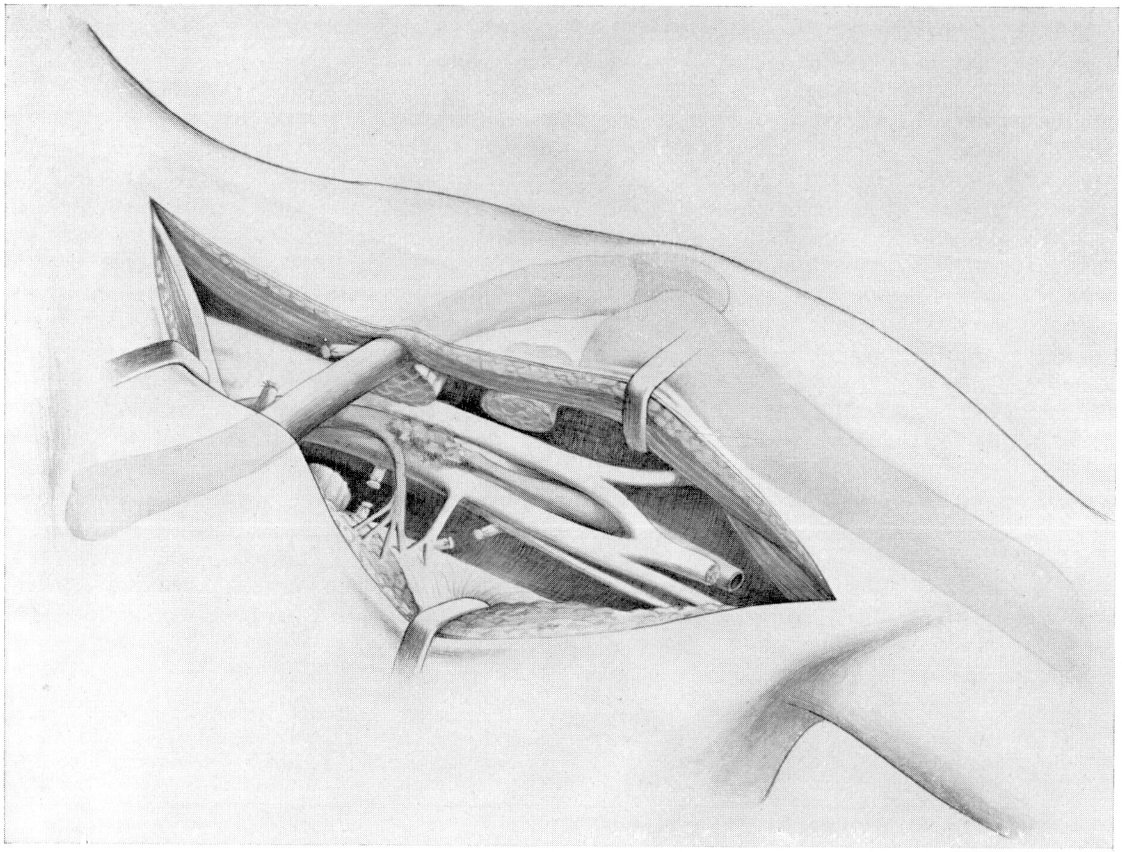

FIG. **15,** 3. Exposure of the infraclavicular brachial plexus.

tissues round the bone are cut through, including the subclavius. There is always brisk bleeding, and some time may be spent in controlling it. All the soft tissues are stripped subperiosteally, laterally and medially. The bare clavicle now spans a ravine, and the surgeon may find it no hindrance to his subsequent manoeuvres. If he does, the middle third of the clavicle is excised and discarded. I soon abandoned oblique osteotomy with subsequent internal fixation of the bone.

If, after defining the extent of the lesion, the operator finds that separation of the nerve and vessels is going to be a delicate affair, he must decide whether the lesion is one in which resection and suture will be necessary, or whether the continuity of nervous tissue is such that spontaneous recovery is probable. In other words he must make a decision which, in other situations, is not usually taken until the damaged part has been completely freed by dissection. The various steps described on page 262 under 'Identification of the Nature of the Damage' are taken without the nerve trunks being first separated from the axillary vessels. If it is obvious that resection and suture will be required, the dissection between vessels on the one hand and nerve trunks on the other is then carried out in such a way that if dangerously close adhesions are encountered some of the nerve tissue is left adherent to the vessels; the dissection is made at the expense of the nerve trunks. Although there are no ill effects after ligating the axillary vein above and below the area of damage, it is unjustifiable to endanger the axillary artery. If there is reasonable continuity of the cords of the plexus, and especially if there is a positive response on electrical stimulation, the operation is brought to a close.

Exploration of the infraclavicular region may be dictated as much by damage to blood vessels as by injury of the plexus, in which case the caveat given above does not apply; for examples of such neurovascular injuries see Figures **6**, 2 and **6**, 3 (pp. 93 and 94).

Musculocutaneous nerve. In exploring the infrequent lesions of this nerve the approach is from above; it is the same as for exposure of the lower part of the axillary plexus, and the pectoralis major is cut as much as is required to expose the outer cord of the plexus in normal surroundings.

Radial nerve. It is fortunate that injuries of the proximal part of this nerve are uncommon because the exposure is difficult. Two incisions are required. The first is inside the axilla, in the line of the plexus, at which level the posterior cord is identified. The nerve to the medial head of the triceps is found in the distal part of the wound. The second incision is on the outer side of the arm, following the usual line of exposure of the radial nerve in the spiral groove; but it is carried higher and farther back than usual, along the posterior border of the deltoid near its insertion. The lateral head of the triceps is reflected posteriorly. A useful guide to the line of detachment is provided by the posterior cutaneous nerve of the forearm which, along with small branches of the profunda artery, emerges at the anterior border of the lateral head. The reflection of this muscle is continued until the radial nerve is found in the spiral groove. The nerve is then traced[1] proximally, and the operator is plagued by bleeding from small branches of the profunda vessels if not by the main vessels themselves. As the nerve is followed upwards it is found to emerge from a tunnel, the familiar *triangular space* of anatomical textbooks, which is bounded posteriorly by the long head of the triceps, superiorly by the teres major and latissimus dorsi as they approach their insertions, and anteriorly by the shaft of the humerus. In this region the nerve supplying mainly the outer head of the triceps is encountered. Gentle teasing of the connective tissue inside the tunnel —which can be difficult and not so gentle if there is much scarring—leads to the medial exposure. If the nerve is found to be severed inside the tunnel it is impossible to repair it there. Because little is gained by mobilization of the nerve, even down to the elbow, anterior transposition of its distal part is obligatory. The nerve is freed well down to the elbow, its cutane-

[1] It is, perhaps, desirable to define this word. *Tracing* a nerve is exposing it just sufficiently to reveal its course. *Freeing* or *mobilizing* a nerve means severing everything that tethers it, except its essential branches. The latter operation is required only as a preliminary to repair. Mobilization impairs the blood supply of the nerve and upsets its axial orientation. The manoeuvre is fully discussed on page 267.

ous branches being sacrificed, and then drawn up through an anterior tunnel made by burrowing between the anterior surface of the brachialis and the deep surface of the biceps. After closure of the postero-lateral incision the repair is carried out on the medial side of the upper arm with the elbow flexed about 90 degrees and the shoulder abducted no more than is necessary to allow sufficient access. Unless it is possible to suture the nerve without difficulty it is best not to attempt it, provided that the muscles required for extensor tendon transplantation are available.

The commonest type of damage to the radial nerve is in the spiral groove. The site of injury is, as usual, approached from each end and the proximal part of the approach is the postero-lateral exposure that has just been described. The lateral head of the triceps is reflected posteriorly until the nerve is found winding round the shaft of the humerus. The distal part of the exposure follows the anterior border of the brachioradialis and the nerve is discovered here by dissecting along the deep surface of this muscle. The two reaches of the nerve are then traced towards the site of damage, where the scarring is often formidable.

The exposure for injuries of the radial nerve near the elbow and for those of the posterior interosseous nerve differ in one important respect. The proximal part of the incision (Fig. **15**, 4) follows the lateral supracondylar ridge; it continues distally straight down the forearm along the dorsal border of the radial extensor muscles, ending some 9 to 10 cm below the epicondyle. The origins of brachioradialis and the long radial extensor of the wrist are detached from the humerus and turned antero-medially, care being taken not to get lost in the fibres of the underlying brachialis. If on account of extensive scarring there is a risk of this, the incision should be extended proximally until the radial nerve is exposed in normal surroundings; it is then traced distally. The septum that separates the short from the long radial extensor of the wrist can be recognized without difficulty and the incision is deepened on the anterior (volar) surface of the septum. This brings the fibres of the supinator into view.

In exploration of the posterior interosseous nerve it is particularly important to stimulate the main trunk—that is to say the most distal part of the radial nerve—before the damaged part of the nerve is exposed. Contraction of the long radial extensor will show where its posterior border is situated, and it is along this line that the distal part of the incision is made. Stimulation may also provide evidence of re-innervation of some of the apparently paralysed muscles. The distal part of the nerve is exposed by following the surface of the supinator proximally and medially, and there is no objection to incising this muscle delicately, at right angles to the direction of its fibres, in the line of the nerve as it winds round the neck of the radius. The nerve will speedily become visible. Dissection of the nerve from above downwards is straightforward

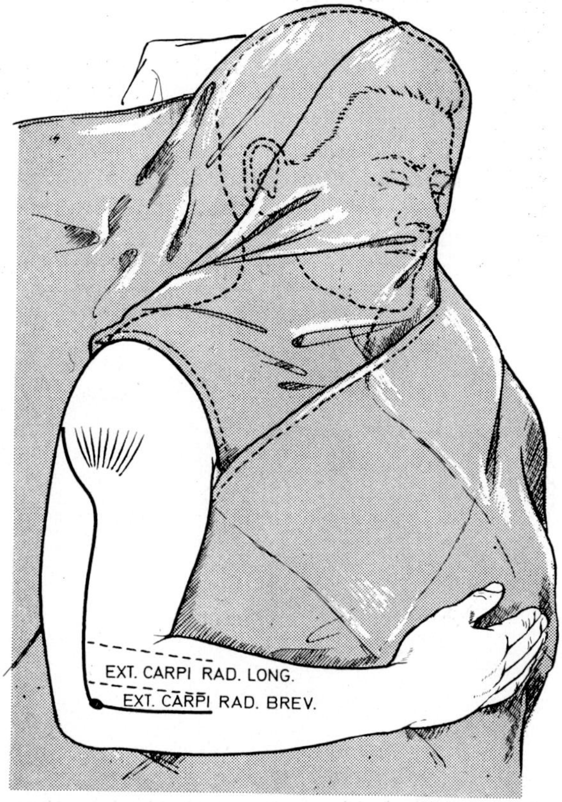

FIG. **15,** 4. Incision for exposure of the lower two-thirds of the radial nerve and, distally, of the posterior interosseous nerve. The distal dissection should pass posterior to the brachioradialis and extensor carpi radialis longus if the site of suture is near the elbow. Otherwise it may follow the anterior border of the brachioradialis.

though care may be needed to avoid injuring the branches to the radial extensors. If the nerve has been severed everything depends on the state of the distal stump: can an appropriate resection of it be made proximal to the tunnel in the supinator? If this is possible then repair will be satisfactory because closure of the gap by mobilization of the proximal stump will present no difficulty.

The final step in the operation, the nerve

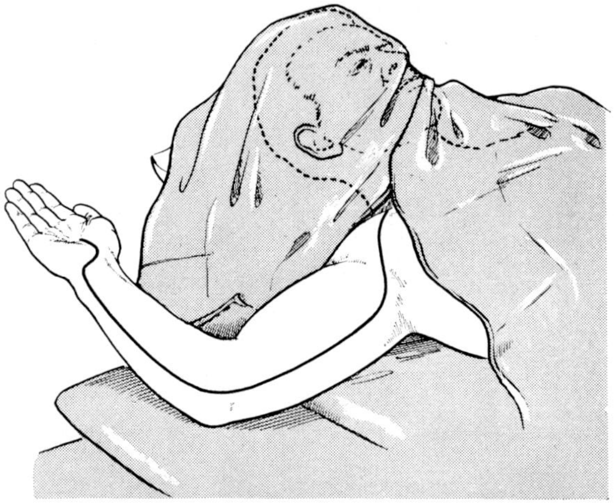

FIG. **15,** 5. The incision, only part of which is required in any one operation, for exposure of the median and ulnar nerves and of the infraclavicular brachial plexus. Although the lateral skin flap must be elevated to expose the median nerve in the forearm, the extra trouble is often repaid by the ease of closure and always by the cosmetic result.

suture, is carried out in comfort with the elbow flexed 90 degrees and the wound held wide open with two self-retaining retractors.

Median nerve. The extensile incision is shown in Figure **15**, 5. Exposure of the median nerve in the arm is straightforward and calls for no comment.

Difficulties can arise at the elbow and in the upper third of the forearm, and here it is necessary to describe the forearm dissection. This is another 'tunnel' situation, the median nerve diving deeply between the superficial, fleshy part of the pronator teres and the deep, tendinous head of the muscle which takes origin from the coronoid process of the ulna. This deep head must be severed. If the median nerve is injured near the elbow it should be exposed first in the arm, then in normal surroundings in the mid-forearm. Beneath the flexor carpi radialis lies the thin radial origin of the flexor digitorum superficialis, the fibres of which run transversely. Longitudinal incision of this thin sheet of muscle exposes the median nerve, which is then traced proximally. The question is what to do with the main, superficial part of pronator teres. It can be detached from the radius in Z fashion as shown in Figure **15**, 6; or, with the elbow flexed, a tunnel can be made beneath the muscle. If the median nerve is injured at the elbow it is best to detach pronator teres from its insertion so that the nerve, which at this level has many branches, can be brought to the surface.

If the median nerve is injured in the mid-forearm it is first exposed beneath the pronator teres, the deep, ulnar head of which is divided; the superficial head also if there is much scarring. The median nerve is exposed distally at the wrist and traced proximally, the radial origin of the flexor digitorum superficialis being cut across, as already described. As the dissection is continued proximally a watch is kept for the nerve supply to the part of the superficial flexor that moves the index finger; it is separate and leaves the main nerve trunk near the middle of the forearm. Every effort should be made to conserve it.

Exposure of the median nerve at and distal to the wrist is so familiar as not to require description.

Ulnar nerve. The only point about this nerve if injured in the arm is that the branch of the radial nerve supplying the medial head of the triceps runs close to the ulnar nerve throughout most of its course. But if the medial head of the triceps is paralysed no time need be devoted to hunting for its nerve supply.

Repair of the ulnar nerve at the elbow generally involves anterior transposition. This operation may also be required for the repair of lesions at other levels because it greatly shortens the course of the nerve. Anterior transposition is also an operation in its own right, for the relief of the various forms of traumatic ulnar neuritis (p. 114).

Anterior transposition of the ulnar nerve. There are three ways of doing this operation. The nerve may be placed superficial to the common flexor origin; it may be laid in a groove cut in the muscle; and the whole common flexor mass, except the flexor carpi ulnaris, may be lifted away from its origin, so that the transposed ulnar nerve finally lies deep to it, not very far medial to the median. The first method has given satisfactory results for traumatic ulnar neuritis, though it is best to reserve it for patients who have a good covering of fat. It is essential to resect the septum that runs proximally from the medial epicondyle; otherwise the nerve will pass over its sharp edge. Some care is also required to ensure that the distal part of the nerve is not kinked where it dips down between the flexor carpi ulnaris and the flexor digitorum superficialis. The second method, laying the nerve in a groove cut in the muscle, should be abandoned completely. There is a risk of the intermuscular septa becoming adherent to the nerve and setting up an irritative disturbance which may be far more serious than the traumatic neuritis for which the operation was undertaken. An example of this is shown in Figure 7, 4 (p. 117). The third method, devised by Learmonth (1942), is by far the best and is equally applicable in traumatic ulnar neuritis and in nerve repair. The whole of the flexor carpi ulnaris is reflected medially; it is best to begin this dissection distally where the

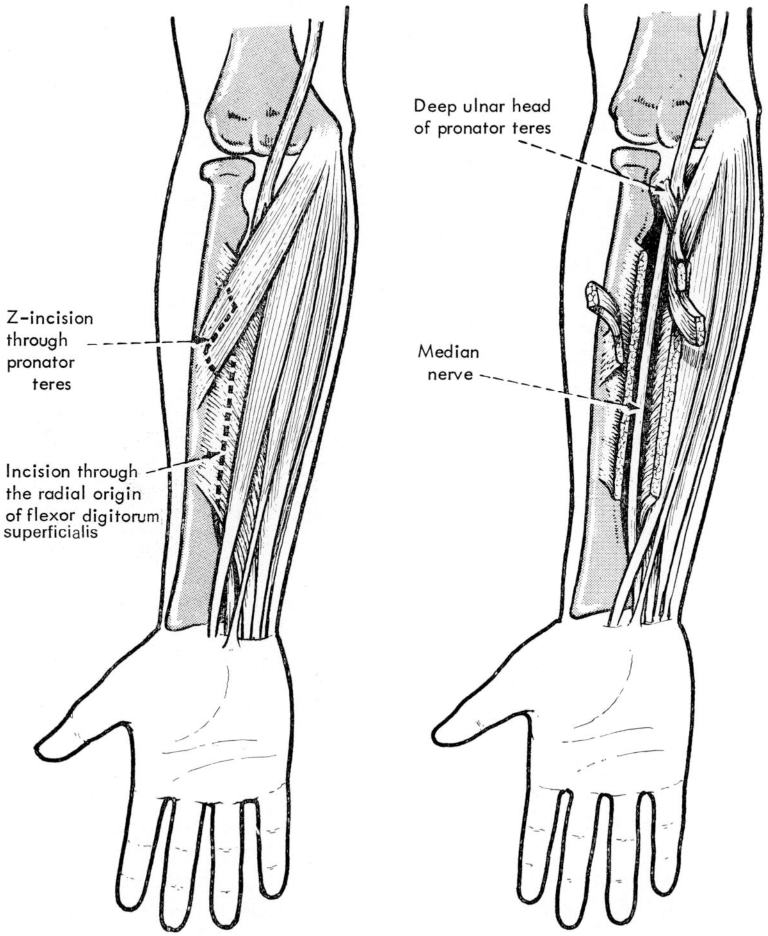

FIG. **15,** 6. If it is necessary to expose the median nerve throughout its course in the forearm the radial origin of flexor digitorum superficialis is cut in the line of the nerve, and pronator teres is severed in Z fashion near its insertion. The deep, ulnar origin of the pronator is severed too.

plane of cleavage between this muscle and the flexor digitorum superficialis is easily identifiable. This is particularly important in injuries of the ulnar nerve near the elbow, so that one may approach the lesion from normal surroundings. At the finish, the fishtail origin of the flexor carpi ulnaris is turned medially, exposing the ulnar nerve as it lies between the two heads of origin of the muscle. Next, the upper border of the pronator teres is defined; closed scissors are then pushed beneath the common flexor origin so as to emerge in the bed of the ulnar nerve. After the scissors have been opened a little the common flexor mass is severed with a knife about 1·5 cm distal to the epicondyle. The common flexor mass is dissected distally until the nerve has a straight course beneath the muscle across the front of the elbow. It is as necessary in this operation as in the others to resect the septum above the epicondyle. When the nerve has been placed in its new bed—a suture may have been performed too—the common flexor origin is re-attached with the elbow flexed 90 degrees and the forearm pronated. This position should be maintained in plaster-of-Paris for three weeks. Whichever type of transposition is used, some mobilization of the branches supplying the flexor carpi ulnaris will be required.

For the commonest of all ulnar nerve injuries, those just proximal to the wrist, mobilization in the forearm gives a depressingly small return. If there is any difficulty in getting the nerve ends together with the wrist flexed not more than 30 degrees no hesitation should be felt in carrying the dissection proximally and transposing the ulnar nerve anteriorly.

Ulnar nerve lesions in the hypothenar eminence. The approach to these injuries is much the same as for decompression of the nerve when it is stretched over a ganglion arising from a carpal joint (p. 122). The incision is like a question mark, the straight part being proximal and the convexity of the curve facing the centre of the palm. The nerve is first traced from the proximal side; if there is difficulty in finding where it leads the deep branch of the ulnar nerve may be uncovered by retracting the long flexor tendons of the fingers laterally, so as to expose the nerve where it lies in close contact with the metacarpals and the palmar interossei.

If both *median and ulnar nerves* require exposure at the elbow or in the upper forearm they are first exposed proximally and distally. The flexor carpi ulnaris is reflected medially, and the origin of the other muscles arising from the medial epicondyle of the humerus is detached in the manner described for anterior transposition of the ulnar nerve. The lateral reflection of the common flexor mass is continued until the median nerve and its branches come into view. The deep head of the pronator teres is severed.

Lower Limb

Sciatic nerve. The incision shown in Figure **15**, 7 would expose the sciatic nerve and its terminal divisions from end to end; the extent of the

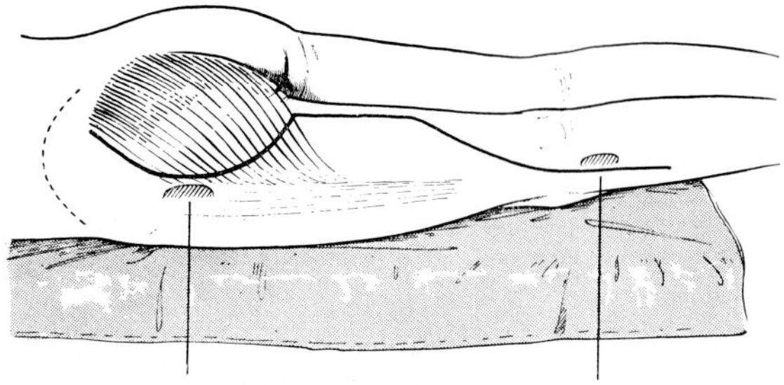

Fig. **15**, 7. The extensile incision for exposure of the sciatic nerve and of its divisions. Gluteus maximus is transected laterally and turned medially.

incision used in an individual case depends on the level of the lesion and on the bulkiness of the thigh and buttock.

If the nerve has been injured in the buttock the insertion of the gluteus maximus is exposed through the proximal part of the incision. The sciatic nerve is first found beneath the long head of the biceps femoris, which overlaps it from the medial side. As the nerve is traced proximally, the lower border of the gluteus maximus is lifted away from it. This is best done with the gloved finger which is pushed beneath the muscle and laterally. The lower part of the insertion of the gluteus maximus is severed along a line about 2 cm from its attachment to the femur and to the fascia lata. This deep probing, followed by further detachment of the gluteus maximus, is continued until the site of damage is revealed. The two divisions of the sciatic nerve are sometimes separate, and it may be found that the common peroneal division emerges through instead of below the piriformis. If the nerve has been injured close to its point of emergence from the pelvis the exposure can be extended a little by nibbling away the upper rim of the greater sciatic notch, care being taken to avoid injury to the superior gluteal vessels.

If the nerve is injured in the mid-thigh its

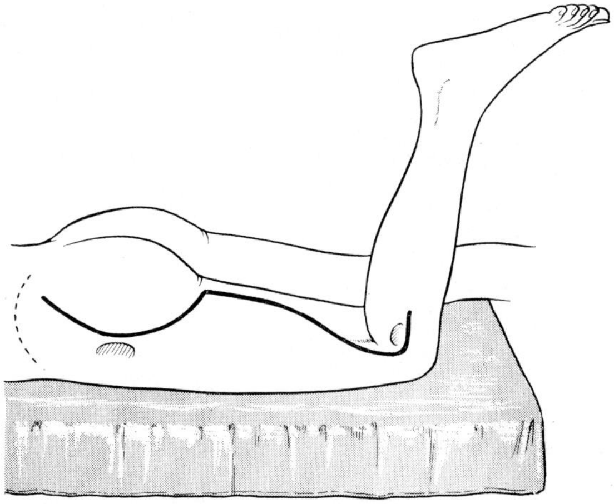

FIG. **15,** 8. Even if the knee is flexed to a right angle there is no difficulty in closing the incision.

proximal part is exposed, as already described, just distal to the gluteus maximus and lateral and deep to the long head of the biceps. The distal part of the nerve is exposed well below the site of injury. The best guide to it is the biceps which on its deep surface is hugged by the common peroneal division of the nerve. The latter is followed proximally to the bifurcation, and the main nerve is beneath the belly of the long head of the biceps. Although this is yet another 'tunnel' situation there is no need to cut through the biceps; it is justifiable to do so only if the injury has destroyed the muscle. Adequate exposure of the sciatic nerve can be obtained by elevation of the long head, which can be retracted to one side or the other, depending on the level of damage.

If either division of the sciatic nerve is injured in the lower third of the thigh or level with the knee the exposure is through the lower part of the incision shown in Figure **15**, 7 which, it will be noted, runs laterally. This is important because the incision may have to be closed with the knee flexed 90 degrees (Fig. **15**, 8), which is well-nigh impossible if an incision has been made in the mid-line. Although the nerve proximal to the lesion is deeply placed its exposure in normal surroundings in the mid-thigh presents no difficulty. In order to find the distal parts of the nerve—the tibial and common peroneal divisions—the head of the fibula and the cleft between the two origins of the gastrocnemius are exposed. The common peroneal nerve is found just distal to the first, the tibial nerve deep to and embraced by the two heads of the gastrocnemius.

Common peroneal nerve. If injured near the neck of the fibula the distal part of this nerve may be found by antero-medial reflection of the peronei, the dissection starting about 10 cm below the site of injury. The branches of the nerve—it breaks up near the neck of the fibula—will be exposed on the deep surface of the flap. Repair may be facilitated by resection of the upper end of the fibula.

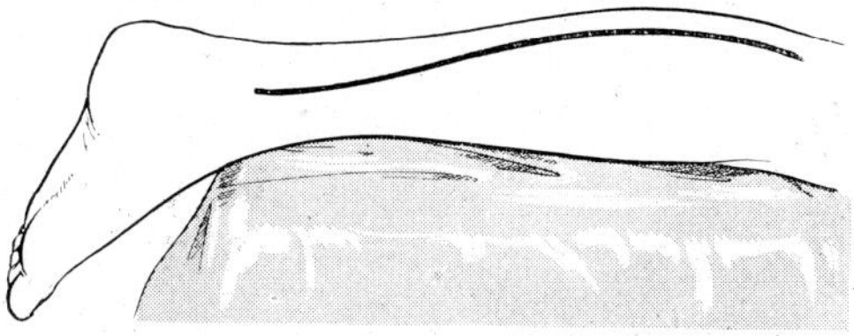

FIG. **15,** 9. The incision for complete exposure of the posterior tibial nerve.

Posterior tibial nerve. Because of the huge mass of muscle overlying this nerve there is only one satisfactory way of exposing it in the mid-calf (Fig. **15**, 9). The nerve is first found where it lies between the heads of the gastrocnemius, then exposed distally on the medial side of the leg where the calcaneal tendon merges with its muscles. The gastrocnemius and the underlying soleus are split in the mid-line and the cleavage is continued distally for as far as the situation requires. If the posterior tibial nerve is injured in the lower third of the leg the calf-splitting operation can be avoided by making an incision along the postero-medial margin of the tibia and detaching the soleus from it. Yet this can be difficult if the patient has an unusually bulky leg; so this exposure should be employed only if local conditions are favourable.

Identification of the Nature of the Damage

If there is obvious division of the nerve and the gap is not so great that end-to-end suture is impossible, sutures of fine black silk are attached forthwith to corresponding points on the nerve sheath proximally and distally, at levels where the funiculi are normal. It is unwise to attach any instrument to these loosely tied guide sutures because they can so easily be pulled out accidentally. It may be that the nerve is known to be severed, and that its ends have been approximated. The guide sutures are inserted as described. If there is an obvious end-bulb, but it is connected with the distal part of the nerve by a bridge of tissue, there can equally be no doubt that the nerve has been severed.

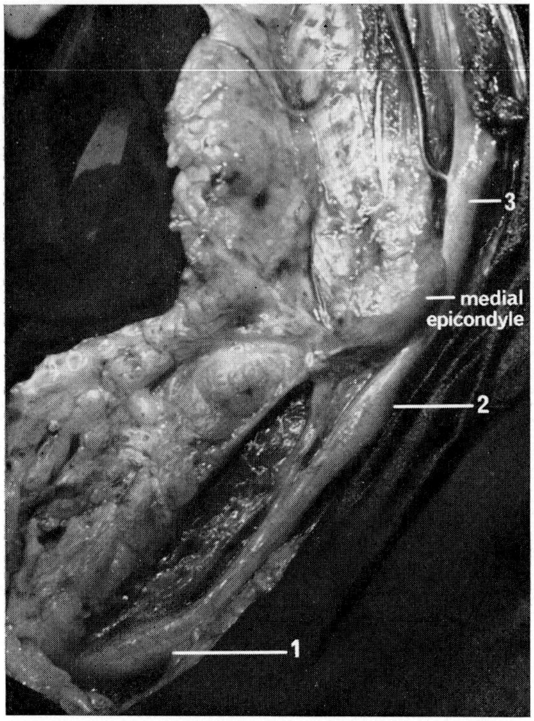

Fig. **15,** 10. The ulnar nerve nine months after a multiple missile injury: three fusiform neuromata. Clinically, complete paralysis: at operation contraction in flexor carpi ulnaris and flexor digitorum profundus on electrical stimulation. Fair spontaneous recovery: intrinsic muscles of the hand 3, considerable impairment of tactile sensibility. If the damage had been complete at the site of the proximal lesion it is unlikely that the two more distal swellings would have developed (cf. Fig. **2,** 3, p. 11).

These findings are straightforward; but some lesions present considerable difficulty, particularly if multiple (Fig. **15**, 10). It is important to identify those in which there is a prospect of good spontaneous recovery; if resection and suture are performed unnecessarily the surgeon has injured his patient, because recovery after surgical repair is at best always inferior to that occurring after axonotmesis. On the other hand, valuable time can be wasted in waiting for recovery that may never occur; so it is improper, when there is an element of doubt, to close the wound and hope for the best. The surgeon must take other steps to enable him to make up his mind.

Electrical stimulation. The nerve will have been stimulated before the lesion was exposed. But even when a positive response has been obtained it may yet be justifiable to proceed to full exploration if the evidence, both clinical and that derived from electrical stimulation, points to a partial division. The cause of the injury has to be borne in mind too; an incised wound can cause partial severance of the nerve which calls for partial repair.

Dissection of the lesion. It is sometimes necessary, as in the case illustrated in Figure **5**, 10 (p. 72), to free the nerve from scar tissue so that the nature of the damage becomes more apparent.

Inspection and palpation. If the nerve appears and feels *almost normal* (Fig. **15**, 11), if there is

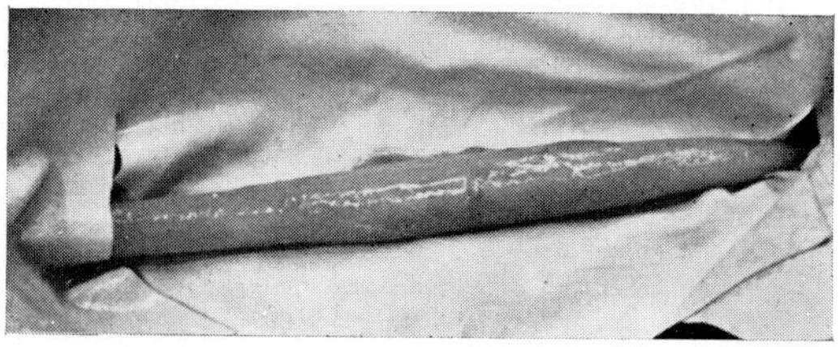

Fig. **15,** 11. A high-velocity missile just missed the median nerve in the upper arm. Complete motor and incomplete sensory paralysis. Exploration required to discover whether there was a partial division of sufficient severity to warrant resection and suture. The swelling was uniformly soft, and it was therefore concluded that the lesion was probably an axonotmesis. Recovery was most satisfactory except in the thenar muscles. (Reproduced by kind permission from *Br. J. Surg.* War Surgery Supplement No. 2, 1948.)

no more than slight swelling, only a little roughening of the sheath, and no intraneural induration, the lesion is almost certainly an axonotmesis and good spontaneous recovery may be expected. There is an exception to this. In some traction lesions the appearance of the nerve is very nearly normal and there may be no change in consistence. But the funiculi cannot be seen through the epineurium over a considerable length of the nerve. Yet because the

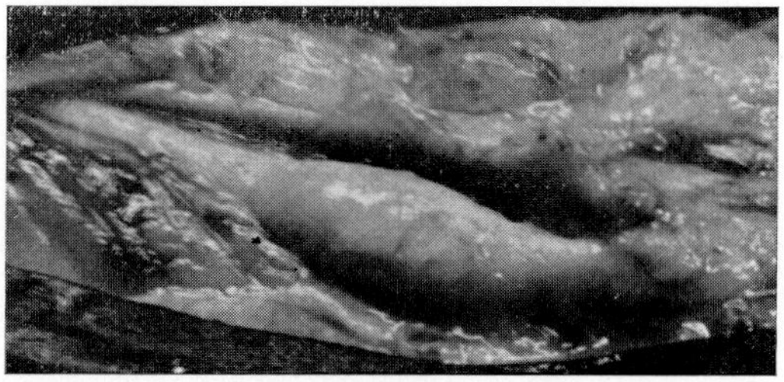

FIG. **15**, 12. A 42-year-old soldier suffered an open dislocation of the elbow with immediate ulnar paralysis. When the nerve was explored seven and a half months later this large fusiform neuroma was found a little way proximal to the medial epicondyle. Two funiculi, destined for flexor carpi ulnaris and flexor digitorum profundus, were distinguishable, and when these funiculi were stimulated electrically the muscles contracted. Trial incisions revealed much scar tissue. It was decided that resection and suture were required, but because the consequent gap would have been at least 8 cm it seemed, on second thoughts, best to leave the neuroma alone in the hope that there would be some spontaneous regeneration. There was none: the second thoughts were wrong. (Reproduced by kind permission from *Spec. Rep. Ser. med. Res. Coun.* (*Lond.*) No. 282, 1954.)

longitudinal extent of traction lesions is almost always such as to preclude successful resection and suture, nothing radical can be done. All one can say then is that some recovery is possible and, indeed, in a case of this sort, probable.

The gross shrinkage and pallor of nerves involved in Volkmann's ischaemia have already been described (p. 99).

The nerve may show a smooth symmetrical swelling, a *fusiform neuroma* (Fig. **15**, 12). These swellings are usually little firmer than normal nerve and although the nature of the damage is obscure—it may be the result of intraneural bleeding—the quality of spontaneous regeneration is such that it may be regarded as predominantly an axonotmesis. If there is no palpable intraneural scarring no radical treatment is required; the prospect of spontaneous recovery is good. If, however, some induration can be felt further investigation is necessary (p. 265).

Sometimes there is little change in the calibre of the nerve—perhaps no more than slight swelling or constriction, or a little thickening of the sheath on one side—yet there is a palpable intraneural scar. The temptation is to leave such a lesion alone. A certain number will exhibit spontaneous regeneration, but only of poor quality. The prognosis is so uncertain—in many cases it proved bad—that further investigation is always necessary (p. 265).

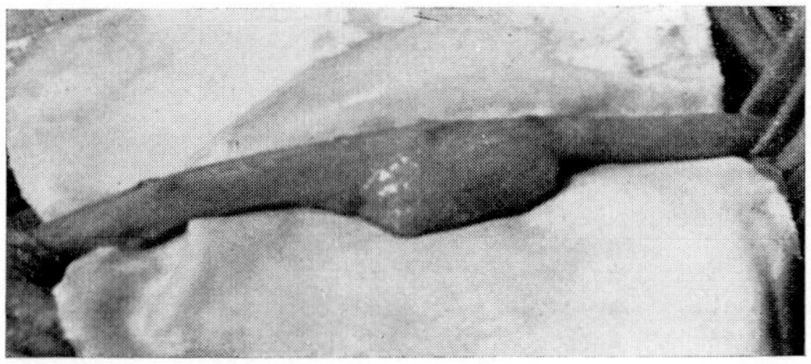

FIG. **15**, 13. Lateral neuroma in which the two humps are fused. Missile injury above the elbow, partial paralysis of the median nerve with general weakness of all muscles supplied by it and loss of cutaneous sensibility limited to the terminal one and a half segments of the thumb and index. The decision to leave the nerve alone was determined largely by the mildness of the paresis. Two years later recovery was so good that even two-point discrimination was normal.

A lateral neuroma is easily recognizable, and indicates partial division. In Chapter 5 (p. 67) we considered the incidence of partial division of the median and ulnar nerves. The question here is what is to be done when exploration reveals this sort of damage. The following figures give some guidance:

In 71 per cent of the cases of partial division the paralysis was known to be partial. In just over half of this group it was decided that the nerve required repair. In those cases in which the nerve was left alone (Fig. **15**, 13 and Fig. **2**, 19, p. 23) recovery was at least as good as if the nerve had been repaired.

In 29 per cent of the cases the clinical picture was that of complete paralysis. In just over four out of five of them the nerve was repaired. In the remainder, recovery was as good as if the nerve had been repaired.

First, let us consider the patients with partial

paralysis. If the disability is small, or if the level of the lesion is so far proximal—for example, an injury of the ulnar nerve just distal to the axilla—that the prospect of obtaining a satisfactory result after suture is poor, then there is no justification even for exploration. There must be a reasonable possibility of doing something useful when, as has just been shown, there is an even chance of satisfactory recovery if nothing is done. Having concluded that exploration is warranted, how does one decide whether to leave the exposed nerve alone or to repair it? Here again the clinical assessment of the degree of nerve involvement is relevant. If it is known that function that has been lost is more important than the function that has been spared—for example, a partial injury of the median nerve near the wrist causing complete loss of sensibility but with retention of power in the thenar muscles—then the inclination is towards repair. If the nerve presents the 'Bactrian camel' appearance (Figs **15**, 14, **15**, 15 and **15**, 16), which indicates separation of the severed funiculi, repair is necessary. If on the other hand there is a single lateral swelling (Fig. **15**, 13), indicating minimal separation of the damaged funiculi, there is a good prospect of spontaneous recovery.

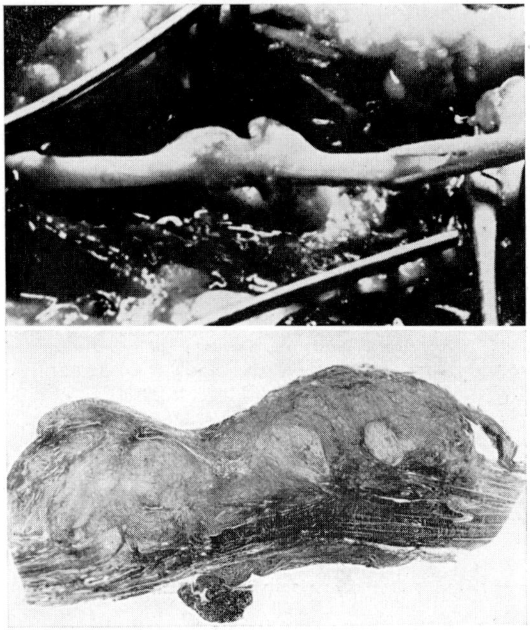

FIG. **15,** 14. A lateral neuroma with a double hump. Four months after the bullet wound that injured the radial nerve there was a little action in extensor carpi radialis longus. But no other muscles recovered and this is why the nerve was explored, resected and sutured. The serious damage involves at least five-sixths of the cross-section of the nerve. (Reproduced by kind permission from *Spec. Rep. Ser. Med. Res. Coun.*, No. 282, 1954.)

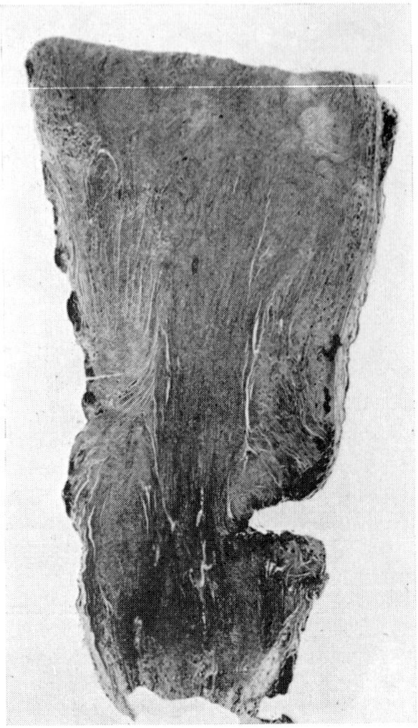

FIG. **15,** 15. Here the notch is due more to the missile that injured the nerve than to the formation of cellular humps. (This figure and Fig. **15,** 16 reproduced by kind permission of Dr. William Blackwood.)

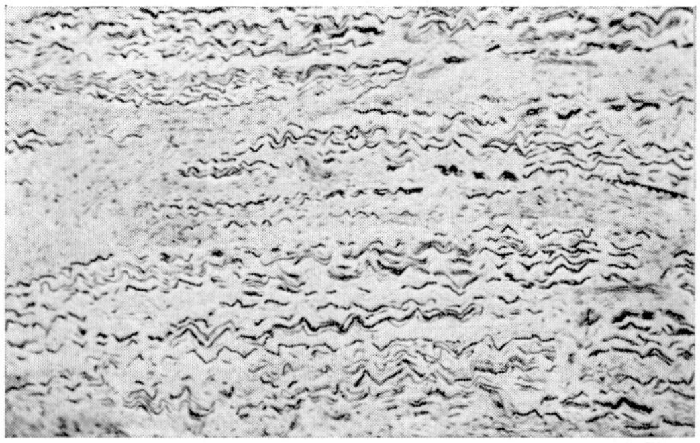

FIG. **15,** 16. A longitudinal section through the part of the nerve (Fig. **15,** 15) that was in continuity. There are no normal fibres, only fine regenerating ones. It is arguable – but only just – that a partial repair would have sufficed.

But Figure **15**, 17 shows a single hump, though the nerve is totally disorganized. The swelling was so uniformly hard that no trial incision was made; total resection and suture were performed without hesitation. We had learned our lesson from the case illustrated in Figure **15**, 12. further investigation. In our earlier experience of these lesions we sometimes closed the wound and hoped for the best. We came to regret this, and the results of the long-delayed repairs that had to be performed were mostly poor. When there is an element of doubt that cannot be otherwise dispelled trial incision of the lesion (see below) is required.

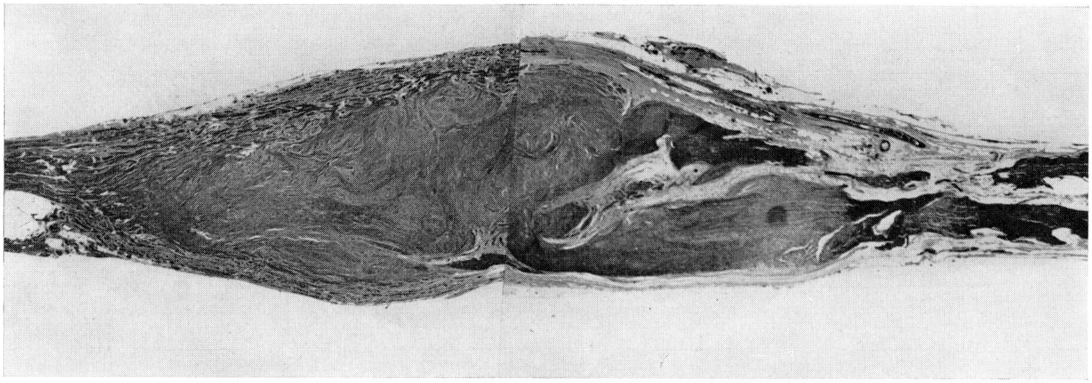

FIG. **15**, 17. A single hump – a lateral neuroma – due to total internal disruption of the nerve.

Partial suture of a nerve, except as a primary procedure, is technically unsatisfactory (Fig. **15**, 34, p. 279). If anything is done it should be total resection and suture or, if the intact funiculi can be conserved, an autologous inlay graft (Fig. **16**, 16, p. 298).

Patients who present with complete paralysis require exploration anyway, because there is no other means of knowing whether the nerve has been completely severed. Discovering it to be in continuity is fortuitous (Fig. **15**, 18). The debate then centres on finding reasons why resection and suture should *not* be performed. The injury has probably been produced by a high-velocity missile; and as has been explained (p. 78), it is almost certain that the funiculi still in continuity have been so disorganized by the pressure wave produced by the missile that no spontaneous recovery is possible. Only if the damage is marginal, and only if most of the nerve appears and feels normal is it safe to leave it alone. If repair is deemed necessary it should be by complete resection and suture rather than by an inlay graft.

Whether or not the paralysis is complete the decision, in the borderline case, to leave the lesion alone in the hope that spontaneous recovery will occur ought not to be taken without

Injection of saline and contrast media. If normal saline solution is injected into the nerve near a lesion in continuity its diffusion will be arrested

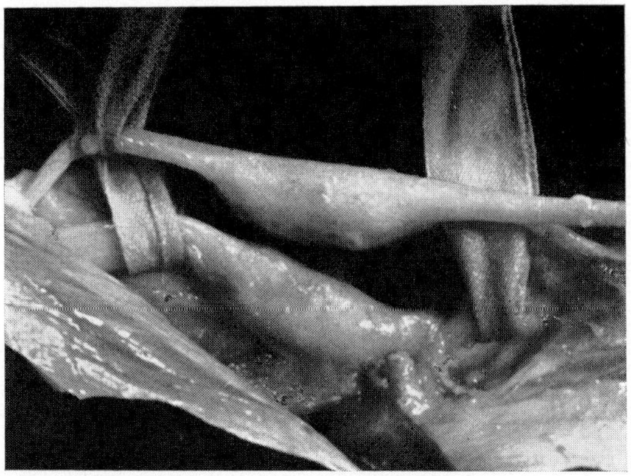

FIG. **15**, 18. Partial paralysis of the tibial (lower) and total paralysis of the common peroneal nerve (upper) produced by a missile. On exploration, eleven months after the injury, both nerves responded on electrical stimulation, so in spite of the large size of the lateral neuromata they were left alone. The final recovery in both nerves was good, better than that seen after the most successful suture of either nerve. (Reproduced by kind permission from *Br. J. Surg.* War Surgery Supplement, No. 2, 1948.)

if scar tissue is present; otherwise, the liquid (which may be tinted with a harmless dye) will spread freely between the funiculi and beneath the sheath. The test, although an entertaining one, gives less certain information than can be obtained by other means. Reference has already been made (p. 56) to the injection of a contrast medium into a damaged nerve, with a view to radiographic demonstration of an intraneural obstruction to its passage.

Trial incision. Three types of lesion in continuity have been described in which there may be a palpable intraneural scar: (1) the fusiform neuroma, (2) the nerve that is of normal calibre or even indented, and (3) the lateral neuroma.

The best way of determining the depth of the scarring is to incise the nerve transversely,[1] beginning at the point where the damage is greatest, where the induration is most easily palpable. Guide sutures are inserted above and below the lesion in case the incision finishes as a transection. If the biopsy is not being conducted in a bloodless field, oozing from the exploratory cut is prevented by using retracting tapes very gently as tourniquets, or, better, by the equally gentle application of Crile's clamps usually employed in operations on arteries. The incision starts where the scarring is nearest to the surface of the nerve. If fibrous tissue is encountered it is deepened, and the scar is sometimes found to involve most of the thickness of the nerve. If more than two-thirds is affected then no hesitation need be felt in proceeding to resection and suture. On the other hand, if funiculi are disclosed at a point near the centre of the nerve there is a case for inlay grafting. Figure **15**, 12 illustrates a case in which a disastrous error was made in dealing with a fusiform neuroma.

The surgeon has now made one of four decisions: that the nerve should be left alone; that it should be repaired by suture; that on account of the magnitude of the gap, repair by grafting is required; or that the damage is such that no form of repair is possible.

[1] A transverse incision is preferable to a longitudinal one. The little wound gapes in a way that a longitudinal one does not. As soon as more or less undamaged funiculi are reached the more superficial fibrotic tissue retracts, and the funiculi are immediately recognizable. If an inlay graft is a possibility the plane for the partial resection of the nerve (Fig. **16**, 16, p. 298) is thus revealed. Because there is almost invariably considerable proliferation of the perineurium, even around relatively healthy funiculi, there is a risk of getting lost in between them if a longitudinal incision is used.

SUTURE

Secondary Suture

We have first to consider what can be done to bring the ends of the nerve together, short of autologous grafting. There are three possibilities: mobilization of the proximal or distal part of the nerve, or of both; bulb suture; and bone shortening. The second and third may be dismissed briefly.

Bulb Suture

When the estimated gap after resection of the proximal and distal end-bulbs slightly exceeds the closure that can be achieved by mobilization and flexion of the appropriate joint, bulb suture may be used (Fig. **15**, 20). After full mobilization of the nerve the end-bulbs are stitched together with strong silk, with the neighbouring joint—elbow or knee—in sufficient flexion. Gradual, controlled extension of the joint is started immediately, and when full extension has been achieved the nerve is exposed again; and it may be found that suture is then possible. Hoen and Brackett (1956) modified this preliminary stretching by attaching a metal shell, like a torpedo head, to the proximal end-bulb and pulling on it by a wire that came out through the skin.

The disadvantage of bulb suture is that two explorations of the nerve are required. It has been superseded by autologous nerve grafting.

Bone Shortening

Shortening of an intact bone is unjustifiable because it is not without hazard. There is one situation in which moderate shortening of a bone and closure of a large gap in a nerve may properly be performed: that is, when there is non-union of a fracture of the humerus and severe injury of a neighbouring nerve. The osteosynthesis is planned in such a way that the resected ends of the nerve can be brought together comfortably, after appropriate mobilization. The osteosynthesis is completed before the

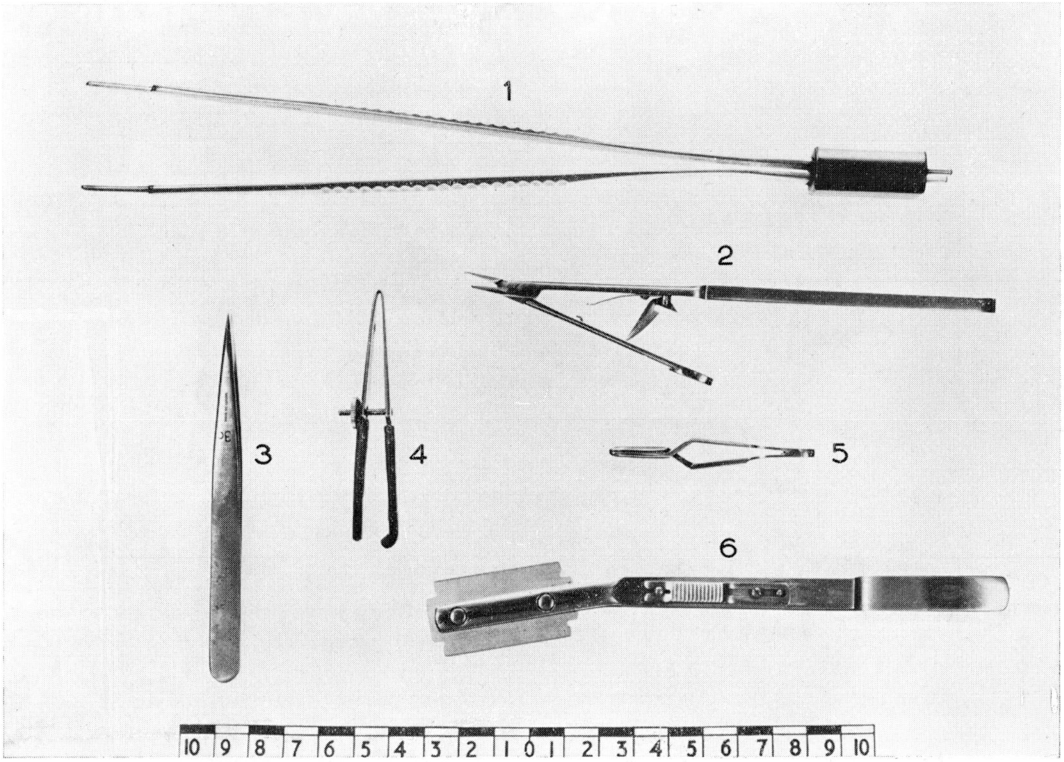

FIG. **15**, 19. Instruments used in nerve suture.
1. Bipolar stimulator: a smaller model is often convenient.
2. Ophthalmic needle holder.
3. Watchmaker's forceps.
4. Crile's arterial clamp for controlling the circulation in a nerve.
5. Carrel's arterial clamp, used for securing the two first stitches in suture of a nerve.
6. Razor-blade holder.

nerve is sutured. The time required for this formidable combined operation is four to five hours.

Mobilization of the Nerve

This procedure was the greatest contribution to repair of peripheral nerves during the First World War.

The price paid for it is destruction of the collateral blood supply of the nerve and reliance for its survival on the longitudinally disposed blood vessels. These are more adequate in the proximal part of the severed nerve than in the distal, so that if there is any choice proximal mobilization is preferable. Nevertheless, Nicholson and Seddon (1957) found that extensive mobilization of the median nerve in the forearm,

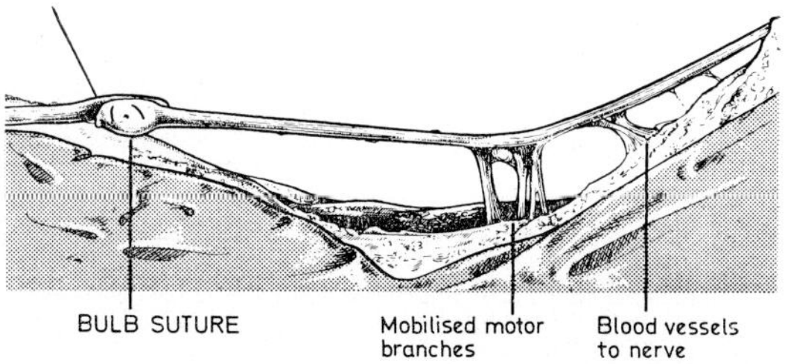

FIG. **15**, 20. Drawing from a photograph taken at operation. Bulb suture of the median nerve in the mid-forearm. The motor branches are just distal to the elbow, which is to the right.

to permit the closure of sizable gaps at the wrist, impaired recovery a little. On the other hand we may take comfort from the fact that free grafts of a nerve up to the size of the ulnar, which must perforce be completely revascularized, may be used with success.

In its simplest terms mobilization is no more than freeing the stumps of a nerve from their bed so that when the neighbouring joint is flexed they can be approximated with no bowstringing across the flexure. If the gap in the nerve is distal to the flexed joint mobilization is very effective, because whatever branches may be present proximally can alter course so that they run in retrograde fashion (Fig. **15**, 21). On the other hand, if the nerve injury is proximal to the flexed joint the same branches tether the distal stump of the nerve (Fig. **15**, 22) and so hinder closure of the gap.

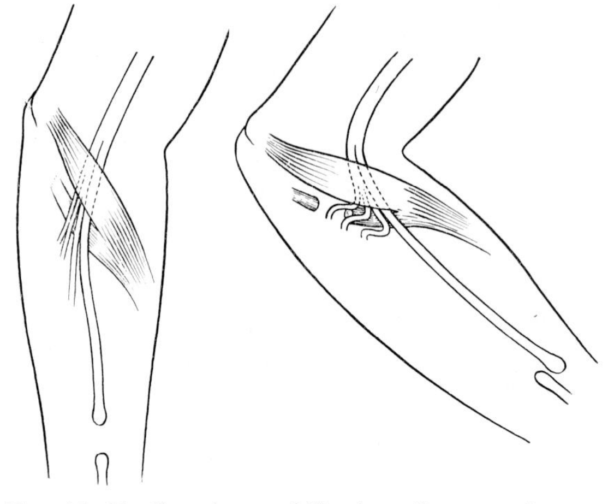

FIG. **15**, 21. Complete mobilization of a nerve is most effective when the lesion is distal to the branches that have been freed from the main nerve.

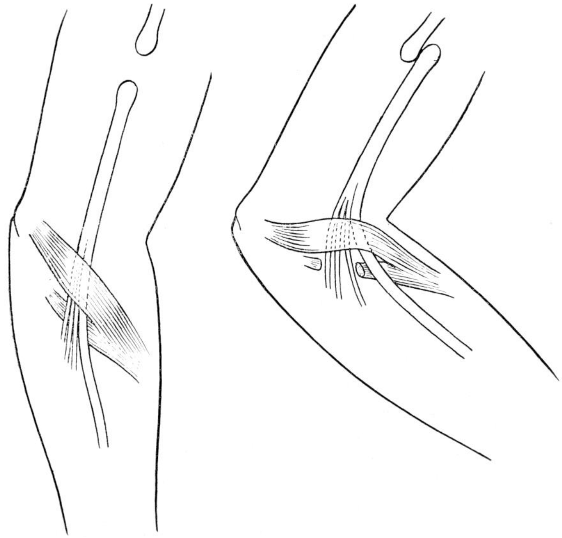

FIG. **15**, 22. If the lesion is proximal to the branches the nerve is still tethered by them even though they have been mobilized. Yet stripping them up is still worth while.

Mobilization is even more effective if some of the branches are gently dissected away from the main nerve trunk; their funiculi are separable over a length of several centimetres before the branches actually part from the parent nerve. Sunderland (1945*a*) has shown over what distances branches of all the main nerves may safely be mobilized in the adult arm. The results of this work and of our own observations are shown in Figure **15**, 23.

Occasionally it is justifiable to take the even more drastic step—required only when the gap in the nerve is proximal to the joint to be flexed —of sacrificing a few branches, usually motor, that are restricting mobilization. This may be warranted in repair of the median nerve proximal to the elbow; sacrifice of the branches to pronator teres and flexor carpi radialis is less important than restoration of function in the hand.

Bunnell (1964, p. 363) had an excellent manoeuvre which I learned from Joseph Boyes. In repairing the common injury of the median nerve at the wrist one may be in need of a few centimetres of extra length to obtain a comfortable suture. The incision is extended to the middle of the forearm, though even the lower third may suffice. The proximal end of the median nerve is grasped firmly with gauze and gentle traction is applied. The nerve slides distally in the most obliging fashion: all that has happened is that the areolar tissue around it in the upper third of the forearm has given way: nothing else is damaged.

The best form of mobilization is transposition of a nerve, commonplace in repair of the ulnar and rare in repair of the radial nerve (see p. 258 and p. 256 respectively). Somewhat akin to transposition is the division of structures that tether a nerve, of which the most important is the deep origin of pronator teres; release of it permits the median nerve to jump forward and so to shorten its course in front of the elbow.

Whatever is done to the stumps of a nerve its blood supply should be imperilled as little as possible; above all, the longitudinal vessels must be respected. Any major vessels joining the nerve should, if possible, be preserved and when collaterals have to be divided they should be cut at a little distance from the nerve so that the extraneural longitudinal vessels are not interrupted (Sunderland, 1945*d*).

Peripheral nerves have a certain elasticity (p. 4); what happens when this limit has been reached? That the suture line will not necessarily come asunder—though Lyons and Woodhall (1949) have described cases in which it did—is shown by the case illustrated in Figure **2**, 16, p. 19.

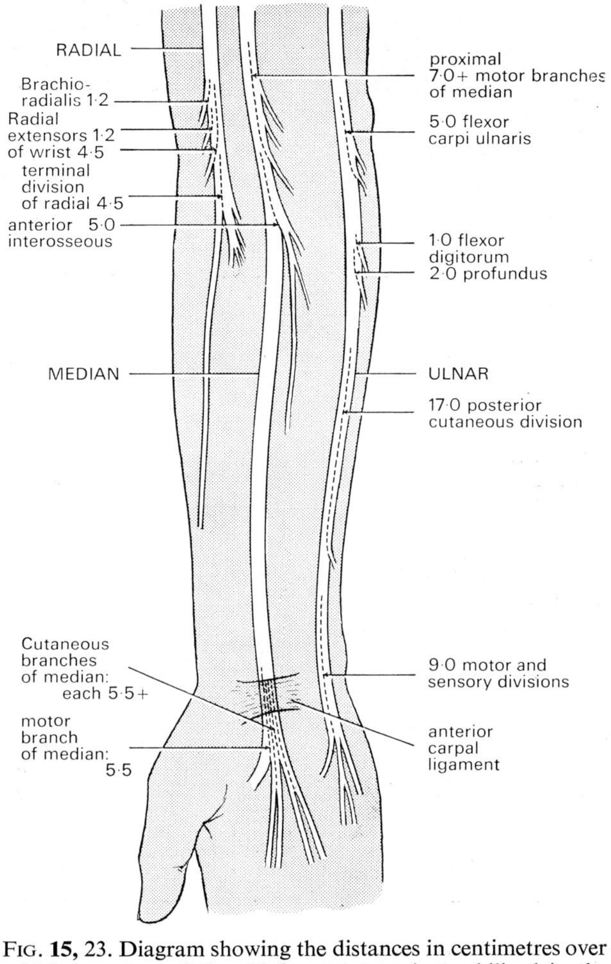

FIG. **15,** 23. Diagram showing the distances in centimetres over which branches of the chief nerves can be mobilized in the upper limb of an adult. Figures based on Sunderland's (1945*a*) and on measurements made during the course of operations.

Limitations of Mobilization

It is remarkable what large gaps can be closed by this technique, and the most impressive figures are those given by Babcock (1927). In certain situations, notably in repair of the common peroneal nerve, I have closed gaps of up to 17 cm; this means flexing a joint acutely. But we found (Highet and Holmes, 1943) that when a large gap had been closed, recovery did not take place. This was investigated experimentally by Highet and Sanders (1943). The reason for failure was extensive collagenization of the nerve, a consequence of what amounted to a slow traction injury. Excessive stretching of the nerve had devascularized it. Hence it emerges that an operation that is technically possible can be none the less undesirable; the biological limit for the closure of large gaps is stricter than the anatomical, however carefully and slowly extension of the flexed joint is carried out after the nerve suture.

Critical Resection Length

Babcock (1927) and others of the same period were concerned with the extent of gaps that it was anatomically possible to close. At that time this was reasonable enough because there was no acceptable alternative to end-to-end suture. Now that autografting can be employed with a reasonable prospect of success we need other figures: it has already been explained that what is anatomically feasible may be positively harmful. Grantham, Pollard and Brabson (1948) published valuable figures, setting out what defects could 'be repaired with ease' as well as the maximum defects. But it was not until Zachary (M.R.C.R., 1954) published his results that we possessed figures based on *recovery* in relation to the extent of the gap closed. However, the correspondence between Zachary's figures (Table XLI) and the maxima of Grantham *et al.* is fairly close. Both are for adults. Any defect in excess of these must not be repaired by end-to-end suture, even though it is technically possible.

There are no corresponding figures for children; one would need many cases to provide adequate information at various ages. However, there is a good working rule that is applicable regardless of stature: *mobilization of a nerve that permits end-to-end suture with the elbow or knee joint flexed not more than 90 degrees is compatible with satisfactory recovery.* Flexion of a joint beyond this 90 degrees limit is dangerous, and one has then to consider closing the remaining gap by autologous nerve grafting. Even this limit is too great at the wrist; because the normal range of extension of this joint is 65 degrees or more, only 30 degrees of flexion or less is permissible.

TABLE XLI—Gaps that it is permissible to close: in centimetres, after resection of end-bulbs. Male adults of average stature (Zachary).

MEDIAN		
proximal to branches to pronator teres		7
between branches to pronator teres and those to flexor pollicis longus		9
distal to the above		7
ULNAR		
proximal to elbow		9·5
upper third of forearm	with anterior transposition	13
distal to the above		10
RADIAL		
proximal to mid-point of spiral groove		8
between this point and the terminal branches		8
posterior interosseous nerve		7·5
TIBIAL DIVISION OF SCIATIC		
in buttock		11
in thigh		11
in popliteal fossa		7
COMMON PERONEAL DIVISION OF SCIATIC		
in buttock		
in thigh		9
in popliteal fossa		

Resection of the End-bulbs

Before the end-bulbs are resected it is wise to satisfy oneself that the mobilization has been adequate; with the limb in its final position there should be a generous overlap of the stumps, because the aim is to suture the nerve without tension.

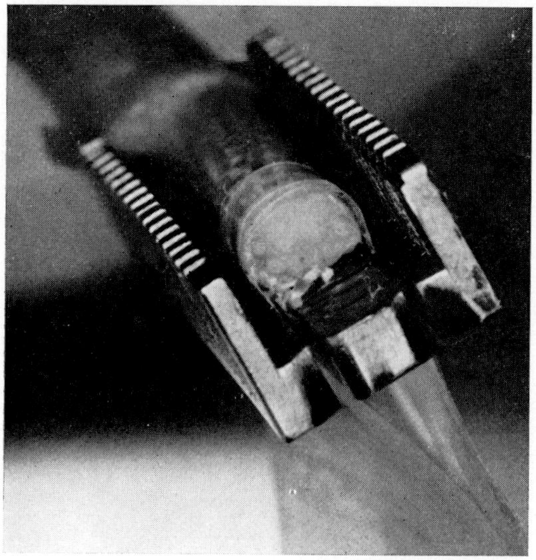

FIG. **15,** 24. The neurotome devised by Gabrielsson and Stenström. It is like two combs mounted vertically and in parallel. The plastic film, which secures the nerve, passes through two longitudinal slots. The razor blade is guided by the teeth of the combs. (Reproduced by kind permission of the inventors and of the Williams and Wilkins Company.)

If the surgeon is working in a bloodless field the resection is done before the pneumatic tourniquet is deflated. The best instrument for cutting across the nerve is a new safety-razor-blade of the highest quality (I have inspected several makes under a low-power microscope) which may, though it is not essential, be mounted in a special holder (Fig. **15**, 19, p. 267). The difficulty, as Edshage (1964) has shown, is to cut the nerve so as to obtain a perfectly plane surface, and to achieve this neurotomes have been devised. Edshage has one, and I have had encouraging experience with the instrument (Fig. **15**, 24) devised by Gabrielsson and Stenström (1966). However, with practice, a clean cut can be made free-hand. This is certainly more convenient if exploratory incisions are necessary (Fig. **15**, 25). Two important points have to be recalled. The first is that the funiculi are lax—if you wish, too long—inside the epineurium, and after one clean sweep of the razor blade the funiculi pout out. The second is that an ideal suture leaves the apposed funiculi barely in contact (p. 15). Thus, if epineural

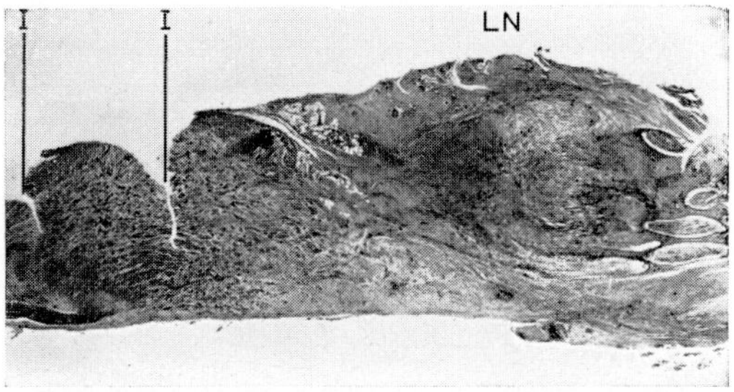

FIG. **15,** 25. A young man suffered a missile injury in continuity of the ulnar nerve. The lateral neuroma (LN) was very firm; there was no response on proximal electrical stimulation. It was certain that resection and suture were required and exploratory incisions (1-1) were made on the proximal side of the swelling. The final transection was well to the left of the incisions shown.

suture is performed after a single sweep of the razor blade the funiculi are bound to be crowded together by the stitches. There are two ways of avoiding this. If the razor is used free-hand the epineurium alone is first cut all round. It retracts, exposing the underlying funiculi; these can then be cut flush with the epineurium. If a neurotome is used there must be a similar final cut after healthy funiculi have been exposed.

There is rarely any risk of inadequate resection of the proximal stump because the very existence of a neuroma is an indication that it contains healthy axons. Resection at the upper limit of the neuroma generally exposes bundles that have not been affected by retrograde degeneration, and the junction of neuroma with the proximal nerve-trunk is, therefore, the site of election. When the neuroma is buried in scar there is still no difficulty; on cutting the nerve across one can easily recognize the translucent mobile bundles of a healthy proximal stump. Unfortunately, the distal stump cannot be approached with the same confidence; there may be serious collagenization within its funiculi (Holmes, 1947) that cannot always be recognized by the naked eye. The distal resection should, therefore, err on the side of generosity, especially in the digital nerves. **Immediate histological examination.** We have used this (MacKenzie and Woods, 1961), but I am not fully convinced of its necessity. Figure **15**, 26 shows an abnormality in one funiculus

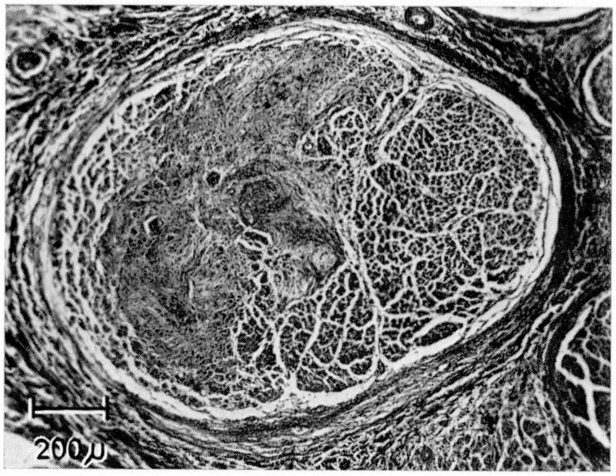

FIG. **15**, 26. A degree of intra-funicular damage that cannot be detected except by formal microscopy.

that would certainly elude the naked eye, but it would not be revealed in a frozen section. The routine histological examination of the resected piece or pieces of nerve is, however, essential; a note on the appearances revealed by various staining methods, for which I am indebted to Miss Kathleen Page, is appended to this chapter (pp. 282-285).

Haemostasis

The pneumatic tourniquet is now released. All bleeding is arrested, and it may be necessary to deal with a small vessel spurting from the proximal cut surface of the nerve. No effort should be spared to ensure that bleeding from the nerve ends is fully controlled; a suture may be ruined by a haematoma separating the cut surfaces (Lyons and Woodhall, 1949, p. 232). The wound is closed except for the part in which the nerve suture will take place.

Opaque Markers

Small pieces of inert metal are attached to the epineurium on each stump so that one can determine whether any separation occurs subsequently (Figs **15**, 27 and **15**, 28). We use gold, 99·9 per cent pure, obtained in strips 15 cm long, 4 mm wide, perforated with holes 0·75 mm in diameter, these holes being 5 mm apart.[1] The thickness of the metal is 0·05 mm; it can be cut with the greatest ease and flattened out conveniently on the surface of the epineurium. As might be expected it produces a moderate fibrous but not a cellular reaction.

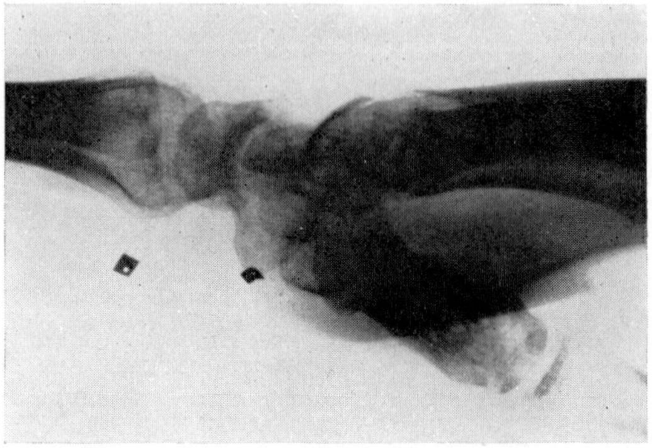

FIG. **15**, 27. Gold markers on the median nerve: no separation.

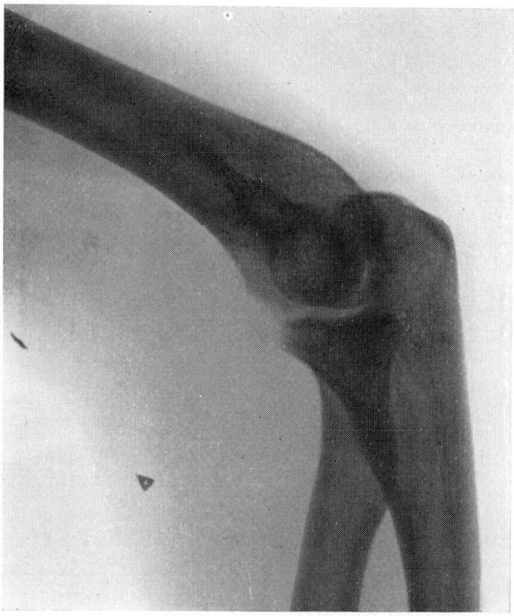

FIG. **15**, 28. Wide separation of markers discovered 18 weeks after repair of the median nerve at the elbow, though it may have occurred earlier. The nerve was resutured, and recovery was fairly satisfactory.

[1] Obtainable from Johnson, Matthey and Company, 73/83 Hatton Garden, London, E.C.1.

Suture Materials

There are three reasons for the unabating popularity of this topic: new filamentous materials are becoming available, and more delicate needles; in some quarters interest is shifting from the standard epineural suture to funicular suture; and with this microsurgery, formerly the forte of the ophthalmic surgeon and the otologist, is now being employed in the repair of nerves.

The discussion so far has been leading up to secondary repair and this, I am persuaded, should be by epineural, not funicular suture. The reason for this is that in patients requiring secondary suture more or less of the substance of the nerve has been lost, or has deliberately to be sacrificed. The internal topography of a nerve changes from one centimetre length to another, and it is unrealistic to employ funicular suture to approximate faces of a nerve whose patterns are not exactly congruous. Funicular suture can be considered only in primary repair, though I am not aware that even here its superiority to epineural suture has yet been convincingly demonstrated. The line between the classical type of suture and funicular suture is a little blurred. If one has to unite, say, several digital nerves in the palm to the stump of the median nerve, as a secondary procedure, this is coming close to funicular suture. But the important point is that here the suture material is still epineural, whereas in funicular suture it is not. Indeed, herein lies danger of the latter.

The position is simplified if we now confine ourselves to the standard epineural suture; a discussion of funicular suture will be found on page 278. Mukherjee and Douglas (1951) point out that suture material need be no stronger than the epineurium; and in general the finer the material the less the reaction that it provokes. They measured the tensile strength of normal human epineurium (sometimes, as a consequence of the nerve injury, it is thicker and tougher than usual, but as this cannot be counted on we must ignore it here), and found that although there were inevitable variations as between the same nerve in different subjects and between different nerves, the tensile strengths ranged from 310 to 510 g with means ranging from 389 to 423 g. We may, therefore, limit our choice to the finest threads having a tensile strength of about this order; moreover, the strength of a knotted loop is twice that of a single thread (Edshage, 1964). Metal filaments, particularly stainless steel, have great tensile strength and provoke little tissue reaction. It should, therefore, be possible to use very fine steel wire. The trouble is its tendency to kink, and so to tear the epineurium; it is brittle too and so breaks easily (Mukherjee and Douglas, 1951; Edshage, 1964; personal observations). Plain catgut, although it has been recommended (Sunderland and Smith, 1950), is regarded by others (Guttmann, 1943; Edshage, 1964) as provoking too violent a reaction: it is, after all, an absorbable suture. Synthetic fibres, Nylon and Terylene, have been examined (Mukherjee and Douglas); the trouble with them is that the knots slip.

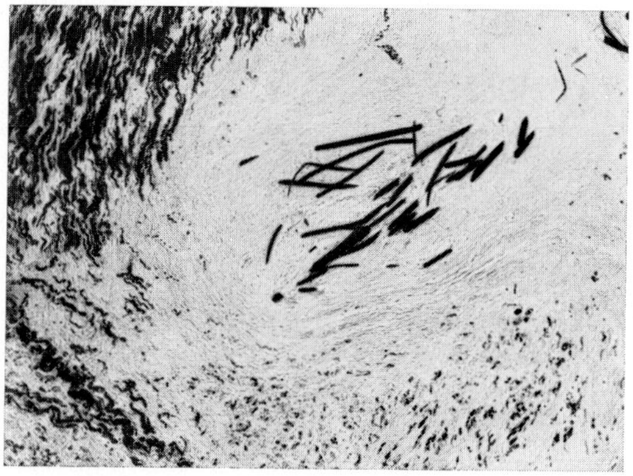

FIG. **15**, 29. Fibrous reaction round a stitch of dyed silk that is breaking up. (Reproduced by kind permission from Blackwood, W. 1954, in *Spec. Rep. Ser. med. Res. Coun. (Lond.)* No. 282.)

We are therefore left, for the present, with human hair and silk. If the latter is not perfectly pure, if it is dyed (Fig. **15**, 29), waxed, or otherwise sophisticated it provokes unfavourable reactions (Guttmann; Edshage); but pure silk is now obtainable with a 8/0 calibre and is ordinarily the material of choice.

Human hair has been commended (Guttmann; Sunderland and Smith), and its defects pointed out by others (Edshage). Its calibre is small—50 to 75 microns—but its tensile strength is less than half that of the epineurium of a main nerve.

I use silk for main trunk sutures and human hair (brunette) for small nerves. All material is mounted in small eyeless needles.

It is possible to suture nerves without using any filamentous material. Plasma-clot suture was devised by Young and Medawar (1940). It is unsuitable for uniting the larger nerve trunks because it cannot be relied on to hold the epineural sleeves together with the same accuracy as stitches do. We limit its use to the fixation of small autologous grafts (pp. 297-298).

All kinds of devices, various sorts of sleeves, have been employed in place of stitches; they do not warrant discussion.

The Suture

A fine needle holder, such as is used in ophthalmic surgery, is essential. Some form of magnifying apparatus adds greatly to the accuracy of nerve suture. Spectacles have the advantage of being cheap, they move with the operator and with some models he can look over the top of the magnifying lenses. There are two disadvantages; low magnification and the short distance between the surgeon's face and the site of operation. Excellent operating microscopes are now available, and the *diploscope* enables the assistant as well as the surgeon to view the nerve ends. The magnification is up to 40 diameters and the working distance is 20 cm. But anyone who has neither the inclination nor the resources to obtain an operating microscope should certainly use spectacles. A wide range of delicate instruments is available, as are fine suture material and minute cutting-edge needles.

The insertion of the first two stitches is crucial. The guide sutures will have been accurately placed, and the first stitch picks up the epineurium on each side exactly in line with them. If the gap to be closed is small one may look hopefully at the cut surfaces of the nerve, because they may show almost identical funicular patterns, which are the best possible guide to the points of insertion of this first stitch. The second one is inserted diametrically opposite. This is equally important. It may be that owing to the lapse of time since the injury there has been enough shrinkage of the distal part of the nerve to reduce its calibre, and the disparity, which has to be accepted, must be shared equally by the two lines of suture. Very small clamps—Carrel's little arterial compressors (Fig. **15**, 19, p. 267) are ideal—are attached to these main approximating sutures, which are left long. Interrupted stitches are placed along the superficial surface of the nerve, between the two approximating sutures, and no more than are required to bring the epineurium together without any pouting of the funiculi. Every knot is tied with just sufficient tension to approximate the epineurium; a continuous suture is undesirable because the tendency is to make it too tight. Then the nerve is turned over by reversing the sides on which the little clamps lie—this is why these instruments must be small because one of them is passed beneath the nerve—and what was the under surface of the nerve now lies superficially. It may be found, as with the median nerve at the wrist, that this torsion of the nerve through 180 degrees is resisted because of insufficient mobilization of one stump; there should be no hesitation in freeing it so that the rotation of the nerve is unimpeded. The deep line of suture must be as neat as the superficial one.

The guide sutures are now removed.

Wrapping the Suture Line

This topic has been discussed in Chapter 2 (pp. 18-20). The natural protection of the funiculi is the epineurium, which heals with astonishing rapidity producing a beautifully smooth surface. The invasion of the suture line by fibrocytes coming from outside the nerve is a myth, though it dies hard.

The wound is now closed appropriately over the nerve. Suction drainage may be considered desirable, though if haemostasis has been thorough oozing should be minimal.

Post-operative Management

Plaster-of-Paris bandages are applied to hold the limb in the correct degree of flexion, which is maintained for three weeks. This encasement of the limb limits the treatment of the paralysed part (see Chap. 13), but as much should be done as is possible: the patient can at least be encouraged to keep his fingers or toes moving with such muscles as are not paralysed. The limb is kept elevated for about 10 days. If the patient has suffered a nerve injury in the lower limb and is in a plaster hip spica, with the knee flexed, he should spend at least half of his time lying prone.

At the end of the third week the plaster is removed and a radiograph is taken to demonstrate the distance between the gold plates. Its extent at the time of operation will have been noted. We have found that if separation occurs—a rare event—it usually happens during this period. There is no mistaking the separation; the gap increases considerably, and small changes may safely be disregarded. A second, precautionary radiograph is taken when extension of the flexed joint has been achieved. The markers may prove informative later (p. 272).

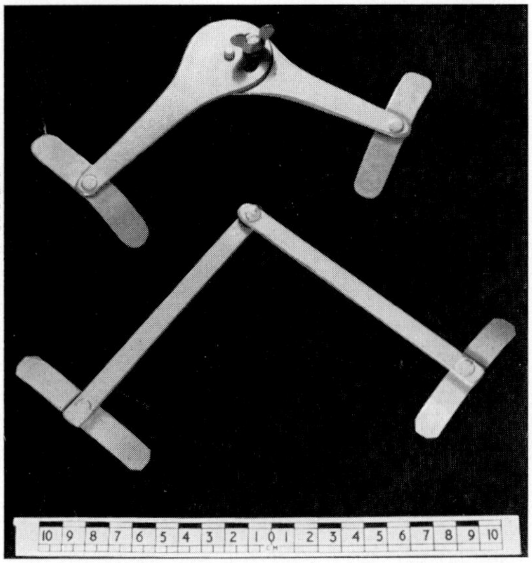

FIG. **15**, 30. Hinges for incorporation in plaster. One, with a stop, may suffice at the elbow. If a second hinge is necessary it need not have a stop device.

After removal of the stitches a new plaster case is applied with a hinge (Fig. **15**, 30), or in the lower limb a pair of them, at the flexed joint. This hinge permits unrestricted flexion, which should be encouraged, so that the nerve is not being stretched all the time. Extension is limited by the placement of the controlling screw, and if there are three or four screw holes, the screw may be shifted at intervals of about two weeks.

The extent of this second plaster is determined by the site of suture. If in the lower limb, a hip spica is almost always applied post-operatively, for comfort and to avoid the risk of inadvertent flexion of the hip when the patient is turned from the supine to the prone position. Unless the sciatic nerve has been sutured in the buttock or high in the thigh, the hip may be left free when the second plaster is applied, and the patient may be allowed up on crutches. If the median or ulnar nerve has been repaired near the elbow the plaster need not include the wrist. If either of these nerves has been repaired near the wrist, and approximation has depended on mobilization at the elbow—in the case of the ulnar nerve, anterior transposition—the wrist may also be liberated, provided the patient is reliable and understands that extension of the wrist must be increased very gradually.

When the plaster is finally removed and a further, precautionary radiograph has been taken, the patient is supplied with whatever form of apparatus is appropriate (see p. 234 *et seq.*); the full regime of treatment of the paralysed part, rehabilitation and resettlement (Chap. 13) is instituted.

Primary Suture

The debate about the relative merits of primary and secondary suture still continues. This is because no one, so far as I am aware, has yet had either the time or the patience to conduct a strictly controlled clinical trial (For discussion of this topic, see Preface, p. x and also p. 314).

Sherren (1908), a great pioneer, reported favourably on the results of primary suture. Thorburn (1922), in his history of British surgery during the First World War, regarded it as the ideal. Platt and Bristow (1924) speak of the 'extreme perfection attained after many so-called primary sutures'; one could not ask for more than that. However, surgeons became increasingly conscious of the nature of the wound in determining which type of repair was preferable, as is evident from the writings of Pollock and Davis (1933), Platt (1937) and Gallie (1942). During the Spanish Civil War, Jolly (1942) abandoned primary suture in favour of secondary repair. In 1946 Zachary and Holmes reported on our own cases; we came to favour secondary suture. Rank, Wakefield and Hueston (1973), whose results were reported in detail by McEwan (1962), were even more emphatic about the virtues of primary suture; but they were clearer than anyone else had been about the importance of the kind of wound, and this alone has clarified the debate. Bunnell (1964) favours primary suture in recent incised wounds. Michon and Masse (1964) still prefer secondary suture. These are but a few of the views that have been published.

In addition to a better understanding of the sort of injury that may be dealt with by primary suture two other points have emerged. The first is the remarkable capacity for recovery in children, no matter how a nerve is repaired (Fig. **16**, 15, p. 296; Fig. **17**, 2, p. 305). The other (see, for example, Gosset and Michon, 1965) is the need for primary suture of certain nerves, such as those in the hand, that would be difficult or impossible to identify if any attempt were made to repair them secondarily.

Before we discuss the various factors involved, let us recall the conditions which Rank and Wakefield regard as essential for the successful outcome of a primary suture. There are four. The wound must be what they call 'tidy', by which is meant a clean gash produced by something sharp. In peace time most open wounds involving nerves are caused by glass. Broken glass has an edge sharper than a razor's; electron microscopists use glass for section cutting. The second condition is the ready availability of a surgeon experienced in the repair of nerves. The third is that the conditions for operating are wholly satisfactory; this means, *inter alia*, that an operation room and its staff can be brought into action at any time of the day or night, for the performance of an operation likely to be time-consuming. These last two conditions embrace the fourth which is that the operation should be performed well within the time limit for the possible supervention of infection. An illustrative case is described on page 277. We come now to the structure that has to be repaired.

The epineurium. Elsewhere (Seddon, 1944) I have drawn attention to the state of the epineurium. It may be found that in what appears to be a 'tidy', incised wound the epineurium shows rents. This is a certain indication that whatever caused the damage was not razor-sharp, and to that extent the wound is in fact 'untidy'. It is not possible to suture a nerve neatly if there are tears in this delicate membrane; resection clear of the tears is needed. We have repeatedly observed that the epineurium becomes thickened and tougher after nerve injury and the tears have healed. Thus if a secondary suture is performed one is dealing with an unbroken membrane that holds the stitches much more readily.

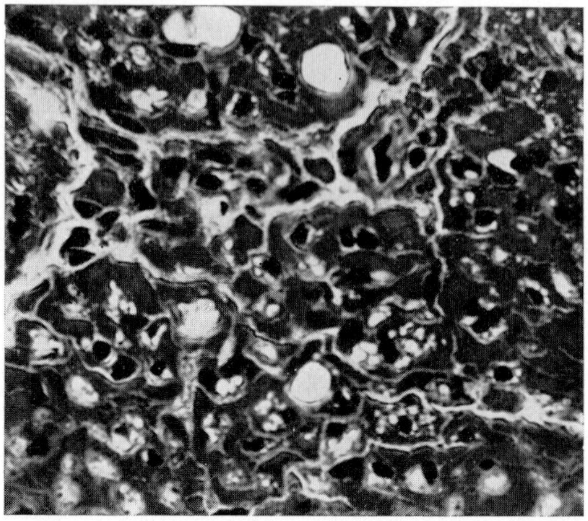

FIG. **15**, 31. A simple wound at the wrist severed the ulnar nerve and several tendons. Four months after primary suture there was no sign of recovery. Over a length of 10 mm distal to the suture line there was impenetrable collagenization of all the funiculi: $\times 390$. (By kind permission from Zachary, R. B. and Holmes, W. 1946. *Surg. Gynec. Obstet.* **82**, 682.)

The nerve. It is accepted that a missile wound damages the substance of a nerve for a considerable distance on either side of the point of severance, and for this reason alone primary suture is contraindicated. The wound is always untidy. But the sort of incised wound that tears the epineurium, although supposedly tidy, can also cause intraneural damage over a distance of perhaps a few millimetres. We have ample histological evidence of this (Fig. **15**, 31). One may hopefully snip a small piece off each end; the chances are that the part damaged intraneurally will thus be circumvented, but there is no certainty about it. And it was the unpredictability of primary suture as compared with secondary that worried us so much. If the nerve ends are tacked together with a view to the later performance of a secondary repair the extent of the intraneural damage becomes manifest as fibrosis, which may be palpable and is always easily detectable when the nerve is cut across. There is no guesswork here.

The points against secondary suture have also to be considered. If the aim is funicular suture, or at least epineural suture so accurately performed that the apposed faces of the nerve are almost exactly congruous, the chances of achieving this are greater with primary repair. If there is a partial lesion of a nerve, primary repair may be manifestly superior, as in the following case.

Late one Sunday afternoon (the time is significant) one of our nurses cut her wrist on sharp glass. She was seen within 10 minutes and was found to have a median paralysis that was complete except for the index finger, in which sensibility was normal (Fig. **15**, 32). It was imperative to preserve one of the most important sensory areas in the body. Operation revealed that the whole of the median nerve except for one plump funiculus had been neatly severed. Primary suture was carried out and the girl made a good recovery. It is almost certain that identification of this one funiculus would have been impossible had a secondary repair been performed.

This story (one could give other examples) is in line with what should be done with small nerves such as those in the hand; primary repair is necessary not only because of ease of identification, but to avoid a hazard that may be peculiar to digital nerves (see p. 278).

Another argument against secondary repair is the progressive shrinkage of the nerve distal to the injury; but it is not a strong one because it hardly becomes significant within the period required to obtain satisfactory healing of a clean incised wound. Lastly, the patient has to submit to two operations.

Mobilization. In order to obtain satisfactory apposition, even at a primary operation, some flexion of the neighbouring joint is necessary. At the wrist this must be minimal because the wrist can be extended 65 degrees, in some people more. This can cause separation of the suture line. So a certain amount of mobilization is necessary, which is carried out through an extension of the incision caused by the wound; there is no objection to this if the latter is clean and if the operation is performed early. A difficulty arises with wounds remote from a joint, say in the mid-forearm. In order to get the nerve ends together comfortably the incision may need to be prolonged up to the elbow, and the deep dissection described on page 258 carried out. One hesitates a little to do this in the presence of an accidental wound that might just conceivably be infected.

If tendons are injured as well as nerves they may be repaired at the same time, though I myself prefer to repair the tendons, tack the nerve ends together and repair the latter when mobility of the tendons is well on the way to recovery.

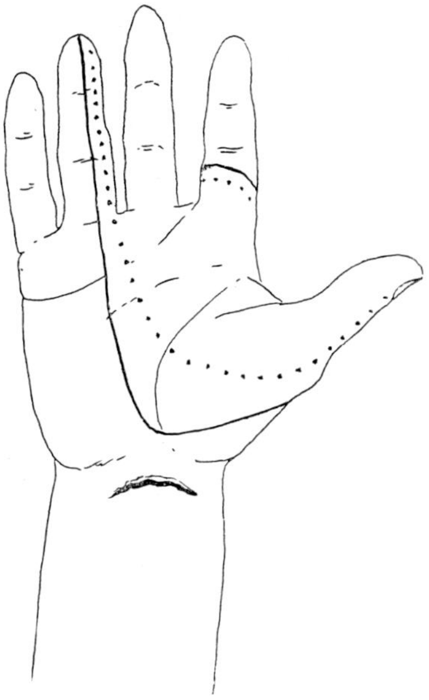

FIG. **15**, 32. Glass cut at the wrist. Total median paralysis except in the index finger. Primary suture: one funiculus found to be intact.

Concomitant vascular injury. If a neighbouring artery has been severed and has not been repaired, the state of the distal part of a divided nerve is different immediately after the injury from what it is a few weeks later. The tip of the distal stump of the nerve may be completely avascular, and as a result of this shows devastating endoneurial fibrosis (Holmes, 1947; Fig. **15**, 33). It differs from a free nerve graft, which is also completely avascular, in that its immediate environment is ischaemic too. This phenomenon is well seen after digital nerve injuries. The probable reason why primary repair can give a good result in spite of severance of the digital vessels is that the distal reach of the nerve is quickly revascularized from the proximal stump. But in larger nerves (Holmes, 1947) this may not apply: so if a main artery has been cut and ligated it is probably wiser simply to tack the nerve ends together. By the time the patient is ready for secondary suture the extent of the ischaemic damage will be readily recognizable and the collateral circulation is fully established. White (1969) found that in the re-implantation of severed limbs this risk of ischaemic nerve damage is considerable, and for this reason he advised secondary repair of the nerves.

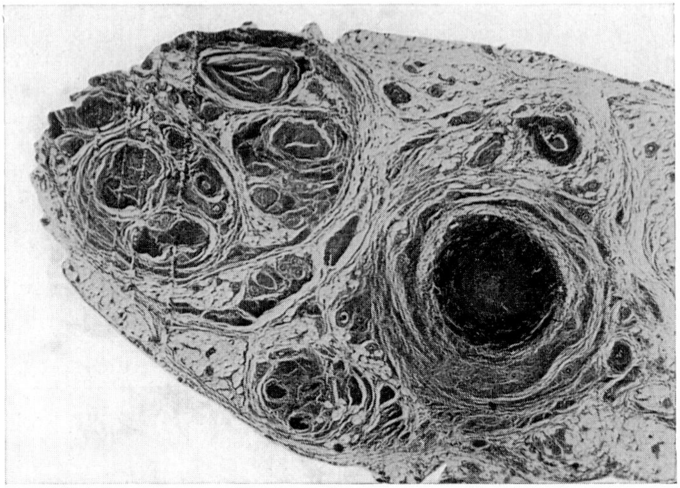

FIG. **15,** 33. Thrombosis of a digital artery. The funiculi of the distal stump of the digital nerve (top left) are collagenized throughout. Specimen obtained at operation. (Reproduced by kind permission from Holmes, W. 1947, *Brit. J. Surg.* **35,** 167.)

The scar. A primary operation leaves a scar traversing all the tissues that have been severed, with the nerve suture line in the centre of it. Thus, when movement of the part begins this scar tethers and possibly damages the nerve where it has been repaired. It is not uncommon to find a slightly tender neuroma developing, which indicates a little separation, though not enough to be revealed by the metal markers. When a secondary operation is performed the incision, although sometimes following the scar of the original wound in part or wholly, is mainly longitudinal. Moreover, if time has been allowed for the tissues to become supple the scarring is minimal by the time the nerve is explored; thus the development of possibly dangerous adhesions at the suture line is diminished.

Availability of an expert surgeon. In everyday surgical practice nerve injuries are not common. The flow of cases, even to a centre specializing in work of this kind, is sporadic. If a policy of primary repair is followed the surgeon or surgeons concerned must consider the price to be paid. They must have a proper understanding with clinicians throughout their catchment area, and be prepared to undertake a possibly prolonged operation at any time of the day or night. However, this has been facilitated by the development of accident services and particularly of departments dedicated to repair of the hand. These cover most of the nerve injuries encountered in civil practice.

FUNICULAR SUTURE

It is the haphazard character of nerve regeneration (pp. 15-17) that sets a limit to what may be achieved by nerve suture; this is the compelling reason for endeavouring to repair a nerve as accurately as possible. It is common practice to respect the cross-sectional orientation of the resected nerve stumps. Smith (1964) showed that by employing moderate magnification, 6 to 40 diameters, the standard epineural suture could be performed much more accurately. If the loss of nerve substance has been minimal the consequence of this is something approaching congruous apposition of the proximal and distal funiculi. The next development, if it is technically feasible, is funicular suture. But however fine the suture material most surgeons are hesitant to leave it embedded in the substance of the nerve; it always provokes some reaction. Hakstian (1968) has got round this by employing pull-out funicular sutures which are withdrawn through the skin one week or even less after the operation. Funicular suture is applicable only to primary repair with little or no loss of tissue. Hakstian has devised an ingenious method for identifying the motor and sensory funiculi. The operation is started under local anaesthesia. The funiculi in the distal stump are stimulated electrically; the motor ones produce muscular contraction, and these funiculi are labelled with small drops of methylene blue. The proximal bundles are stimulated in turn, the patient recording his sensations; it appears that they are not always well localized, so it may be difficult to distinguish one sensory funiculus from another. The sensory funiculi are labelled with dye too, and on the basis of this information the funicular suture is performed. Hakstian uses a very fine unipolar stimulating electrode which, in the circumstances, is probably justifiable.

Autologous Grafting

Although this topic belongs in the next chapter it must be mentioned here because Millesi and others often use autologous grafting in place of direct suture. This may be justifiable, but it requires demonstration—as does funicular suture—by strictly controlled clinical trial, a subject discussed on page 314.

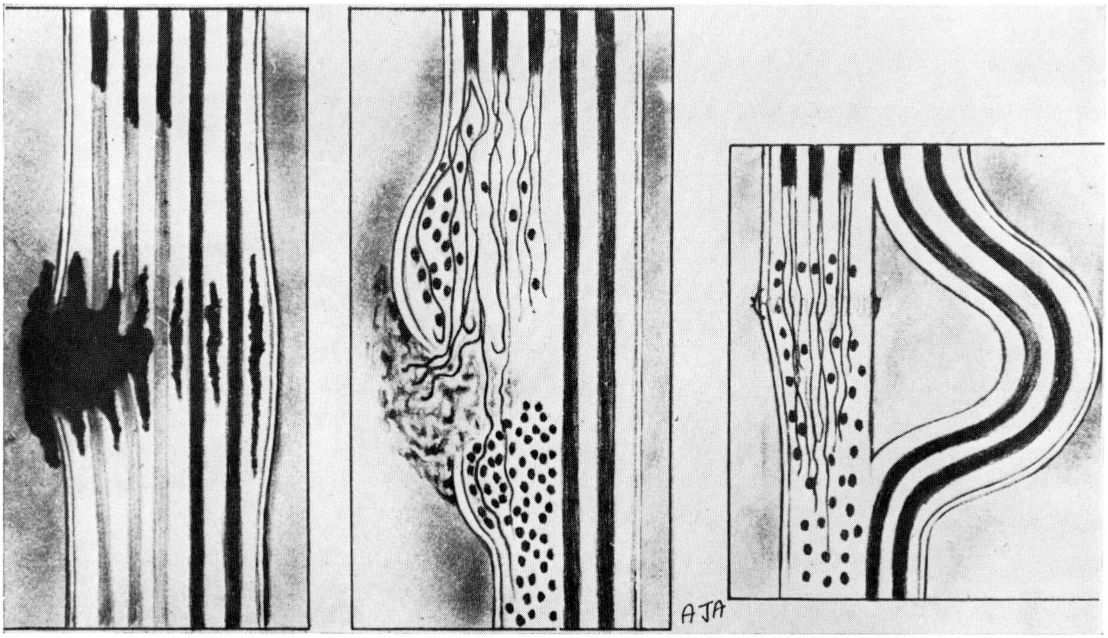

FIG. **15**, 34. Loop suture for repair of a partial division: not recommended.

Partial Suture

It has already been noted that if a clean incised wound has partially divided a nerve primary suture is the ideal. Secondary repair involves separating the normal funiculi from those that have been severed. This can be difficult, sometimes so much so that I thought it wiser to leave the nerve alone in the hope that some sort of unaided union would occur. If separation is possible the nerve can be dealt with by what has been called a loop suture (Fig. **15**, 34). On paper this appears satisfactory, and it is so if the separated part is in fact a separate nerve such, for example, as one division of the sciatic. But otherwise it is an awkward operation because there is no complete epineural sleeve; on the margin where it is lacking funicular stitches are essential. A better and simpler operation is the inlay graft described on page 298.

Severance of the Nerve in Two or More Places

Very rarely this occurs as a result of a missile injury or glass cuts (Fig. **2**, 3, p. 11; Fig. **15**, 10, p. 262). The surgeon should endeavour to close the gaps; at the worst the nerve between the sites of injury approximates to a free graft, which is not to be despised (p. 295).

Failure of the First Suture

This has sometimes been demonstrated by separation of the gold markers. In one case in which, regrettably, they were not used, doubt did not arise until signs of recovery failed to appear at the expected time. There should be no hesitation in re-suturing the nerve; we have not found this difficult, and the results were passably good.

NEUROLYSIS

This term is used to describe the operation in which an injured nerve is freed from scar or other neighbouring tissue to facilitate its recovery. It is not customarily applied—although semantically reasonable—to the relief of those disorders, almost all chronic, in which a nerve, initially normal, has been damaged solely by some derangement of its immediate environment. Familiar examples of this are traumatic ulnar neuritis and compression of the median nerve in the carpal tunnel. Similarly, endoneurolysis, a much more ambitious procedure, is used to describe the removal of scar tissue from within the nerve; it is not applied to the enucleation of a neurilemmoma, or to the treatment of an intraneural ganglion.

When a nerve is injured the neighbouring structures suffer too. Scar tissue forms. If the nerve injury is due to a fracture there may be a mass of callus as well, or some protuberance of healed bone. The question is whether spontaneous recovery of a nerve injured in continuity can be prevented, or at least impeded, by the presence of these extraneural abnormalities. Their noxious influence is sometimes patent. A missile injures a nerve and a neighbouring artery. The nerve could regenerate spontaneously, but is prevented from doing so by the gradual enlargement of an aneurysm, removal of which is essential. A nerve is trapped between the fragments of a fracture; it must be freed: see, for example, the case referred to on p. 80. A nerve is tethered by the bony protrusion of a fracture that has united in imperfect position (see p. 81). It may be that in Volkmann's ischaemia (p. 109) the initial paralysis produced by the ischaemia persists because of compression of the nerve by fibrosis of the surrounding muscle, though here there is an element of doubt.

But these are all rare events. Neurolysis is usually performed for the removal of scar tissue which is supposed to be strangulating or otherwise embarrassing the nerve. Here are some instructive examples.

A man aged 35 years suffered a severe open fracture-dislocation of the ankle and also complained of painful numbness of the foot. An operation was performed an hour after the accident, and so far as the skeletal injury was concerned he made a good recovery. The second plaster was removed after 95 days. But the pain in the foot had persisted and after about the 105th day—by which time he was walking, which was probably significant—it became worse. We saw him five months after the accident. Part of the sole of the foot was insensitive, part of it hypersensitive. There was no sweating. The muscles of the sole were paralysed and showed a reaction of degeneration. The nerve was explored and there was an enormous mass of scar tissue posterior to the medial malleolus and beneath the flexor retinaculum. The scar involved the nerve slightly, but I felt certain that the trouble was compression. Division of the retinaculum released the nerve which, apart from a little epineural thickening and a few adhesions, looked and felt normal. Stimulation produced no motor response. The scar was excised as liberally as possible.

A few hours after the operation sensibility returned in the sole of the foot, but it did not become normal until four months later, by which time the muscles of the sole were regaining their power.

This was a successful neurolysis, but it may well have been that the flexor retinaculum was a greater source of embarrassment to the nerve than the scar (cf. the tarsal tunnel syndrome, p. 126). The aggravation of the pain when the man began to walk lends some support to this suggestion.

A man aged 25 years received a deep and complex wound of the forearm, which severed the median nerve 14 cm distal to the elbow. Because of the skeletal injuries he was not sent to us for repair of the nerve until almost a year later. In the course of this the neighbouring muscles were found to be scarred extensively. Periodic radiographic examination showed that the metal plates near the suture line, though not separated, were immobile. Because of this, but far more because there were no signs of recovery at the expected time, the nerve was re-explored 11 months after the suture. The scarring was most extensive, but the only point of adhesion to the nerve was at the site of the gold plate proximal to the suture line.

However, stimulation of the nerve produced contraction in the thenar muscles; so evidently recovery was well advanced. The startling point of interest was that although these muscles were paralysed before the operation and there was no sign of sensory recovery, the muscles were acting feebly on the day after the neurolysis and there was some return of sensibility in the hand.

Was this coincidental? The element of coincidence is stronger in the following two cases.

A man aged 25 years suffered multiple injuries in a motor-cycle accident, which included an open fracture of the humerus with immediate radial paralysis. The fracture was treated conservatively and united with some deformity. On account of the latter the radial nerve, which showed no sign of recovery, was explored 53 days after the accident. It was damaged at the site of the fracture 15 cm above the elbow, so there had not been time for regenerating fibres to reach the most proximal muscle, the brachioradialis. The nerve exhibited a fusiform neuroma and was firmly stuck to a mass of soft callus. A graph (Fig. **15**, 35) showing when the muscles began to contract voluntarily (strictly speaking the line should not be straight) suggested that the neurolysis initiated the recovery, which ultimately was very good.

But in the light of later experience we came to the conclusion that this operation (which I did) was unnecessary, indeed meddlesome. We should have waited until signs of spontaneous recovery could be expected, that is, about 150 days after the accident.

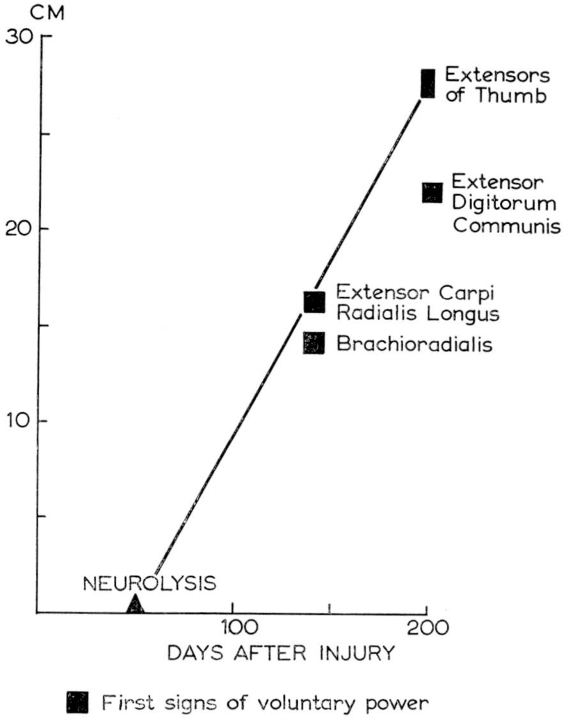

FIG. **15**, 35. Neurolysis that appeared to be effective, but was probably unnecessary.

A young man suffered a fracture of the shaft of the humerus and there was immediate radial paralysis. Because spontaneous recovery occurs so frequently (p. 79), the fracture was treated in the usual way. After an appropriate interval—which had been worked out from knowledge of the level of the fracture (see p. 246)—the more proximal muscles began to recover. But after what seemed to be an adequate lapse of time there was no evidence of recovery in the more distal extensors; I wondered whether a bony protuberance, clearly visible radiographically in the line of the radial nerve, was hindering regeneration in part of the nerve. I therefore explored it; the nerve was a little stretched over a hump of bone, which was removed. Sure enough, recovery of the distal muscles began shortly afterwards.

Yet when the times of recovery were plotted in relation to the distances of the various muscles from the nerve lesion (Fig. **15**, 36), by the method described on page 28, it became clear that regeneration—which unfortunately had eluded detection electromyographically—had been regular throughout and that, for all we knew, the removal of the bony mass had been undertaken just at the time when regeneration was about to reveal itself as clinically detectable recovery.

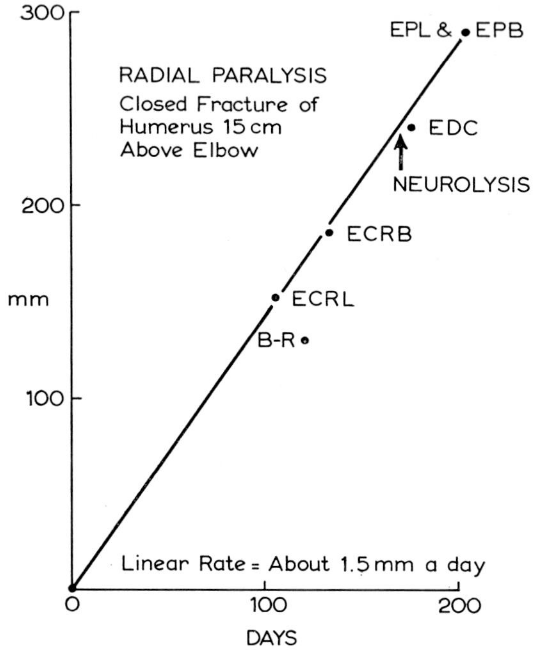

FIG. **15**, 36. A case in which neurolysis of the radial nerve may have been unnecessary.

These successes—which are few, and there is a large element of doubt about the third—are far outnumbered by the dismal failures. Neurolysis is too often undertaken as a *pis-aller*, particularly after unsatisfactory nerve suture at the wrist. I cannot share Bateman's (1962) enthusiasm for the operation. Of course if it is performed with sufficient frequency there are bound to be a fair number of apparent successes; as in the third case I have described, regeneration may be well advanced though not evident at the time of intervention. When recovery becomes manifest the patient is delighted; so is the uncritical surgeon.

ENDONEUROLYSIS

Whereas neurolysis has its place I can see none for this operation. Examination of many sections of damaged nerves shows that the funiculi and their contents can exist in a healthy state even when there is a great increase in the perineurium due to post-traumatic collagenization. All that the most dexterous surgeon can hope to achieve is removal of some of this tissue without injuring the funiculi, though he must necessarily damage their blood supply. What matters is the intrafunicular collagenization, and this is irremediable. Harmful intraneural scarring does not spare the endoneurium. Yet, incredible as it may seem, the term *intrafascicular* neurolysis is used (Bateman, 1962, p. 168) and it need hardly be added that the correlative adjective is 'meticulous'.

This scepticism about endoneurolysis is illustrated by a case history.

The common peroneal nerve illustrated in Figure **15**, **37** was injured as a result of a gunshot wound. Apart from good power in the peronei the paralysis was complete. The nerve was explored four months after the injury in the hope that a partial repair could be undertaken.

The nerve was damaged over a length of 5 cm and there were two bulges on its anterior (dorsal) aspect, that is in the deep (anterior tibial) division. This part of the nerve was indurated whereas in the posterior—in the drawing, lower—part, the superficial peroneal division, the consistence was normal. Electrical stimulation provoked a response only in the peronei. The nerve was injected with normal saline solution which passed easily along the superficial peroneal component but was held up by the anterior scar, which was impenetrable.

I was not sure that I could undertake a partial resection and repair without endangering the part of the nerve that was conducting. Here was a case that some would have dealt with by endoneurolysis, but I lacked confidence and decided to leave the nerve alone. This patient made an almost perfect recovery.

HISTOLOGY IN PERIPHERAL NERVE SURGERY

By KATHLEEN M. PAGE

Department of Morbid Anatomy
Institute of Orthopaedics
London

Because the validity of histological examination depends on the correct sectioning of pieces of nerve that are often small, the specimens have

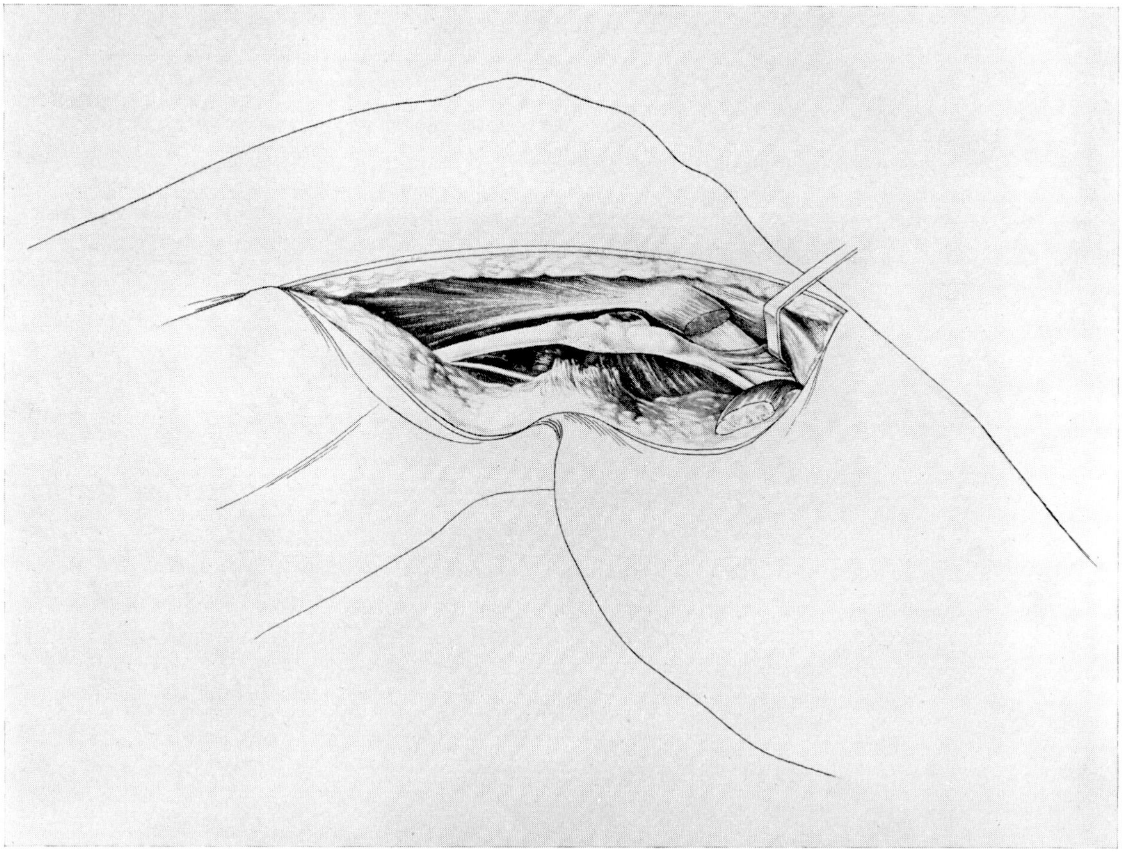

FIG. **15,** 37. An injury in continuity of the common peroneal nerve produced by a missile. Paralysis was complete except for the peronei. Five months after injury the nerve was explored under local anaesthesia. There was a dense scar in the anterior (in the diagram, the upper) half of the nerve, which supplied the paralysed muscles in the anterior compartment of the leg. Electrical stimulation produced no response and an intraneural injection of normal saline solution could not be forced past the scar. The posterior (lower) half of the nerve, supplying the peroneal muscles was softer, it permitted the passage of saline and, of course, responded on electrical stimulation. Was partial repair indicated or 'endoneurolysis'?

to be handled with precision from first to last. If a damaged nerve is in some sort of continuity there is usually only one excised piece; otherwise there are two, sometimes more. They must be clearly identifiable. Never more than one piece of nerve should be placed in one bottle of the standard fixative, which is 10 per cent formol saline; and the labelling should be done immediately. Some surgeons follow the commendable practice of mounting each piece on a small rectangle of dry, sterile postcard; if the nerve has not been bathed in normal saline solution it will usually adhere firmly. But it is disheartening if a small slice of nerve arrives squashed flat on unsuitable card, from which it cannot be detached (Page, 1970).

Sometimes specimens arrive in the laboratory encircled by a silk stitch that secures them to the card. Some surgeons even go so far as to snip the card at one corner to indicate which end of the specimen is the site of resection.

Yet these good techniques are not free from hazard. The plane of resection will have been exactly transverse; the plane of histological section must be the same and show the whole thickness of the nerve. The pressure applied to

TABLE XLII—Histological methods, and the appearances revealed

	METHOD	FIXATION	PROCESSING	STAIN
GENERAL STRUCTURE	1.	Formalin	Paraffin	Haematoxylin and eosin
	2. Frozen section	None	Freezing	None
AXONS	1.	Formalin	Paraffin	*Palmgren* (4)
	2.	Formalin	Freezing	*Schofield's* (1) modification of *Bielschowsky*
MYELIN Normal	1.	Formalin	Paraffin	*Page* (2)
	2.	Chromic acid and osmium tetroxide: not precluded by previous formalin fixation.	Paraffin	*Fleming-Kultschitsky* (3)
	3. Frozen section	None	Freezing	*Page* (2)
MYELIN Degenerate	1.	Chromic acid and osmium tetroxide: not precluded by previous formalin fixation	Paraffin	*Fleming-Kultschitsky* (3)
	2.	Potassium chlorate and osmium tetroxide	Paraffin	*Swank-Davenport* (5): Marchi type stain
COLLAGEN		Formalin, preferably followed by secondary fixative containing mercuric chloride	Paraffin	*Masson*

(1) Drury, R. A. B. and Wallington, E. A. (1967). *Carleton's Histological Technique*, 4th edition. London: Oxford University Press.
(2) Page, K. M. (1965). A stain for myelin using solochrome cyanin. *Journal of Medical Laboratory Technology*, **22**, 224.
(3) Page, K. M. (1970 and 1971). Histological methods for peripheral nerves. *Journal of Medical Laboratory Technology*, **27**, 1 and **28**, 44.

APPEARANCES: those that are specific are shown in ***Heavy type***					
		Cells			
Axons	Myelin	Nuclei	Cytoplasm	Collagen	Reticulin
	Shades of red	Purple	Red	Pink	
	Anisotropic			Anisotropic	Anisotropic
Dark Brown to Black	Sometimes brownish	Sometimes brown		Faint to golden brown	Faint to golden brown
		Sometimes brown		More or less golden brown	More or less golden brown
	Blue	May be counterstained with neutral red			
	Black				
	Blue				
	Black				
	Black (only if degenerate)				
	If normal shades of red	Dark red to dark blue	Red	***Blue or Green,*** depending on the stain used—aniline blue or light green	

(4) Palmgren, A. (1948). A rapid method for selective silver staining of nerve fibres and nerve endings in mounted paraffin sections. *Acta Zoologica*, **29**, 377.
(5) Swank, R. L. and Davenport, H. A. (1935). Chlorate-osmic-formalin method for staining degenerating myelin. *Stain Technology*, **10**, 87.

the specimen to make it adhere to the card, or a tight encircling stitch, can distort the surface of resection—the funiculi being mobile within the epineurium—and the specimen then arrives in the laboratory with its cut surface making an oblique angle with the epineurium. The consequence is that a fair number of sections may have to be cut before obtaining one that shows the whole thickness of the nerve. This loss of a few millimetres of tissue is immaterial if the resection has been made well clear of the lesion. But if, as is sometimes the case, the surgeon has been obliged to make a minimal resection the section-cutting required to correct for obliquity of the resected surface, consequent on faulty mounting, may encroach on pathological tissue. Thus the appearance revealed may be less favourable than it would have been had there been no distortion.

Information is required on four components of a nerve: (1) nerve fibres, (2) myelin sheaths, (3) cellular elements, in particular Schwann cells and fibrocytes, often difficult to distinguish because of the pleomorphism of Schwann cells, and (4) collagen. In peripheral nerve surgery there is rarely need to examine a specimen for degenerate myelin; nor is there much to be gained from the demonstration of reticulin fibres. However, for the sake of completeness, both of these elements are mentioned in Table XLII. Moreover, alternative methods of staining are given in most cases.

If rapid-frozen sections are required during the course of an operation a slice 2 or 3 mm thick is cut from the relevant end of the specimen, frozen and cut on the cryostat. Sections are taken at close intervals until the whole circumference of the nerve is included in the section. All the sections are examined, either unstained in polarized light, or after staining.

The rapidity of the procedure is variable, depending partly on the number of sections that have to be cut. Although it should take no more than 10 to 15 minutes to complete, half an hour may easily be consumed by technical difficulties.

If the result of histological examination is not required immediately the tissue is fixed in formalin before pieces are cut from the ends for sectioning. These are embedded so as to ensure that the sections are cut from the correct surfaces. Sections are cut at close intervals until the outline of the nerve is complete. Conventional staining procedures are employed.

It is sometimes desirable to make longitudinal sections (see Fig. **5**, 16, p. 74). If, as is usually the case, the specimen is more than 1 cm long it is best first to remove a slice from each end for transverse section and then embed the main mass of tissue separately.

16. Nerve Grafting and Kindred Procedures

THE HISTORY OF attempts to repair large gaps in peripheral nerves goes back almost to the dawn of Listerian surgery. In November 1886, Lister himself (Cameron, 1944) wrote a letter to his friend, Sir Hector Cameron, about a patient with an apparently innocent tumour of the sciatic nerve, and suggested that if removal of it left a sizable gap in the nerve 'it would, I think, be worthwhile to try whether regeneration of nerve-fibres might be brought about by connecting the ends of the nerve by means of several very fine catgut stitches . . . so as to form a channel along which new nerve-tissue might develope' (*so spelt*). That same month Assaky (1886) reported experiments in which he had performed this *suture à distance*. But already, in 1870, Philipeaux and Vulpian had performed a far more significant experiment in which a graft taken from the lingual nerve was used to bridge a gap in the hypoglossal. This was not to bear good fruit in clinical practice until over half a century later. And Albert (1885) had, without success, implanted a human homograft.

The whole subject is well reviewed by Sanders (1942), and here we may content ourselves by considering trends of thought and action, and noting a few milestones along a road that still stretches ahead of us. Discussion may be confined to only two sorts of the many ingenious methods that have been devised. The first is direct and is the chief focus of interest today: nerve grafting. The other, now relegated to the background, though not discarded, is indirect: nerve anastomosis—that is, using a healthy nerve to activate a more important neighbouring one that has been extensively damaged. And with this may be mentioned the neurovascular island flap.

NERVE GRAFTING

There are three types of nerve graft: heterograft, homograft and autograft. The first may be dismissed as foreign material that is treated as such by the body; at best it could provide no more than the same sort of bridge for outgrowing axons as Assaky's strands of catgut. Homografts are still debatable. The autograft alone has an established place in nerve repair, and will therefore be described first.

AUTOGRAFTS

Experimental work on nerve regeneration and on various types of grafting ran parallel with the development of surgery and gathered momentum early in this century, though long bedevilled by the notion that regeneration of nerve fibres could originate distal to the site of damage. But in spite of some encouraging evidence from animal experiment, British surgeons concluded, at the end of the First World War, that autologous grafting had been a failure.

Interest revived as a result of the work of Bunnell (1927) on digital nerve grafting; of Ballance and Duel (1932) on repair of the facial nerve; and of Bunnell and Boyes (1939) on repair of major nerves in the limbs. In Britain the encouraging results of Sanders and Young (1942) in animals prompted a further attempt to use autografts in the treatment of patients whose injuries were otherwise irremediable. Five years later it was evident that autologous nerve grafting was worth while (Seddon, 1947*b*), and by 1963 (Seddon) we were able to report a fair measure of success in over 100 patients. In some of them recovery was remarkable, as in the following case.

The 13-year-old girl who is the subject of Figures **16**, 1 to 4 suffered a deep glass cut that severed all the important structures in the right axilla, in particular the musculocutaneous, median, ulnar and radial nerves. Six weeks later P. M. Yeoman explored the nerves and discovered the state of affairs shown in Figure **16**, 1A. The gaps in the musculocutaneous, median and radial nerves, after appropriate resection, were 5·5, 8·0 and 5·5 cm respectively. He decided to use the distal part of the ulnar nerve to repair the musculocutaneous and radial; it was possible to perform end-to-end suture of the median after mobilization of its distal stump.

Sander's (1942) review of the dismal results of operations performed during the First World

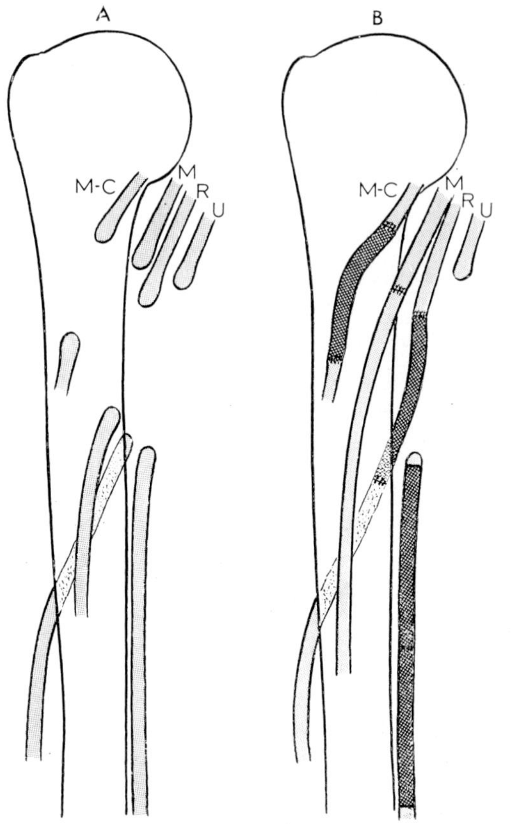

FIG. **16,** 1. A, The nerve damage. B, The repair.

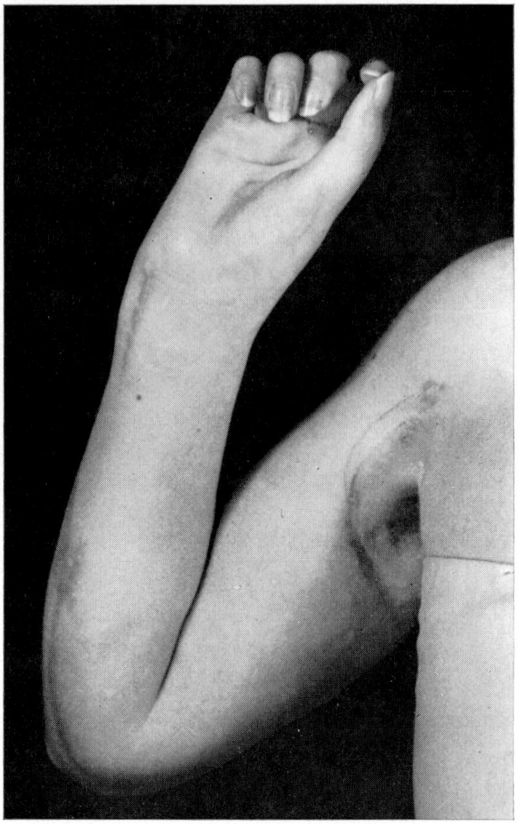

FIG. **16,** 2. Powerful flexion of the elbow.

War suggested that they were largely due to the techniques employed. We have, therefore, to consider the factors that make for success.

Survival of the Graft

Survival of a graft depends on its revascularization. Here the evidence from animal experiment is of little help. In clinical practice we are concerned with the transplantation not only of cutaneous nerves but of major nerve trunks as well, which are larger than the main nerves in any of the animals that have been used. It was proved (Seddon, Young and Holmes, 1942) that a human cutaneous nerve graft could be fully re-innervated, presenting an appearance barely distinguishable from normal. In 1945 Barnes, Bacsich and Wyburn reported the result of an important experiment. A patient had an irreparable lesion of the ulnar nerve, and at the conclusion of the exploration that established this, a piece of the distal stump of the nerve was removed and sutured to the proximal stump after the end-bulb had been resected, exposing healthy bundles. This was, therefore, a predegenerate autograft. It had the same chances of survival as a graft implanted therapeutically, except that it could not be revascularized from the distal part of the nerve. Thus, the state of a similar graft used for repair of a nerve would, if anything, be marginally better than what was revealed by this specimen. There was no necrosis. The graft was re-innervated throughout, but there was no myelination of the fibres. It seemed probable that as in Holmes and Young's (1942) animal experiments, in which long-delayed repairs were performed, this lack of myelination was due to endoneurial collagenization, with consequent narrowing of the Schwann tubes which prevented the nerve fibres from attaining their proper diameter. In 1947 Holmes reported the results

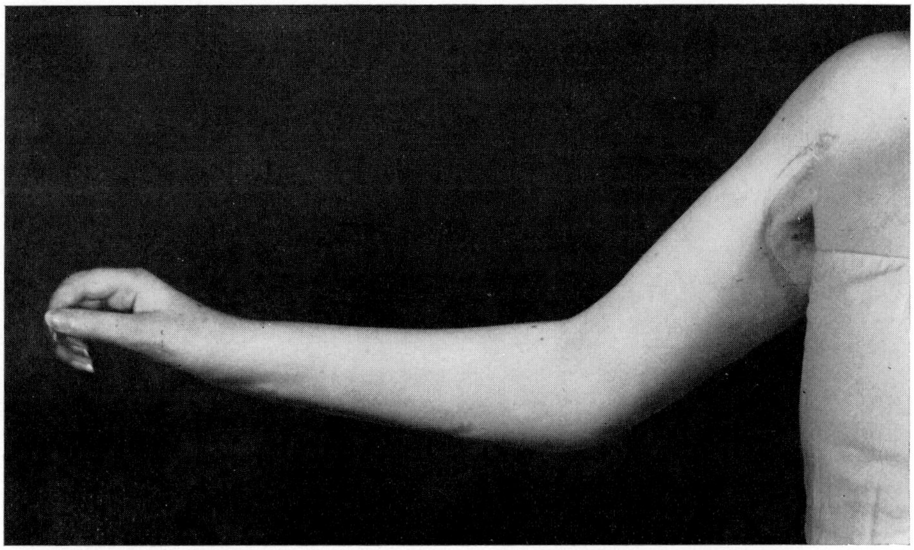

FIG. **16,** 3. Extension of the wrist and of the metacarpophalangeal joints.

of examination of material obtained in somewhat similar ways, and found good re-innervation of three predegenerate grafts taken from the (human) common peroneal nerve, though unfortunately he made no comment on the myelination of the fibres. But another graft, taken from the *proximal* part of the common peroneal nerve, the twin of one of the predegenerate grafts, was necrotic (Figs **16**, 5 and **16**, 6). In cases of irreparable damage of the radial nerve the proximal part of the nerve was cut across and then, after being completely freed, was left lying in soft tissues away from the nerve, or re-attached to the cut surface of the proximal stump. Some explants were, therefore, severely tested, for they could not be revascularized from the proximal or the distal part of the host nerve. A graft from the proximal part of the posterior interosseous nerve that was re-attached to the parent stump was removed five weeks later; it presented a normal appearance of re-innervation. Two entirely free grafts—explants from the radial nerve, placed in the subcutaneous tissues and hence in a poorly vascularized bed—were examined at 49 and 84 days after explantation. In the first, Wallerian degeneration was patchy and in places greatly retarded. The 84 days' specimen showed complete Wallerian degeneration. Both specimens showed some excess of collagen both

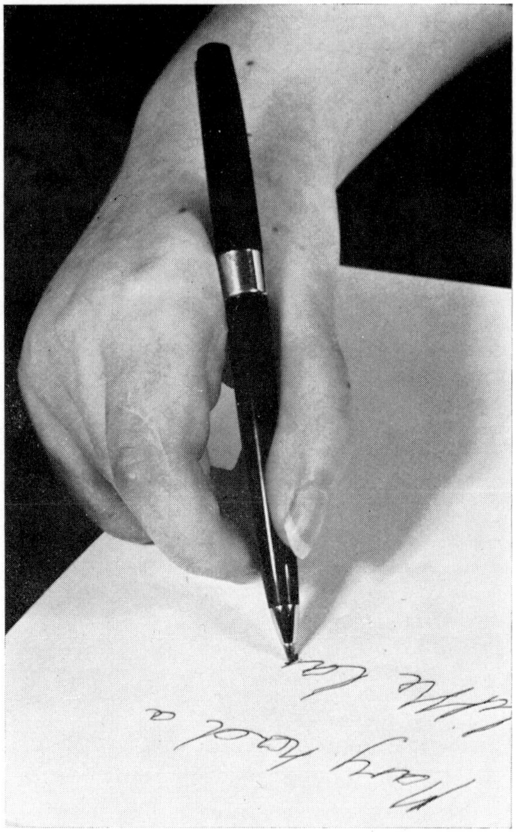

FIG. **16,** 4. Function of the hand.

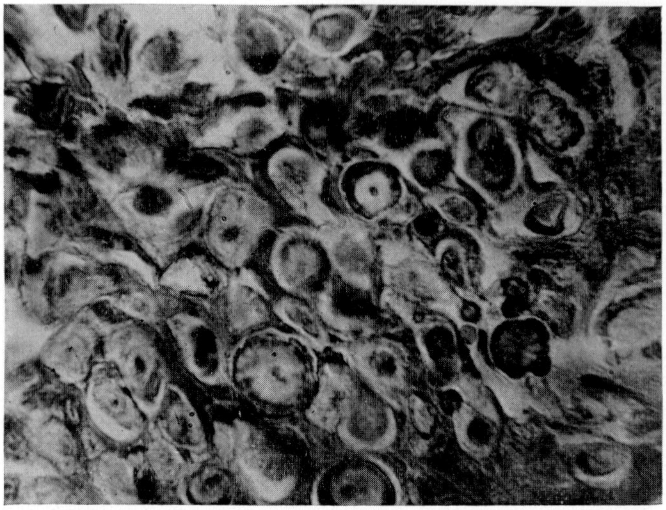

FIG. **16,** 5. Total necrosis of a graft taken from the proximal part of a severed common peroneal nerve. The Schwann cells are missing. There has been no Wallerian degeneration, and even after 17 months the axons and their myelin sheaths are easily distinguishable. (This figure and Fig. **16,** 6 reproduced by kind permission from Holmes, W. 1947. *Brit. J. Surg.* **35,** 167.)

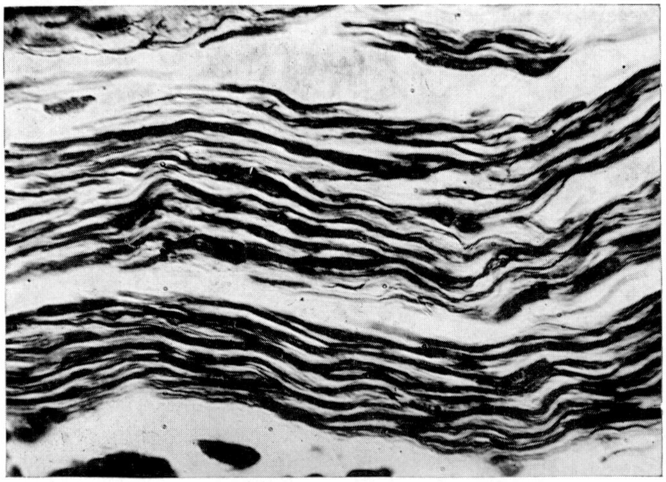

FIG. **16,** 6. A graft taken from the distal and therefore degenerate part of the same nerve. There is abundant re-innervation.

in the endoneurium and in the perineurium, but in Holmes's opinion (and he was examining all our nerve-repair material) not sufficient to hinder re-innervation. In none of these specimens from the radial or posterior interosseous nerve was there any necrosis. Since that time I have had opportunity of repeating these experiments and they have yielded similar results (Figs **16**, 7 and **16**, 8).

We may accept cutaneous nerve grafts unhesitatingly; they survive, and are satisfactory conductors of regenerating fibres. Of the larger grafts, one the size of the posterior interosseous, taken from the proximal part of the nerve, survives and undergoes normal Wallerian degeneration, followed by abundant re-innervation. Grafts the size of the radial nerve, even bereft of vascular connection with the proximal or distal part of the nerve, do not necrose; Wallerian degeneration is retarded though ultimately complete; and there is a certain amount of collagenization, though not enough to prevent re-innervation. A graft taken from the proximal part of the

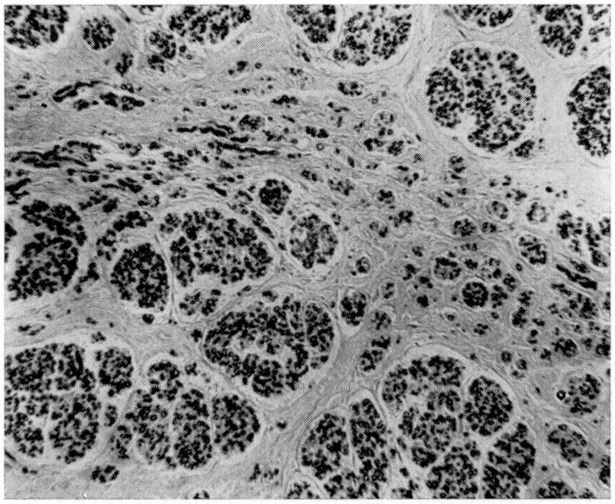

FIG. **16,** 7. The distal part of the proximal stump of an ulnar nerve, which could not be repaired, was severed and reattached. This photomicrograph shows the condition of the free graft 459 days later. There are, as after any nerve repair, some fibres that have wandered between the funiculi. Myelin stain.

common peroneal nerve becomes necrotic, whereas one taken from the distal part of that nerve, and therefore predegenerate, not only survives but acts as a channel for new fibres. If a graft has been degenerate for a long time—over 600 days in Barnes's case—the new nerve fibres that have grown into it are unmyelinated. We do not know what happened in the grafts that had been degenerate for shorter periods—215 and 338 days in the specimens that Holmes examined—because he did not comment on myelination.

It appears that there is a critical diameter for survival of a graft taken from normal nerve: the radial nerve falls within the limit, the common peroneal nerve beyond it. We also know that predegeneration ensures survival even of a very thick graft. There is nothing surprising in this. Wallerian degeneration involves intense metabolic activity; but if it is already past, the metabolic requirements of the degenerate nerve are, presumably, minimal. So we come to a question that has long exercised laboratory workers and clinicians: is predegeneration helpful in free autologous nerve grafting?

Huber (1920), Bentley and Hill (1936), Bunnell and Boyes (1939) and Sanders and Young (1942) thought it made no difference. On the other hand Duel (1933) found that fibres grow through predegenerate grafts faster than through non-degenerate ones; and clinicians interested in repair of the facial nerve—Ballance and Duel (1932) and Collier (1940), as well as others—

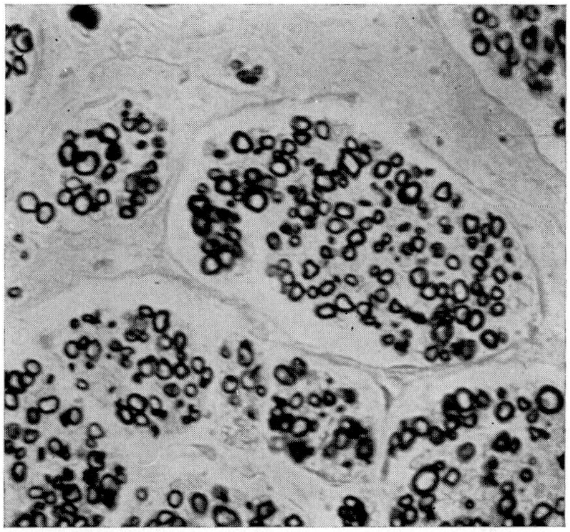

FIG. **16,** 8. A higher magnification, showing good maturation of many fibres in spite of the nerve's being devoid of peripheral connections. There is very little endoneurial collagenization.

favoured predegenerate grafts. Apart from the question of survival of the graft (which hardly arises in repair of the facial nerve) there is the activity of the Schwann cells on which the union of sutured nerves and of grafts chiefly depends. Abercrombie and Johnson (1942) showed that between 15 and 25 days after severance of a nerve the Schwann cells in the degenerating part reach the peak of their activity.

There appears to be a case for predegeneration, more particularly if grafts of large calibre are used. However, in one case of mine, in which predegenerate grafts were taken from the distal part of the common peroneal nerve for repair of the tibial division of the sciatic nerve 338 days after injury, there was no useful recovery two and a half years after operation; it was for this reason that biopsies were performed and were reported on by Holmes (1947). It is probable that the period of degeneration should be a matter of a few weeks rather than months. In repairing the facial nerve it is simple enough to prepare a predegenerate graft to order; in the surgery of the limbs it would add very considerably to the complexity of operations that are invariably delicate.

Fortunately another remedy was found by Barnes and his colleagues in 1945 and at about the same time, independently, by Strange (1947; 1950)—the nerve-pedicle operation which is illustrated in Figure **16**, 9. The blood supply of the graft is preserved, and as a result of ligation of the donor nerve at an appropriate level Wallerian degeneration occurs too. The excellence of this procedure is attested by the results (Table LIV, p. 311); there have been no failures. A similar operation for repair of the tibial division of the sciatic nerve was devised by MacCarty (1951; Fig. **16**, 10). I have used it for a patient with a neurosarcoma but, alas, death from metastasis occurred before there was time for evidence of recovery to become apparent. A happier experience is illustrated in Fig. **16**, 11.

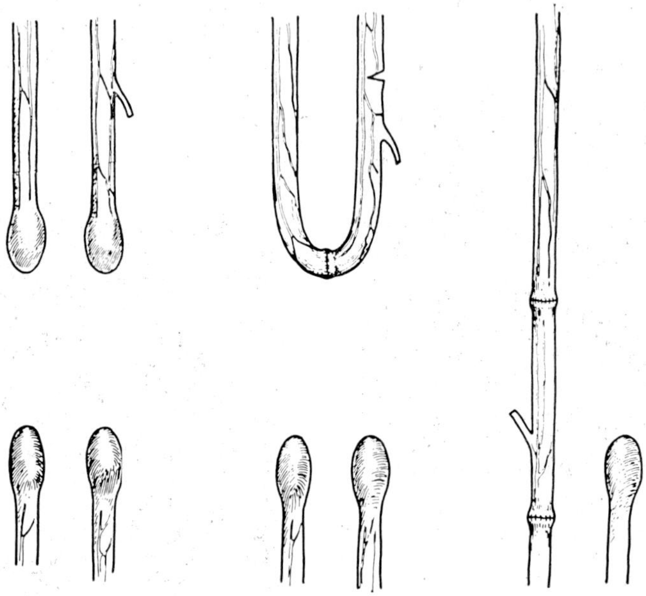

FIG. **16**, 9. Left: the two damaged nerves. Centre: after transection through healthy funiculi the proximal parts of the median and ulnar nerves are united. The latter is cut across or ligated at an appropriate level so that it will degenerate, but the longitudinal blood vessels are disturbed as little as possible. The second stage, swinging down the graft (right), is carried out six weeks later: it is usual to find that the detached end of the graft oozes blood.

The Length of the Graft

Tarlov and Epstein (1945) and Hiller (1951) have drawn attention to the significance of revascularization of a graft throughout its length. It has often been supposed that there is a limit to the length of a graft that can be successfully implanted, but good regeneration has occurred through grafts up to and over 15 cm in length (Seddon, 1963; Figs **16**, 12 and **16**, 13). It seems clear from this as well as from animal experiment that vascularization from the bed of the graft is most important. Hence every effort should be made to remove scars that would hinder revascularization of the graft or to implant it in healthy surroundings, making a detour if possible, and if the supply of material permits.

The Calibre of the Graft or Grafts

The implanted main trunk graft or cable graft should have about the same calibre as the recipient nerve. Anything less, or any alternative that may have given encouraging results in animal experiments, is useless. In Britain, during the First World War, the surgeon who came nearest to achieving success was Joyce (1919, 1920); he used two or (for the sciatic nerve) three strands of a cutaneous nerve to bridge a gap, but they were wrapped in Cargile membrane. Kirk and Lewis (1915), in the United States, had found that in dogs a tube of fascia lata would conduct nerve fibres across a gap of a centimetre or two in the sciatic nerve. No nerve graft was used. The fascial tube tended to shrink: Platt (1920), in his clinical application of this method, prevented this by filling the tube with petroleum jelly. The tube encased a small graft which was inserted, it appeared, *pour encourager les autres*. The failure of these operations (Stopford, 1920; Platt, 1921) and the indifferent results of those in which a slender graft alone was used led to condemnation of nerve grafting (M.R.C.R., 1920). This antipathy—for that is what it became—continued into the first half of the Second World War. The only progress made in this field by the British was in repair of the facial nerve.

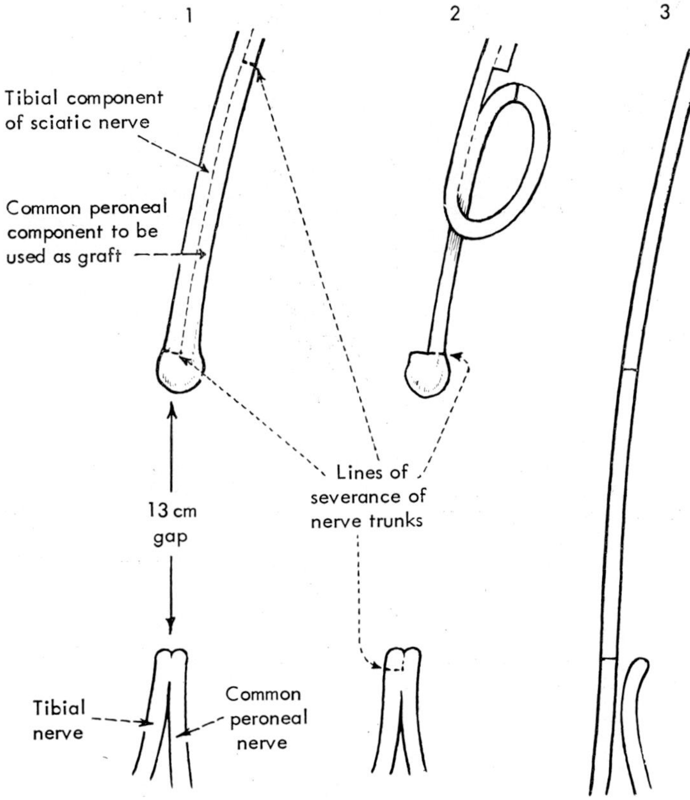

FIG. **16,** 10. MacCarty's nerve-pedicle operation for repair of the tibial division of the sciatic nerve.
1. A large gap in the nerve.
2. Proximal end of the tibial division sutured to the common peroneal division at an appropriate level.
3. The graft swung distally to bridge the gap.

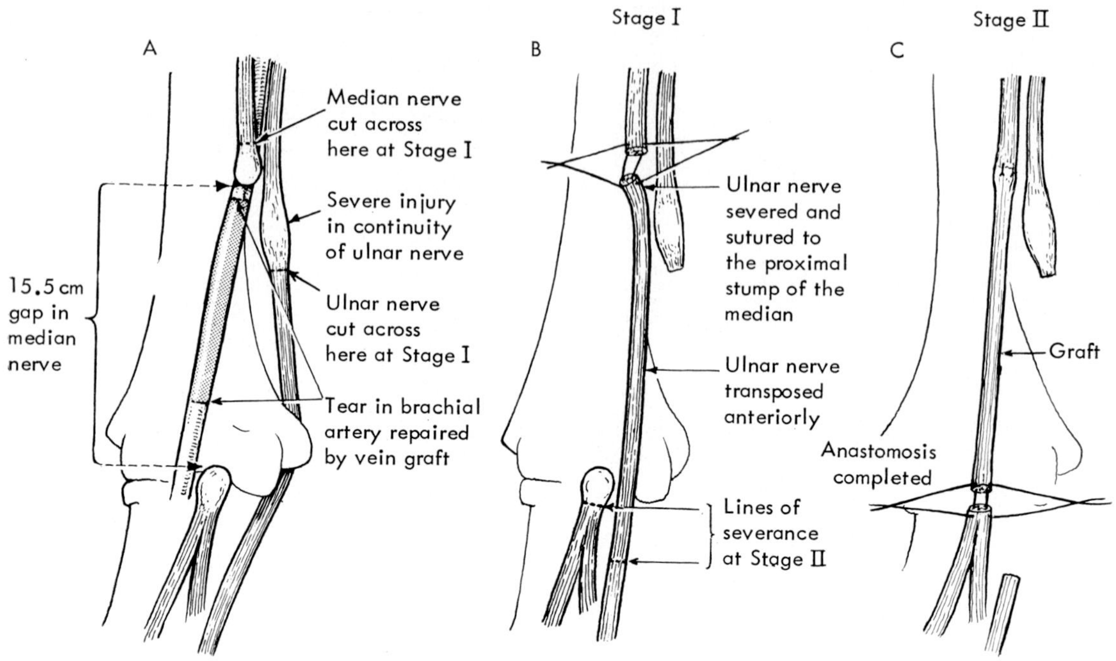

FIG. **16**, 11. A. Missile injury of right arm which destroyed the brachial vessels and the median nerve and injured the ulnar nerve in continuity. Complete median and ulnar paralysis. Immediate repair of the brachial artery with a vein graft from the leg.
B. Three months later first stage of an ulnar-to-median nerve-pedicle graft, with anterior transposition of the ulnar nerve.
C. After a further two months bridging operation completed. Fourteen months after the injury: all median-innervated muscles 4 except pronator teres and abductor pollicis brevis, both 0. Sensibility 3+. A section of the fusiform neuroma on the ulnar nerve is shown in Fig. **5**, 9, p. 71.

Shrinkage of the Graft

It was shown by Sanders and Young (1942) that a graft shrinks, and allowance must be made for this. It may have been shrinkage of the graft that led Davis and Cleveland (1934) to recommend resection and resuture of the distal junction at about the time when regenerating axons might be expected to have reached it. They thought that invasion of the distal junction by fibrocytes obstructed the passage of axons from the graft into the distal stump. The junction may have separated.

Delay

Delay between injury and repair is as harmful in nerve grafting as in ordinary suture (Fig. **16**, 14).

Age of the Patient

Up to the age of 15 years the results are excellent; after that the prognosis is less satisfactory (Fig. **16**, 15).

Sources of Material

This is the chief limiting factor in autografting. If two main nerve trunks have been damaged so extensively that there is no hope of repairing either by suture, one can usually repair the more important by means of a graft taken from the other, though I have not yet succeeded in applying this to the main divisions of the sciatic nerve (p. 293). When only one nerve is damaged, as for example in an ischaemic lesion of the median nerve in the forearm, one part of the nerve may

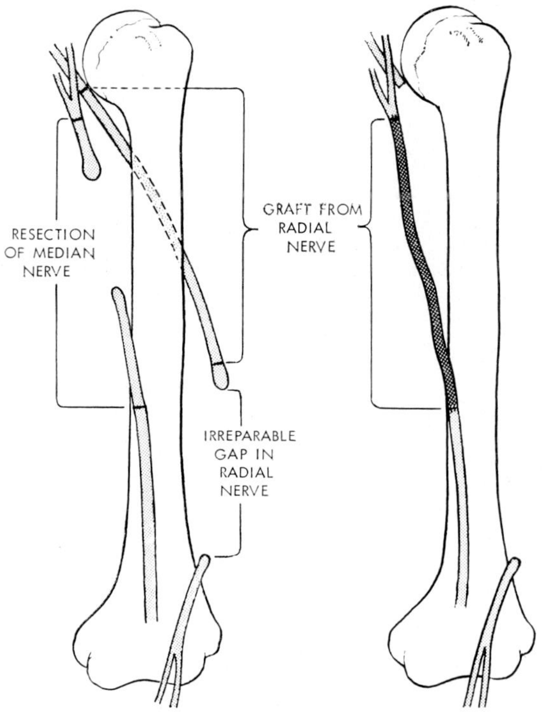

FIG. **16,** 12. The patient broke his humerus. This severed the radial nerve, as it turned out irreparably. As a result of his being dragged violently there were traction injuries of the musculocutaneous, ulnar and median nerves; of these the first two recovered, but the median had snapped and was badly damaged over a length of 14 cm. Repair was carried out in the manner shown. He made a good recovery; the radial paralysis was treated by arthrodesis of the wrist and transplantation of the flexor carpi ulnaris into the extensors of the digits. The result, 25 years later, is still satisfactory.

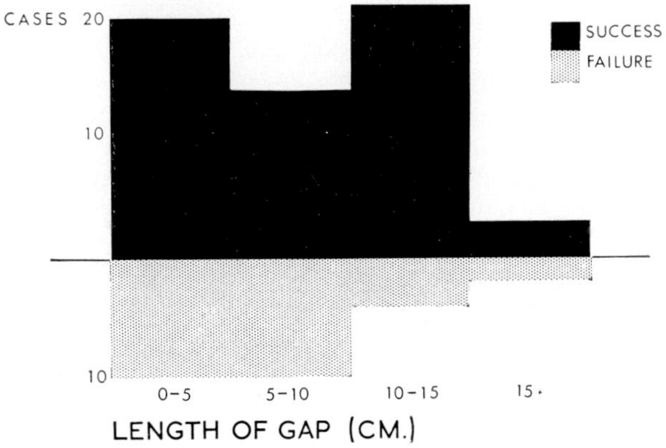

FIG. **16,** 13. The results of nerve grafting in relation to the extent of the gaps repaired. Partial successes and successes have been run together. Author's series. Cases of digital nerve grafting have been excluded as too complex for satisfactory representation, leaving 83 cases. (Figs **16,** 13 to **16,** 15, reproduced from Seddon, H. J. 1963. *J. Bone Jt Surg. B.*)

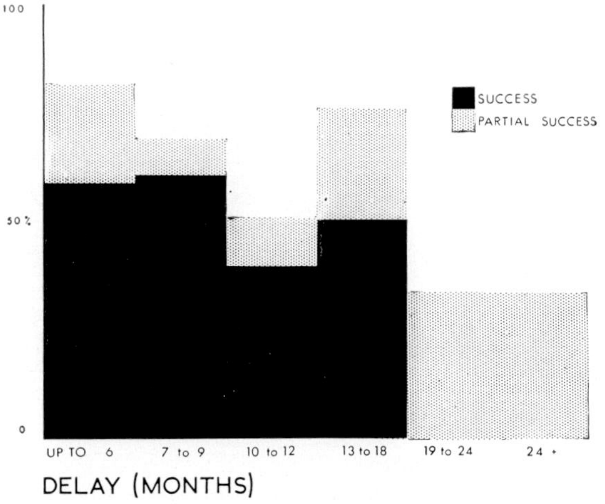

FIG. **16,** 14. Histogram showing the proportion of successes and partial successes after autologous nerve grafting in relation to the interval between injury and repair

be used for repair of the other (Fig. **6,** 18, p. 105). But more often the problem is finding enough material from a cutaneous nerve, making appropriate allowance for shrinkage and the number of grafts required to match the calibre of the recipient nerve. This is how choices were made in 122 cases (Table XLIII).

If a cutaneous nerve is to be used it should not be one that has entered its area of distribution—for example, the lateral cutaneous nerve of the thigh below the anterior superior iliac spine, or the posterior cutaneous nerve of the thigh. Nerves such as these give off branches throughout their course, with the result that the peripheral diameter is much smaller than the proximal. There are four ideal cutaneous nerves; the medial cutaneous of the forearm proximal to its bifurcation at the elbow, the available length ranging from 20 to 27 cm; the superficial radial nerve between the elbow and the wrist, yielding a length of 20 to 25 cm; the sural between its origin and the lateral malleolus, yielding a length of 25 to 40 cm; and the saphenous in the thigh, up to 40 cm, but dissecting it out is laborious. The superficial radial nerve should not be used for repair of the median unless the donor nerve is irreparably damaged. If the superficial radial nerve is excised on the injured side the patient is deprived of such benefits as would result from sensory overlapping from the superficial radial into the median area. If the contralateral superficial radial nerve is used the patient will then have two subnormal hands instead of one.

All four nerves recommended have much the same diameter, about 2 by 3 mm.

There is a theoretical objection to using cutaneous nerves for the repair of nerves containing motor fibres (Gutmann and Sanders, 1943; Sunderland, Lavarack and Ray, 1949). The largest nerve fibres are the motor and proprioceptive, and the fibres present in cutaneous

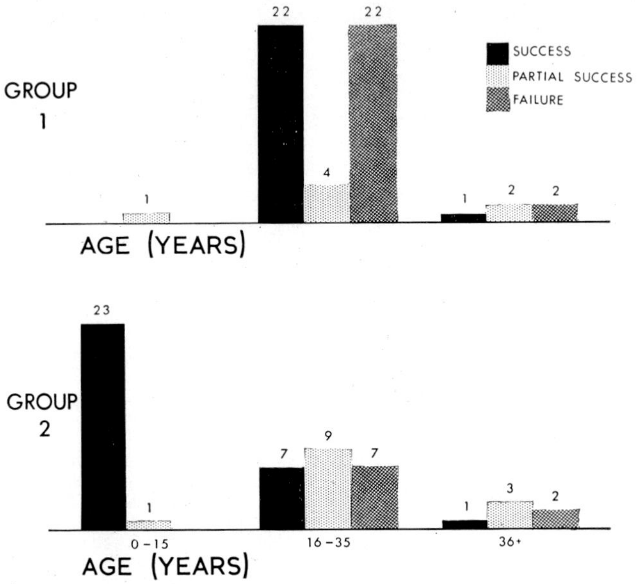

FIG. **16,** 15. The influence of age on the quality of recovery. Patients in Group 1 were treated during the Second World War, those in Group 2 were treated subsequently and are therefore representative of what may be expected in normal surgical practice.

TABLE XLIII—Sources of material used for grafting

Cutaneous Nerves	
Medial cutaneous of forearm	51
Superficial radial	8
Sural	9
Others	4
Main Trunk	
Ulnar	29
Half-thickness median	8
Common peroneal	5
Radial	4
Others	4
	122

nerves are never of a size equal to that of the largest fibres in a mixed or motor nerve. It might therefore be thought that motor recovery through a cutaneous nerve graft would be appreciably inferior to the sensory recovery. The evidence presented by our series of cases shows that this possible objection has little substance; and Simpson and Young (1945) have shown that large fibres in the proximal stump have no difficulty in inflating rather smaller distal Schwann tubes, and so attaining a diameter sufficient for their effective function.

The favourite cutaneous nerve is the medial cutaneous nerve of the forearm, and the ulnar provides the favourite large-calibre graft.

Technique of Operation

Cutaneous scarring. Because the wounds of nerves that call for repair by grafting are usually extensive, the need for the replacement of skin scars by healthy tissue often arises. Nothing less than a full-thickness flap or tube-pedicle graft will suffice because it is important that the graft should lie, so far as possible, in healthy well-vascularized tissue. When the first operation for plastic repair of the skin is undertaken the stumps of the divided nerve should be exposed. This will enable the surgeon to determine the extent of the gap and so to estimate whether the nerve can be repaired by secondary suture or by grafting. If the gap is too great to be closed by any means, there may be no need for an elaborate plastic skin repair; replacement of the scar by a split-skin graft will suffice. The plastic repair, if indicated, should be carried to a conclusion as rapidly as possible so as not to add unduly to the delay between the injury and repair of the nerve.

Exposure of the nerve. The technique is the same as for secondary suture, except that there will be no need to prolong the incision for mobilization of the stumps unless the gap is so great that, with the supply of graft material at the surgeon's disposal, it cannot be closed by grafting alone. He must then consider whether reduction of the gap by mobilization of the stumps will bring grafting within the range of possibility. If there is a reasonable prospect of success, full mobilization of the stumps is carried out and, after they have been approximated as much as possible, the neighbouring joint being flexed to a convenient degree, the remaining gap is bridged by grafting.

Suture possible but undesirable. No joint should be flexed more than 90, better 70, degrees in order to get the nerve ends comfortably together. When the median and/or ulnar nerve has been severed at the wrist the latter should not be flexed; proximal mobilization is used and the elbow alone is flexed. In any situation some remaining gap may need to be bridged by grafts, and at the wrist there is much to be said in favour of Millesi's technique (p. 298).

Resection of end-bulbs. This is done in the fashion described for secondary suture (p. 271).

Suture of a main-trunk graft. This is done with stitches; fibrin suture is disadvantageous, because it is difficult to close the epineurium completely.

Inlay grafting. The technique is illustrated in Figure **16**, 16.

Fibrin suture. For the fixation of grafts of small calibre fibrin suture is a great convenience (Seddon and Medawar, 1942). Young and Medawar's (1940) original preparation was cockerel plasma, fortified by dissolving fibrinogen in it so that its normal concentration was increased up to tenfold. This was superseded by human material, which in Britain is obtainable from the Blood Products Laboratory, the Lister Institute, Elstree, Hertfordshire. The human fibrinogen comes as a sterile powder in an ampoule containing about 130 mg of protein of which three-quarters forms the clot. If kept in an ordinary refrigerator it may be stored for up to three years. The human thrombin comes in similar form, 250 units in the ampoule.

Preparation of the grafts to form a cable. The grafts are cut to the correct length, which should be about 15 per cent greater than the gap to be bridged, and the cross-sectional area of the assembled grafts should, if possible, equal that of the proximal stump. Although grafts should be kept moist, it is best to avoid using normal saline solution; a blood-soaked swab is better. The ends of the recipient nerve may, if necessary, be tacked to convenient places with one or two epineural sutures. The bed for the graft should be of healthy and preferably vascular tissue, muscle being ideal. If scar tissue at the site of implantation cannot be excised almost completely it is sometimes possible to fold the scarred area on itself and suture the tissues so that the presenting surface is free of scar.

Before the grafts are implanted the bed for them is made horizontal; it is going to be a little lake, and temporary damming here and there with small pieces of bone wax or fibrin foam is often useful. The grafts may now be implanted. If normal saline solution has been avoided their ends are tacky and will stick to the cut surfaces of the recipient nerve. This obviates having to hold the more superficial grafts in position with watchmaker's forceps. There is no difficulty in withdrawing the latter from the clot; but the delicate task of the member of the team, who, while these manoeuvres were in progress, has been preparing the solutions for the clot and who will apply the mixture of them to the two

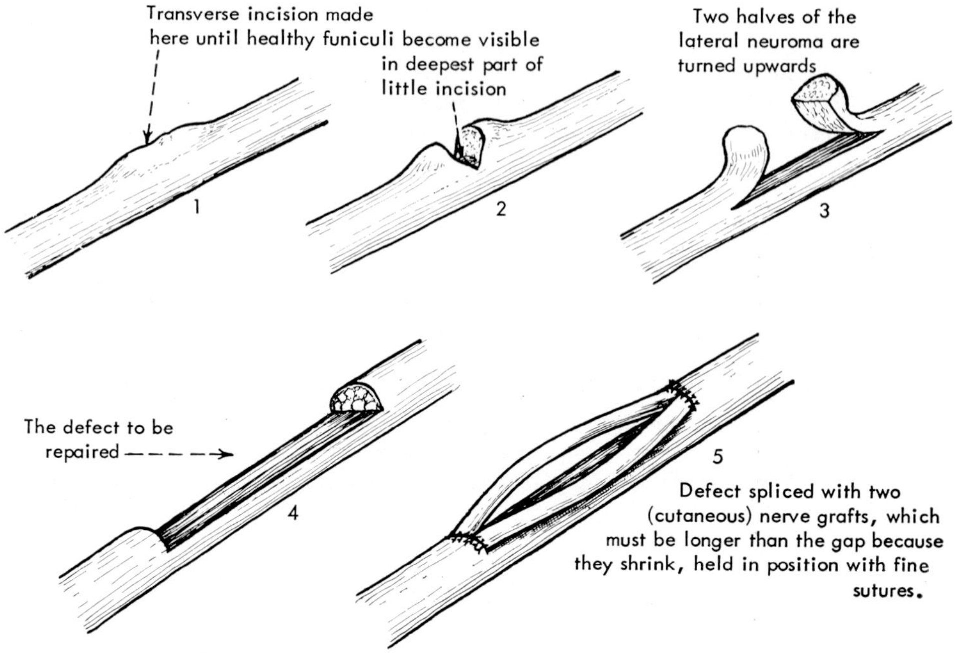

FIG. **16,** 16. Repair of a partially divided nerve—the lateral neuroma is shown in 1-3—by inlay grafting.

suture lines, is happier if he has the field of operation to himself.

The clotting solutions. The ampoule containing the fibrinogen is filled up to the 10 ml mark with sterile pyrogen-free distilled water. The powder is dissolved by gentle rotation, *not by shaking*. All but a few flakes dissolve in 10 minutes; these will dissolve within an hour to give a cloudy solution that will keep for weeks in a refrigerator.

The thrombin is dissolved rapidly in 2 ml of sterile pyrogen-free normal saline solution. It cannot be stored cold for more than a week.

Application of the fibrinogen. Sterile pipettes, teats and test-tubes are in readiness; a fresh one must be used for each application; not the smallest trace of thrombin must be allowed to get into the fibrinogen bottle. Two drops of the thrombin solution are placed in each of three or four tubes. With a fresh pipette, about 1 ml of fibrinogen is drawn up and then placed in a tube containing the two drops of thrombin: 20 drops of fibrinogen are correct and it is mixed rapidly with the thrombin by sucking it into and expelling it from the pipette. The solution is then dropped on to one suture line. It is likely to have clotted before there is time to apply it to the other suture line, and a second lot is prepared for this.

If the application has been too generous so that there is a nerve-in-aspic appearance, vascularization of the grafts could be retarded. The clot is so firm that the superfluity can be trimmed away with a small very sharp scalpel.

Results

The tabulated results are recorded in the following chapter. Unusual applications of nerve grafting have been mentioned on page 106, Fig. **6**, 19, and page 295, Fig. **16**, 12.

Grafting as a Routine Procedure

An impressive development of autologous nerve grafting comes from Millesi and his colleagues (1967; 1969; 1972*a* and *b*) in Vienna. Their arguments are based on animal experimental and clinical trial. There is no doubt that a sutured nerve subjected to great tension may be so damaged that recovery will be prevented by intraneural collagenization. Millesi goes further than this and says that any degree of tension after suture is harmful, although he accepts primary repair of a nerve where there is virtually no loss of substance. In all other cases repair by grafting—using strands from the sural nerve—is recommended. It is particularly desirable in injuries of the median and ulnar nerves at the wrist where (though this point is not specifically mentioned) allowance should be made for a range of 65 degrees of extension or more. Thus, at one sweep, he dispenses with all the surgical acrobatics required to reduce the size of a gap in a nerve. He condemns suture under tension, which is not practised by any knowledgeable surgeon today, he has no use for stretching in moderation *after* suture. The normal elasticity of nerve—at the very least 6 per cent—is ignored and so are the well-documented results of closure of, for example, gaps at the wrist of more than 2·5 cm by ordinary mobilization and suture.

An additional merit claimed for this form of repair, although applicable chiefly to distal lesions and where the gap is comparatively small, is that the nerve grafts may be inserted in such a way as to conform with the funicular pattern and thereby enhance the quality of regeneration.

To expose the funiculi the epineurium is resected. Each obvious group of funiculi is cut across above and below, where it appears healthy; the gap in each is measured and a strand of sural nerve rather longer than is required to bridge it is attached at each end with one stitch of 10/0 Nylon, the stickiness of the cut funicular surfaces being sufficient to complete the union. For the ulnar nerve 4, for the radial nerve 4–5 and for the median 5–6 grafts are required. The amount of suture material required is small; and because the resections are not at the same levels these few stitches are widely dispersed.

The reported results are on the whole good and the assessment of them seems to have been carried out with great care.

Homografts

In a number of species of animals used experimentally homografting has been successful. It may be, though it is unlikely, that the reaction that leads to rejection is less pronounced than in man. The more probable explanation is that the gaps bridged have been small, usually 2 to 3 cm. Moreover, we have already commented (p. 9) on the increased capacity for nerve regeneration, the lower one goes in the mammalian scale; regenerating fibres jump considerable gaps whatever is interposed. But this is not the whole story, as has been shown by well-controlled experiments. Thanks to Medawar we are now well informed about the phenomenon of acquired immunity to the implantation of homologous tissue, the heart of the tissue—and organ—transplantation problem. It takes time for this immunity and the reaction consequent on it to develop. If a homograft has been used to fill a small gap in a nerve it can act as a bridge for the outgrowing axons, which are able to reach the distal part of the nerve—home ground, so to speak—before the immune reaction destroys the stroma of the graft. But if the gap is extensive, and if the immune reaction provoked by nerve tissue is anything like that produced by skin, then the storm breaks long before the outgrowing axons have reached the other side. This, as we have found from examination of material from the six cases in which homografts were used—all failures—is exactly what happens.

We must be clear about our aims. Although Campbell, Bassett and Böhler (1963) used homografts in the treatment of patients who presented large gaps, in some there were gaps of the order of 3 cm that could have been bridged by other methods of proven reliability. Prepackaged, deep-freeze homografting could revolutionize the repair of peripheral nerve injuries; much tedious work would be eliminated. But most of us have set our sights lower; we would be content to use homografts only to bridge gaps that could not possibly be repaired by other means; that is to say, gaps of the order of 10 cm or more, in an adult. But this is to ask for a homograft that will succeed in the most testing conditions.

The reaction provoked by the implantation of homologous tissue is of two kinds, humoral and cellular, the latter being by far the more important. A fresh homograft (Sanders and Young, 1942) provokes a brisk cellular reaction, quite unlike that seen after implantation of an autograft. The failure of homografts in man (Seddon and Holmes, 1944; Spurling, Lyons, Whitcomb and Woodhall, 1945; Barnes, Bacsich, Wyburn and Kerr, 1946) was complete; some of them were even necrotic.

The immune reaction may be avoided by its

suppression in the host or by reducing the antigenicity of the graft. Although immunosuppressive agents have been used, even for homologous grafting in inactive neural leprosy (Gye *et al.*, 1972), it must be remembered that repair of a nerve is not a life-saving operation. Attention has, therefore, wisely been concentrated on treatment of the graft, and for this various methods are under investigation not one of which has yet met with unqualified success.

Irradiation has been a favourite method of reducing antigenicity. The grafts, stored at low temperature (−24·5°C), and perhaps dessicated were exposed to 1·66–2·5 megarads which had the added advantage of sterilizing them (Campbell *et al.*, 1963; Marmor, 1964; Gye *et al.*, 1972).

Predegeneration. It may well be that because axoplasm and myelin are absent from degenerate nerve it is less antigenic. Lewis and McLaurin (1969) used predegenerate irradiated homografts in rabbits with good results. But predegeneration would need to be a uniformly successful prerequisite in higher mammals before it could possibly be considered clinically; the ethical and technical difficulties of securing predegenerate homologous material are daunting.

Millipore is a synthetic membrane (Campbell *et al.*, 1956) with pores not exceeding 0·45 microns in diameter. When wrapped around a graft it excludes all cells from surrounding tissues and therefore all blood vessels, but permits the diffusion of extracellular body fluid. Yet obviously it cannot prevent cellular invasion of the graft from the stumps of the host nerve or the ingrowth of blood vessels from them. Millipore has the disadvantage of being inelastic, wrinkling when bent or compressed; it fragments fairly easily and this provokes fibrosis and even calcification. Nevertheless Campbell, Bassett and Böhler (1963) reported encouraging results from its use in animals. In its clinical application it was found desirable to ensheath a graft more than 5 cm long with a number of Millipore cylinders which were imbricated. It proved desirable too to remove it later, perhaps replacing it by a non-irritant wrapping material such as Silastic.

Cialit. Suitable sources of irradiation are not universally available and some surgeons have taken to storing homologous nerve grafts in a solution of an organic mercury compound, sodium 2-(ethylmercuri-mercaptyl)-benzoxazol-5-carboxylate, Cialit for short, which has the following formula:

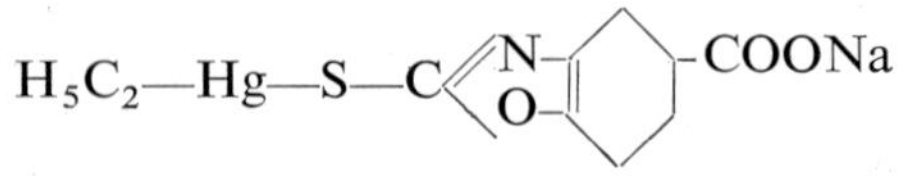

It first came into use for the storage of homologous bone and tendon and, like irradiation, it is said to sterilize material as well as reduce its antigenicity, at a concentration of 1 in 5,000. Irradiation followed by storage in Cialit has been used by Morotomi and Hirasawa (1973).

It is not yet possible confidently to recommend homologous nerve grafting. The animal experimental work on which it is based is encouraging, but as we have already had occasion to observe what works well in a small or medium-sized mammal may not prove satisfactory in man.

This is not to say that no successes have been reported. Böhler (1967), using irradiated homografts and Millipore, got some good results, but a fair proportion of failures; Marmor (1967), using irradiated grafts without Millipore, tells a similar story. A fair test is for a sufficiently experienced surgeon, following directions precisely, and using grafts in patients presenting no adverse local features other than the size of the gap to be bridged, to obtain at least passable results. It fell to my lot to meet two patients, one with an extensive traction injury of the median nerve in the arm and another with a similar lesion of the ulnar nerve. Scarring of the bed of the nerve was minimal and no major blood vessels were damaged. In these two patients I implanted grafts 16 cm and 9 cm long respectively, observing Marmor's directions precisely. No recovery occurred in either patient. The appearance of the graft in one of them, 15 months after implantation, is shown in Figure **16**, 17; it was much the same in the other patient. Examination of biopsy specimens in one case, and of the whole of the graft in the other, showed that the grafts had been transformed into fibrous tissue, in which even a ghost of normal nerve structure was barely detectable. Hiles (1972), equally careful in his technique, gives two discouraging reports.

Afanassieff (1967) is enthusiastic about his experiences with homografts preserved in Cialit. But he does not present his results in detail and he makes the extraordinary statement that what-

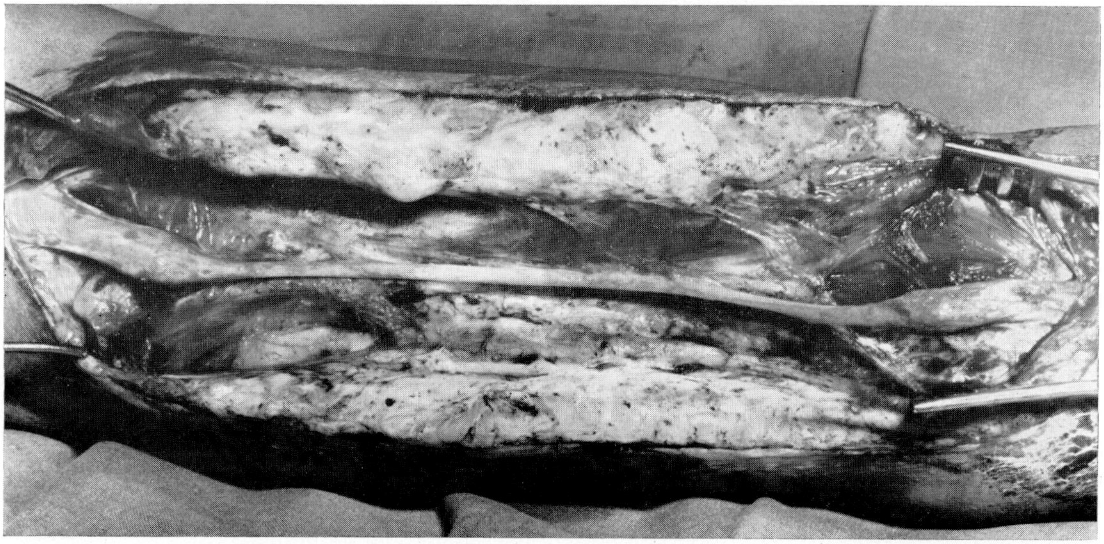

FIG. **16,** 17. A 20-year-old patient suffered a severe traction injury of the median nerve in the arm. Six months later (after an exploratory operation) the defect was repaired with a 16-cm frozen irradiated graft of appropriate diameter. Fifteen months after this there were no signs of recovery. Exploration revealed an avascular shrunken graft. Small pieces of nerve were removed from each junction and from the middle of the graft. They all showed fibrous replacement of the graft and no trace of re-innervation.

ever the length of the graft the obstruction (*barrage*) that it represents is traversed in two months irrespective of its length. It has been my good fortune to meet Tsuneichi Egawa, one of whose assistants, Teruo Doi (1970), has made a dispassionate study of the subject both experimentally and clinically. Egawa gave me an up-to-date list of his cases (all male except No. 8) which is reproduced here in tabular form.

List of Cases prepared by Tsuneichi Egawa and Teruo Doi

CASE NUMBERS	1	2	3	4	5	6	7	8	9	10
Age (years)	22	35	15	36	19	34	48	20	22	32
Interval before operation (months)	19	13	2	5	9	11	72	5	11	36
Level of injury	forearm	forearm	digit	forearm	elbow	axilla	upper arm	elbow	elbow	forearm
Cause of injury	machine	machine	saw	glass	machine	machine	wire	surgical operation	machine	machine
Nerve repaired by grafting	median	ulnar	digital	median	median	ulnar	ulnar	radial	median	ulnar
Length of graft (cm)	8	11	2	7	8	12	6.5	4	12	7
Associated damage										
Nerve	+	+	—	+	+	+	—	—	+	—
Artery	+	—	—	—	+	+	—	—	+	—
Ischaemic contracture	+	—	—	—	+	+	—	—	+	—
Muscle and tendon	+	+	+	+	+	+	—	—	+	—
Bone	+	—	—	—	+	—	—	—	+	+
Post-operative observation (months)	96	75	64	62	62	34	31	28	7	5
Result (MRC grades)										
Sensory	0	2	4	3	0	1	fibrous replacement	absorbed	0	0
Motor	0	2	—	2	0	1			0	0

When a method of treatment is *sub judice* no report less detailed than this is acceptable. It is, for example, immediately apparent that in cases 1, 5 and 9 the failure may have been due to the graft's traversing an ischaemic part of the forearm; likewise, in cases 9 and 10 insufficient time has elapsed to permit of any definite conclusion being drawn. But the result in case 3 was excellent, two-point discrimination being 8 mm at 64 months, with no possibility of overlap from an area of normal sensibility; and case 4 was satisfactory too.

NERVE ANASTOMOSIS

Before the days of nerve grafting, anastomosis between the proximal end of a normal, appropriately severed hypoglossal nerve and the distal end of a damaged facial nerve was a well-recognized remedy for facial paralysis. Today there is insufficient interest in operations of this kind in the limbs. They are of two kinds.

Sensory. In irremediable paralysis of the median nerve crude but useful sensibility in the median area of the hand can follow union of an intact superficial radial nerve with the median at the wrist (Harris, 1920; Turnbull, 1948, 1963), but Sunderland (1974) makes a better case, that merits careful study, for using the dorsal cutaneous branch of the intact ulnar nerve.

Motor. Opportunities for using the facio-hypoglossal type of anastomosis in the limbs are rare, but perhaps we are not sufficiently on the lookout for them. In a case of traumatic tetraplegia extending up to the fifth cervical segment Benassy and Robart (1966) helped the patient very considerably by severing an intact musculocutaneous nerve and uniting it to the neighbouring totally paralysed median. A similar type of operation for total brachial plexus paralysis has been mentioned on page 296, and has proved popular in Japan (Kotani, Matsuda and Suzuki, 1973; Tsuyama and Hara, 1973).

NEUROVASCULAR-CUTANEOUS TRANSFERENCE

This is a valuable palliative operation, spatially more limited in its effects than sensory-nerve anastomosis, but giving the patient a limited area of normal sensibility in an otherwise totally insensitive part (Moberg, 1955; Tubiana and Duparc, 1959, 1961; Littler, 1960). It is used for restoration of sensibility at the gripping surfaces of the index finger and thumb. An island of skin, with a pedicle composed of a digital nerve and its accompanying vessels, is taken from a relatively unimportant digit and transposed to the desired area.

17. Results of Repair of Nerves

THE NUMBER OF nerve lesions submitted to detailed analysis is shown in Table XLIV. The total appears impressive, but because no repair was performed in many cases the series is inadequate for certain purposes. For the study of some of the factors influencing the outcome of nerve suture we must turn to much larger series such as the collected results analysed by Zachary in the Medical Research Council Report (M.R.C.R., 1954); and those presented by Woodhall and Beebe (1956) in the American Veterans' monograph entitled *Peripheral Nerve Regeneration*. But both the American and British reports are concerned almost exclusively with war injuries suffered by young men in the armed forces; we must look for other evidence to obtain a balanced picture. The series of cases considered here has the merit of spanning a period of almost 25 years; five years of war, and 20 years of peace.

TABLE XLIV

Number of patients		2,229
with a single nerve lesion	1,620	
with two nerve lesions	527	
with three nerve lesions	73	
with four nerve lesions	8	
with five nerve lesions	1	
Total number of nerve lesions		2,930

Earlier series of results of nerve suture have been reported, but even to summarize them would be a fruitless exercise, largely because there have been no universally agreed criteria for assessment.

The system of grading introduced by the Nerve Injuries Committee of the (British) Medical Research Council (M.R.C.R., 1954) was a step forward. It is as follows:

MOTOR RECOVERY

- M0 No contraction.
- M1 Return of perceptible contraction in the proximal muscles.
- M2 Return of perceptible contraction in both proximal and distal muscles.
- M3 Return of function in both proximal and distal muscles of such degree that all *important* muscles are sufficiently powerful to act against resistance.
- M4 Return of function as in Stage 3 with the addition that all synergic and independent movements are possible.
- M5 Complete recovery.

SENSORY RECOVERY

- S0 Absence of sensibility in the autonomous area.
- S1 Recovery of deep cutaneous pain sensibility within the *autonomous area* of the nerve.
- S2 Return of some degree of superficial cutaneous pain and tactile sensibility within the autonomous area of the nerve.
- S3 Return of superficial cutaneous pain and tactile sensibility throughout the autonomous area with disappearance of any previous over-reaction.
- S3+ Return of sensibility as in Stage 3 with the addition that there is some recovery of two-point discrimination within the autonomous area.
- S4 Complete recovery.

DEFINITION OF PROXIMAL AND DISTAL MUSCLES

RADIAL NERVE

Proximal muscles	*Distal muscles*
Brachioradialis	Abductor pollicis longus
Extensor carpi radialis longus	Extensor pollicis longus
Extensor carpi radialis brevis	Extensor pollicis brevis
Extensor digitorum communis	Extensor indicis
Extensor carpi ulnaris	

Median Nerve

Proximal muscles	*Distal muscles*
Pronator teres	Thenar muscles
Flexor carpi radialis	
Flexor digitorum superficialis	
Flexor digitorum profundus	
Flexor pollicis longus	

Ulnar Nerve

Proximal muscles	*Distal muscles*
Flexor carpi ulnaris	Hypothenar muscles
Flexor digitorum profundus	Interossei

Common Peroneal Nerve

Proximal muscles	*Distal muscles*
Tibialis anterior	Extensor digitorum brevis
Extensor digitorum longus	
Extensor hallucis longus	
Peronei	

Tibial Nerve

Proximal muscles	*Distal muscles*
Gastrocnemius and soleus	Intrinsic muscles of the sole
Tibialis posterior	
Long flexors of the toes	

This seemed attractive, but there are difficulties.

1. For each nerve there is a particular value that must be attached to each rating: for example sensibility is of no importance in radial nerve lesions and of little importance in ulnar nerve lesions. It is motor recovery that counts. But the median nerve supplies two of the most important sensory areas in the body, the tips of the thumb and the index finger. Thus we have to change the elevation of our sights in studying this or that nerve.

2. We must also decide what grade of recovery constitutes *success:* in Figure **17**, 1 for example, do we content ourselves with S3, or raise our sights and aim at S3 + ?

3. The time taken for recovery to reach its final grade varies according to the level of the nerve lesion. The plateau shown in Figure **17**, 9 is reached three years after suture of the median nerve at or near the wrist; more time must be allowed for recovery after more proximal suture of the nerve. We shall return to this topic in considering the results of repair of the sciatic nerve (p. 309).

4. It is not possible to apply this system of grading to injuries of the brachial plexus, and Brooks (1949) was obliged to devise a more elaborate system. Neither is it applicable without modification to the sciatic nerve, particularly its tibial division.

5. For grading motor recovery the system is satisfactory, but less so for sensory recovery.

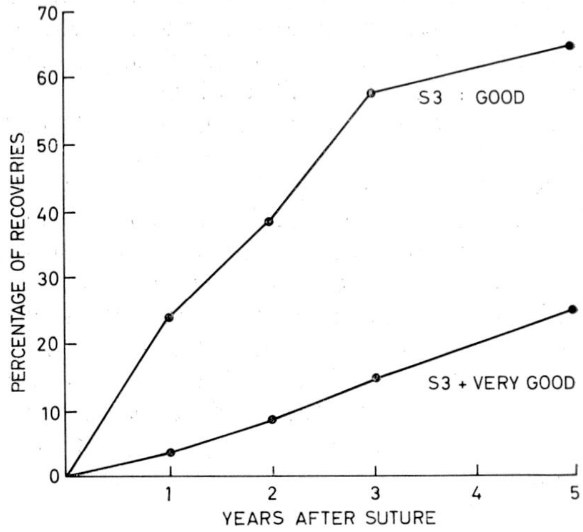

Fig. **17**, 1. Sensory recovery after suture of the median nerve at the wrist. S3: return of superficial pain and light tactile sensibility throughout the median area: no over-reaction. S3+ : the same, but with some return of tactile localization and two-point discrimination of the order of one cm or less (Nicholson and Seddon, 1957).

For the latter Moberg's tests (pp. 45 and 53) are better, in that they are more objective and one, the *picking up test*, is based on function. They apply only to the hand, but this is hardly a serious objection because injuries of the median and ulnar nerves are by far the commonest and the most important. For all other nerves the Medical Research Council system may be retained, or Sunderland's (1949) elaborate variant.

Unfortunately, the information conveyed by these systems of grading is difficult to digest, though the tables such as appear in the Medical Research Council Report, in Nicholson and Seddon's (1957) paper and in McEwan's (1962) are scientifically indispensable.

In all of our cases the M.R.C. system of grading was used, but for present purposes results will be presented in a simplified form to which the following is the key:

M4 or better	good
M3	fair
M2	poor
M1 & 0	bad
S4 (normal) or S3+	good
S3	fair
S2	poor
S1 & 0	bad

Motor and sensory results have been combined with appropriate weighting according to which nerve is under consideration. For example, sensibility is so important in median nerve paralysis that S4 or S3+ : M3 is counted as good. In ulnar nerve paralysis it is the other way round. In radial paralysis the sensory component is ignored.

We have now to consider the purposes served by presenting the results of nerve repair.

The first is to indicate whether the operation is worth undertaking. In traction injuries of the fifth and sixth cervical trunk it is doubtful. By contrast, the results of nerve repair in children of 15 years or less (Table XLV: Fig. **17**, 2) are in general so good that adverse factors, such as proximal situation of the lesion, may be largely discounted. The second purpose is to provide the patient with reliable information about his expectations, not only the chances of repair succeeding but what we surgeons mean by success. A man's ability to return to his occupation may be at stake.

Lastly, detailed results can provide the basis for judging the efficacy of one form of repair in comparison with another. But no yardstick by

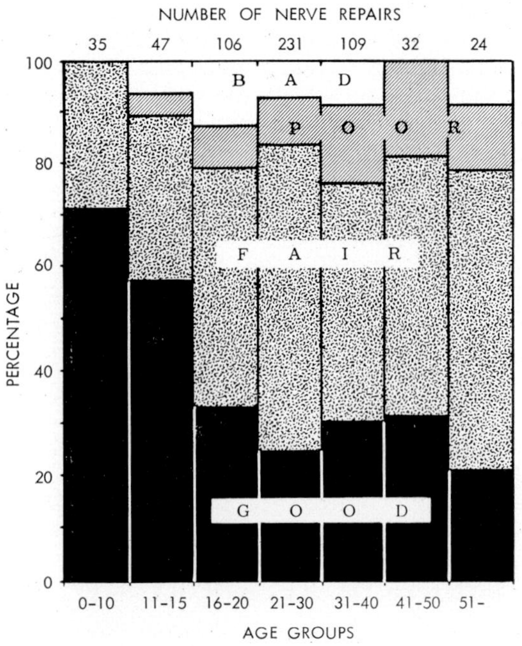

FIG. **17**, 2. Influence of age on recovery after nerve suture (Table XLV).

TABLE XLV—Influence of age on regeneration after repair of median and ulnar nerves: all levels

AGE-GROUP	TOTAL IN EACH AGE-GROUP	GRADE OF RECOVERY AFTER REPAIR							
		Good		Fair		Poor		Bad	
		Number	%	Number	%	Number	%	Number	%
0-10	35	25	71	10	29	—	—	—	—
11-15	47	27	57·6	15	32	2	4·2	3	6·4
16-20	106	35	33	49	46	9	8·5	13	12·2
21-30	231	57	24·7	137	59·2	20	8·6	17	7·7
31-40	109	33	30·3	50	45·8	17	15·6	9	8·2
41-50	32	10	31·3	16	50	6	18·8	—	—
51-	24	5	20·8	14	58	3	12·5	2	8·3
TOTAL	584								

itself suffices unless certain conditions are observed. A criterion may be brutally simple; in the treatment of bone sarcoma it is survival, *tout court*. Yet even this is useless unless the scheme of treatment is so planned that in all respects except the treatment given, the groups of patients dealt with by method A or method B are comparable.

In the study of nerve repair this means (at least) comparable age-groups (see Fig. **17**, 2), the same type of wound, the same nerve injured at the same level and the application of a uniform degree of skill in the performance of the operations under consideration.

It is valuable, too, if results are assessed by clinicians who had been in no way responsible for the essential treatment: for example, Lena McEwan (1962) in the Melbourne cases, and O. R. Nicholson and C. Schuler in my own (Nicholson and Seddon, 1957); likewise D. K. Clawson (Clawson and Seddon, 1960*a*, *b*). Yet it is doubtful whether valid comparisons can be made—high church clinical investigators would say impossible—unless the same observer assesses the results of treatment in *both* of the groups of cases that are to be compared.

RESULTS OF REPAIR BY SUTURE

Accessory Nerve

The results of repair of this motor nerve ought to be as good as those of the posterior interosseous and musculocutaneous nerves. They are not. The dismal story is told on pages 172 to 174.

Musculocutaneous Nerve

The results of repair, whether by secondary suture or grafting, are excellent. Thirteen injuries of the musculocutaneous nerve were seen. Three were due to glass cuts and seven to missiles: secondary suture was performed in six of these cases, with very good results in five, and a fair result in one; three lesions were repaired by grafting (see Fig. **6**, 3 p. 94 and Figs **16**, 1 and **16**, 2, p. 288) with satisfactory results in all.

Radial Nerve

(Table XLVI; Fig. **17**, 3)

There were only four primary sutures; of the secondary sutures, some undertaken for the repair of severe missile injuries, three out of four

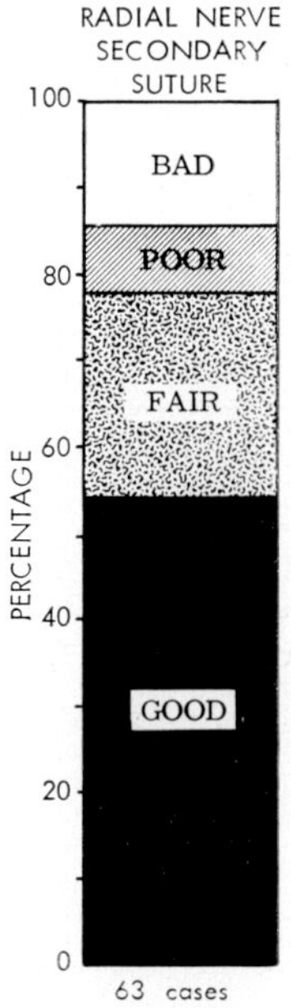

FIG. **17**, 3. Recovery after secondary suture of the radial nerve. Good = M4.

TABLE XLVI—Radial nerve

	SECONDARY SUTURE		PRIMARY SUTURE
	Number	%	Number
Bad	9	14·3	—
Poor	5	7·9	—
Fair	15	23·8	2
Good	34	54·0	2
TOTAL	63		

TABLE XLVII—Median nerve: secondary suture

	AXILLA		ARM AND ELBOW		FOREARM		WRIST	
	Number	%	Number	%	Number	%	Number	%
Bad	—	—	2	4·9	1	1·8	5	4·5
Poor	—	—	4	9·7	2	3·6	5	4·5
Fair	2	67	20	48·8	39	69·6	52	47·3
Good	1	33	15	36·6	14	25	48	43·6
TOTALS	3		41		56		110	

TABLE XLVIII—Median nerve: primary suture

	ARM AND ELBOW	FOREARM	WRIST
Bad	—	—	—
Poor	—	2	3
Fair	1	1	8
Good	—	—	6
TOTALS	1	3	17

Good = M3 : S3+ or, in children, almost 4.

(54 per cent plus 23·8 per cent) were worth while. In the patients whose results are described as *good*, function was barely distinguishable from normal.

POSTERIOR INTEROSSEOUS NERVE

The case for exploration of this nerve, in appropriate circumstances, with a view to repair if it is found to be severed and the gap is small, has been presented on page 203. Fifteen explorations were performed. In seven cases the nerve was sutured; in five restoration of function was almost complete, in one case there was fair recovery, and in one the late result is unknown.

MEDIAN NERVE

(Tables XLVII and XLVIII; Fig. **17**, 4)

The thoroughly satisfactory results were those shown as good: in those listed as fair, supplementary operations—such, for example, as tendon transplantation for loss of opposition of the thumb—were necessary in some cases.

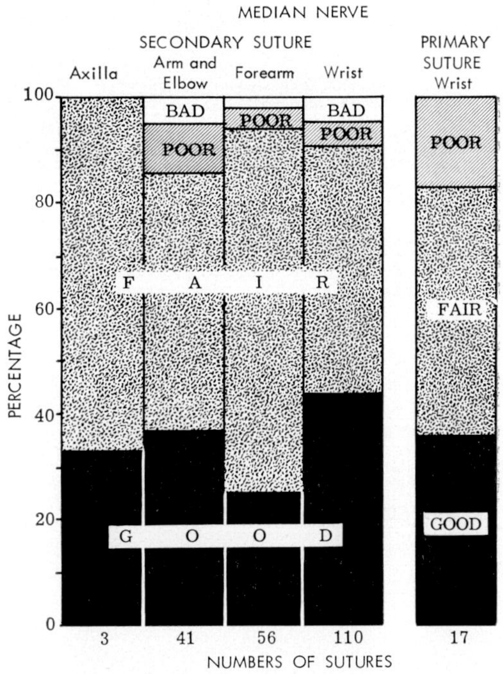

FIG. **17**, 4. Recovery after secondary suture of the median nerve: and after primary suture at the wrist. Good = M3: S3+ or better.

No significance can be attached to the three cases of suture of the median nerve in the axilla; all were in children, which is why the results were fair or good. At the wrist the results were better than at more proximal levels. The results of primary suture and secondary suture at the wrist were much the same, and the injuries in these two

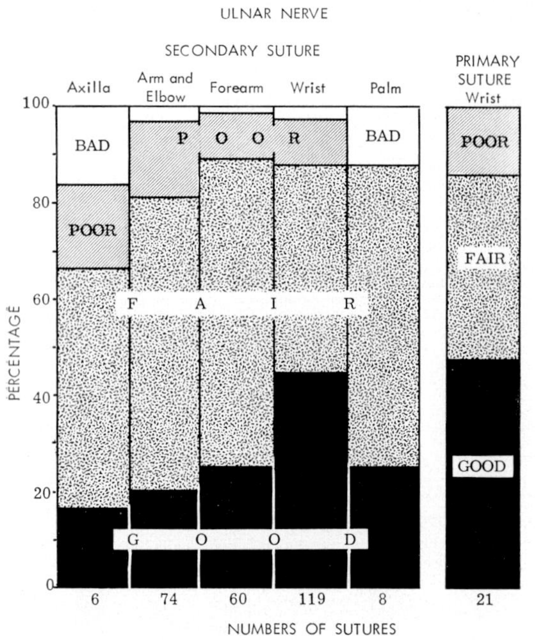

FIG. **17**, 5. Recovery after secondary suture of the ulnar nerve: and after primary suture at the wrist. Good = M3 or better: S3 or better.

groups were roughly comparable. There were only four more proximal primary repairs.

No injuries of the median nerve in the palm were repaired by suture: all were grafted.

ULNAR NERVE

(Tables XLIX and L; Fig. **17**, 5)

The ulnar nerve is repaired more often than any other. There were a few repairs in the palm, that is to say, in the hypothenar region. There were rather more primary sutures than in the case of the median nerve: 33 out of a total of 300 = 11 per cent, as compared with 21 out of a total of 231 = 9 per cent. At the wrist the results were much the same whether the nerve had been repaired primarily or secondarily.

DIGITAL NERVES

The superiority of primary suture over secondary suture (Table LI; Fig. **17**, 6) or autogenous grafting (Table LIV, p. 311) is unmistakable. In some cases of secondary repair the collagenization of the distal stump was such that resection

TABLE XLIX—Ulnar nerve: secondary suture

	AXILLA		ARM AND ELBOW		FOREARM		WRIST		PALM	
	Number	%	Number	%	Number	%	Number	%	Number	%
Bad	1	16·6	2	2·7	1	1·5	3	2·5	1	12·5
Poor	1	16·6	12	16·2	6	10	12	10	—	—
Fair	3	50	45	61·1	38	63·5	51	43	5	62·5
Good	1	16·6	15	20	15	25	53	44·5	2	25
TOTALS	6		74		60		119		8	

TABLE L—Ulnar nerve: primary suture

	AXILLA	ARM AND ELBOW	FOREARM	WRIST
Bad	—	—	—	—
Poor	—	1	3	3
Fair	—	3	1	8
Good	1	—	3	10
TOTALS	1	4	7	21

Good = M3 or better: S3.

TABLE LI—Digital nerves: excluding those in the palm

	PRIMARY SUTURE		SECONDARY SUTURE	
	Number	%	Number	%
Bad	—	—	1	12·5
Poor	1	7·7	1	12·5
Fair	5	38·5	4	50
Good	7	53·8	2	25
TOTALS	13		8	

was inadequate. We do not know how far this noxious change can extend, but there is little doubt that it is due to severance of the adjoining digital artery (see Fig. **15**, 33, p. 278). The best hope for the survival of a digital nerve is primary suture, even though the wound may be untidy; there is then at least a chance that revascularization of the distal stump will take place across the suture line. Autologous grafting is better than secondary suture.

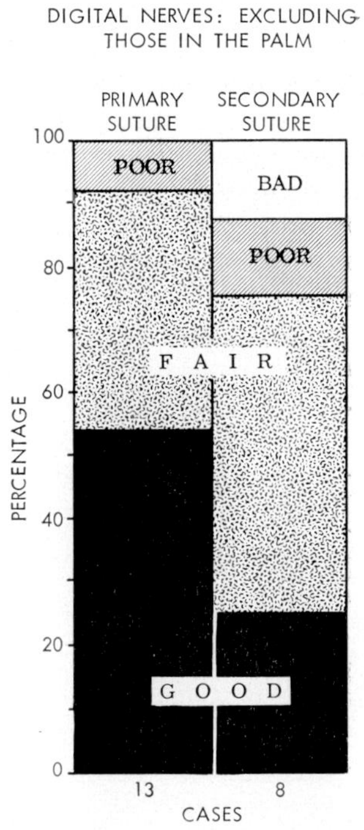

FIG. **17**, 6. Primary and secondary suture of the digital nerves, excluding those injured in the palm. Good =S3+or better.

SCIATIC NERVE: COMMON PERONEAL NERVE: TIBIAL NERVE

(Tables LII and LIII)

Injury of these nerves being in the proximal part of the limb, the results of repair are like those of repair of proximally situated lesions of the median and ulnar nerves: poor at the periphery. We have never seen recovery in the intrinsic muscles of the foot, though it has been reported in 21·3 per cent of the cases in the American series (Woodhall and Beebe, 1956). Recovery even in the long muscles of the leg—apart from the triceps surae, which behaves well—is usually disappointing; so much so that it is necessary to introduce a separate grading to indicate the power in Category M1: thus contraction against gravity and resistance in the proximal muscles, but no recovery in the intrinsic muscles of the foot, is designated as M1 (3), and in the tibial nerve this is often limited to the triceps surae. Indeed, in Tables LII and LIII all reference to distal recovery has been omitted.

The common peroneal nerve and the tibial nerve must be considered separately; functionally and sometimes anatomically they are separate nerves. Thus, no distinction is made between an injury limited to, say, the common peroneal nerve where it is anatomically separate and injury of this nerve as part of the main sciatic trunk.

The figures are taken direct from the report of Clawson and Seddon (1960*a*). So few additional cases have been seen, and followed over an adequate period, since Clawson carried out his survey that nothing is gained by including them. The levels of injury are given in the 1960*a* paper, but little useful can be gleaned from them, because few nerves were repaired at the level of the hip or at the knee: most of them were in the thigh; so these anatomical subdivisions have been excluded.

The number of nerves repaired, mostly by secondary suture, was 145. We lost touch with a number of patients who had moved to remote parts of Britain or to other countries, and the report of results is based on the findings in the 70 or so who returned for re-examination and a smaller number who completed and returned detailed questionnaires. There were then 119 nerve sutures and 13 autologous grafts.

Common Peroneal Nerve
(Table LII)

Seventy-two nerves were sutured: in 35 per cent of the cases, recovery in the proximal muscles was such that the chief aim of repair—correction of foot-drop—was achieved. The proportion of successes is much the same as is given in the American Report (29·4 per cent) and in the British Report (36 per cent).

Sensory recovery is unimportant, and has been omitted from the Table. Recovery was observed in 74 per cent of the cases.

Table LII—Suture of common peroneal nerve

MOTOR RECOVERY		
M0	19	
M1 (1-3)	27	
M1 (4-5)	21	good: 34·7% (M1 (4-5) and M2 or more)
M2 or more	5	
	—	
	72	

Tibial Nerve
(Table LIII)

Forty-seven nerves were repaired. In 79 per cent there was functionally useful motor recovery, though usually only in the triceps surae. In half of the cases showing motor recovery there was return of power in the tibialis posterior, but in only a minority was it functionally useful. Still fewer cases showed recovery in the long flexors of the toes, and in none was it useful. These results are rather better than those given in the British Report (M.R.C.R., 1954), and it is possible that this is because Clawson and I saw our patients again after a much longer period.

Table LIII—Suture of tibial nerve

MOTOR RECOVERY		
M0	5	
M1 (1-3)	5	
M1 (4-5)	37	fair 78·7% (M1 (4-5) and M2)
M2	0	
SENSORY RECOVERY		
S0	12	
S1	6	
S2	26	fair to good 61·7% (S2–S4)
S3	3	
S4	0	

Sensory recovery is important and is recorded in Table LIII. It was functionally useful in 62 per cent of the patients whose progress we had been able to follow. It was in no way dependent on whether the whole sciatic nerve or only its tibial component had been repaired. It is a great advance on the 27 per cent recorded in the British Report. But this may be a consequence of the passage of time, for in the British Report it was noted that in 80·5 per cent there was some response to pin-prick in the sole. The American figure is much the same as ours.

RESULTS OF NERVE GRAFTING

The precise grade of neurological recovery after autologous nerve grafting was determined in all except a few cases and reported in detail (Seddon, 1947*b*). In a later report (Seddon, 1963) the details were omitted, and the results were given simply as success, partial success (which meant that the operation had been worth while), and failure. Table LIV has been brought up to date, with the grading altered to that used for nerve suture in the first part of this Chapter, namely good, fair and bad.

The following points emerge. The results were fair in the repair of digital nerves in the palm. Figure **17**, 7 shows what was done for repair of the awkward lesion illustrated in Figure **11**, 51; p. 209. The grafting of nerve lesions in the digits —18 cases—was rather better; certainly more

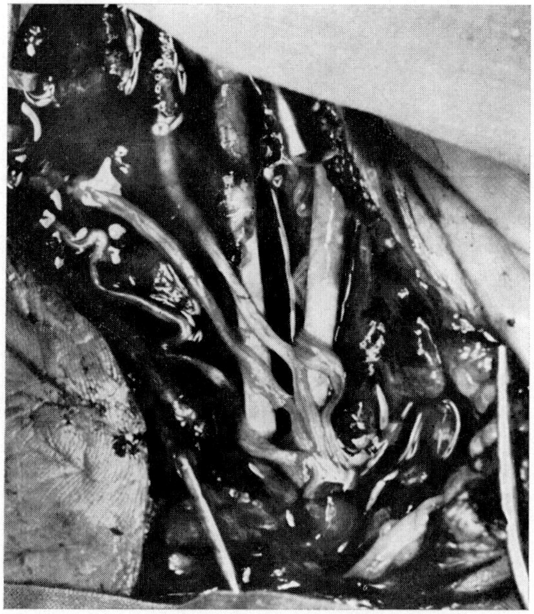

FIG. **17**, 7. Four median digital nerve grafts: repair of the palmar lesion shown in Figure **11**, 51, p. 209. They are even more lax than is necessary to allow for shrinkage because they cross the flexor tendons. Plasma clot suture; hence the dazzling reflections.

successful than secondary suture, probably because the resection of the distal stump could be more generous.

Main-trunk grafting in the upper limb was rewarding, ulnar-to-median nerve-pedicle grafting most of all.

Repair of the tibial division of the sciatic nerve with free grafts taken from the common peroneal

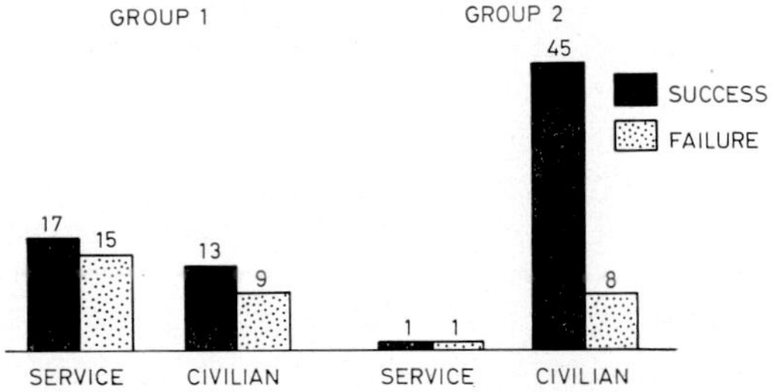

FIG. **17**, 8. Group 1: patients treated by autologous grafting during the Second World War. Group 2: those operated on subsequently. Total up to 1963: 109. (Reproduced by kind permission from *J. Bone Jt Surg.*, 1963, **45B**, 447.)

nerve was disappointing: here the best hope may be McCarty's (1951) nerve-pedicle operation (Fig. **16**, 10, p. 293).

Inlay grafts were used exclusively for repair of partial lesions of the median and ulnar nerves, and there was only one failure out of 11 cases.

During the war years we made mistakes, such as attempting to repair proximally situated lesions which anyway respond badly after end-to-end suture. Our later experience (Fig. **17**, 8, Group 2) was more encouraging. In adults the rate of failure declined from 45 to 31 per cent, but it was nerve grafting in children, with their remarkable capacity for recovery, that chiefly accounted for the better figures.

GENERAL OBSERVATIONS ON NERVE REPAIR

1. Age. It is firmly established that recovery in children is far better than in adults and there

TABLE LIV

CUTANEOUS NERVES USED AS GRAFTS			
TYPE OF REPAIR	BAD	FAIR	GOOD
Digital: in palm	2	5	1
in digits	6	2	10
Others: single strand	3	1	3
Cable	9	4	9
Inlay	1	4	6
MAIN NERVE TRUNKS USED AS GRAFTS			
	BAD	FAIR	GOOD
Upper limb			
Free	6	2	17
Pedicle	—	5	8
Lower limb. Free: all common peroneal to tibial	4	5	—

should, therefore, be no hesitation in embarking on the repair of proximally situated lesions in the young.

2. Level of lesion. In general the more proximal the lesion the worse the prognosis (Fig. **17**, 9).

3. Delay. The longer the delay before repair is undertaken the worse the prognosis, until a time is reached—the *critical delay* (p. 242)—when it is futile to consider repairing a nerve; an example of this is shown in Figure **17**, 10, in which even

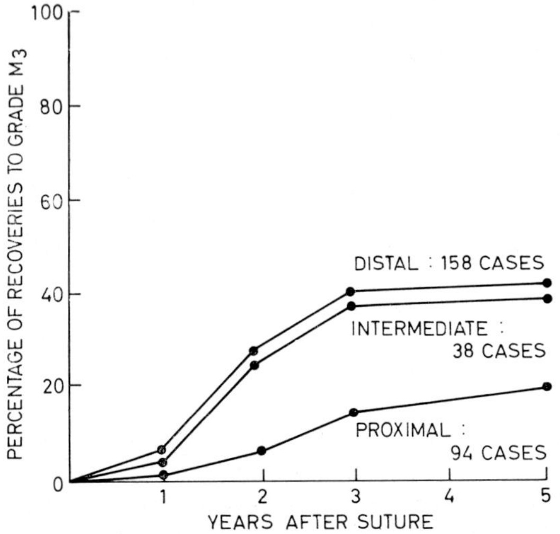

FIG. **17**, 9. Results of repair of the median nerve in relation to the level of the lesion. (Reproduced by kind permission from *Peripheral Nerve Injuries*, Spec. Rep. Ser. Med. Res. Coun. (Lond.) No. 282, 1954.)

the youth of the patient was no help. Regeneration of the nerve occurred, but the muscle atrophy was irreversible.

4. Extent of the gap closed by end-to-end suture. Zachary (M.R.C.R., 1954) found that the greater the gap the worse the prognosis. The success of autologous grafting has taken much of the sting out of this, but Nicholson and Seddon (1957) found that recovery was poorer when there had been extensive mobilization of the proximal stump of the median nerve—with consequent devascularization—in order to permit easy closure of even a moderate gap at the wrist.

The results that have been presented are for the whole series of patients. War injuries are far more destructive than most of those encountered in peace time, and repair is correspondingly difficult; it may be impossible. So it is desirable to ascertain the prognosis after nerve repair—usually suture—in civilian practice. The most important injuries are those of the median and ulnar nerves, especially at the wrist.

A survey of these civilian injuries was carried out in 1956 by O. R. Nicholson, assisted by Constantin Schuler. Three hundred and five nerve repairs were performed in 277 patients. The period of post-operative observation was three years or more in two-thirds of the cases;

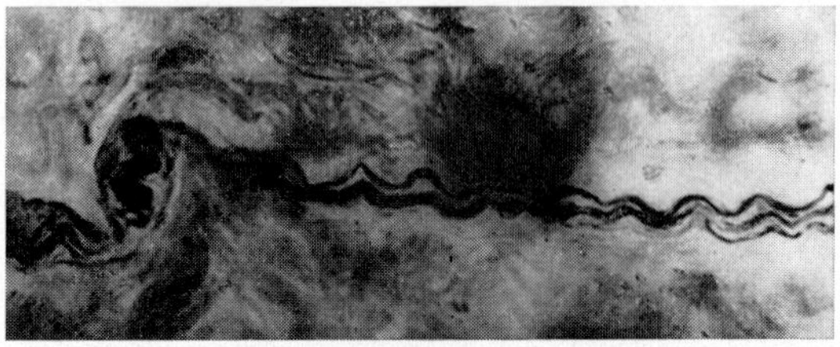

FIG. **17**, 10. A child of 3 suffered a complete transection of the radial nerve. Seven and a half years later the nerve was sutured. Clinically there was no recovery but later, when a tendon transplantation was performed, the grossly atrophic muscle was found to contain numerous nerve fibres. A few fibres are shown here: the blotchy background of atrophic muscle fibres lacks distinguishable features.

only the five-year results are shown in Table LV. Ninety-four per cent of the injuries were caused by broken glass. The same methods of examination and recording were used as in Zachary's classical study, and as in my own recent analysis, though in this chapter I have attempted to present the results by single categories embracing motor and sensory function.

The results of suture of nerves at the wrist (Nicholson and Seddon, 1957) are appreciably better than in series including war injuries, of which Zachary's in the Medical Research Council Report (1954) is the most authoritative.

Before we consider the implications of Table LV, some preliminary observations are necessary. The percentages assigned to Lena McEwan's figures are my own; the criteria are the same as those used in my own series to indicate good results. A difficulty is that McEwan uses Sunderland's (1949) grading for sensibility; and it seems likely that her category 4 includes patients with correct localization of touch to within 2 cm which is spreading the net fairly wide.

Although these figures are less meaningful

TABLE LV—Results of repair of lesions of the median and ulnar nerves at the wrist

REFERENCES	NERVE	SERIES	AGE-GROUPS	Number of cases studied	Percentage of satisfactory recoveries	
SERIES A Medical Research Council Report: 1954.	MEDIAN: Motor	A	All	158	39·8	Grade M3 or better
		B	All	52	65·4	
		C	Children	26	92	
			Adults	15	60	
SERIES B Nicholson and Seddon: 1957.	MEDIAN: Sensory	A	All	145	11	Grade S3+or better
In Series A and B all cases followed for less than five years have been excluded.		B	All	53	24·6	
		C	Children	28	93	
			Adults	18	67	
SERIES C Melbourne, Australia: reported by McEwen: 1962	ULNAR: Motor	A	All	93	16	Grade M4
		B	All	60	35	
		C	Children	24	71	
			Adults	22	23	
	ULNAR: Sensory	A	All	155	38	Grade S3 or better
		B	All	57	68·5	
		C	Children	22	100	
			Adults	25	84	

than they appear, a few firm conclusions may be drawn from them.

1. McEwan is right in listing children separately from adults. Her age-limit of 14 years is the upper limit for admission of patients to the Royal Children's Hospital in Melbourne. Table XLV and Figure **17**, 2 show a *progressive* decline with age in the quality of recovery, the 11 to 15 age-group being inferior to the 0 to 10, but much better than the 16 to 20 group. However, 14 or 15 years seems to be as good a limit as any.

2. Series B shows that civilian injuries are more favourable than those in Series A, which includes war injuries.

3. The Melbourne results, even allowing for any error I have made in the interpretation of them, are extremely good.

It is open to discussion whether my attempt to grade recovery by means of a single figure, to cover both motor and sensory function, is warranted. The patient is not interested in disquisitions on muscle power and sensibility. He asks—to give the commonest example—what are the chances of getting the best possible hand, one barely short of normal, after repair of one or both nerves at the wrist. It is good enough if we can tell him that the probability is—with us—a little under an even chance, something well over it for a child, and something better than an even chance if the injury is a clean gash across the wrist.

Bowden and Napier (1961) performed a useful service in analysing manual skills in relation to nerve injuries. Function can be quantified; it can provide a chart to monitor rehabilitation (Wynn Parry, 1973, pp. 253-258). But the documentation is formidable and unsuited to our present problem.

For the comparison of one form of treatment with another there is much to be said for retaining the motor : sensory grading. But we are still far from being able to make these comparisons with any degree of accuracy. The Medical Research Council grading suffices for nerves other than the median and ulnar. But something must be done about the assessment of nerve regeneration in the hand. There is no great difficulty in assessing muscle power and the ability to move digits independently. Sensibility is the problem. Societies dedicated to the surgery of the hand are now well established; it would be valuable if their collective wisdom could be applied to the selection of the best methods of sensory examination and the notation required to express results.

Yet when an agreed system has been found the battle will hardly have begun. Let us consider one old and one new situation that could be resolved by a controlled clinical trial, and in no other way. First, primary suture.

Primary Suture

The Melbourne School, headed by Rank and Wakefield, advocates primary repair if there is a recent incised wound—one which they aptly describe as tidy—if an experienced surgeon is immediately available, and if conditions for operating are irreproachable. Their results are outstandingly good; yet they throw no clear light on the relative merits of primary as opposed to secondary suture. McEwan's paper describes the results of 62 primary and 35 secondary repairs; so primary suture was dominant. Yet even if the results had been separated, no valid comparison is possible because primary suture was reserved for the favourable, the tidy injuries.

Michon and Masse (1964) give figures to support their view that early secondary suture is preferable, but their two groups of cases are not comparable either. Their 36 secondary sutures of the median, ulnar and radial nerves were performed by them and their team. Of the 22 primary sutures some were performed by the same group of surgeons, and for good reasons, which they give; but others had been dealt with elsewhere, and possibly indifferently.

Although Rank and his colleagues may be right in advocating primary suture in favourable circumstances (pp. 275 to 278) proof of its superiority is still lacking. Our own former condemnation of primary suture (Zachary and Holmes, 1946) had no more secure foundation.

Yet maybe this hoary controversy can now be laid to rest, the choice of primary or secondary suture being determined by circumstances. But Millesi's claims deserve the impartial test of a controlled clinical trial.

Surgery is sometimes too important to be left entirely to surgeons. They do the work: others have a duty to assess their results. The forms of treatment—in this case autologous grafting and, for simplicity, secondary suture—are applied to roughly comparable groups of cases. There ought to be fair agreement on technique among the surgeons participating, who must necessarily rid their minds of bias in favour of one operation or the other.

The random allocation—*not alternation of cases*—is arranged by an understanding statistician.

The assessment of the results of a controlled clinical trial follows a well-established technique.

1. The assessor must not have been personally involved in the treatment of the patients.

2. He, or she, must be kept unaware of which form of treatment has been given. Telltale evidence (in this case scars) must be concealed.

3. Two heads are not better than one. If two or more assessors differ, the most experienced, voluble, or assertive—but not necessarily the most dispassionate—usually wins. The single assessor, being human, is prone to err, but if he has any qualifications for the job the errors will be small and *almost always in the same direction*. Thus such error as there is will have the same incidence in both groups of cases. The assessments, here and there fall short of absolute values, but they form a sound basis for comparative study.

Some reader may regard an exercise of this kind as too rarified, or at any rate impracticable—though there is monumental evidence that it is not. The modern chemotherapy of pulmonary tuberculosis, now within the means of very poor countries, rests on the renowned Madras experiments originated by Wallace Fox. It has been my privilege to be associated with him in the conduct of controlled clinical trials in a kindred surgical field, the treatment of tuberculosis of the spine (M.R.C.R. 1973*a* and *b* and 1974 *a* and *b*. My only regret is that I did not subject myself to this sort of discipline earlier in my career.

References

Abbot, L. C. and Saunders, J. B. de C. M. (1933). Injuries of the median nerve in fractures of the lower end of the radius. *Surgery, Gynec. Obstet.*, **57**, 507.

Abercrombie, M. and Johnson, M. L. (1942). The outwandering of cells in tissue cultures of nerves undergoing Wallerian degeneration. *J. exp. Biol.*, **19**, 266.

Abercrombie, M. and Johnson, M. L. (1946*a*). Quantitative histology of Wallerian degeneration. I. Nuclear population in rabbit sciatic nerve. *J. Anat.*, **80**, 37.

Abercrombie, M. and Johnson, M. L. (1946*b*). Collagen content of rabbit sciatic nerve during Wallerian degeneration. *J. Neurol. Neurosurg. Psychiat.*, **9**, 113.

Abercrombie, M. and Johnson, M. L. (1947). The effect of reinnervation on collagen formation in degenerating sciatic nerves of rabbits. *J. Neurol. Neurosurg. Psychiat.*, **10**, 89.

Abercrombie, M., Johnson, M. L. and Thomas, G. A. (1949). The influence of nerve fibres on Schwann cell migration investigated in tissue culture. *Proc. R. Soc. Ser. B.*, **136**, 448.

Adams, J. C. (1964). Vulnerability of the sciatic nerve in closed ischio-femoral arthrodesis by nail and graft. *J. Bone Jt Surg.*, **46B**, 748.

Adams, W. E. (1943). The blood supply of nerves. 2. The effects of exclusion of its regional sources of supply on the sciatic nerve of the rabbit. *J. Anat.*, **77**, 243.

Adrian, E. D. and Bronk, D. W. (1929). The discharge of impulses in motor nerve fibres. Part II. The frequency of discharge in reflex and voluntary contractions. *J. Physiol., Lond.*, **67**, 119.

Afanassieff, A. (1967). Premiers résultats de 20 homogreffes de nerfs conservés par le cialit (Main et avant-bras). *Presse méd.*, **75**, 1409.

Aitken, J. T., Sharman, N. and Young, J. Z. (1947). Maturation of regenerating nerve fibres with various peripheral connections. *J. Anat.*, **81**, 1.

Aitken J. T. and Thomas P. K. (1962). Retrograde changes in fibre size following nerve section. *J. Anat.*, **96**, 121.

Albert, E. (1885). Einige Operationen an Nerven. *Wien. med. Presse*, **26**, 1285.

Allbrook, D. B. and Aitken, J. T. (1951). Reinnervation of striated muscle after acute ischaemia. *J. Anat.*, **85**, 376.

American Academy of Orthopedic Surgeons (1966). *Joint Motion, Method of Measuring and Recording.* Edinburgh: Churchill Livingstone

Antoni, N. R. E. (1920). *Ueber Rückenmarkstumoren und Neurofibrome; Studien zur pathologischen Anatomie und Embryogenese; mit einem klinishen Anhang.* Munich: J. E. Bergmann.

Assaky, G. (1886). De la suture des nerfs à distance. *Archs gén. Méd.*, **2**, 529.

Babcock W. W. (1927). A standard technique in operations on peripheral nerves with especial reference to the closure of large gaps. *Surgery, Gynec. Obstet.*, **45**, 364.

Bacsich, P. and Wyburn, G. M. (1945*a*). The vascular pattern of peripheral nerve during repair after experimental crush injury. *J. Anat.*, **79**, 9.

Bacsich, P. and Wyburn, G. M. (1945*b*). The effect of interference with the blood supply on the regeneration of peripheral nerves. *J. Anat.*, **79**, 74.

Bacsich, P. and Wyburn, G. M. (1945*c*). Degenerative and regenerative changes at the site of trauma after experimental crush injury of peripheral nerves. *Proc. R. Soc. Edinb.*, **62**, 182.

Ballance, C. and Duel, A. B. (1932). Operative treatment of facial palsy by the introduction of nerve grafts into fallopian canal and by other intratemporal methods. *Archs Otolar.*, **15**, 1.

Bardeen C. R. (1906). Development and variation of nerves and musculature of inferior extremity and of the trunk in man. *Am. J. Anat.*, **6**, 259.

Barker, D. and Young, J. Z. (1947). Recovery of stretch reflexes after nerve injury. *Lancet*, **1**, 704.

Barnes, R. (1949). Traction injuries of the brachial plexus in adults. *J. Bone Jt Surg.*, **31B**, 10.

Barnes, R. (1953). The role of sympathectomy in the treatment of causalgia. *J. Bone Jt Surg.*, **35B**, 172.

Barnes, R., Bacsich, P. and Wyburn, G. M. (1945). A histological study of a pre-degenerated nerve graft. *Br. J. Surg.*, **33**, 130.

Barnes, R., Bacsich, P., Wyburn, G. M. and Kerr, A. S. (1946). A study of the fate of nerve homografts in man. *Br. J. Surg.*, **34**, 34.

Bateman, J. E. (1947). A miniature galvanic stimulator. *J. Bone Jt Surg.*, **29**, 241.

Bateman, J. E. (1962). *Trauma to Nerves in Limbs.* Philadelphia: Saunders.

Benassy, J. and Robart, J. (1966). Un cas de transposition du nerf musculo-cutané sur le nerf médian. *Annls Chir. plast.*, **11**, 187.

Benjamin, A. (1957). The relief of traumatic arterial spasm in threatened Volkmann's ischaemic contracture. *J. Bone Jt Surg.*, **39B**, 711.

Bentley, F. H. and Hill, M. (1936). Experimental surgery. Nerve grafting. *Br. J. Surg.*, **24**, 368.

Bentley, F. H. and Schlapp, W. (1943). Experiments on the blood supply of nerves. *J. Physiol., Lond.*, **102**, 62.

Bernhardt, M. (1895). Über isolirt im Gebiete des Nervus cutaneus femoralis externus vorkommende Parästhesien. *Neurol. Zentbl.*, **14**, 242.

Betts, L. O. (1940). Morton's metatarsalgia: neuritis of the fourth digital nerve. *Med. J. Aust.* **1**, 514.

Black, A. N., Burns, B. D. and Zuckerman, S. (1941). An experimental study of the wounding mechanism of high-velocity missiles. *Br. med. J.*, **2**, 872.

BLACKWOOD, W. and RUSSELL, H. (1945). Further experiments in the study of immersion foot. *Edinb. med. J.*, **52**, 160.

BLUNT, M. J. and STRATTON, K. (1956). The development of a compensatory collateral circulation to nerve trunk. *J. Anat.*, **90**, 508.

BÖHLER, J. (1967). Nerventransplantation und Tubilisation von Nervennähten und Nerventransplantation. *10th Int. Congr. Soc. int. Chir. orthop. Traumat.*, p. 755. Brussels: Acta Medica Belgique.

BONNEY, G. (1954). The value of axon responses in determining the site of lesion in traction injuries of the brachial plexus. *Brain*, **77**, 588.

BONNEY, G. (1959). Prognosis in traction lesions of the brachial plexus. *J. Bone Jt Surg.*, **41B**, 4.

BONNEY, G. and GILLIATT, R. W. (1958). Sensory nerve conduction after traction lesion of the brachial plexus. *Proc. R. Soc. Med.*, **51**, 365.

BOURGUIGNON, G. (1923). *La chronaxie chez l'homme.* Paris: Masson.

BOWDEN, R. E. M. and GUTMANN, E. (1944). Denervation and re-innervation of human voluntary muscle. *Brain*, **67**, 273.

BOWDEN, R. E. M. and GUTMANN, E. (1945). Clinical value of muscle biopsies. *Lancet*, **2**, 768.

BOWDEN, R. E. M. and NAPIER, J. R. (1961). The assessment of hand function after peripheral nerve injuries. *J. Bone Jt Surg.*, **43B**, 481.

BOWDEN, R. E. M. and SHOLL, D. A. (1950). The advance of functional recovery after radial nerve lesions in man. *Brain*, **73**, 251.

BOWEN, T. L. and STONE, K. H. (1966). Posterior interosseous nerve paralysis caused by a ganglion at the elbow. *J. Bone Jt Surg.*, **48B**, 774.

BRAIN, W. R., WRIGHT, A. D. and WILKINSON, M. (1947). Spontaneous compression of both median nerves in the carpal tunnel. Six cases treated surgically. *Lancet*, **1**, 277.

BRAND, P. W. (1964). In *Leprosy in Theory and Practice*, ed. Cochrane, R. G. and Davey, T. F. 2nd ed. Bristol: Wright.

BROOKS, D. M. (1949). Open wounds of the brachial plexus. *J. Bone Jt Surg.*, **31B**, 17.

BROOKS, D. M. (1952). Nerve compression by simple ganglia. *J. Bone Jt Surg.*, **34B**, 391.

BROWN, H. and FLYNN, J. E. (1973). Abdominal pedicle flap for hand neuromas and entrapped nerves. *J. Bone Jt Surg.*, **55A**, 575.

BUCHTHAL, F., KNAPP, G. G. and LINDHARD, J. (1936). Die Struktur der quergestreiften, lebenden Muskelfaser des Froches in Ruhe und während der Kontraktion. *Skand. Arch. Physiol.*, **73**, 163.

BÜDINGER, F. and KOLMER, H. (1943). Beitrag zur Behandlung der Schmerzsyndrome Nervenschussverletzten. (Treatment of the pain syndrome in gun-shot injuries of nerves.) *Nervenarzt*, **16**, 67.

BUFALINI, C. and PESCATORI G. (1969). Posterior cervical electromyography in the diagnosis and prognosis of brachial plexus injuries. *J. Bone Jt Surg.*, **51B**, 627.

BUNNELL, S. (1927). Surgery of nerves of the hand. *Surgery, Gynec. Obstet.*, **44**, 145.

BUNNELL, S. (1964). *Surgery of the Hand*, 4th ed. Revised by Boyes, J. H. Montreal: Pitman Medical; Philadelphia: Lippincott.

BUNNELL, S. and BOYES, J. H. (1939). Nerve grafts. *Am. J. Surg.*, **44**, 64.

BURRATI, G. (1972). Electrodiagnosis of denervation of skin. *Hand*, **4**, 68.

Byers, P.D. and Darby A.T. Personal communication.

CAJAL, S. RAMON Y. *See* RAMON Y CAJAL, S.

CALVET, LEROY and LACROIX (1941-42). Luxations de l'épaule et lésions vasculaires. *J. Chir., Paris*, **58**, 337.

CAMERON, H. C. (1944). Lord Lister on nerve repair. *Br. Med. J.*, **2**, 833.

CAMPBELL, A. W. (1905). *Histological Studies on the Localisation of Cerebral Function.* London: Cambridge University Press.

CAMPBELL, J. B., BASSETT, C. A. L. and BÖHLER, J. (1963). Frozen, irradiated homografts shielded with microfilter sheaths in peripheral nerve surgery. *J. Trauma*, **3**, 302.

CAMPBELL, J. B., BASSETT, C. A. L., GIRALDO, J. M., SEYMOUR, R. J. and ROSSI, J. P. (1956). Application of monomolecular filter tubes in bridging gaps in peripheral nerves and for prevention of neuroma formation. *J. Neurosurg.*, **13**, 635.

CANNON, B. W. and LOVE, J. G. (1946). Tardy median palsy; median neuritis; median thenar neuritis amenable to surgery. *Surgery, St. Louis*, **20**, 210.

CAPENER, N. L. (1956). The hand in surgery. *J. Bone Jt Surg.*, **38B**, 128.

CAVE, L., FUSTEC, R. and BASSET, A. (1965). Radiologie de la lepre. *Annales de Radiologie*, **8**, 61.

CHAPMAN, L., RAMOS, A. O, GOODELL, H. and WOLFF H. G. (1961). Neurohumoral features of afferent fibers in man. *Archs Neurol., Chicago*, **4**, 617.

CHLENOV, L. G. (1944). On the pathogenesis of causalgia. *Vop. Neurokhir.*, **8**, 7.

CIBA FOUNDATION SYMPOSIUM (1966). *Touch, Heat and Pain.* London. J. and A. Churchill.

CLARK, J. M. P. (1946). Reconstruction of biceps brachii by pectoral muscle transplantation. *Br. J. Surg.*, **34**, 180.

CLARK, K. (1961) Ganglion of the lateral popliteal nerve. *J. Bone Jt Surg.*, **43B**, 778.

CLARK, W. E. LE GROS and BLOMFIELD, L. (1945). The efficiency of intramuscular anastomoses, with observations on the regeneration of devascularized muscles. *J. Anat.*, **79**, 15.

CLAWSON, D. K. and SEDDON, H. J. (1960*a*). The results of repair of the sciatic nerve. *J. Bone Jt Surg.*, **42B**, 205.

CLAWSON, D. K. and SEDDON, H. J. (1960*b*). The late consequences of sciatic nerve injury. *J. Bone Jt Surg.*, **42B**, 213.

CODMAN, E. A. (1934). *The Shoulder.* Boston, Mass.: Privately published.

COLLIER, J. (1940). Facial paralysis and its operative treatment. *Lancet*, **1**, 91.

CRAGG B. G. and THOMAS P. K. (1957). Changes in conduction velocity and fibre size proximal to peripheral nerve lesions. *J. Physiol., Lond.* **157**, 315.

CRAGG, B. G. and THOMAS, P. K. (1964). The conduction velocity of regenerated peripheral nerve fibres. *J. Physiol., Lond.*, **171**, 164.

CRAIG, W. S. and CLARK, J. M. P. (1958). Of peripheral nerve palsies in the newly born. *J. Obstet. Gynaec. Br. Commonw.*, **65**, 229.

CRAIG, W. S. and CLARK, J. M. P. (1961). Radial palsy simulating Volkmann's contracture in a newly born baby. *J. Obstet. Gynaec. Br. Commonw.*, **68**, 130.

CROWE, F. W., SCHULL, W. J. and NEEL, J. W. (1956). *Multiple Neurofibromatosis.* Springfield, Ill.: Thomas.

CURTIS, R. M. and EVERSMANN, W. W. (1973). Internal neurolysis as an adjunct to the treatment of the carpal-tunnel syndrome. *J. Bone Jt Surg.*, **55A**, 733.

DALE, R. H. (1954). Electrical accidents. *Br. J. plast. Surg.*, **7**, 44.

DAVIS, D. R. (1949). Some factors affecting the results of treatment of peripheral nerve injuries. *Lancet*, **1**, 877.

DAVIS, L. and CLEVELAND, D. A. (1934). Experimental studies in nerve transplants. *Ann. Surg.*, **99**, 271.

DAVIS, L., SCARFF, J. E., ROGERS, N. and DICKINSON, M. (1943). High altitude frostbite. *Surgery, Gynec. Obstet.*, **77**, 561.

DAWSON, G. D. and SCOTT, J. W. (1949). The recording of nerve action potentials through skin in man. *J. Neurol. Neurosurg. Psychiat.*, **12**, 259.

De BAKEY, M. E., and SIMEONE, F. A. (1946). Battle injuries of the arteries in World War II. *Ann. Surg.*, **123**, 534.

DÉJERINE, J. Mme DÉJERINE and MOUZON, J. (1915). Les lésions des gros troncs nerveux des membres par projectiles de guerre, les différents syndromes cliniques et les indications opératoires. *Presse méd.*, **23**, 153.

DELBET, P. and CAUCHOIX, A. (1910). Les paralysies dans les luxations de l'épaule. *Revue Chir.*, **41**, 327.

DENMARK, A. (1813). An example of symptoms resembling tic douloureux produced by a wound in the radial nerve. *Med. chir. Trans.*, **4**, 48.

DENNY-BROWN, D. E. (1946). Importance of neural fibroblasts in regeneration of nerve. *Archs Neurol. Psychiat.*, **55**, 171.

DENNY-BROWN, D. E. and BRENNER, C. (1944*a*). Paralysis of nerve induced by direct pressure and by tourniquet. *Archs Neurol. Psychiat.*, **51**, 1.

DENNY-BROWN, D. E. and BRENNER, C. (1944*b*). Lesion in peripheral nerve resulting from compression by spring clip. *Archs Neurol. Psychiat.*, **52**, 1.

DENNY-BROWN, D. E. and DOHERTY, M. M. (1945). Effects of transient stretching of peripheral nerve. *Archs Neurol. Psychiat.*, **54**, 116.

DENNY-BROWN, D. E., ADAMS, R. D., BRENNER, C. and DOHERTY, M. M. (1945). The pathology of injury to nerve induced by cold. *J. Neuropath. exp. Neurol.*, **4**, 305.

DESMEDT, J. E. (1973). *New Developments in Electromyography and Clinical Neurophysiology.* (In three volumes.) Basel: S. Karger.

DIVINCENTI F. C., MONCRIEF, J. A. and PRUITT, B. A. (1969). Electrical injuries: a review of 65 cases. *J. Trauma*, **9**, 497.

DODGE, H. W., Jr. and CRAIG, W. MCK. (1957). Benign tumours of peripheral nerves and their masquerade. *Minn. Med.*, **40**, 294.

DOI, T. (1970). Experimental study and clinical use of peripheral nerve homografts. Med. J. Osaka Univ., **22**, 395.

DOINIKOW, B. (1913). Histologische und histopathologische Untersuchungen am peripheren Nervensystem mittels vitaler Färbung. *Folia neurobiol.*, **7**, 731.

DOTT, N. M. (1935). Personal communication.

DOUPE, J., BARNES, R. and KERR, A. S. (1943). Studies in denervation: effect of electrical stimulation on circulation and recovery of denervated muscle. *J. Neurol. Psychiat., Lond.*, **6**, 136.

DOUPE, J., CULLEN, C. H. and CHANCE, G. Q., (1944). Post-traumatic pain and causalgic syndrome. *J. Neurol. Psychiat., Lond.*, **7**, 33.

DUEL, A. B. (1933). History and development of surgical treatment of facial palsy. *Surgery, Gynec. Obstet.*, **56**, 382.

DUNHAM, E. C. (1955). *Premature Infants*, p. 223. London: Cassell.

EAMES, R. A. and GAMBLE, H. J. (1970). Schwann cell relationships in normal human cutaneous nerves. *J. Anat.*, **106**, 417.

EARL, C. J., FULLERTON, P. M., WAKEFIELD, G. S. and SHUTTA, H. S. (1964). Hereditary neuropathy with liability to pressure palsies. *Q. Jl Med.* **33**, 481.

EBELING, P., GILLIATT, R. W. and THOMAS, P. K. (1960). A clinical and electrical study of ulnar nerve lesions in the hand. *J. Neurol. Neurosurg. Psychiat.* **23**, 1.

ECHLIN, F., OWENS, F. M. and WELLS, W. L. (1949). Observations on "major" and "minor" causalgia. *Archs Neurol. Psychiat.*, **62**, 183.

ECKER, A. D. and WOLTMAN, H. W. (1938). Meralgia paraesthetica: a report of 150 cases. *J. Am. med. Ass.*, **110**, 1650.

EDEN, R. C. (1939). Vascular complications of cervical ribs and first thoracic rib abnormalities. *Br. J. Surg.*, **27**, 111.

EDSHAGE, S. (1964). Peripheral nerve suture. A technique for improved intraneural topography. Evaluation of some materials. *Acta chir. scand.*, Suppl. **331**.

EHRENFEST, H. (1931). *Birth Injuries of the Child*, 2nd ed., p. 307. New York: Appleton.

ELKIN, D. C. and WOODHALL, B. (1944). Combined vascular and nerve injuries of warfare. *Ann. Surg.*, **119**, 411.

ENGEL, A. G. and SANTA, T. (1973). Motor endplate fine structure in Desmedt, **1**, 196.

ERB, W. (1876). Diseases of the peripheral cerebro-spinal nerves. Vol. XI of *Cyclopedia of the Practice of Medicine*, ed. Ziemssen, H. von. London: Samson Low, Marston, Searle and Rivington.

EWING, M. R. (1950). Postoperative paralysis in the upper extremity. *Lancet*, **1**, 99.

FAHLGREN, H., HED, R. and LUNDMARK, C. (1957). Myonecrosis and myoglobinuria in alcohol and barbiturate poisoning. *Acta med. scand.*, **158**, 405.

FAHRNI, W. H. (1950). Neonatal sciatic palsy. *J. Bone Jt Surg.*, **32B**, 42.

FALCONER, M. A. (1953). Surgical treatment of intractable phantom-limb pain. *Br. med. J.*, **1**, 299.

FALCONER, M. A. (1966). In *Pain*, ed. Knighton, R. S. and Dumke, P. R. Boston: Little, Brown and Co.

FALCONER, M. A. and LI, F. W. P. (1962). Resection of the first rib in costo-clavicular compression. *Lancet*, **1**, 59.

FALCONER, M. A. and WEDDELL, G. (1943). Costo-clavicular compression. *Lancet*, **2**, 539.

FAWCETT, K. J. and DAHLIN, D. C. (1967). Neurilemmoma of bone. *Am. J. clin. Path.*, **47**, 759.

FEARN, C. B. d'A. and GOODFELLOW, J. W. (1965). Anterior interosseous nerve palsy. *J. Bone Jt Surg.*, **47B**, 91.

FEINSTEIN, B., PATTLE, R. E. and WEDDELL, G. (1945). Metabolic factors affecting fibrillation in denervated muscle. *J. Neurol. Neurosurg. Psychiat.*, **8**, 1.

FISCHER, E. (1939). The effect of faradic and galvanic stimulation upon the course of atrophy in denervated skeletal muscles. *Am. J. Physiol.*, **127**, 605.

FLETCHER, I. (1967). New developments in splintage of the upper limb. *Physiotherapy.*, **53**, 362.

FLETCHER, I. (1969). Traction injuries of the brachial plexus. *Hand*, **1**, 129.

FOERSTER, O. (1927). *Die Leitungsbahnen des Schmerzgefuehls und die chirurgische Behandlung der Schmerzzustände*. Berlin and Vienna: Urban and Schwarzenberg.

FREEMAN, N. E. (1947). The treatment of causalgia arising from gunshot wounds of the peripheral nerves. *Surgery, St. Louis*, **22**, 68.

FRIEDMAN, N. B. (1946). The reactions of tissue to cold. *Am. J. clin. Path.*, **16**, 634.

FROMME, A. (1917). Über Kriegsaneurysmen. *Beitr. klin. Chir.*, **105**, 293.

FRYKMAN, G. (1967). Fracture of the distal radius including sequelae—shoulder-hand-finger syndrome, disturbance in the distal radio-ulnar joint and impairment of nerve function. *Acta orthop. scand.*, Suppl. 108.

FULLERTON, P. M. (1963). The effect of ischaemia on nerve conduction in the carpal tunnel syndrome. *J. Neurol. Neurosurg. Psychiat.*, **26**, 385.

GABRIELSSON, G. J. and STENSTRÔM, S. J. (1966). A contribution to peripheral nerve suture technique. *Plastic reconstr. Surg.*, **38**, 68.

GAILLAND, L. A. (1967). Rappels de corde en 'S' et en '8': causes possibles d'accidents. *Bull. mens. Club Alpin Suisse*, **43**, 121.

GALLIE, W. E. (1942). Some lessons learned in the Great War. *Surgery, Gynec. Obstet.*, **74**, 370.

GAMBLE, H. J. (1964). Comparative electron-microscopic observations on the connective tissues of a peripheral nerve and a spinal root in the rat. *J. Anat.*, **98**, 17.

GARDNER, W. J. and TURNER, O. (1940). Bilateral acoustic neurofibromas. *Archs Neurol. Psychiat.*, **44**, 76.

GARLAND, H. and MOORHOUSE, D. (1952). Compressive lesions of the external popliteal (common peroneal) nerve. *Br. med. J.*, **2**, 1373.

GHENT, W. R. (1959). Meralgia paraesthetica. *Can. med. Ass. J.*, **81**, 631.

GIBSON, J. M. C. (1962). Rupture of the axillary artery. *J. Bone Jt Surg.*, **44B**, 114.

GILLIATT, R. W. (1961). Nerve conduction: Motor and sensory. In *Electrodiagnosis and Electromyography*, 2nd ed. Ed. Licht, S. H., New Haven, Conn: Licht.

GILLIATT, R. W. (1962). Electrodiagnosis and electromyography in clinical practice. *Br. med. J.*, **2**, 1073.

GILLIATT, R. W. and HJORTH, R. J. (1972). Nerve conduction during Wallerian degeneration in the baboon. *J. Neurol. Neurosurg. Psychiat.*, **35**, 335.

GILLIATT, R. W., LE QUESNE, P. M., LOGUE, V. and SUMNER, A. J. (1970). Wasting of the hand associated with a cervical rib or band. *J. Neurol. Neurosurg. Psychiat.*, **33**, 615.

GILLIATT, R. W. and SEARS, T. A. (1958). Sensory nerve action potentials in patients with peripheral nerve lesions. *J. Neurol. Neurosurg. Psychiat.*, **21**, 109.

GILLIATT, R. W. and THOMAS, P. K. (1960). Changes in nerve conduction with ulnar lesions at the elbow. *J. Neurol. Neurosurg. Psychiat.*, **23**, 312.

GOODFELLOW, J. W. FEARN, C. B. d'A. and MATTHEWS, J. M. (1967). Iliacus haematoma. *J. Bone Jt Surg.*, **49B**, 478.

GOODMAN, H. V. and GILLIATT, R. W. (1961). The effect of treatment on median nerve conduction in patients with the carpal tunnel syndrome. *Ann. phys. Med.*, **6**, 137.

GOSSET, J. and MICHON, J. (1965). Les plaies récentes de la main et des doigts. *J. Chir., Paris*, **90**, 205.

GRANIT, R., LEKSELL, L. and SKOGLUND, C. R. (1944). Fibre interaction in injured or compressed region of nerve. *Brain*, **67**, 125.

GRANTHAM, E. G., POLLARD, C. and BRABSON, J. A. (1948). Peripheral nerve surgery. Repair of nerve defects. *Ann. Surg.*, **127**, 696.

GREENFIELD, A. D. M., SHEPHERD, J. T. and WHELAN, R. F. (1951). The part played by the nervous system in the response to cold of the circulation through the finger-tip. *Clin. Sci.*, **10**, 347.

GRENET, H., ISAAC-GEORGES, P. and LADET, Mlle (1937). Paralysie radiculaire du plexus brachial et paralysie diaphragmatique. *Bull. Soc. Pédiat. Paris*, **35**, 146.

GRIFFITHS, D. Ll. (1940). Volkmann's ischaemic contracture. *Br. J. Surg.*, **28**, 239.

GRIFFITHS, D. Ll. Personal communication.

GUNTHER, H. (1921). Zur Pathogenese der Kohlenoxydvergiftung. *Z. klin. Med.*, **92**, 41.

GUNTHER, H. (1940). Die kryptogenen Myopathien. *Ergebn. inn. Med. Kinderheilk.*, **58**, 331.

GUTMANN, E. and GUTTMANN, L. (1944). Effect of galvanic exercise on denervated and reinnervated muscles in rabbit. *J. Neurol. Neurosurg. Psychiat.*, **7**, 7.

GUTMANN, E., GUTTMANN, L., MEDAWAR, P. B. and YOUNG, J. Z. (1942). The rate of regeneration of nerve. *J. exp. Biol.*, **19**, 14.

GUTMANN, E. and HOLUBAR, J. (1951). Atrophy of nerve fibres in the central stump following nerve section and the possibilities of its prevention. *Archo int. Studi neurol.* **1**, 3.

GUTMANN, E. and SANDERS, F. K. (1943). Recovery of fibre numbers and diameters in the regeneration of peripheral nerves. *J. Physiol., Lond.*, **101**, 489.

GUTMANN, E. and YOUNG, J. Z. (1944). The reinnervation of muscle after various periods of atrophy. *J. Anat.*, **78**, 15.

GUTTMANN, L. (1933). Motorische und vegetative Grenzzonenreflexe bei Läsionen peripherer und zentraler Abschnitte des Nervensystems. *Z.ges.Neurol. Psychiat.*, **147**, 291.

GUTTMANN, L. (1940). Topographical studies of disturbances of sweat secretion after complete lesions of peripheral nerves. *J. Neurol. Psychiat., Lond.*, **3**, 197.

GUTTMANN, L. (1943). Experimental study of nerve suture with various suture materials. *Br. J. Surg.*, **30**, 370.

GUTTMANN, L. and MEDAWAR, P. B. (1942). Chemical inhibition of fibre regeneration and neuroma formation in peripheral nerves. *J. Neurol. Psychiat., Lond.*, **5**, 130.

GYE, R. S., MCLEOD, J. G., HARGRAVE, J. C., POLLARD, J. D., LOEWENTHAL, J. and BOOTH, G. C. (1972). Use of immuno-suppressive agents in human nerve grafting. *Lancet*, **1**, 647.

HAFTEK, J. (1967*a*). Influence of heat on the regeneration of sensory nerve fibres. *Neurologia Neurochir. pol.*, **1**, 239.

HAFTEK, J. (1967*b*). Wartość diagnosyczna mielografii w zamkniętych urazach splotu barkowego. *Polski Przegl. radiol. Med. nuklear.*, **31**, 179.

HAFTEK, J. (1970). Stretch injury of peripheral nerve. *J. Bone Jt Surg.*, **52B**, 354.

HAFTEK, J. and THOMAS, P. K. (1968). Electron microscope observations on the effects of localized crush injuries on the connective tissues of peripheral nerves. *J. Anat.*, **103**, 233.

HAKSTIAN, R. W. (1968). Funicular orientation by direct stimulation. *J. Bone Jt Surg.*, **50A**, 1178.

HALPERN, L. (1949). Disturbance of dermatokinesthesis in cerebral and spinal diseases. *J. nerv. ment. Dis.*, **109**, 1.

HARRIS, R. (1952). Variations in strength duration curves and excitability indices in normal subjects. *Ann. phys. Med.*, **1**, 126.

HARRIS, R. I. (1920). An operation for the relief of median anaesthesia. *J. orthop. Surg.*, **2**, 519.

HART, M. S. and BASOM, W. C. (1958). Neurilemmoma involving bone. *J. Bone Jt Surg.*, **40A**, 465.

HARVEY, E. N., BUTLER, E. G., MCMILLEN, J. H. and PUCKETT, W. O. (1945). Mechanism of wounding. *War Med., Chicago*, **8**, 91.

HAUCH, E. and OTTSEN, M. (1939). Radialislähmung bei Neugeborenen. *Acta obstet. gynec. scand.*, **19**, 345.

HEAD, H. and HOLMES, G. (1911). Sensory disturbances from cerebral lesions. *Brain*, **34**, 102.

HEARD, G. (1962). Nerve sheath tumours and von Recklinghausen's disease of the central nervous system. *Ann. R. Coll. Surg.*, **31**, 229.

HEARD, G. (1963). Malignant disease in von Recklinghausen's neurofibromatosis. *Proc. R. Soc. Med.*, **56**, 502.

HENDERSON, W. R. (1948). Clinical assessment of peripheral nerve injuries. Tinel's test. *Lancet*, **2**, 801.

HENRY, A. K. (1927). An operation for slinging a dropped shoulder. *Br. J. Surg.*, **15**, 95.

HIGHET, W. B. (1942). Procaine nerve block in investigation of peripheral nerve injuries. *J. Neurol. Psychiat., Lond.*, **5**, 101.

HIGHET, W. B. and HOLMES, W. (1943). Traction injuries to the lateral popliteal nerve and traction injuries to peripheral nerves after suture. *Br. J. Surg.*, **30**, 212.

HIGHET, W. B. and SANDERS, F. K. (1943). The effects of stretching nerves after suture. *Br. J. Surg.*, **30**, 355.

HILES, R. W. (1972). Freeze dried irradiated nerve homograft. *Hand*, **4**, 79.

HILLER, F. (1951). Nerve regeneration in grafts. *J. Neuropath. clin. Neurol.*, **1**, 5.

HINES, H. M., THOMPSON, J. D. and LAZERE, B. (1943). Physiologic basis for treatment of paralysed muscle. *Archs phys. Ther.*, **24**, 69.

HIRSCHMANN, J. (1943). Der Nervenschussschmerz und seine Behandlung. *Nervenarzt*, **16**, 82.

HOADLEY, A. E. (1893). Six cases of metatarsalgia. *Chicago med. Rec.*, **5**, 32.

HOARE, J. R. (1968). Solitary neural tuberculoid leprosy. *Proc. R. Soc. Med.*, **61**, 672,

HODES, R. R., LARRABEE, M. C. and GERMAN, W. (1948). The human electromyogram in response to nerve stimulation and the conduction velocity of motor axons. *Archs Neurol. Psychiat.*, **60**, 340.

HOEN, T. I. and BRACKETT, C. E. (1956). Peripheral nerve lengthening. *J. Neurosurg.*, **13**, 43.

HOFFMAN, H. (1950). Local re-innervation in partially denervated muscle: a histo-physiological study. *Aust. J. exp. Biol. med. Sci.*, **28**, 383.

HOFFMAN, H. (1951). A study of the factors influencing innervation of muscles by implanted nerves. *Aust. J. exp. Biol. med. Sci.*, **29**, 289.

HOLMES, W. (1947). Histological observations on the repair of nerves by autografts. *Br. J. Surg.*, **35**, 167.

HOLMES, W. and YOUNG, J. Z. (1942). Nerve regeneration after immediate and delayed suture. *J. Anat.*, **77**, 63.

HOLMES, W. and ZACHARY, R. B. (1946). Nerve biopsy. *J. Neurol. Psychiat., Lond.*, **9**, 93.

HOLMES, W., HIGHET, W. B. and SEDDON, H. J. (1944). Ischaemic nerve lesions occurring in Volkmann's contracture. *Br. J. Surg.*, **32**, 259.

HOLSTEIN, A. and LEWIS, G. B. (1963). Fractures of the humerus with radial nerve paralysis. *J. Bone Jt Surg.*, **45A**, 1382.

HOSOI, K. (1931). Multiple neurofibromatosis (von Recklinghausen's disease) with special reference to malignant transformation. *Archs Surg., Chicago*, **22**, 258.

HOWARD, F. M. (1961). Ulnar nerve palsy in wrist fractures. *J. Bone Jt Surg.*, **43A**, 1197.

HOWSE, A. J. G. and SEDDON, H. J. (1966). Ischaemic contracture of muscle associated with carbon monoxide and barbiturate poisoning. *Br. med. J.*, **1**, 192.

HUBER, G. C. (1920). Repair of peripheral nerve injuries. *Surgery, Gynec. Obstet.*, **30**, 464.

HUDSON, F. P., MCCANDLESS, A. and O'MALLEY, A. G. (1950). Sciatic paralysis in newborn infants. *Br. med. J.* **1**, 223.

HUNT, J. R. (1908). Occupation neuritis of the deep palmar branch of the ulnar nerve. *J. nerv. ment. Dis.*, **35**, 673.

HUNT, J. R. (1909). *Trans. Am. neurol. Ass.*, **35**, 184.

HUNT, J. R. (1911). The thenar and hypothenar types of neural atrophy of the hand. *Am. J. med. Sci.*, **141**, 224.

HUNT, J. R. (1914). The neural atrophy of the muscles of the hand, without sensory disturbances. *Rev. Neurol. Psychiat.*, **12**, 137.

INTERNATIONAL UNION AGAINST CANCER (1965). *Illustrated Tumour Nomenclature*. Berlin: Springer.

JACKSON, E. S. C. (1945). The role of galvanism in the treatment of denervated voluntary muscle in man. *Brain*, **68**, 300.

JAHNKE, E. J. Jr. and SEELEY, S. F. (1953). Acute vascular injuries in the Korean War. *Ann. Surg.*, **138**, 158.

JASIŃSKI, B. and BRÜTSCH, H. (1952). Zur Pathogenese, Prognose und Therapie traumatischer Myoglobinurien. *Schweiz. med. Wschr.*, **82**, 29.

JASPER, H. (1946). The rate of re-innervation of muscle following nerve injuries in man as determined by the electromyogram. *Trans. R. Soc. Can.*, **40**, 81.

JEFFERSON, G. (1934). Arterial embolectomy. *Br. med. J.*, **2**, 1090.

JENKINS, S. A. (1952). Solitary tumours of peripheral nerve trunks. *J. Bone Jt Surg.*, **34B**, 401.

JHA, B. D., GOLDBY, F. and GAMBLE, H. J. (1959). The effect of temperature on the maturation of regenerating peripheral nerves in the rat. *J. Anat.*, **93**, 436.

JOHNSON, R. J. and BONFIGLIO, M. (1969). Lipofibromatous hamartoma of the median nerve. *J. Bone Jt Surg.*, **51**A, 984.

JOLLY, D. W. (1942). *Field Surgery in Total War*. London: Hamilton.

JONES, F. WOOD (1919). Voluntary muscular movements in cases of nerve lesions. *J. Anat.*, **54**, 41.

JOYCE, J. L. (1919). A study of a series of peripheral nerve injuries from a surgical aspect. *Br. J. Surg.*, **6**, 418.

JOYCE, J. L. (1920). Late results of operation. *Br. med. J.*, **2**, 468.

KAHN, E. A. (1951). Direct observation of sweating in peripheral nerve lesions. *Surgery, Gynec. Obstet.*, **92**, 22.

KARABARBOUNIS, L. A. (1973). La neurographie. In *Les Lésions Traumatiques des Nerfs Périphériques*. Ed. Michon, J. and Möberg, E. Paris: Expansion Scientifique.

KECK, C. (1962). The tarsal-tunnel syndrome. *J. Bone Jt Surg.*, **44**A, 180.

KEITH, A. (1919). *Menders of the Maimed*. London: Oxford Medical Publications.

KIBEL, M. A., MATHESON, A. T. and STEWART K. S. (1961). Neonatal sciatic palsy. *Cent. Afr. J. Med.*, **7**, 399.

KILOH, L. G. (1950). Brachial plexus lesions after cholecystectomy. *Lancet*, **1**, 103.

KILOH, L. G. and NEVIN, S. (1952). Isolated neuritis of anterior interosseous nerve. *Br. med. J.*, **1**, 850.

KILVINGTON, B. (1940). Note on distribution of myelinated nerve fibres within nerve bundles. *Aust. J. exp. Biol. med. Sci.*, **18**, 367.

KINMONTH, J. B. (1952). The physiology and relief of traumatic arterial spasm. *Br. med. J.*, **1**, 59.

KINMONTH, J. B., HADFIELD, G. J., CONNOLLY, J. E., LEE, R. H. and AMOROSO, E. C. (1956). Traumatic arterial spasm. *Br. J. Surg.*, **44**, 164.

KINMONTH, J. B. and SIMEONE, F. A. (1952). Motor innervation of large arteries. *Br. J. Surg.*, **39**, 333.

KIRK E. G. and LEWIS, D. (1915). Fascial tubulization in the repair of nerve defects. *J. Am. med. Ass.*, **65**, 486.

KIRKER, J. R. (1952). Dislocation of the shoulder complicated by rupture of the axillary vessels. *J. Bone Jt Surg.*, **34B**, 72.

KIRKLIN, J. W., CHENOWETH, A. I. and MURPHEY, F. (1947). Causalgia: a review of its characteristics, diagnosis and treatment. *Surgery, St. Louis*, **21**, 321.

KLINE, D. G., HAYES, G. J. and MORSE, A. S. (1964). A comparative study of response of species to peripheral nerve injury. I. Severance. II. Crush and severance with primary suture. *J. Neurosurg.*, **21**, 968; 980.

KOPELL, H. P. and THOMPSON, W. A. L. (1963). *Peripheral Entrapment*. Baltimore: Williams and Wilkins Company.

KOTANI, P. T., MATSUDA, H. and SUZUKI, T. (1973). Trial surgical procedures of nerve transfer to avulsion injuries of plexus brachialis. In *Orthopaedic Surgery and Traumatology*. Ed. Delchef, J., De Marneffe, R. and Vander Elst, E. Amsterdam: Excerpta Medica.

KUGELBERG, E., EDSTRÖM, L. and ABBRUZZESE, M. (1970). Mapping of motor units in experimentally reinnervated rat muscle. *J. Neurol. Neurosurg. Psychiat.*, **33**, 319.

LAM, S. J. S. (1962). A tarsal-tunnel syndrome. *Lancet*, **2**, 1354.

LANCE, M. (1937). Paralysie obstétricale des membres inférieurs. *Bull. Soc. Pédiat. Paris*, **35**, 25.

LANGEN, P. (1930). Radialislähmungen bei Neugeborenen. *Arch. Gynaek.*, **139**, 560.

LANGLEY, J. N. and HASHIMOTO, M. (1917). On the suture of separate nerve bundles in a nerve trunk and on internal nerve plexuses. *J. Physiol., Lond.*, **51**, 318.

LANGLEY, J. N. and ITAKAGI, M. (1917). The oxygen use of denervated muscle. *J. Physiol., Lond.*, **51**, 202.

LARREY, D. J. (1812). *Mémoires de Chirurgie Militaire et Campagnes*, vol. III, p. 13. Paris: Smith and Buisson.

LEACH, P. and CUTHBERT, H. (1972). Brachial plexus lesions associated with traumatic asphyxia. *Br. J. Surg.*, **59**, 527.

LEARMONTH, J. R. (1933). The principle of decompression in the treatment of certain diseases of peripheral nerves. *Surg. Clin. N. Am.*, **13**, 905.

LEARMONTH, J. R. (1942). Technique for transplanting the ulnar nerve. *Surgery, Gynec. Obstet.*, **75**, 792.

LEBEDENKO, V. V. (1943). The time element in restorative surgery of peripheral nerve lesions. *Am. Rev. sov. Med.*, **1**, 23.

LEFFERT, R. D. and SEDDON, H. J. (1965). Infraclavicular brachial plexus injuries. *J. Bone Jt Surg.*, **47B**, 9.

LETTIN, A. W. F. (1965). Carpal tunnel syndrome in childhood. *J. Bone Jt Surg.*, **47B**, 556.

LEWIN, W. (1943). Pressure palsy in the paralysed limb. *Lancet*, **2**, 756.

LEWIS, H. P. and MCLAURIN, R. L. (1969). Application of tissue transplant technique to experimental nerve grafting. *J. Trauma*, **9**, 227.

LEWIS, T. (1942). *Pain*. New York: The Macmillan Company.

LEWIS, T. and LANDIS, E. M. (1930). Some physiological effects of sympathetic ganglionectomy in the human being and its effect in a case of Raynaud's malady. *Heart*, **15**, 151.

LIPSCOMB, P. R. and BURLESON, R. J. (1955). Vascular and neural complications in supracondylar fractures of the humerus in children. *J. Bone Jt Surg.*, **37**A, 487.

LITTLER, W. (1960). Neurovascular skin island transfer in reconstructive hand surgery. *Trans. int. Soc. plast. Surg.* p. 175. 2nd congress, London 1959.

LIU, C. T., BENDA, C. E. and LEWEY, F. H. (1948). Tensile strength of human nerves: experimental physical and histologic study. *Archs Neurol. Psychiat.*, **59**, 322.

LIVINGSTON, W. K. (1947*a*). Evidence of active invasion of denervated areas by sensory fibres from neighbouring nerves in man. *J. Neurosurg.*, **4**, 140.

LIVINGSTON, W. K. (1947*b*). *Pain Mechanisms*. New York: The Macmillan Company.

LIVINGSTON, W. K., DAVIS, E. W. and LIVINGSTON, K. E. (1945). 'Delayed recovery' in peripheral nerve lesions caused by high-velocity projectile wounding. *J. Neurosurg.*, **2**, 170.

LOHR, W. and JACOBI, W. (1932). Die Darstellung der peripheren Nerven. *Arch. klin. Chir.*, **171**, 538.

LYONS, W. R. and WOODHALL, B. (1949). *Atlas of Peripheral Nerve Injuries*. Philadelphia: Saunders.

MCCARROLL, H. R. (1950). Clinical manifestations of congenital neurofibromatosis. *J. Bone Jt Surg.*, **32A**, 601.

MACCARTY, C. S. (1951). Two-stage autograft for repair of extensive damage to sciatic nerve. *J. Neurosurg.*, **8**, 319.

MCEWAN, L. E. (1962). Median and ulnar nerve injuries. *Aust. N.Z. J. Surg.*, **32**, 89.

MCGOWAN, A. J. (1950). The results of transposition of the ulnar nerve for traumatic ulnar neuritis. *J. Bone Jt Surg.*, **32B**, 3.

MACKENZIE, I. G. and WOODS, C. G. (1961). Causes of failure after repair of the median nerve. *J. Bone Jt Surg.*, **43B**, 465.

MCKINLEY, J. C. (1921). The intraneural plexus of fasciculi and fibers in the sciatic nerve. *Archs Neurol. Psychiat.*, **6**, 377.

MACKINNON, P. C. B. (1964). Plastic paint and eccrine sweat glands. *Med. biol. Illust.*, **14**, 13.

MCQUILLAN, W. M., NEILSON, J. M. M., BOARDMAN, A. K. and HAY, R. L. (1971). Sensory evaluation after median nerve repair. *Hand*, **3**, 101.

MAKINS, G. H. (1919). *On Gunshot Injuries to the Blood Vessels*. Bristol: Wright.

MALT, R. A. and MCKHANN, C. F. (1964). Replantation of severed arms. *J. Am. med. Ass.*, **189**, 716.

MANNERFELT, L. (1964). Studies on an anastomosis between the median and ulnar nerves in the forearm. *Acta Univ. lund.*, Section 2, No. 6.

MANNERFELT, L. (1968). Median nerve entrapment after dislocation of the elbow. *J. Bone Jt Surg.*, **50B**, 152.

MARIE, P. and FOIX, C. (1913). Atrophie isolée de l'eminence thénar d'origine névritique. *Revue Neurol.*, **26**, 647.

MARMOR, L. (1964). Regeneration of peripheral nerves by irradiated homografts. *J. Bone Jt Surg.*, **46A**, 383.

MARMOR, L. (1967). *Peripheral Nerve Regeneration Using Nerve Grafts*. Springfield, Ill.: Thomas.

MARTIN, C. and MASSE, P. (1958). Le syndrome du canal carpien chez l'enfant. *Archs fr. Pédiat*, **15**, 930.

MARTIN, R. (1763). *Tal om Nervers allmänna Egenskaper i Människans kropp*. Stockholm: Salvius.

MARWAH, V. (1964). Compression of the lateral popliteal (common peroneal) nerve. *Br. med. J.*, **2**, 1367.

MASSON, P. (1932). Experimental and spontaneous schwannomas (peripheral gliomas). *Am. J. Path.*, **8**, 367.

MAURER, A. (1939). Note sur les plaies vasculaires récentes et leur traitment d'après 444 observations. *Mém. Acad. Chir.*, **65**, 1156.

MAURER, P., TOMENO, B. and COMITI, V. (1973). Traumatismes des nerfs périphériques. Traitement médico-chirurgical des séquelles douloureuses. *Revue de Chirurgie Orthopédique*, **59**, 189.

MEDICAL PROTECTON SOCIETY (1968). *Annual Report*.

MEDICAL RESEARCH COUNCIL (1920). The diagnosis and treatment of peripheral nerve injuries. *Spec. Rep. Ser. med. Res. Coun.*, No. 54. London: H.M.S.O.

MEDICAL RESEARCH COUNCIL (1975) *Aids to the Examination of the Peripheral Nervous System*. London: H.M.S.O.

MEDICAL RESEARCH COUNCIL (1954). Peripheral nerve injuries. *Spec. Rep. Ser. med. Res. Coun.*, No. 282. London: H.M.S.O.

MEDICAL RESEARCH COUNCIL. (1973). A controlled trial of ambulant outpatient treatment and inpatient rest in bed in the management of tuberculosis of the spine in young Korean patients on standard chemotherapy. A study in Masan, Korea. *J. Bone Jt Surg.*, **55B**, 678.

MEDICAL RESEARCH COUNCIL. (1973). A controlled trial of plaster-of-Paris jackets in the management of ambulant outpatient treatment of tuberculosis of the spine in children on standard chemotherapy. A study in Pusan, Korea. *Tubercle*, **54**, 261.

MEDICAL RESEARCH COUNCIL. (1974). A controlled trial of débridement and ambulatory treatment in the management of tuberculosis of the spine in patients on standard chemotherapy. A study in Bulawayo, Rhodesia. *J. trop. Med. Hyg.*, **77**, 72.

MEDICAL RESEARCH COUNCIL. (1974). A controlled trial of anterior spinal fusion and débridement in the surgical management of tuberculosis of the spine in patients on standard chemotherapy. A study in Hong Kong. *Br. J. Surg.*, **61**, 853

MERLE d'AUBIGNÉ, R. and DEBURGE, A. (1967). Etiologie, évolution et pronostic des paralysies traumatiques du plexus brachial. *Revue Chir. orthop. répar. Appar. moteur*, **53**, 23.

MERLE d'AUBIGNÉ, R., MAURER, P. and BOMBART, M. (1961). Séquelles douloureuses des traumatismes des nerfs périphériques. *Mém. Acad. Chir.*, **88**, 425.

MICHON, J. and MASSE, P. (1964). Le moment optimum de la suture nerveuse dans les plaies du membre supérieur. *Revue Chir. orthop. répar. Appar. moteur*, **50**, 205.

MICHON, J. and MOBERG, E. and others. (1973). *Les Lésions Traumatiques des Nerfs Périphériques*. Paris: Expansion Scientifique Francaise.

MICHON, J. and MOBERG, E. (1975). *Traumatic Nerve Lesions of the Upper Limb*. Edinburgh: Churchill Livingstone.

MILLENDER, L. H., NALEBUFF, E. A. and HOLDSWORTH, D. E. (1973). Posterior interosseous nerve syndrome secondary to rheumatoid arthritis. *J. Bone Jt Surg.*, **55A**, 753.

MILLESI, H. (1969). Wiederherstellung durchtrennter peripherer Nerven und Nerventransplantation. *Münch. med. Wschr.* **111**, 2669.

MILLESI, H., GANGLBERGER, J. and BERGER, A. (1967). Erfahrungen mit der Mikrochirurgie peripherer Nerven. *Chirurgia Plastica Reconstructiva*, **3**, 47.

MILLESI, H., BERGER, A. and MEISSL, G. (1972*a*). Experimentelle Untersuchungen zu Heilung durchtrennter peripherer Nerven. *Chirurgia Plastica*, **1**, 174.

MILLESI, H., MEISSL, G. and BERGER, A. (1972*b*). The interfascicular nerve-grafting of the median and ulnar nerves. *J. Bone Jt Surg.*, **54A**, 727.

MITCHELL, J. K. (1895). *Remote Consequences of Injuries of Nerves and their Treatment*. Philadelphia: Lea.

MITCHELL, S. W. (1872). *Injuries of Nerves*. Philadelphia: Lippincott.

MITCHELL, S. W., MOREHOUSE, G. R. and KEEN, W. W. (1864). *Gunshot Wounds and other Injuries of Nerves*. Philadelphia: Lippincott.

MOBERG, E. (1955). Transfer of sensation. *J. Bone Jt Surg.*, **37A**, 305.

MOBERG, E. (1958). Objective methods for determining the functional value of sensibility in the hand. *J. Bone Jt Surg.*, **40B**, 454.

MOBERG, E. (1964). Aspects of sensation in reconstructive surgery of the upper extremity. *J. Bone Jt Surg.*, **46A**, 817.

MOBERG, E. (1965). Relation of touch and deep sensation to hand reconstruction. *Am. J. Surg.*, **109**, 353.

MORLEY, G. H. (1964). Intraneural lipoma of the median nerve in the carpal tunnel. *J. Bone Jt Surg.*, **46B**, 734.

MOROTOMI, T. and HIRASAWA, Y. (1973). Clinical experience in peripheral nerve homografting. In *Orthopaedic Surgery and Traumatology*. Ed. Delchef, J., De Marneffe, R. and Vander Elst, E. Amsterdam: Excerpta Medica.

MORTON, T. G. (1876). A peculiar and painful affection of the fourth metatarsophalangeal articulation. *Am. J. med. Sci.*, **71**, 37.

MOSER, H. (1943). Zur Beurteilung kausalgischer Beschwerden nach Verwundung. *Münch. med. Wschr.*, **90**, 705.

M.R.C.R. (1920). *See* Medical Research Council (1920).

M.R.C.R. (1954). *See* Medical Research Council (1954).

MUKHERJEE, S. R. and DOUGLAS, D. M. (1951). An investigation into the value of nylon and terylene as nerve sutures. *Br. J. Surg.*, **39**, 271.

MULDER, D. S., GREENWOOD, F. A. H. and BROOKS, C. E. (1973). Post-traumatic thoracic outlet syndrome. *J. Traum.*, **13**, 706.

MULDER, J. D. (1951). The causative mechanism in Morton's metatarsalgia. *J. Bone Jt Surg.*, **33B**, 94

MULHOLLAND, R. C. (1966). Non-traumatic paralysis of the posterior interosseous nerve. *J. Bone Jt Surg.*, **48B** 781.

MURPHEY, F., HARTUNG, W. and KIRKLIN, J. W. (1947). Myelographic demonstration of avulsing injury of the brachial plexus. *Am. J. Roentg. Radium Ther.*, **58**, 102.

MURRAY, M. R. and STOUT, A. P. (1940). Schwann cell versus fibroblast as the origin of the specific nerve sheath tumour: observations upon normal nerve sheaths and neurilemmomas *in vitro*. *Am. J. Path.*, **16**, 41.

NAPIER, J. R. (1949). The significance of Tinel's sign in peripheral nerve injuries. *Brain*, **72**, 63.

NARAKAS, A. (1972). Plexo braquial. Terapéutica quirurgica directa. *Revista de orthopedia y traumatologia*, **16**, 855.

NATHAN, P. W. (1947). On the pathogenesis of causalgia in peripheral nerve injuries. *Brain*, **70**, 145.

NATHANIEL, E. J. H. and PEASE, D. C. (1963). Collagen and basement membrane formation by Schwann cells during nerve regeneration. *J. Ultrastruct. Res.*, **9**, 550.

NICHOLSON, O. R. and SEDDON, H. J. (1957). Nerve repair in civil practice: results of treatment of median and ulnar nerve lesions. *Br. med. J.*, **2**, 1065.

NICOL, J. A. C. (1948). The giant nerve-fibres in the central nervous system of Myxicola (Polychaeta, Sabellidae). *Q. Jl microsc. Sci.*, **89**, 1.

NICOL, J. A. C. and YOUNG, J. Z. (1946). Giant nerve fibre of *Myxicola infundibulum* (Grube). *Nature*, **158**, 167.

NISSEN, K. I. (1948). Plantar digital neuritis: Morton's metatarsalgia. *J. Bone Jt Surg.*, **30B**, 84.

NISSEN, K. I. (1959). Pain in the arm and the carpal tunnel syndrome (editorial). *Post-grad. med. J.*, **35**, 379.

NOBEL, W. (1966). Peroneal palsy due to haematoma in the common peroneal nerve sheath after distal torsional fractures and inversion ankle sprains. *J. Bone Jt Surg.*, **48A**, 1484.

OCHOA, J., DANTA, G., FOWLER, T. J. and GILLIATT, R. W. (1971). Nature of the nerve lesion caused by a pneumatic tourniquet. *Nature*, **233**, 265.

O'CONNELL, J. E. A. (1944). Maternal obstetrical paralysis. *Surgery Gynec. Obstet.*, **79**, 374.

ÖNNE, L. (1962). Recovery of sensibility and sudomotor activity in the hand after nerve suture. *Acta chir. scand.*, suppl. 300.

ÖNNE, L. (1964). Sensibility of the hand. *Current Practice in Orthopaedic Surgery*. Vol. 2. p. 41. St Louis: Mosby.

OSBORNE, G. V. (1959). Ulnar neuritis. *Post-grad. med. J.*, **35**, 392.

OSBORNE, G. V. (1970). Compression neuritis of the ulnar nerve at the elbow. *Hand*, **2**, 10.

OTTOLENGHI, C. E. (1961). Die ischämische Kontractur nach supracondylären Ellbogenbrüchen bei Kindern. Vorbeugung und Behandlung. *Wiederherst. Chir. Traumat.*, **6**, 60.

OTTOW, B. (1932). Eine unter der Geburt entstandene doppelseitige Radialislähmung beim Neugeborenen. *Zentbl. Gynäk.*, **56**, 2714.

PAGE, K. M. (1970). Histological methods for peripheral nerves. *J. med. Lab. Tech.* **27**, 1.

PAGET, J. (1864). Clinical lecture on some cases of local paralysis. *Med. Times, Lond.*, **1**, 331.

PARKES, A. R. (1945). Traumatic ischaemia of peripheral nerves, with some observations on Volkmann's ischaemic contracture. *Br. J. Surg.*, **32**, 403.

PARKES, A. R. (1961). Intraneural ganglion of the lateral popliteal nerve. *J. Bone Jt Surg.*, **43B**, 784.

PATTERSON, F. P. and MORTON, K. S. (1973). Neurological complications of fractures and dislocations of the pelvis. *J. Traum.*, **12**, 1013.

PENFIELD, W. (1949). Late spinal paralysis after avulsion of the brachial plexus. *J. Bone Jt Surg.*, **31B**, 40.

PHILIPEAUX, J.-M. and VULPIAN, A. (1870). Note sur des essais de greffe d'un tronçon du nerf lingual entre les deux bouts du nerf hypoglosse. *Archs Physiol. norm. path.*, **3**, 618.

PHILIPPIDES, D. (1942). Das Wesen und die Behandlung der Kausalgie. *Chirurg*, **14**, 481.

PINNER-POOLE, B., TOMASULA, J. J. and CAMPBELL, J. B. (1967). *Tenth International Congress. Société Internationale de Chirurgie Orthopédique et de Traumatologie*. p. 782. Symposium on nerve suture and nerve grafts in the upper limb. Brussels: Acta Medica Belgica.

PLATT, H. (1920). Results of bridging gaps in injured nerve trunks by autogenous fascial tubulization and autogenous nerve grafts. *Br. J. Surg.*, **7**, 384.

PLATT, H. (1921). *The Surgery of the Peripheral Nerve Injuries of Warfare*. Bristol: Wright.

PLATT, H. (1926). The pathogenesis and treatment of traumatic neuritis of the ulnar nerve in the post-condylar groove. *Br. J. Surg.*, **13**, 409.

PLATT, H. (1928). On the peripheral nerve complications of certain fractures. *J. Bone Jt Surg.*, **10**, 403.

PLATT, H. (1937). Discussion on injuries of peripheral nerves. *Proc. R. Soc. Med.*, **30**, 863.

PLATT, H. (1940). Traction lesions of the external popliteal nerve. *Lancet*, **2**, 612.

PLATT, H. and BRISTOW, W. R. (1924). The remote results of operations for injuries of the peripheral nerves. *Br. J. Surg.*, **11**, 535.

POLLOCK, L. J. and DAVIS, L. (1933). *Peripheral Nerve Injuries*. New York: Hoeber.

PORTER, R. W. (1966). New test for finger-tip sensation. *Br. med. J.*, **2**, 927.

POTH, E. J., FERNANDEZ, E. B. and DRAGER, G. A. (1945). Prevention of formation of endbulb neuromata. *Proc. Soc. exp. Biol. Med.*, **60**, 200.

PRESTON, F. W., WALSH, W. S. and CLARKE T. H. (1952). Cutaneous neurofibromatosis (von Recklinghausen's disease): clinical manifestations and incidence of sarcoma in 61 male patients. *Archs Surg. Chicago.*, **64**, 813

PRINCETEAU, ABADIE and DESQUEYROUX (1913). Paralysies du membre supérieur après emploi de la bande d'Esmarch. *J. Méd. Bordeaux*, **43**, 85.

PUCKETT, W. O., GRUNDFEST, H., MCELROY, W. D. and MCMILLEN, J. H. (1946). Damage to peripheral nerves by high velocity missiles without direct hit. *J. Neurosurg.*, **3**, 294.

PULVERTAFT, R. G. (1964). Unusual tumours of the median nerve. *J. Bone Jt Surg.*, **46B**, 731.

PURCELL, F. H. and GURDJIAN, E. S. (1935). Haemangiomata of peripheral nerves. *Am. J. Surg.*, **30**, 541.

RAMON Y CAJAL, S. (1928). *Degeneration and Regeneration of the Nervous System*. London: Milford.

RANK, B. K., WAKEFIELD, A. R. and HUESTON, J. T. (1973). *Surgery of Repair as applied to Hand Injuries*. 4th edition. Edinburgh: Churchill Livingstone.

RASMUSSEN, T. B. and FREEDMAN, H. (1946). Treatment of causalgia. An analysis of 100 cases. *J. Neurosurg.* **3**, 165.

RAZEMOTH, J.-P., PETYT, B. and BONTE, G. (1973). La neurographie dans les lésions des nerfs périphériques. In *Les Lésions Traumatiques des Nerfs Périphériques*. Ed. Michon, J. and Moberg, E. Paris: Expansion Scientifique.

RECKLINGHAUSEN, F. VON (1882). Ueber die multiplen Fibrome der Haut und ihre Beniehung zu den multiplen Neuromen. In *Festschrift zu Rudolf Virchow*. Berlin: Hirschwald.

REUSS, A. R. VON (1920). *Diseases of the Newborn*, p. 189. London: John Bale, Sons & Danielsson.

RICHARDS, R. L. (1967). Causalgia, a centennial review. *Archs Neurol. Chicago.*, **16**, 339.

RICHTER, C. P. and KATZ, D. T. (1943). Peripheral nerve injuries determined by the electrical skin resistance method. *J. Am. med. Ass.*, **122**, 648.

RIDDOCH, G. (1941). Phantom limbs and body shape. *Brain*, **64**, 197.

ROAF, R. (1963). Lateral flexion injuries of the cervical spine. *J. Bone Jt Surg.*, **45B**, 36.

ROLES, N. C. and MAUDSLEY, R. H. (1972). Radial tunnel syndrome. *J. Bone Jt Surg.*, **54B**, 499.

ROPER, B. A. (1972). External rotation palsy of the shoulder. Proc. Roy. Soc. Med. **65**, 375.

ROTH, W. K. (1895). Meralgia paraesthetica. *Medskoe Obozr. Sprimona*. **43**, 678.

ROWNTREE, T. (1949). Anomalous innervation of the hand muscles. *J. Bone Jt Surg.*, **31B**, 505.

RUSSELL, D. S. and RUBINSTEIN, L. J. (1971). *Pathology of Tumours of the Nervous System*. 3rd edition, p. 284. London: Edward Arnold.

RUSSELL, W. R. and WHITTY, C. W. M. (1947). Traumatic neuritis of deep palmar branch of ulnar nerve. *Lancet*, **1**, 828.

SAITO, M., KAMIZAWA, K. and KATO, S. (1933). Roentgenologic visualization of peripheral nerves; neurography in vivo. *Am. J. Surg.*, **22**, 78.

SAKURAI, M. and MONTAGNA, W. (1964). The skin of primates. *J. invest. Derm.*, **42**, 411.

SANDERS, F. K. (1942). The repair of large gaps in the peripheral nerves. *Brain*, **65**, 281.

SANDERS, F. K. and YOUNG, J. Z. (1942). The degeneration and re-innervation of grafted nerves. *J. Anat.*, **76**, 143.

SCHIFF, M. (1851). Ueber motorische Lähmung der Zunge. Heilkunde. *Arch. Anat. Physiol* (*physiol. Abt.*) **10**, 579, 665.

SEDDON, H. J. (1930). Haemophilia as a cause of lesions in the nervous system. *Brain*, **53**, 306.

SEDDON, H. J. (1942). A classification of nerve injuries. *Br. med. J.*, **2**, 237.

SEDDON, H. J. (1943). Three types of nerve injury. *Brain*, **66**, 237.

SEDDON, H. J. (1944). The early management of peripheral nerve injuries. *Practitioner*, **157**, 101.

SEDDON, H. J. (1947*a*). Nerve lesions complicating certain closed bone injuries. *J. Am. med. Ass.*, **135**, 691.

SEDDON, H. J. (1947*b*). The use of autogenous grafts for the repair of large gaps in peripheral nerves. *Br. J. Surg.*, **35**, 151.

SEDDON, H. J. (1948). Brachial Plexus. In *British Surgical Practice*. Ed. Carling, E. R. and Ross, J. P. London: Butterworth.

SEDDON, H. J. (1952). Carpal ganglion as a cause of paralysis of the deep branch of the ulnar nerve. *J. Bone Jt Surg.*, **34B**, 386.

SEDDON, H. J. (1956). Volkmann's contracture. Treatment by excision of the infarct. *J. Bone Jt Surg.*, **38B**, 152.

SEDDON, H. J. (1963). Nerve grafting. *J. Bone Jt Surg.*, **45B**, 447.

SEDDON, H. J. (1964). Volkmann's ischaemia. *Br. med. J.*, **1**, 1587.

SEDDON, H. J. (1966). Volkmann's ischaemia in the lower limb. *J. Bone Jt Surg.*, **48B**, 627.

SEDDON, H. J. (1967). Nerve suture and nerve grafts in the upper limb. *Tenth International Congress: Société Internationale de Chirurgie Orthopédique et de Traumatalogie*. p. 739. Brussels: Acta Medica Belgica.

SEDDON, H. J. and HOLMES, W. (1944). Late condition of nerve homografts in man. *Surgery Gynec. Obstet.*, **79**, 342.

SEDDON, H. J. and HOLMES, W. (1945). Ischaemic damage in the peripheral stump of a divided nerve. *Br. J. Surg.*, **32**, 389.

SEDDON, H. J. and MEDAWAR, P. B. (1942). Fibrin suture of human nerves. *Lancet*, **2**, 87.

SEDDON, H. J., MEDAWAR, P. B. and SMITH, H. V. (1943). Rate of regeneration of peripheral nerves in man. *J. Physiol. Lond.*, **102**, 191.

SEDDON, H. J., YOUNG, J. Z. and HOLMES, W. (1942). The histological condition of a nerve autograft in man. *Br. J. Surg.*, **29**, 378.

SEVER, J. W. (1925). Obstetric paralysis; report of eleven hundred cases. *J. Am. med. Ass.*, **85**, 1862.

SHARRARD, W. J. W. (1966). Posterior interosseous neuritis. *J. Bone Jt Surg.*, **48B**, 777.

SHARRARD, W. J. W. and KNOWELDEN, J. (1956). The ineffectiveness of splinting in the treatment of abductor paralysis at the shoulder. *Lancet*, **1**, 9.

SHAWE, G. D. H. (1955). On the number of branches formed by regenerating nerve-fibres. *Br. J. Surg.*, **42**, 474.

SHEPHERD, R. H., SHOLL, D. A. and VIZOSO, A. D. (1949). Size relationships subsisting between body length, limbs and jaws in man. *J. Anat.*, **83**, 296.

SHERREN, J. (1908). *Injuries of Nerves and their Treatment*. London: Nisbet.

SIDEY, J. D. (1969). Weak ankles. A study of common peroneal entrapment neuropathy. *Br. med. J.*, **3**, 623.

SIEGEL, R. S. and WEIDEN, I. (1968). Combined median and ulnar nerve lesions complicating fractures of the distal radius and ulna. *J. Trauma*, **8**, 1114.

SIMPSON, S. A. and YOUNG, J. Z. (1945). Regeneration of fibre diameter after cross-unions of visceral and somatic nerves. *J. Anat.*, **79**, 48.

SLESSOR, A. J. (1948). Causalgia: a review of 22 cases. *Edinb. med. J.*, **55**, 563.

SMITH, J. W. (1964). Microsurgery of peripheral nerves. *Plastic reconstr. Surg.*, **33**, 317.

SMITH, J. W. (1966). Factors influencing 'nerve' repair 1. Blood supply of peripheral nerves. *Archs Surg. Chicago*, **A3**, 335.

SMITH, R. W. (1849). *A Treatise on the Pathology, Diagnosis and Treatment of Neuroma*. Dublin: Hodges and Smith.

SMITHWICK, R. H. (1940). Rationale and technic of sympathectomy for relief of vascular spasm of extremities. *New Engl. J. Med.*, **222**, 699.

SORREL, E. and SORREL-DÉJERINE, Y. (1938). Les lésions nerveuses dans les fractures fermées récentes de l'extrémité inférieure de l'humérus. *Revue Orthop.*, **25**, 609.

SPEIGEL, I. J. and LEWIN, P. (1945). Tourniquet paralysis: analysis of three cases of surgically proved peripheral nerve damage. *J. Am. med. Ass.*, **129**, 432.

SPINNER, M. (1972). *Injuries to the major branches of peripheral nerves of the forearm*. Philadelphia, London, Toronto: W. B. Saunders Company.

SPITZER, A. G. and PATERSON, D. C. (1973). Acute nerve involvement in supracondylar fractures of the humerus in children. *J. Bone Jt Surg.*, **55B**, 227.

SPRUNG, R. (1943). Ueber die neurotische Dystrophie im Röentgenbild bei Nervenschussverletzungen. *Arch. klin Chir.*, **204**, 564.

SPURLING, R. G. (1930). Causalgia of the upper extremity. Treatment by dorsal sympathetic ganglionectomy. *Archs Neurol. Psychiat.*, **23**, 748.

SPURLING, R. G., LYONS, W. R., WHITCOMB, B. B. and WOODHALL, B. (1945). Failure of whole fresh homogenous nerve grafts in man. *J. Neurosurg.*, **2**, 79.

STAAL, A. (1970). The entrapment neuropathies. In *Handbook of Clinical Neurology*, vol. 7, chap. 11. Ed. Vinken, P. J. and Bruyn, G. W. Amsterdam: North Holland Publishing Company.

STEVENS, H. (1957). Meralgia paresthetica. *Archs Neurol. Psychiat.*, **77**, 557.

STEVENSON, T. M. (1966). Carpal tunnel syndrome. *Proc. R. Soc. Med.*, **59**, 824.

STOFFEL, A. (1913). Beiträge zu einer rationeller Nervenchirurgie. *Münch. med. Wschr.*, **60**, 175, 1365.

STOFFEL, A. (1915). Ueber die Behandlung verletzter Nerven im Kriege. *Münch. med. Wschr.*, **62**, 201.

STOPFORD, J. S. B. (1918). The variation in distribution of the cutaneous nerves of the hand and digits. *J. Anat.*, **53**, 14.

STOPFORD, J. S. B. (1920). The treatment of large defects in peripheral nerve injuries. *Lancet*, **2**, 1296.

STOUT, A. P. (1949). *Atlas of Tumor Pathology*. Section II, Fascicle 6. Tumors of the Peripheral Nervous System. Washington, D.C: Armed Forces Institute of Pathology.

STRANGE, F. G. ST. C. (1947). An operation for nerve pedicle grafting: preliminary communication. *Br. J. Surg.*, **34**., 423.

STRANGE, F. G. ST. C. (1950). Case report on pedicled nerve graft. *Br. J. Surg.*, **37**, 331.

SUNDERLAND, S. (1945*a*). The intraneural topography of the radial, median and ulnar nerves. *Brain*, **68**, 243.

SUNDERLAND, S. (1945*b*). The blood supply of the nerves of the upper limb in man. *Archs Neurol. Psychiat.*, **53**, 91.

SUNDERLAND, S. (1945*c*). The blood supply of the sciatic nerve and its popliteal divisions in man. *Archs Neurol. Psychiat.*, **54**, 280.

SUNDERLAND, S. (1945*d*). Blood supply of peripheral nerves: practical considerations. *Archs Neurol. Psychiat.*, **54**, 283.

SUNDERLAND, S. (1946). The innervation of the first dorsal interosseous muscle of the hand. *Anat. Rec.*, **95**, 7.

SUNDERLAND, S. (1947). Rate of regeneration in human peripheral nerves: analysis of interval between injury and onset of recovery. *Archs Neurol. Psychiat.*, **58**, 251.

SUNDERLAND, S. (1949). Observations on the course of recovery and late end results in series of cases of peripheral nerve suture. *Aust. N.Z. J. Surg.*, **18**, 4.

SUNDERLAND, S. (1952). The multiple motor innervation of individual muscle fibres in man. *Acta anat.*, **16**, 167.

SUNDERLAND, S. (1965). The connective tissues of peripheral nerves. *Brain*, **88**, 841.

SUNDERLAND, S. (1968). *Nerves and Nerve Injuries*. Edinburgh: Livingstone.

SUNDERLAND, S. (1974). The restoration of median nerve function after destructive lesions which preclude end-to-end repair. *Brain*, **97**, 1.

SUNDERLAND, S. and BRADLEY, K. C. (1949). The cross sectional area of peripheral nerve trunks devoted to nerve fibres. *Brain*, **72**, 428.

SUNDERLAND, S. and BRADLEY, K. C. (1950). Endoneurial tube shrinkage in the distal segment of a severed nerve. *J. comp. Neurol.*, **93**, 411.

SUNDERLAND, S. and BRADLEY, K. C. (1961*a*). Stress-strain phenomena in human peripheral nerve trunks. *Brain*, **84**, 102.

SUNDERLAND, S. and BRADLEY, K. C. (1961*b*). Stress-strain phenomena in human spinal nerve roots. *Brain*, **84**, 120.

SUNDERLAND, S. and BRADLEY, K. C. (1961*c*). Stress-strain phenomena in denervated peripheral nerve trunks. *Brain*, **84**, 125.

SUNDERLAND, S. and KELLY, M. (1948). The painful sequelae of injuries to peripheral nerves. *Aust. N.Z. J. Surg.*, **18**, 75.

SUNDERLAND, S., LAVARACK, J. O. and RAY, L. J. (1949). The caliber of nerve fibers in human cutaneous nerves. *J. comp. Neurol.*, **91**, 87.

SUNDERLAND, S. and RAY, L. J. (1947). The selection and use of autografts for bridging gaps in injured nerves. *Brain*, **70**, 75.

SUNDERLAND, S. and RAY, L. J. (1948). The intraneural topography of the sciatic nerve and its popliteal divisions in man. *Brain*, **71**, 242.

SUNDERLAND, S. and RAY, L. J. (1952). The effect of denervation on nail growth. *J. Neurol. Neurosurg. Psychiat.*, **15**, 50.

SUNDERLAND, S. and SMITH, G. K. (1950). The relative merits of various suture materials for the repair of severed nerves. *Aust. N.Z. J. Surg.*, **20**, 85.

SUTARMAN and THOMSON, M. L. (1952). A new technique for enumerating active sweat glands in man. *J. Physiol.*, **117**, 51 P.

TARLOV, I. M. and EPSTEIN, J. A. (1945). Nerve grafts: importance of adequate blood supply. *J. Neurosurg.*, **2**, 49.

TAVERNIER, L., DECHAUME, J. and POUZET, F. (1936). Infarctus musculaires et lésions nerveuses dans le syndrome de Volkmann. *J. Méd. Lyon.*, **17**, 815.

TAYLOR, A. S. (1920). Brachial birth palsy and injuries of similar type in adults. *Surgery, Gynec. Obstet.*, **30**, 494.

TELFORD, E. D. and MOTTERSHEAD, S. (1948). Pressure at the cervico-brachial junction. *J. Bone Jt Surg.*, **30B**, 249.

THOMAS, P. K. (1960). Motor nerve conduction in the carpal tunnel syndrome. *Neurology, Minneap.*, **10**, 1045.

THOMAS, P. K. (1963). The connective tissue of peripheral nerve: an electron microscope study. *J. Anat.*, **97**, 35.

THOMAS, P. K. (1964). The deposition of collagen in relation to Schwann cell basement membrane during peripheral nerve regeneration. *J. Cell Biol.*, **23**, 375.

THOMAS, P. K. (1966). The cellular response to nerve injury, 1. The cellular outgrowth from the distal stump of transected nerve. *J. Anat.*, **100**, 287.

THOMAS, P. K. and FULLERTON, P. M. (1963). Nerve fibre size in the carpal tunnel syndrome. *J. Neurol. Neurosurg. Psychiat.*, **26**, 520.

THOMAS, P. K. and JONES, D. G. (1967). The cellular response to nerve injury 2. Regeneration of the perineurium after nerve section. *J. Anat.*, **101**, 45.

THOMAS, T. T. (1916). Obstetrical or brachial birth palsy. *Am. J. Obstet. Dis. Wom.*, **73**, 577.

THOMSON, A. (1900). *On Neuroma and Neuro-fibromatosis.* Edinburgh: Turnbull and Spears.

THORBURN, W. (1922). Injuries to the peripheral nerves. *Official History of Great War. Medical Services: Surgery of the War.* Vol. **2**, p. 145. London: H.M.S.O.

TILESIUS, W. G. (1793). *Historia Pathologica Singularis Cutis Turpitudinis.* Leipzig: S. L. Crusius.

TILLMAN, A. J. B. (1935). Traumatic neuritis in the puerperium. *Am. J. Obstet. Gynec.*, **29**, 660.

TINEL, J. (1917). *Nerve Wounds.* p. 34. London: Baillière, Tindall and Cox.

TINEL, J. (1919). Les paresthésies précoces après suture ou greffe nerveuse. *Rev. neurol.*, **26**, 521.

TÖNNIS, W. and GÖTZE, W. (1942). Zur operativen Behandlung der Schussverletzungen der peripheren Nerven und ihre Erfolgsaussichten. *Dte. Militärarzt.*, **7**, 245.

TOUZÉ, J. and THIERRY, M. (1952). Hémoglobinurie due à une attrition musculaire localisée. *Bull. Mém. Soc. méd. Hôp. Paris*, **68**, 971.

TOWER, S. S. (1939). The reaction of muscle to denervation. *Physiol. Rev.*, **19**, 1.

TOWER, S. S. (1940). Unit for sensory reception in cornea, with notes on nerve impulses from sclera, iris and lens. *J. Neurophysiol.*, **3**, 486.

TROTT, A. W., NESLINE, M. D. and GREEN, W. T. (1958). The chronology of circulatory changes in poliomyelitis. *J. Bone Jt Surg.*, **40A**, 245.

TSUYAMA, N. and HARA, T. (1973). Intercostal nerve transfer in the treatment of brachial plexus injury of root-avulsion type. In *Orthopaedic Surgery and Traumatology*. Ed. Delchef, J., De Marneffe, R. and Vander Elst, E. Amsterdam: Excerpta Medica.

TUBIANA, R. and DUPARC, J. (1959). Opération palliative pour paralysie sensitive à la main. (Rapport de R. Merle d'Aubigné.) *Mém. Acad. Chir.*, **85**, 666.

TUBIANA, R. and DUPARC, J. (1961). Restoration of sensibility in the hand by neurovascular skin island transfer. *J. Bone Jt Surg.*, **43B**, 474.

TUCK, W. H. (1957). Drop-foot appliance with concealed spring. *J. Bone Jt Surg.*, **39B**, 335.

TUCK, W. H. (1962). Drop-foot appliance with rubber torsion socket. *J. Bone Jt Surg.*, **44B**, 896.

TUCK, W. H. (1966). The use of Ortholen for a concealed toe-raising appliance. *Physiotherapy*, **52**, 442.

TURNBULL, F. (1948). Radial-median anastomosis. *J. Neurosurg.*, **5**, 562.

TURNBULL, F. (1963). Restoration of digital sensation after transference of nerves. *J. Neurosurg.*, **20**, 238.

UNGLEY, C. C. and BLACKWOOD, W. (1942). Peripheral vasoneuropathy after chilling: 'immersion foot and immersion hand'. *Lancet*, **2**, 447.

VAINIO, K. and RITAMA, V. (1956). Morton's metatarsalgia in rheumatoid arthritis. *Ann. Chir. Gynaec. Fenn.*, **45**, 197.

VEROCAY, J. (1910). Zur Kenntnis der "Neurofibrome". *Beitr. path. Anat.*, **48**, 1.

VIAL, J. D. (1958). The early changes in the axoplasm during Wallerian degeneration. *J. biophys. biochem. Cytol.*, **4**, 551.

VIZOSO, A. D. (1950). The relationships between internodal length and growth in human nerves. *J. Anat.*, **84**, 342.

VIZOSO, A. D. and YOUNG, J. Z. (1948). Internode length and fibre diameter in developing and regenerating nerves. *J. Anat.*, **82**, 110.

WADSTEIN, T. (1931). Two cases of ganglia in the sheath of the peroneal nerve. *Acta orthop. Scand.*, **2**, 221.

WADSWORTH, T. G. (1972). Injuries of the capitular (lateral humeral condylar) epiphysis. *Clinical Orthopaedics and Related Research*, **85**, 127.

WADSWORTH, T. G. and WILLIAMS, J. R. (1973). Cubital tunnel external compression syndrome. *Br. med. J.*, **1**, 627.

WALLER, A. (1862). On the sensory, motor and vasomotor symptoms resulting from refrigeration of the ulnar nerve. *Proc. R. Soc.*, **11**, 436.

WALTERS, A. (1959). The differentiation of causalgia and hyperpathia. *Can. med. Ass. J.*, **80**, 105.

WARREN, J. D., (1963). Anterior interosseous nerve palsy as a complication of forearm fractures. *J. Bone Jt Surg.*, **45B**, 511.

WATSON-JONES, R. (1949). Léri's pleonosteosis, carpal tunnel compression of the median nerves and Morton's metatarsalgia. *J. Bone Jt Surg.*, **31B**, 560.

WATSON-JONES, R. (1964). Encapsulated lipoma of the median nerve at the wrist. *J. Bone Jt Surg.*, **46B**, 736.

WEDDELL, G. (1961). In *Brain and Behaviour*, ed. vol. 1. p. 13. Brazier, M. A. B. Washington, D.C.: American Institute of Biological Sciences.

WEDDELL, G., GUTTMANN, L. and GUTMANN, E. (1941). The local extension of nerve fibres into denervated areas of skin. *J. Neurol. Psychiat.*, **4**, 206.

WEDDELL, G. and MILLER S. (1962). Cutaneous sensibility. *A. Rev. Physiol.*, **24**, 199.

WEISS, P. and EDDS, M. V. (1946). Spontaneous recovery of muscle following partial denervation. *Am. J. Physiol.* **145**, 587.

WEISS, P., EDDS, M. V. and CAVANAUGH, M. (1945). Effect of terminal connections on caliber of nerve fibres. *Anat. Rec.*, **92**, 215.

WERTHEMANN, A. (1952). Die Entwicklungsstörungen der Extremitäten. In *Handbuch der Speziellen Pathologischen Anatomie und Histologie*. Vol. 9/6 p. 378. Ed. Lubarsch, O., Henke, F. and Rössle, R. Berlin: Springer.

WHITE, J. (1968). The results of traction injuries to the common peroneal nerve. *J. Bone Jt Surg.*, **50B**, 346.

WHITE, J. C. (1949). The autonomic nervous system. In *Textbook of Surgery*, ed. Christopher, F. 5th edition, p. 541. London: Saunders.

WHITE, J. C. (1969). Nerve regeneration after replantation of severed arms. *Ann. Surg.*, **170**, 715.

WHITE, J. C. and HANELIN, J. (1954). Myelographic sign of brachial plexus avulsion. *J. Bone Jt Surg.*, **35A**, 113.

WHITE, J. C., HEROY, W. W. and GOODMAN, E. N. (1948). Causalgia following gunshot injuries of nerves. *Ann. Surg.*, **128**, 161.

WHITTAKER, W. G. (1958). Injuries to the sacral plexus in obstetrics. *Can. med. Ass. J.*, **79**, 622.

WICKHAM, C. E. G. (1948). Balanced-pulse galvanism. Application of a new principle avoiding ionization effects. *Br. med. J.*, **1**, 1136.

WICKSTROM, J., HASLAM, E. T. and HUTCHINSON, R. H. (1955). The surgical management of residual deformities of the shoulder following birth injuries of the brachial plexus. *J. Bone Jt Surg.*, **37A**, 27.

WILLIS, R. A. (1960). *Pathology of Tumours*. 3rd edition, p. 842. London: Butterworth.

WILLIS, R. A. (1962). *The Borderland of Embryology and Pathology*. 2nd edition, p. 369. London: Butterworth.

WOLTMAN, H. W. and LEARMONTH, J. R. (1934). Progressive paralysis of the nervus interosseus dorsalis. *Brain*, **57**, 25.

WOODHALL, B. and BEEBE, G. W. (1956). *Peripheral Nerve Regeneration*. (American) Veterans Administration Monograph. Washington, D.C.: United States Government Printing Office.

WORLD HEALTH ORGANISATION (1969). *Histological Typing of Soft Tissue Tumours*; by Enzinger, F. M., Lattes, R. and Torloni, H. (International Histological Classification of Tumours No. 3) Geneva: World Health Organisation.

WORSTER DROUGHT, C. (1921). The relative incidence of injuries by gunshot wounds to peripheral nerves. *Jl R. Army med. Corps*, **37**, 386.

WYNN PARRY, C. B. (1973). *Rehabilitation of the Hand*. 3rd edition. London: Butterworth.

YEOMAN, P. M. (1961). Léri's pleonosteosis. *Proc. R. Soc. Med.*, **54**, 275.

YEOMAN, P. M. (1963). *Traction Injuries of the Brachial Plexus*. Thesis for Doctorate of Medicine, Cambridge. Unpublished.

YEOMAN, P. M. (1964). Fatty infiltration of the median nerve. *J. Bone Jt Surg.*, **46B**, 737.

YEOMAN, P. M. (1968). Cervical myelography in traction injuries of the brachial plexus. *J. Bone Jt Surg.*, **50B**, 253.

YEOMAN, P. M. and SEDDON, H. J. (1961). Brachial plexus injuries: treatment of the flail arm. *J. Bone Jt Surg.*, **43B**, 493.

YOUNG, J. Z. (1942). The functional repair of nervous tissue. *Physiol. Rev.*, **22**, 318.

YOUNG, J. Z. (1950). The determination of the characteristics of nerve fibres. In *Genetic Neurology*, ed. Weiss, P. Chicago: Chicago University Press.

YOUNG, J. Z., HOLMES, W. and SAUNDERS, F. K. (1940). Nerve regeneration. *Lancet*, **2**, 128.

YOUNG, J. Z. and MEDAWAR, P. B. (1940). Fibrin suture of peripheral nerves. *Lancet*, **2**, 126.

ZACHARY, R. B. (1945). Thenar palsy due to compression of the median nerve in the carpal tunnel. *Surgery Gynec. Obstet.*, **81**, 213.

ZACHARY, R. B. and HOLMES, W. (1946). Primary suture of nerves. *Surgery Gynec. Obstet.*, **82**, 632.

Author Index

Subject Index

Page numbers in bold type indicate more important references

D

E

F

M

N

O

T

U

V

W

Printed by T. and A. Constable Ltd, Edinburgh